Springer Texts in Statistics

Series Editors

G. Allen, Department of Statistics, Rice University, Houston, USA

R. De Veaux, Department of Mathematics and Statistics, Williams College, Williamstown, USA

R. Nugent, Department of Statistics, Carnegie Mellon University, Pittsburgh, USA

Statistical Modeling and Computation

Joshua C. C. Chan • Dirk P. Kroese

Second Edition

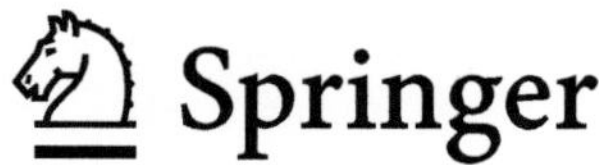 Springer

Joshua C. C. Chan
Purdue University West Lafayette
West Lafayette, IN, USA

Dirk P. Kroese
School of Mathematics and Physics
The University of Queensland
Brisbane, QLD, Australia

Supplementary Information: A Solution Manual to this book can be downloaded from: https://link.springer.com/book/978-1-0716-4132-3

ISSN 1431-875X   ISSN 2197-4136   (electronic)
Springer Texts in Statistics
ISBN 978-1-0716-4134-7   ISBN 978-1-0716-4132-3   (eBook)
https://doi.org/10.1007/978-1-0716-4132-3

To Lesley

Dirk P. Kroese

To Bettina, Basco, and Toffee

Joshua C. C. Chan

Preface

Statistics provides one of the few principled means to extract information from random data, and has perhaps more interdisciplinary connections than any other field of science. However, for a beginning student of statistics the abundance of mathematical concepts, statistical philosophies, and numerical techniques can seem overwhelming. The purpose of this book is to provide a comprehensive and accessible introduction to modern statistics, illuminating its many facets, both from a classical (frequentist) and Bayesian point of view. The book offers an integrated treatment of mathematical statistics and modern statistical computation.

The book is aimed at beginning students of statistics and practitioners who would like to fully understand the theory and key numerical techniques of statistics. It is based on a progression of undergraduate statistics courses at the University of Queensland, the Australian National University, and Purdue University. Emphasis is laid on the mathematical and computational aspects of statistics. No prior knowledge of statistics is required, but we assume that the reader has a basic knowledge of mathematics, which forms an essential basis for the development of the statistical theory. Starting from scratch, the book gradually builds up to an advanced undergraduate level, providing a solid basis for possible postgraduate research. Throughout the text we illustrate the theory by providing working code, rather than relying on black-box statistical packages. Because not all readers will have access to MATLAB, we have switched in this *Second Edition* to the Julia programming language, which is freely available and is very close in syntax to MATLAB. In addition, being a compiled language, Julia is computationally significantly faster than R. We make frequent use of the symbol ☞ in the margin to facilitate cross-referencing between related pages. The book is accompanied by the website https://people.smp.uq.edu.au/DirkKroese/statbook/ from which the Julia code and data files can be downloaded. In addition, we provide MATLAB and R versions for each Julia program.

The book is structured into three parts. In Part I we introduce the fundamentals of probability theory. We discuss models for random experiments, conditional probability and independence, random variables, and probability distributions. Moreover, we explain how to carry out random experiments on a computer.

In Part II we introduce the general framework for statistical modeling and inference, both from a frequentist and Bayesian perspective. We discuss a variety of common models for data, such as independent random samples, linear regression, and ANOVA models. In this *Second Edition* we expanded the modeling framework by adding a section on statistical learning. We discuss the difference between supervised and unsupervised learning, explain training and test loss, and examine prediction accuracy in terms of approximation and statistical error.

Once a model for the data is determined one can carry out a mathematical analysis of the model on the basis of the available data. We discuss a wide range of concepts and techniques for statistical inference, including likelihood-based estimation and hypothesis testing, sufficiency, confidence intervals, and kernel density estimation. We encompass both frequentist and Bayesian approaches, and also highlight popular Monte Carlo sampling techniques.

In Part III we address the statistical analysis and computation of a variety of advanced models, such as generalized linear models, autoregressive and moving average models, Gaussian models, and state space models. This *Second Edition* features two completely new chapters. The first is on shrinkage estimators and regularization techniques, which include ridge and lasso regression, as well as multiple hypothesis testing. The second new chapter is on nonparametric models. This features nonparametric statistical tests, kernel functions, regression and smoothing splines, and Gaussian process regression. Particular attention is paid to fast numerical techniques for frequentist and Bayesian inference on these models. Throughout the book our leading principle is that the mathematical formulation of a statistical model goes hand in hand with the specification of its simulation counterpart.

The book contains a large number of illustrative examples and problem sets (with solutions). To keep the book fully self-contained, we include the more technical proofs and mathematical theory in an appendix. To facilitate the use of Julia we have added a concise introduction to the Julia computing language.

Brisbane, QLD, Australia
West Lafayette, IN, USA
June 11, 2024

Dirk P. Kroese
Joshua C. C. Chan

Acknowledgments

This book has benefited from the input of many people. We thank Zdravko Botev, Tim Brereton, Hyun Choi, Eric Eisenstat, Eunice Foo, Catherine Forbes, Patricia Galvan, Ivan Jeliazkov, Ross McVinish, Gary Koop, Rongrong Qu, Ad Ridder, Leonardo Rojas–Nandayapa, John Stachurski, Rodney Strachan, Mingzhu Sun, Thomas Taimre, Justin Tobias, Elisse Yulian, and Bo Zhang for their valuable comments and suggestions on previous drafts of the book. We also thank Alan Edelman and Evelyne Pelagie Ringoot for their feedback on the Julia code.

Contents

Abbreviations and Acronyms

ANOVA	analysis of variance
AR	autoregressive
ARMA	autoregressive moving average
cdf	cumulative distribution function
EM	expectation–maximization
iid	independent and identically distributed
pdf	probability density function (discrete or continuous)
PGF	probability generating function
KDE	kernel density estimate/estimator
MA	moving average
MCMC	Markov chain Monte Carlo
MGF	moment generating function
ML(E)	maximum likelihood (estimate/estimator)
PRESS	predicted residual sum of squares

Mathematical Notation

Throughout this book we use notation in which different fonts and letter cases signify different types of mathematical objects. For example, vectors $a, b, x, \ldots$ are written in lowercase slanted boldface font, and matrices $\mathbf{A}$, $\mathbf{B}$, $\mathbf{X}$ in uppercase upright boldface font. Euler script fonts $\mathcal{N}$ and $\mathcal{U}$ are used for the normal and uniform distributions, and sans serif fonts for other probability distributions, such as Exp, Gamma and Bin. Probability and expectation symbols are written in black board bold font: $\mathbb{P}$ and $\mathbb{E}$, as well as the identity matrix $\mathbb{I}$. Julia code will always be written in `typewriter` font.

Traditionally, frequentist and Bayesian statistics use a *different* notation system for random variables and their probability density functions. In frequentist statistics and probability theory random variables usually are denoted by uppercase letters $X, Y, Z, \ldots$, and their outcomes by lower case letters $x, y, z, \ldots$. Similarly, for multivariate random variables (i.e., random vectors), we use the notation $X, Y, Z, \ldots$, with outcomes $x, y, z, \ldots$. Observe the notational distinction between a random vector X and a matrix $\mathbf{X}$.

Bayesian statisticians typically use lower case letters for both the random variable/vector and its outcome. More importantly, in the Bayesian notation system it is common to use the *same* letter f (or p) for different probability densities, as in $f(x, y) = f(x)f(y)$. Frequentist statisticians and probabilists would prefer a different symbol for each function, as in $f(x, y) = f_X(x)f_Y(y)$. We will predominantly use the frequentist notation, especially in the first part of the book. However, when dealing with Bayesian models and inference, such as in Chaps. 8 and 13, it will be convenient to switch to the Bayesian notation system. Here is a list of frequently used symbols:

$\approx$	is approximately
$\propto$	is proportional to
∞	infinity
$\otimes$	Kronecker product
$\stackrel{\text{def}}{=}$	is defined as
$\sim$	is distributed as

$\overset{\text{iid}}{\sim},\ \sim_{\text{iid}}$	are independent and identically distributed as
$\overset{\text{approx.}}{\sim}$	is approximately distributed as
$\mapsto$	maps to
$A \cup B$	union of sets A and B
$A \cap B$	intersection of sets A and B
A^c	complement of set A
$A \subseteq B$	A is a subset of or is equal to B
$\emptyset$	empty set
$\|\boldsymbol{x}\|$	Euclidean norm of vector $\boldsymbol{x}$
∇f	gradient of f
$\nabla^2 f$	Hessian of f
$\mathbf{A}^\top,\ \boldsymbol{x}^\top$	transpose of matrix $\mathbf{A}$ or vector $\boldsymbol{x}$
$\operatorname{diag}(\boldsymbol{a})$	diagonal matrix with diagonal entries defined by $\boldsymbol{a}$
$\operatorname{tr}(\mathbf{A})$	trace of matrix $\mathbf{A}$
$\det(\mathbf{A})$	determinant of matrix $\mathbf{A}$
$\|\mathbf{A}\|$	absolute value of the determinant of matrix $\mathbf{A}$. Also, $|A|$ is the number of elements in set A, and $|a|$ the absolute value of real number a
argmax	$\operatorname{argmax} f(x)$ is a value x^* for which $f(x^*) \geq f(x)$ for all x
d	differential symbol
$\mathbb{E}$	expectation
e	Euler's constant $\lim_{n \to \infty}(1 + 1/n)^n = 2.71828\ldots$
i	the square root of -1
$\mathbb{1}_A, \mathbb{1}\{A\}$	indicator function: equal to 1 if the condition/event A holds, and 0 otherwise.
$\mathbb{I}, \mathbb{I}_n$	identity matrix
ln	(natural) logarithm
$\mathbb{N}$	set of natural numbers $\{0, 1, \ldots\}$
φ	pdf of the standard normal distribution
Φ	cdf of the standard normal distribution
$\mathbb{P}$	probability measure
$\mathcal{O}$	big-O order symbol: $f(x) = \mathcal{O}(g(x))$ if $|f(x)| \leq \alpha g(x)$ for some constant α as $x \to a$
o	little-o order symbol: $f(x) = o(g(x))$ if $f(x)/g(x) \to 0$ as $x \to a$
$\mathbb{R}$	the real line = one-dimensional Euclidean space
$\mathbb{R}_+$	positive real line: $[0, \infty)$
$\mathbb{R}^n$	n-dimensional Euclidean space
$\widehat{\boldsymbol{\theta}}$	estimate/estimator
$\boldsymbol{x}, \boldsymbol{y}$	vectors
$\boldsymbol{X}, \boldsymbol{Y}$	random vectors
$\mathbb{Z}$	set of integers $\{\ldots, -1, 0, 1, \ldots\}$

Probability Distributions

Ber	Bernoulli distribution
Beta	beta distribution

Bin	binomial distribution
Cauchy	Cauchy distribution
χ^2	chi-squared distribution
Dirichlet	Dirichlet distribution
DU	discrete uniform distribution
Exp	exponential distribution
F	F distribution
Gamma	gamma distribution
Geom	geometric distribution
InvGamma	inverse-gamma distribution
Mnom	multinomial distribution
$\mathcal{N}$	normal or Gaussian distribution
Poi	Poisson distribution
t	Student's t distribution
TN	truncated normal distribution
$\mathcal{U}$	uniform distribution
Weib	Weibull distribution

Part I
Fundamentals of Probability

In Part I of the book, we consider the *probability* side of statistics. In particular, we will consider how random experiments can be modeled mathematically and how such modeling enables us to compute various properties of interest for those experiments.

Chapter 1
Probability Models

1.1 Random Experiments

The basic notion in probability is that of a **random experiment**: an experiment whose outcome cannot be determined in advance, but which is nevertheless subject to analysis. Examples of random experiments are:

1. Tossing a die and observing its face value
2. Measuring the amount of monthly rainfall in a certain location
3. Counting the number of calls arriving at a telephone exchange during a fixed time period
4. Selecting at random 50 people and observing the number of left-handers
5. Choosing at random ten people and measuring their heights

The goal of *probability* is to understand the behavior of random experiments by analyzing the corresponding *mathematical models*. Given a mathematical model for a random experiment one can calculate quantities of interest such as probabilities and expectations. Moreover, such mathematical models can typically be implemented on a computer, so that it becomes possible to *simulate* the experiment. Conversely, any computer implementation of a random experiment implicitly defines a mathematical model. Mathematical models for random experiments are also the basis of *statistics*, where the objective is to infer which of several competing models best fits the observed data. This often involves the estimation of model parameters from the data.

Example 1.1 (Coin Tossing). One of the most fundamental random experiments is the one where a coin is tossed a number of times. Indeed, much of probability theory can be based on this simple experiment. To better understand how this coin toss experiment behaves, we can carry it out on a computer, using programs such as Julia. The following simple Julia program

© The Author(s), under exclusive license to Springer Science+Business Media, LLC, part of Springer Nature 2025
J. C. C. Chan, D. P. Kroese, *Statistical Modeling and Computation*,
Springer Texts in Statistics, https://doi.org/10.1007/978-1-0716-4132-3_1

simulates a sequence of 100 tosses with a fair coin (i.e., Heads and Tails are equally likely) and plots the results in a bar chart.

```julia
x = rand(100) .< 0.5 # generate a vector of coin tosses
t = 1:100    # range of times
using Plots  # load the plotting library
bar(t,x,legend=false,color=:darkblue)  # plot as a bar chart
```

The function **rand** draws uniform random numbers from the interval $[0, 1]$—in this case a 100-element vector of such numbers. By testing whether the uniform numbers are less than 0.5, we obtain a vector x of logicals (**true** or **false**), indicating, say, Heads and Tails. Typical outcomes for three such experiments are given in Fig. 1.1.

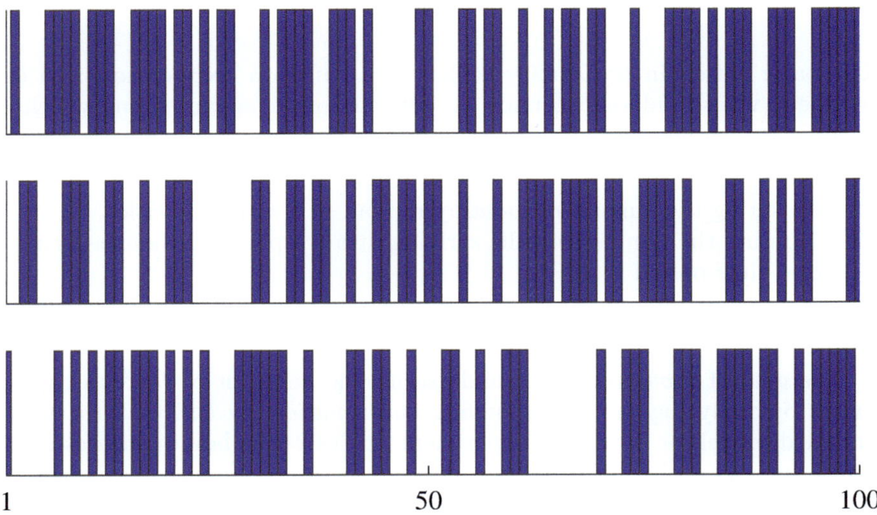

Fig. 1.1 Three experiments where a fair coin is tossed 100 times. The dark bars indicate when "Heads" (=1) appears

We can also plot the average number of Heads against the number of tosses. In the same Julia program, this is accomplished by adding two lines of code:

```julia
y = cumsum(x)./t   # average number of Heads
plot(t,y)          # plot the result in a line graph
```

The result of three such experiments is depicted in Fig. 1.2. Notice that the average number of Heads seems to converge to 0.5, but there is a lot of random fluctuation.

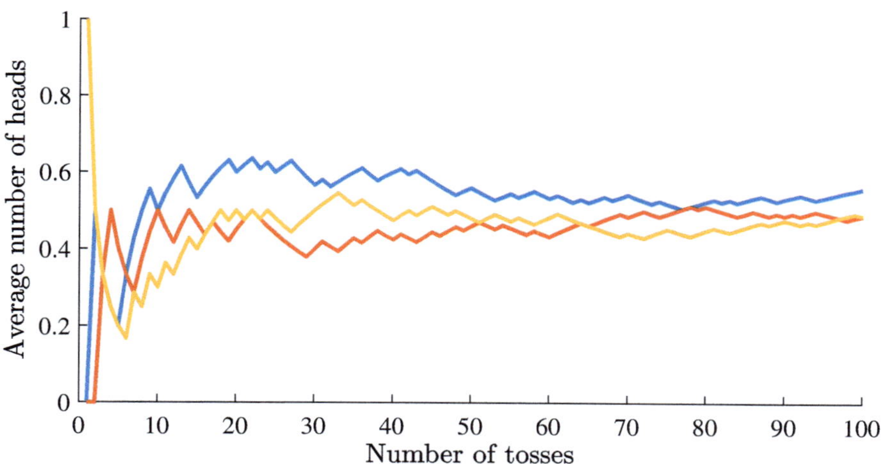

Fig. 1.2 The average number of Heads in n tosses, where $n = 1, \ldots, 100$

Similar results can be obtained for the case where the coin is *biased*, with a probability of, say, Heads of p. Here are some typical *probability* questions.

- What is the probability of x Heads in 100 tosses?
- What is the expected number of Heads?
- How long does one have to wait until the first Head is tossed?
- How fast does the average number of Heads converge to p?

A statistical analysis would start from observed data of the experiment—for example, all the outcomes of 100 tosses are known. Suppose the probability of Heads p is not known. Typical *statistics* questions are:

- Is the coin fair?
- How can p be best estimated from the data?
- How accurate/reliable would such an estimate be?

The mathematical models that are used to describe random experiments consist of three building blocks: a *sample space*, a set of *events*, and a *probability*. We will now describe each of these objects.

1.2 Sample Space

Although we cannot predict the outcome of a random experiment with certainty, we usually can specify a set of possible outcomes. This gives the first ingredient in our model for a random experiment.

Definition 1.1. (Sample Space). The **sample space** Ω of a random experiment is the set of all possible outcomes of the experiment.

Examples of random experiments with their sample spaces are:

1. Cast two dice consecutively and observe their face values.

$$\Omega = \{(1,1),(1,2),\ldots,(1,6),(2,1),\ldots,(6,6)\}\,.$$

2. Measure the lifetime of a machine in days.

$$\Omega = \mathbb{R}_+ = \{\text{ positive real numbers }\}\,.$$

3. Count the number of arriving calls at an exchange during a specified time interval.

$$\Omega = \{0,1,\ldots\}\,.$$

4. Measure the heights of ten people.

$$\Omega = \{(x_1,\ldots,x_{10}) : x_i \geq 0, i = 1,\ldots,10\} = \mathbb{R}_+^{10}\,.$$

Here $(x_1,\ldots,x_{10})$ represents the outcome that the height of the first selected person is x_1, the height of the second person is x_2, and so on.

Notice that for modeling purposes it is often easier to take the sample space larger than is strictly necessary. For example, the actual lifetime of a machine would in reality not span the entire positive real axis, and the heights of the 10 selected people would not exceed 9 feet.

1.3 Events

Often we are not interested in a single outcome but in whether or not one of a *group* of outcomes occurs.

Definition 1.2. (Event). An **event** is a subset of the sample space Ω to which a probability can be assigned.

Events will be denoted by capital letters $A, B, C, \ldots$. We say that event A **occurs** if the outcome of the experiment is one of the elements in A.

Examples of events are:

1. The event that the sum of two dice is 10 or more:

$$A = \{(4,6),(5,5),(5,6),(6,4),(6,5),(6,6)\}\,.$$

2. The event that a machine is functioning for less than 1000 days:

$$A = [0,1000)\,.$$

3. The event that out of a group of 50 people 5 are left-handed:

$$A = \{5\}.$$

Example 1.2 (Coin Tossing). Suppose that a coin is tossed three times, and that we record either Heads or Tails at every toss. The sample space can then be written as

$$\Omega = \{\text{HHH, HHT, HTH, HTT, THH, THT, TTH, TTT}\},$$

where, for instance, HTH means that the first toss is Heads, the second Tails, and the third Heads. An alternative (but equivalent) sample space is the set $\{0,1\}^3$ of binary vectors of length 3; for example, HTH corresponds to (1,0,1) and THH to (0,1,1).

The event A that the third toss is Heads is

$$A = \{\text{HHH, HTH, THH, TTH}\}.$$

Since events are sets, we can apply the usual set operations to them, as illustrated in the *Venn diagrams* in Fig. 1.3.

1. The set $A \cap B$ (*A* **intersection** *B*) is the event that A *and* B both occur.
2. The set $A \cup B$ (*A* **union** *B*) is the event that A *or* B *or* both occur.
3. The event A^c (*A* **complement**) is the event that A does *not* occur.
4. If $B \subseteq A$ (*B* is a **subset** of *A*) then event B is said to *imply* event A.

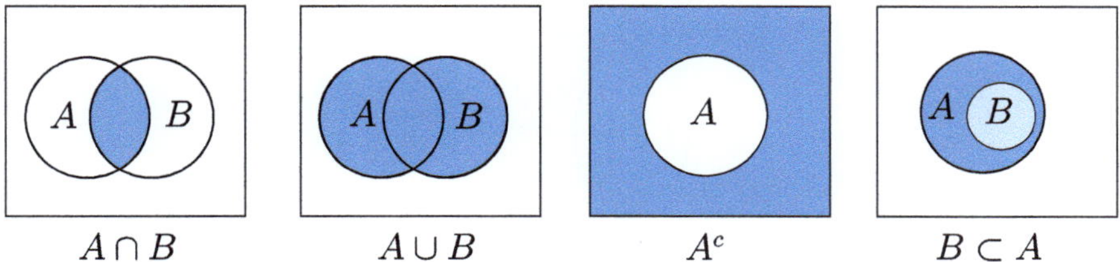

Fig. 1.3 Venn diagrams of set operations. Each square represents the sample space Ω

Two events A and B which have no outcomes in common, that is, $A \cap B = \emptyset$ (empty set), are called **disjoint** events.

Example 1.3 (Casting Two Dice). Suppose we cast two dice consecutively. The sample space is given by $\Omega = \{(1,1),(1,2),\ldots,(1,6),(2,1),\ldots, (6,6)\}$. Let $A = \{(6,1),\ldots,(6,6)\}$ be the event that the first die is 6, and let $B = \{(1,6),\ldots,(6,6)\}$ be the event that the second die is 6. Then $A \cap B = \{(6,1),\ldots,(6,6)\} \cap \{(1,6),\ldots,(6,6)\} = \{(6,6)\}$ is the event that both dice are 6.

Example 1.4 (System Reliability). In Fig. 1.4 three systems are depicted, each consisting of three unreliable components. The *series* system works if all components work; the *parallel* system works if at least one of the components works; and the *2-out-of-3 system* works if at least two out of three components work.

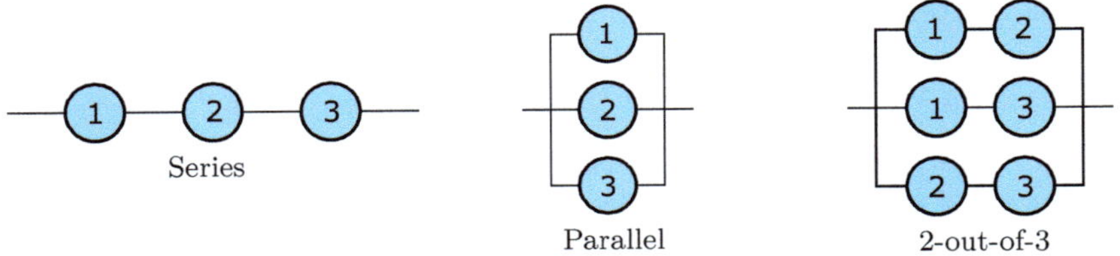

Fig. 1.4 Three unreliable systems

Let A_i be the event that the i-th component is functioning, $i = 1, 2, 3$; and let D_a, D_b, D_c be the events that respectively the series, parallel, and 2-out-of-3 system are functioning. Then, $D_a = A_1 \cap A_2 \cap A_3$ and $D_b = A_1 \cup A_2 \cup A_3$. Also,

$$D_c = (A_1 \cap A_2 \cap A_3) \cup (A_1^c \cap A_2 \cap A_3) \cup (A_1 \cap A_2^c \cap A_3) \cup (A_1 \cap A_2 \cap A_3^c)$$
$$= (A_1 \cap A_2) \cup (A_1 \cap A_3) \cup (A_2 \cap A_3) \,.$$

Two useful results in the theory of sets are the following, due to De Morgan:

Theorem 1.1. (De Morgan's Laws). If $\{A_i\}$ is a collection of sets, then

$$\left(\bigcup_i A_i \right)^c = \bigcap_i A_i^c \tag{1.1}$$

and

$$\left(\bigcap_i A_i \right)^c = \bigcup_i A_i^c \,. \tag{1.2}$$

Proof. If we interpret A_i as the event that component i works in Example 1.4, then the left-hand side of (1.1) is the event that the parallel system is not working. The right-hand side of (1.1) is the event that all components are not working. Clearly these two events are identical. The proof for (1.2) follows from a similar reasoning; see also Problem 1.2. $\square$

1.4 Probability

The third ingredient in the model for a random experiment is the specification of the probability of the events. It tells us how *likely* it is that a particular event will occur.

> **Definition 1.3. (Probability).** A **probability** $\mathbb{P}$ is a function which assigns a number between 0 and 1 to each event and which satisfies the following rules:
>
> 1. $0 \leq \mathbb{P}(A) \leq 1$.
> 2. $\mathbb{P}(\Omega) = 1$.
> 3. For any sequence $A_1, A_2, \ldots$ of *disjoint* events we have
>
> $$\textbf{Sum Rule:} \qquad \mathbb{P}\left(\bigcup_i A_i\right) = \sum_i \mathbb{P}(A_i) . \tag{1.3}$$

The crucial property (1.3) is called the **sum rule** of probability. It simply states that if an event can happen in several distinct ways (expressed as a union of events, none of which are overlapping), then the probability that at least one of these events happens (i.e., the probability of the union) is simply the sum of the probabilities of the individual events. Figure 1.5 illustrates that the probability $\mathbb{P}$ has the properties of a *measure*. However, instead of measuring lengths, areas, or volumes, $\mathbb{P}(A)$ measures the likelihood or probability of an event A as a number between 0 and 1.

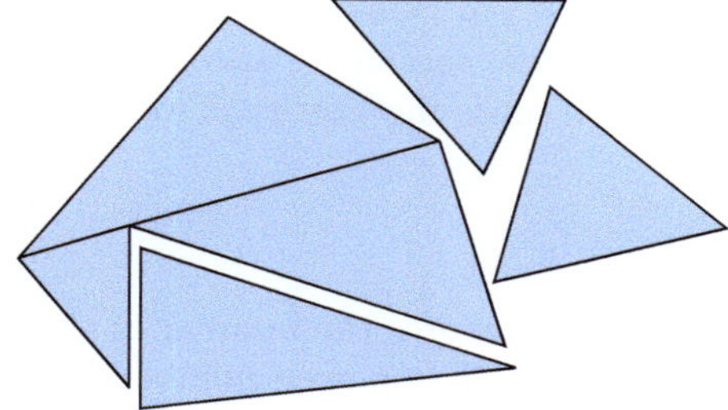

Fig. 1.5 A probability rule $\mathbb{P}$ has exactly the same properties as an area measure. For example, the total area of the union of the non-overlapping triangles is equal to the sum of the areas of the individual triangles

The following theorem lists some important properties of a probability measure. These properties are direct consequences of the three rules defining a probability measure.

Theorem 1.2. (Properties of a Probability). Let A and B be events and $\mathbb{P}$ a probability. Then,

1. $\mathbb{P}(\emptyset) = 0$.
2. if $A \subseteq B$, then $\mathbb{P}(A) \leq \mathbb{P}(B)$,
3. $\mathbb{P}(A^c) = 1 - \mathbb{P}(A)$.
4. $\mathbb{P}(A \cup B) = \mathbb{P}(A) + \mathbb{P}(B) - \mathbb{P}(A \cap B)$.

Proof.

1. Since $\Omega = \Omega \cup \emptyset$ and $\Omega \cap \emptyset = \emptyset$, it follows from the sum rule that $\mathbb{P}(\Omega) = \mathbb{P}(\Omega) + \mathbb{P}(\emptyset)$. Therefore, by Rule 2 of Definition 1.3, we have $1 = 1 + \mathbb{P}(\emptyset)$, from which it follows that $\mathbb{P}(\emptyset) = 0$.
2. If $A \subseteq B$, then $B = A \cup (B \cap A^c)$, where A and $B \cap A^c$ are disjoint. Hence, by the sum rule, $\mathbb{P}(B) = \mathbb{P}(A) + \mathbb{P}(B \cap A^c)$, which (by Rule 1) is greater than or equal to $\mathbb{P}(A)$.
3. $\Omega = A \cup A^c$, where A and A^c are disjoint. Hence, by the sum rule and Rule 2: $1 = \mathbb{P}(\Omega) = \mathbb{P}(A) + \mathbb{P}(A^c)$, and thus $\mathbb{P}(A^c) = 1 - \mathbb{P}(A)$.
4. Write $A \cup B$ as the disjoint union of A and $B \cap A^c$. Then, $\mathbb{P}(A \cup B) = \mathbb{P}(A) + \mathbb{P}(B \cap A^c)$. Also, $B = (A \cap B) \cup (B \cap A^c)$, so that $\mathbb{P}(B) = \mathbb{P}(A \cap B) + \mathbb{P}(B \cap A^c)$. Combining these two equations gives $\mathbb{P}(A \cup B) = \mathbb{P}(A) + \mathbb{P}(B) - \mathbb{P}(A \cap B)$. $\qquad\square$

We have now completed our general model for a random experiment. Of course for any *specific* model we must carefully specify the sample space Ω and probability $\mathbb{P}$ that best describe the random experiment.

Example 1.5 (Casting a Die). Consider the experiment where a fair die is cast. How should we specify Ω and $\mathbb{P}$? Obviously, $\Omega = \{1, 2, \ldots, 6\}$; and common sense dictates that we should define $\mathbb{P}$ by

$$\mathbb{P}(A) = \frac{|A|}{6}, \quad A \subseteq \Omega \, ,$$

where $|A|$ denotes the number of elements in set A. For example, the probability of getting an even number is $\mathbb{P}(\{2, 4, 6\}) = 3/6 = 1/2$.

In many applications the sample space is *countable*: $\Omega = \{a_1, a_2, \ldots, a_n\}$ or $\Omega = \{a_1, a_2, \ldots\}$. Such a sample space is said to be **discrete**. The easiest way to specify a probability $\mathbb{P}$ on a discrete sample space is to first assign a probability p_i to each **elementary event** $\{a_i\}$ and then to define

$$\mathbb{P}(A) = \sum_{i : a_i \in A} p_i \quad \text{for all } A \subseteq \Omega \, .$$

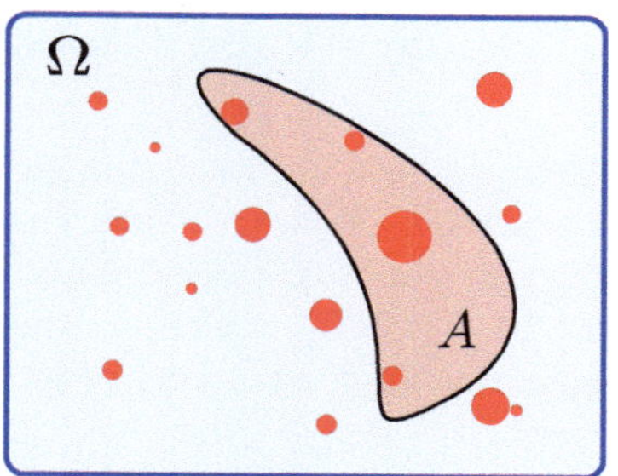

Fig. 1.6 A discrete sample space

This idea is graphically represented in Fig. 1.6. Each element a_i in the sample space is assigned a probability weight p_i represented by a dot—the size of the dot represents the magnitude of p_i. To find the probability of an event A we have to sum up the weights of all the elements in the set A.

Again, it is up to the modeler to properly specify these probabilities. Fortunately, in many applications all elementary events are *equally likely*, and thus the probability of each elementary event is equal to 1 divided by the total number of elements in Ω. In such case the probability of an event $A \subseteq \Omega$ is simply

$$\mathbb{P}(A) = \frac{|A|}{|\Omega|} = \frac{\text{Number of elements in } A}{\text{Number of elements in } \Omega},$$

provided that the total number of elements in Ω is finite. The calculation of such probabilities thus reduces to *counting*; see Problem 1.6. ☞ 19

When the sample space is not countable, for example, $\Omega = \mathbb{R}_+$, it is said to be **continuous**.

Example 1.6 (Drawing a Random Point in the Unit Interval). We draw at random a point in the interval $[0, 1]$ such that each point is equally likely to be drawn. How do we specify the model for this experiment?

The sample space is obviously $\Omega = [0, 1]$, which is a continuous sample space. We cannot define $\mathbb{P}$ via the elementary events $\{x\}$, $x \in [0, 1]$ because each of these events has probability 0. However, we can define $\mathbb{P}$ as follows. For each $0 \le a \le b \le 1$, let

$$\mathbb{P}([a, b]) = b - a.$$

This completely defines $\mathbb{P}$. In particular, the probability that a point will fall into any (sufficiently nice) set A is equal to the *length* of that set.

Describing a random experiment by specifying explicitly the sample space and the probability measure is not always straightforward or necessary. Sometimes it is useful to model only certain *observations* on the experiment. This is where *random variables* come into play, and we will discuss these in Chap. 2. ☞ 23

1.5 Conditional Probability and Independence

How do probabilities change when we know that some event $B \subseteq \Omega$ has occurred? Thus, we know that the outcome lies in B. Then A will occur if and only if $A \cap B$ occurs, and the relative chance of A occurring is therefore $\mathbb{P}(A \cap B)/\mathbb{P}(B)$, which is called the *conditional probability* of A given B. The situation is illustrated in Fig. 1.7.

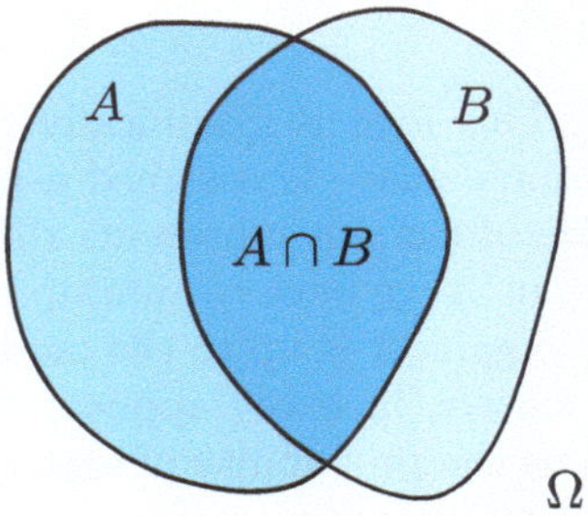

Fig. 1.7 What is the probability that A occurs given that the outcome is known to lie in B?

Definition 1.4. (Conditional Probability). The **conditional probability** of A given B (with $\mathbb{P}(B) \neq 0$) is defined as:

$$\mathbb{P}(A \mid B) = \frac{\mathbb{P}(A \cap B)}{\mathbb{P}(B)} \, . \tag{1.4}$$

Example 1.7 (Casting Two Dice). We cast two fair dice consecutively. Given that the sum of the dice is 10, what is the probability that one 6 is cast? Let B be the event that the sum is 10:

$$B = \{(4,6), (5,5), (6,4)\} \, .$$

Let A be the event that one 6 is cast:

$$A = \{(1,6), \ldots, (5,6), (6,1), \ldots, (6,5)\} \, .$$

Then, $A \cap B = \{(4,6), (6,4)\}$. And, since for this experiment all elementary events are equally likely, we have

$$\mathbb{P}(A \mid B) = \frac{2/36}{3/36} = \frac{2}{3} \, .$$

Example 1.8 (Monty Hall Problem). Consider a quiz in which the final contestant is to choose a prize which is hidden behind one of three curtains (A, B, or C). See Fig. 1.8 for an illustration. Suppose without loss of generality that the contestant chooses curtain A. Now the quiz master (Monty) always opens one of the other curtains: if the prize is behind B, Monty opens C; if the prize is behind C, Monty opens B; and if the prize is behind A, Monty opens B or C with equal probability, e.g., by tossing a coin (of course the contestant does not see Monty tossing the coin!).

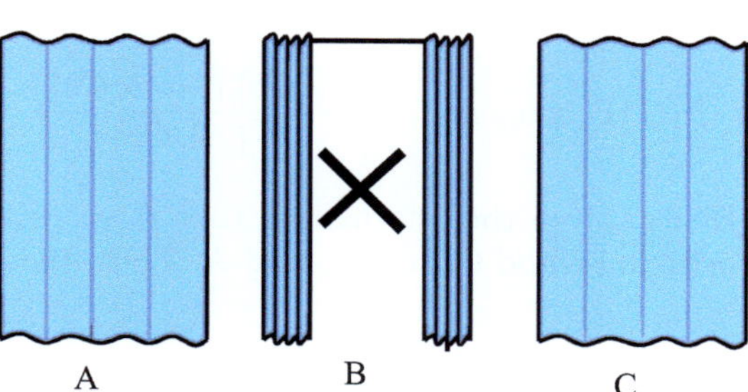

Fig. 1.8 Given that Monty opens curtain B, should the contestant stay with his/her original choice (A) or switch to the other unopened curtain (C)?

Suppose, again without loss of generality, that Monty opens curtain B. The contestant is now offered the opportunity to switch to curtain C. Should the contestant stay with his/her original choice (A) or switch to the other unopened curtain (C)?

Notice that the sample space here consists of four possible outcomes: Ac, the prize is behind A, and Monty opens C; Ab, the prize is behind A, and Monty opens B; Bc, the prize is behind B, and Monty opens C; and Cb, the prize is behind C, and Monty opens B. Let A, B, C be the events that the prize is behind A, B, and C, respectively. Note that $A = \{Ac, Ab\}$, $B = \{Bc\}$, and $C = \{Cb\}$; see Fig. 1.9.

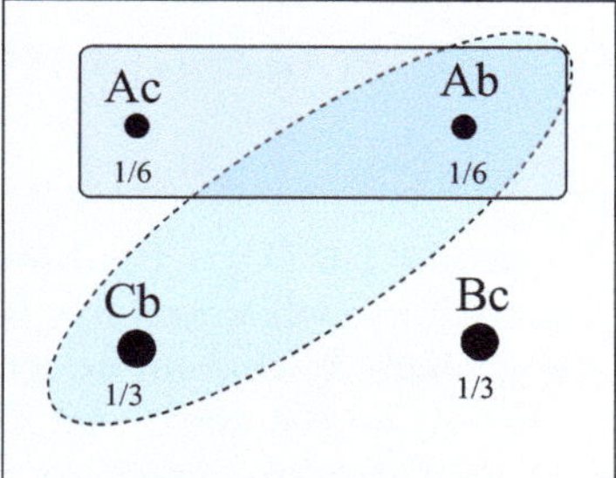

Fig. 1.9 The sample space for the Monty Hall problem

Now, obviously $\mathbb{P}(A) = \mathbb{P}(B) = \mathbb{P}(C)$, and since Ac and Ab are equally likely, we have $\mathbb{P}(\{Ab\}) = \mathbb{P}(\{Ac\}) = 1/6$. Monty opening curtain B means that we have information that event $\{Ab, Cb\}$ has occurred. The probability that the prize is behind A given this event is therefore

$$\mathbb{P}(A \mid \text{B is opened}) = \frac{\mathbb{P}(\{Ac, Ab\} \cap \{Ab, Cb\})}{\mathbb{P}(\{Ab, Cb\})} = \frac{\mathbb{P}(\{Ab\})}{\mathbb{P}(\{Ab, Cb\})} = \frac{\frac{1}{6}}{\frac{1}{6} + \frac{1}{3}} = \frac{1}{3} \, .$$

This is what is to be expected: the fact that Monty opens a curtain does not give any extra information that the prize is behind A. Obviously, $\mathbb{P}(B \mid \text{B is opened}) = 0$. It follows then that $\mathbb{P}(C \mid \text{B is opened})$ must be 2/3, since the conditional probabilities must sum up to 1. Indeed,

$$\mathbb{P}(C \mid \text{B is opened}) = \frac{\mathbb{P}(\{Cb\} \cap \{Ab, Cb\})}{\mathbb{P}(\{Ab, Cb\})} = \frac{\mathbb{P}(\{Cb\})}{\mathbb{P}(\{Ab, Cb\})} = \frac{\frac{1}{3}}{\frac{1}{6} + \frac{1}{3}} = \frac{2}{3} \, .$$

Hence, given the information that B is opened, it is twice as likely that the prize is behind C than behind A. Thus, the contestant should switch!

1.5.1 Product Rule

By the definition of conditional probability (1.4) we have

$$\mathbb{P}(A \cap B) = \mathbb{P}(A)\,\mathbb{P}(B \mid A) \, .$$

It is not difficult to generalize this to n intersections $A_1 \cap A_2 \cap \cdots \cap A_n$, which we abbreviate as $A_1 A_2 \cdots A_n$. This gives the **product rule** of probability. We leave the proof as an exercise; see Problem 1.11.

☞ 20

Theorem 1.3. (Product Rule). Let $A_1, \ldots, A_n$ be a sequence of events with $\mathbb{P}(A_1 \cdots A_{n-1}) > 0$. Then,

$$\mathbb{P}(A_1 \cdots A_n) = \\ \mathbb{P}(A_1)\,\mathbb{P}(A_2 \mid A_1)\,\mathbb{P}(A_3 \mid A_1 A_2) \cdots \mathbb{P}(A_n \mid A_1 \cdots A_{n-1}) \, . \tag{1.5}$$

Example 1.9 (Urn Problem). We draw consecutively three balls from an urn with five white and five black balls, without putting them back. What is the probability that all drawn balls will be black?

Let A_i be the event that the i-th ball is black. We wish to find the probability of $A_1 A_2 A_3$, which by the product rule (1.5) is

$$\mathbb{P}(A_1)\,\mathbb{P}(A_2 \mid A_1)\,\mathbb{P}(A_3 \mid A_1 A_2) = \frac{5}{10}\,\frac{4}{9}\,\frac{3}{8} \approx 0.083 \, .$$

Example 1.10 (Birthday Problem).   What is the probability that in a group of n people all have different birthdays? We can use the product rule. Let A_i be the event that the first i people have different birthdays, $i = 1, 2, \ldots$. Note that $\cdots \subseteq A_3 \subseteq A_2 \subseteq A_1$. Therefore, $A_n = A_1 \cap A_2 \cap \cdots \cap A_n$, and thus by the product rule

$$\mathbb{P}(A_n) = \mathbb{P}(A_1)\,\mathbb{P}(A_2 \mid A_1)\,\mathbb{P}(A_3 \mid A_2) \cdots \mathbb{P}(A_n \mid A_{n-1})\,.$$

Now $\mathbb{P}(A_k \mid A_{k-1}) = (365 - k + 1)/365$, because given that the first $k - 1$ people have different birthdays, there are no duplicate birthdays among the first k people if and only if the birthday of the k-th person is chosen from the $365 - (k - 1)$ remaining birthdays. Thus, we obtain

$$\mathbb{P}(A_n) = \frac{365}{365} \times \frac{364}{365} \times \frac{363}{365} \times \cdots \times \frac{365 - n + 1}{365}, \quad n \geq 1\,. \qquad (1.6)$$

A graph of $\mathbb{P}(A_n)$ against n is given in Fig. 1.10. Note that the probability $\mathbb{P}(A_n)$ rapidly decreases to zero. For $n = 23$ the probability of having no duplicate birthdays is already less than $1/2$.

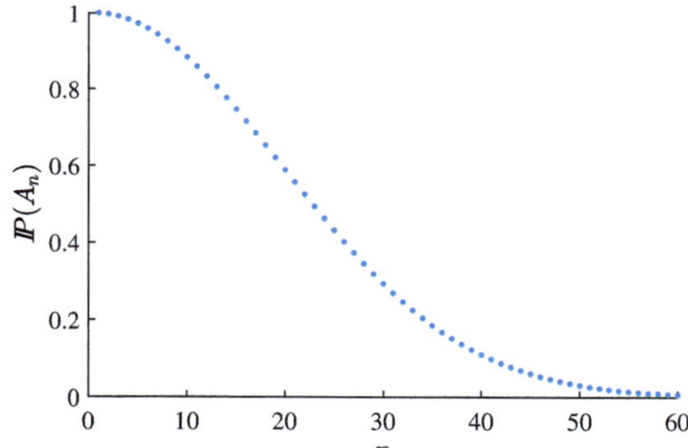

Fig. 1.10 The probability of having no duplicate birthday in a group of n people against n

1.5.2 Law of Total Probability and Bayes' Rule

Suppose that $B_1, B_2, \ldots, B_n$ is a **partition** of Ω. That is, $B_1, B_2, \ldots, B_n$ are disjoint and their union is Ω; see Fig. 1.11.

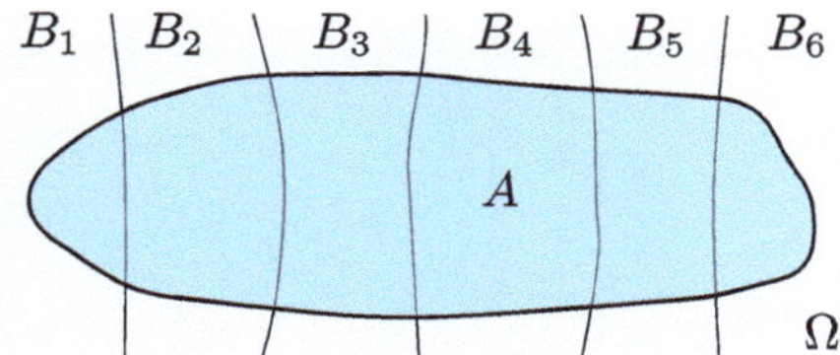

Fig. 1.11 A partition $B_1, \ldots, B_6$ of the sample space Ω. Event A is partitioned into events $A \cap B_1$, $\ldots, A \cap B_6$

A partitioning of the state space can sometimes make it easier to calculate probabilities via the following theorem.

Theorem 1.4. (Law of Total Probability). Let A be an event and let $B_1, B_2, \ldots, B_n$ be a partition of Ω. Then,

$$\mathbb{P}(A) = \sum_{i=1}^{n} \mathbb{P}(A \mid B_i)\, \mathbb{P}(B_i) \,. \tag{1.7}$$

Proof. The sum rule gives $\mathbb{P}(A) = \sum_{i=1}^{n} \mathbb{P}(A \cap B_i)$, and by the product rule we have $\mathbb{P}(A \cap B_i) = \mathbb{P}(A \mid B_i)\, \mathbb{P}(B_i)$. $\square$

Combining the law of total probability with the definition of conditional probability gives **Bayes' Rule**:

Theorem 1.5. (Bayes Rule). Let A be an event with $\mathbb{P}(A) > 0$ and let $B_1, B_2, \ldots, B_n$ be a partition of Ω. Then,

$$\mathbb{P}(B_j \mid A) = \frac{\mathbb{P}(A \mid B_j)\, \mathbb{P}(B_j)}{\sum_{i=1}^{n} \mathbb{P}(A \mid B_i)\, \mathbb{P}(B_i)} \,. \tag{1.8}$$

Proof. By definition, $\mathbb{P}(B_j \mid A) = \mathbb{P}(A \cap B_j)/\mathbb{P}(A) = \mathbb{P}(A \mid B_j)\mathbb{P}(B_j)/\mathbb{P}(A)$. Now apply the law of total probability to $\mathbb{P}(A)$. $\square$

Example 1.11 (Quality Control Problem). A company has three factories (1, 2, and 3) that produce the same chip, each producing 15%, 35%, and 50% of the total production. The probability of a faulty chip at factories 1, 2, and 3 is 0.01, 0.05, and 0.02, respectively. Suppose we select randomly a chip from the total production and this chip turns out to be faulty. What is the conditional probability that this chip has been produced in factory 1?

Let B_i denote the event that the chip has been produced in factory i. The $\{B_i\}$ form a partition of Ω. Let A denote the event that the chip is faulty. We are given the information that $\mathbb{P}(B_1) = 0.15, \mathbb{P}(B_2) = 0.35, \mathbb{P}(B_3) = 0.5$ as well as $\mathbb{P}(A \mid B_1) = 0.01$, $\mathbb{P}(A \mid B_2) = 0.05$, $\mathbb{P}(A \mid B_3) = 0.02$.

We wish to find $\mathbb{P}(B_1 \mid A)$, which by Bayes' rule is given by

$$\mathbb{P}(B_1 \mid A) = \frac{0.15 \times 0.01}{0.15 \times 0.01 + 0.35 \times 0.05 + 0.5 \times 0.02} = 0.052 \,.$$

1.5.3 Independence

Independence is a very important concept in probability and statistics. Loosely speaking it models the *lack of information* between events. We say events A and B are *independent* if the knowledge that B has occurred does not change our assessment of the probability of A. More precisely, A and B are said to be independent if $\mathbb{P}(A \,|\, B) = \mathbb{P}(A)$. Since $\mathbb{P}(A \,|\, B) = \mathbb{P}(A \cap B)/\mathbb{P}(B)$, an alternative definition of independence is: A and B are independent if $\mathbb{P}(A \cap B) = \mathbb{P}(A)\,\mathbb{P}(B)$. This definition covers the case where $B = \emptyset$.

We can extend the definition to arbitrarily many events (compare with the product rule (1.5)):

Definition 1.5. (Independence). The events $A_1, A_2, \ldots,$ are said to be **independent** if for any k and any choice of distinct indices $i_1, \ldots, i_k,$

$$\mathbb{P}(A_{i_1} \cap A_{i_2} \cap \cdots \cap A_{i_k}) = \mathbb{P}(A_{i_1})\,\mathbb{P}(A_{i_2}) \cdots \mathbb{P}(A_{i_k}) . \qquad (1.9)$$

Remark 1.1. In most cases independence of events is a *model assumption*. That is, $\mathbb{P}$ is chosen such that certain events are independent.

Example 1.12 (Coin Tossing and the Binomial Law). We toss a coin n times. The sample space can be written as the set of binary n-tuples:

$$\Omega = \{\underbrace{(0,\ldots,0)}_{n \text{ times}},\ldots,(1,\ldots,1)\} .$$

Here, 0 represents Tails and 1 represents Heads. For example, the outcome $(0,1,0,1,\ldots)$ means that the first time Tails is thrown, the second time Heads, the third times Tails, the fourth time Heads, etc.

How should we define $\mathbb{P}$? Let A_i denote the event of Heads at the i-th throw, $i = 1,\ldots,n$. Then, $\mathbb{P}$ should be such that the following holds.

- The events $A_1,\ldots,A_n$ should be *independent* under $\mathbb{P}$.
- $\mathbb{P}(A_i)$ should be the same for all i. Call this known or unknown probability p $(0 \le p \le 1)$.

These two rules completely specify $\mathbb{P}$. For example, the probability that the first k throws are Heads and the last $n - k$ are Tails is

$$\mathbb{P}(\{(\underbrace{1,1,\ldots,1}_{k \text{ times}},\underbrace{0,0,\ldots,0}_{n-k \text{ times}})\}) = \mathbb{P}(A_1 \cap \cdots \cap A_k \cap A_{k+1}^c \cap \cdots \cap A_n^c)$$

$$= \mathbb{P}(A_1) \cdots \mathbb{P}(A_k)\,\mathbb{P}(A_{k+1}^c) \cdots \mathbb{P}(A_n^c) = p^k(1 - p)^{n-k}.$$

Note that if A_i and A_j are independent, then so are A_i and A_j^c; see Problem 1.12.

Let B_k be the event that k Heads are thrown in total. The probability of this event is the sum of the probabilities of elementary events $\{(x_1, \ldots, x_n)\}$ for which $x_1 + \cdots + x_n = k$. Each of these events has probability $p^k(1-p)^{n-k}$, and there are $\binom{n}{k}$ of these. We thus obtain the **binomial law**:

$$\mathbb{P}(B_k) = \binom{n}{k} p^k (1-p)^{n-k}, \quad k = 0, 1, \ldots, n \ . \tag{1.10}$$

Example 1.13 (Geometric Law). There is another important law associated with the coin toss experiment. Let C_k be the event that Heads appears for the first time at the k-th toss, $k = 1, 2, \ldots$. Then, using the same events $\{A_i\}$ as in the previous example, we can write

$$C_k = A_1^c \cap A_2^c \cap \cdots \cap A_{k-1}^c \cap A_k \ .$$

Using the independence of $A_1^c, \ldots, A_{k-1}^c, A_k$, we obtain the **geometric law**:

$$\begin{aligned} \mathbb{P}(C_k) &= \mathbb{P}(A_1^c) \cdots \mathbb{P}(A_{k-1}^c) \, \mathbb{P}(A_k) \\ &= \underbrace{(1-p) \cdots (1-p)}_{k-1 \text{ times}} \, p = (1-p)^{k-1} \, p \ . \end{aligned}$$

1.6 Problems

1.1. For each of the five random experiments at the beginning of Sect. 1.1, define a convenient sample space.

1.2. Interpret De Morgan's rule (1.2) in terms of an unreliable series system.

1.3. Let $\mathbb{P}(A) = 0.9$ and $\mathbb{P}(B) = 0.8$. Show that $\mathbb{P}(A \cap B) \geq 0.7$.

1.4. Throw two fair dice one after the other.

a. What is the probability that the second die is 3, given that the sum of the dice is 6?
b. What is the probability that the first die is 3 and the second is not 3?

1.5. An "expert" wine taster has to try to match six glasses of wine to six wine labels. Each label can only be chosen once.

a. Formulate a sample space Ω for this experiment.
b. Assuming the wine taster is a complete fraud, define an appropriate probability $\mathbb{P}$ on the sample space.
c. What is the probability that the wine taster guesses four labels correctly, assuming he/she guesses them randomly?

1.6. Many counting problems can be cast into the framework of drawing k balls from an urn with n balls, numbered $1, \ldots, n$; see Fig. 1.12.

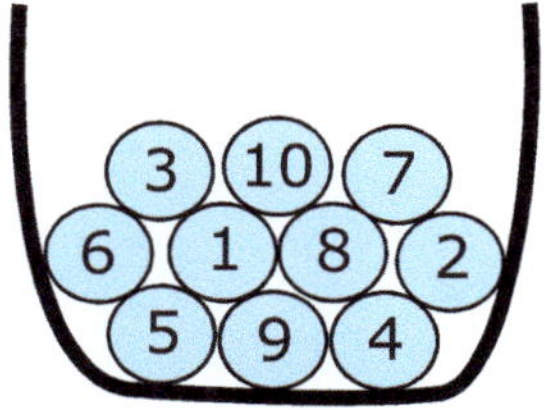

Fig. 1.12 Draw k balls from an urn with $n = 10$ numbered balls

The drawing can be done in several ways. Firstly, the k balls could be drawn one by one or all at the same time. In the first case the **order** in which the balls are drawn can be noted. In the second case we can still assume that the balls are drawn one by one, but we do not note the order. Secondly, once a ball is drawn, it can either be put back into the urn or be left out. This is called drawing with and without **replacement**, respectively. There are thus four possible random experiments. Prove that for each of these experiments the total number of possible outcomes is the following:

1. Ordered, with replacement: n^k.
2. Ordered, without replacement: $^nP_k = n(n - 1) \cdots (n - k + 1)$.
3. Unordered, without replacement: $^nC_k = \binom{n}{k} = \frac{^nP_k}{k!} = \frac{n!}{(n-k)!\,k!}$.
4. Unordered, with replacement: $\binom{n+k-1}{k}$.

Provide a sample space for each of these experiments. Hint: it is important to use a notation that clearly shows whether the arrangements of numbers are ordered or not. Denote ordered arrangements by *vectors*, e.g., $[1, 1, 2]$, and unordered arrangements by *sets*, e.g., $\{1, 2, 3\}$ or *multisets*, e.g., $\{1, 1, 2\}$.

1.7. Formulate the birthday problem in terms of an urn experiment, as in Problem 1.6, and derive the probability (1.6) by counting.

1.8. Three cards are drawn from a full deck of cards, noting the order. The cards may be numbered from 1 to 52.

a. Give the sample space. Is each elementary event equally likely?
b. What is the probability that we draw three Aces?
c. What is the probability that we draw one Ace, one King, and one Queen (not necessarily in that order)?
d. What is the probability that we draw no pictures (no A, K, Q, or J)?

1.9. In a group of 20 people there are 3 brothers. The group is separated at random into two groups of ten. What is the probability that the brothers are in the same group?

1.10. Two fair dice are thrown.

a. Find the probability that both dice show the same face.
b. Find the same probability, using the extra information that the sum of the dice is not greater than 4.

1.11. Prove the product rule (1.5). Hint: first show it for the case of three events:
$$\mathbb{P}(A \cap B \cap C) = \mathbb{P}(A)\,\mathbb{P}(B \mid A)\,\mathbb{P}(C \mid A \cap B) \,.$$

1.12. If A and B are independent events, then A and B^c are also independent. Prove this.

1.13. Select at random three people from a large population. What is the probability that they all have the same birthday?

1.14. In a large population 40% votes for A and 60% for B. Suppose we select at random ten people. What is the probability that in this group exactly four people will vote for A?

1.15. A certain AIDS test has a 0.98 probability of giving a positive result when the blood is infected, and a 0.07 probability of giving a positive result when the blood is not infected (a so-called false positive). Suppose 1% of the population carries the HIV virus.

a. Using the law of total probability, what is the probability that the test is positive for a randomly selected person?
b. What is the probability that a person is indeed infected, *given* that the test yields a positive result?

1.16. A box has three identical-looking coins. However the probability of success (Heads) is different for each coin: coin 1 is fair, coin 2 has a success probability of 0.4, and coin 3 has a success probability of 0.6. We pick one coin at random and throw it 100 times. Suppose 43 Heads come up. Using this information assess the probability that coin 1, 2, or 3 was chosen.

1.17. In a binary communication channel, 0s and 1s are transmitted with equal probability. The probability that a 0 is correctly received (as a 0) is 0.95. The probability that a 1 is correctly received (as a 1) is 0.99. Suppose we receive a 0, what is the probability that, in fact, a 1 was sent?

1.18. A fair coin is tossed 20 times.

a. What is the probability of exactly ten Heads?
b. What is the probability of 15 or more Heads?

1.19. Two fair dice are cast (at the same time) until their sum is 12.

a. What is the probability that we have to wait exactly ten tosses?
b. What is the probability that we do not have to wait more than 100 tosses?

1.20. Independently throw 10 balls into one of three boxes, numbered 1, 2, and 3, with probabilities 1/4, 1/2, and 1/4, respectively.

a. What is the probability that box 1 has two balls, box 2 has five balls, and box 3 has three balls?
b. What is the probability that box 1 remains empty?

1.21. Implement a Julia program that performs 100 tosses with a fair die. Hint: use the **rand** and **ceil** functions, where `ceil(x)` returns the smallest integer larger than or equal to `x`.

1.22. For each of the four urn experiments in Problem 1.6 implement a Julia program that simulates the experiment. Hint: in addition to the functions **rand** and **ceil**, you may wish to use the functions **sortperm** and **sort**.

1.23. Verify your answers for Problem 1.20 with a computer simulation, where the experiment is repeated many times.

Chapter 2
Random Variables and Probability Distributions

Specifying a model for a random experiment via a complete description of the sample space Ω and probability measure $\mathbb{P}$ may not always be necessary or convenient. In practice we are only interested in certain *numerical measurements* pertaining to the experiment. Such random measurements can be included into the model via the notion of a *random variable*.

2.1 Random Variables

Definition 2.1. (Random Variable). A **random variable** is a *function* from the sample space Ω to $\mathbb{R}$.

Example 2.1 (Sum of Two Dice). We throw two fair dice and note the sum of their face values. If we throw the dice consecutively and observe both throws, the sample space is $\Omega = \{(1,1), \ldots, (6,6)\}$. The function X defined by $X(i,j) = i + j$ is a random variable which maps the outcome (i,j) to the sum $i + j$, as depicted in Fig. 2.1.

Note that five outcomes in the sample space are mapped to 8. A natural notation for the corresponding set of outcomes is $\{X = 8\}$. Since all outcomes in Ω are equally likely, we have

$$\mathbb{P}(\{X = 8\}) = \frac{5}{36} \, .$$

This notation is very suggestive and convenient. From a non-mathematical viewpoint we can interpret X as a "random" variable. That is, a variable

J. C. C. Chan, D. P. Kroese, *Statistical Modeling and Computation*, Springer Texts in Statistics, https://doi.org/10.1007/978-1-0716-4132-3_2

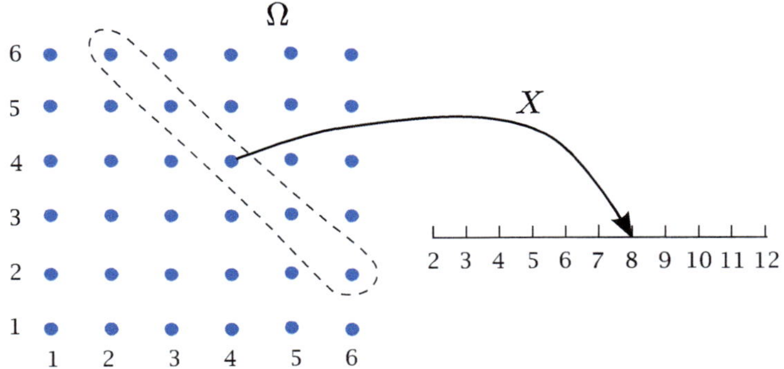

Fig. 2.1 Random variable X represents the sum of two dice

that can take several values with certain probabilities. In particular, it is not difficult to check that

$$\mathbb{P}(\{X = x\}) = \frac{6 - |7 - x|}{36}, \quad x = 2, \ldots, 12 .$$

Although random variables are, mathematically speaking, *functions*, it is often convenient to view them as observations of a random experiment that has not yet taken place. In other words, a random variable is considered as a measurement that becomes available *tomorrow*, while all the thinking about the measurement can be carried out *today*. For example, we can specify today exactly the probabilities pertaining to the random variables.

We often denote random variables with *capital* letters from the last part of the alphabet, e.g., $X, X_1, X_2, \ldots, Y, Z$. Random variables allow us to use natural and intuitive notations for certain events, such as $\{X = 10\}$, $\{X > 1000\}$, $\{\max(X, Y) \leq Z\}$, etc.

☞ 17 **Example 2.2 (Coin Tossing).** In Example 1.12 we constructed a probability model for the random experiment where a biased coin is tossed n times. Suppose we are not interested in a specific outcome but only in the total number of Heads, X, say. In particular, we would like to know the probability that X takes certain values between 0 and n. Example 1.12 suggests that

$$\mathbb{P}(X = k) = \binom{n}{k} p^k (1 - p)^{n-k}, \quad k = 0, 1, \ldots, n , \tag{2.1}$$

providing all the information about X that we could possibly wish to know. To justify (2.1) mathematically, we can reason as in Example 2.1. First, define X as the function that assigns to each outcome $\omega = (x_1, \ldots, x_n)$ the number $x_1 + \cdots + x_n$. Thus, X is a random variable in mathematical terms, that is, a function. Second, the event B_k that there are exactly k Heads in n throws can be written as

$$B_k = \{\omega \in \Omega : X(\omega) = k\} \, .$$

If we write this as $\{X = k\}$, and further abbreviate $\mathbb{P}(\{X = k\})$ to $\mathbb{P}(X = k)$, then we obtain (2.1) directly from (1.10).

We give some more examples of random variables without specifying the sample space.

1. The number of defective transistors out of 100 inspected ones
2. The number of bugs in a computer program
3. The amount of rain in a certain location in June
4. The amount of time needed for an operation

The set of all possible values that a random variable X can take is called the **range** of X. We further distinguish between discrete and continuous random variables:

- **Discrete** random variables can only take *countably many* values.
- **Continuous** random variables can take a continuous range of values, for example, any value on the positive real line $\mathbb{R}_+$.

2.2 Probability Distribution

Let X be a random variable. We would like to designate the probabilities of events such as $\{X = x\}$ and $\{a \leq X \leq b\}$. If we can specify all probabilities involving X, we say that we have determined the **probability distribution** of X. One way to specify the probability distribution is to give the probabilities of all events of the form $\{X \leq x\}$, $x \in \mathbb{R}$. This leads to the following definition.

Definition 2.2. (Cumulative Distribution Function). The **cumulative distribution function** (cdf) of a random variable X is the function $F : \mathbb{R} \to [0, 1]$ defined by

$$F(x) = \mathbb{P}(X \leq x), \ \ x \in \mathbb{R} \, .$$

Note that we have used $\mathbb{P}(X \leq x)$ as a shorthand notation for $\mathbb{P}(\{X \leq x\})$. From now on we will use this type of abbreviation throughout the book. In Fig. 2.2 the graph of a general cdf is depicted.

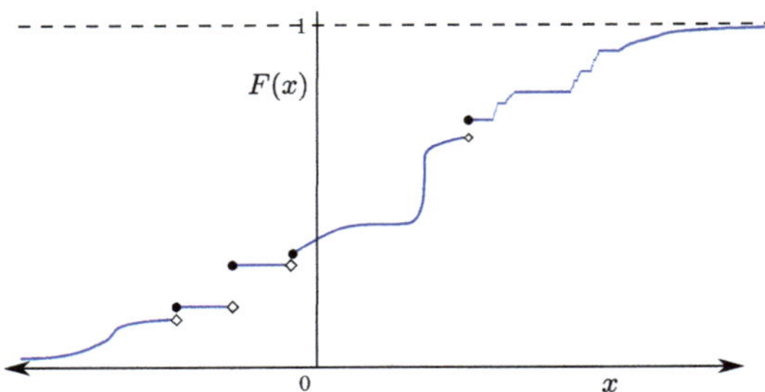

Fig. 2.2 A cumulative
distribution function (cdf)

Theorem 2.1. (Properties of Cdf). Let F be the cdf of a random
variable X. Then,

1. F is bounded between 0 and 1: $0 \leq F(x) \leq 1$.
2. F is increasing: if $x \leq y$, then $F(x) \leq F(y)$.
3. F is right-continuous: $\lim_{h\downarrow 0} F(x+h) = F(x)$.

Proof.

☞ 9

1. Let $A = \{X \leq x\}$. By Rule 1 in Definition 1.3, $0 \leq \mathbb{P}(A) \leq 1$.
2. Suppose $x \leq y$. Define $A = \{X \leq x\}$ and $B = \{X \leq y\}$. Then, $A \subseteq B$,

☞ 10

   and, by Theorem 1.2, $\mathbb{P}(A) \leq \mathbb{P}(B)$.
3. Take any sequence $x_1, x_2, \ldots$ decreasing to x. We have to show that
$\lim_{n\to\infty} \mathbb{P}(X \leq x_n) = \mathbb{P}(X \leq x)$, or, equivalently, $\lim_{n\to\infty} \mathbb{P}(A_n) = \mathbb{P}(A)$, where $A_n = \{X > x_n\}$ and $A = \{X > x\}$. Let $B_n = \{x_{n-1} \geq X > x_n\}$, $n = 1, 2, \ldots$, with x_0 defined as ∞. Then, $A_n = \cup_{i=1}^{n} B_i$ and $A = \cup_{i=1}^{\infty} B_i$. Since the $\{B_i\}$ are disjoint, we have by the sum rule:

$$\mathbb{P}(A) = \sum_{i=1}^{\infty} \mathbb{P}(B_i) \stackrel{\text{def}}{=} \lim_{n\to\infty} \sum_{i=1}^{n} \mathbb{P}(B_i) = \lim_{n\to\infty} \mathbb{P}(A_n) \,,$$

as had to be shown. $\square$

Conversely, any function F with the above properties can be used to specify
the distribution of a random variable X.

If X has cdf F, then the probability that X takes a value in the interval
$(a, b]$ (excluding a, including b) is given by

$$\mathbb{P}(a < X \leq b) = F(b) - F(a) \,.$$

To see this, note that $\mathbb{P}(X \leq b) = \mathbb{P}(\{X \leq a\} \cup \{a < X \leq b\})$, where
the events $\{X \leq a\}$ and $\{a < X \leq b\}$ are disjoint. Thus, by the sum rule:

$F(b) = F(a) + \mathbb{P}(a < X \le b)$, which leads to the result above. Note however that

$$\begin{aligned}
\mathbb{P}(a \le X \le b) &= F(b) - F(a) + \mathbb{P}(X = a) \\
&= F(b) - F(a) + F(a) - F(a-) \\
&= F(b) - F(a-) \,,
\end{aligned}$$

where $F(a-)$ denotes the limit from below: $\lim_{x \uparrow a} F(x)$.

2.2.1 Discrete Distributions

Definition 2.3. (Discrete Distribution). A random variable X is said to have a **discrete distribution** if $\mathbb{P}(X = x_i) > 0$, $i = 1, 2, \ldots$ for some finite or countable set of values $x_1, x_2, \ldots$, such that $\sum_i \mathbb{P}(X = x_i) = 1$. The **discrete probability density function (pdf)** of X is the function f defined by $f(x) = \mathbb{P}(X = x)$.

We sometimes write f_X instead of f to stress that the discrete probability density function refers to the discrete random variable X. The easiest way to specify the distribution of a discrete random variable is to specify its pdf. Indeed, by the sum rule, if we know $f(x)$ for all x, then we can calculate all possible probabilities involving X. Namely,   ☞ 9

$$\mathbb{P}(X \in B) = \sum_{x \in B} f(x) \tag{2.2}$$

for any subset B in the range of X, as illustrated in Fig. 2.3.

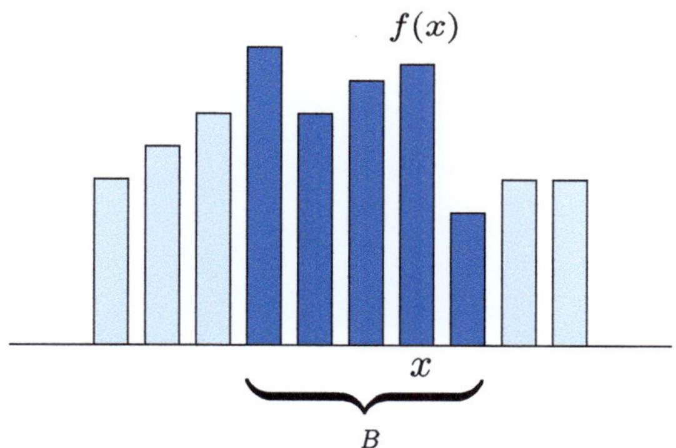

Fig. 2.3 Discrete probability density function

Example 2.3 (Sum of Two Dice, Continued). Toss two fair dice and let X be the sum of their face values. The discrete pdf is given in Table 2.1, which follows directly from Example 2.1.

Table 2.1 Discrete pdf of the sum of two fair dice

x	2	3	4	5	6	7	8	9	10	11	12
$f(x)$	$\frac{1}{36}$	$\frac{2}{36}$	$\frac{3}{36}$	$\frac{4}{36}$	$\frac{5}{36}$	$\frac{6}{36}$	$\frac{5}{36}$	$\frac{4}{36}$	$\frac{3}{36}$	$\frac{2}{36}$	$\frac{1}{36}$

2.2.2 Continuous Distributions

Definition 2.4. (Continuous Distribution). A random variable X with cdf F is said to have a **continuous distribution** if there exists a positive function f with *total integral 1* such that for all $a < b$,

$$\mathbb{P}(a < X \le b) = F(b) - F(a) = \int_a^b f(u)\,\mathrm{d}u . \tag{2.3}$$

Function f is called the **probability density function (pdf)** of X.

Remark 2.1. Note that we use the *same* notation f for both the discrete and the continuous pdf, to stress the similarities between the discrete and continuous case. We will even drop the qualifier "discrete" or "continuous" when it is clear from the context with which case we are dealing. Henceforth we will use the notation $X \sim f$ and $X \sim F$ to indicate that X is distributed according to pdf f or cdf F.

In analogy to the discrete case (2.2), once we know the pdf, we can calculate any probability of interest by means of integration:

$$\mathbb{P}(X \in B) = \int_B f(x)\,\mathrm{d}x , \tag{2.4}$$

as illustrated in Fig. 2.4.

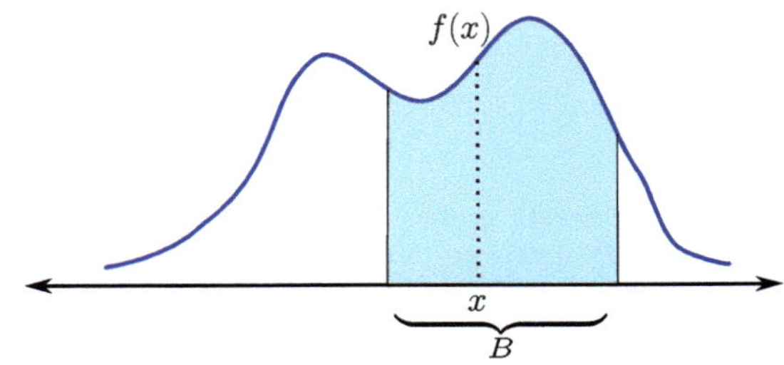

Fig. 2.4 Probability density function (pdf)

Suppose that f and F are the pdf and cdf of a continuous random variable X, as in Definition 2.4. Then F is simply a *primitive* (also called anti-derivative) of f:

$$F(x) = \mathbb{P}(X \le x) = \int_{-\infty}^{x} f(u)\,\mathrm{d}u\ .$$

Conversely, f is the *derivative* of the cdf F:

$$f(x) = \frac{\mathrm{d}}{\mathrm{d}x}F(x) = F'(x)\ .$$

It is important to understand that in the continuous case $f(x)$ is not equal to the probability $\mathbb{P}(X = x)$, because the latter is 0 for all x. Instead, we interpret $f(x)$ as the *density* of the probability distribution at x, in the sense that for any small h,

$$\mathbb{P}(x \le X \le x + h) = \int_{x}^{x+h} f(u)\,\mathrm{d}u \approx h\,f(x)\ . \tag{2.5}$$

Note that $\mathbb{P}(x \le X \le x + h)$ is equal to $\mathbb{P}(x < X \le x + h)$ in this case.

Example 2.4 (Random Point in an Interval). Draw a random number X from the interval of real numbers $[0, 2]$, where each number is equally likely to be drawn. What are the pdf f and cdf F of X? Using the same reasoning as in Example 1.6, we see that

☞ 11

$$\mathbb{P}(X \le x) = F(x) = \begin{cases} 0 & \text{if } x < 0, \\ x/2 & \text{if } 0 \le x \le 2, \\ 1 & \text{if } x > 2. \end{cases}$$

By differentiating F we find

$$f(x) = \begin{cases} 1/2 & \text{if } 0 \le x \le 2, \\ 0 & \text{otherwise.} \end{cases}$$

Note that this density is *constant* on the interval $[0, 2]$ (and zero elsewhere), reflecting the fact that each point in $[0, 2]$ is equally likely to be drawn.

2.3 Expectation

Although all probability information about a random variable is contained in its cdf or pdf, it is often useful to consider various numerical characteristics of a random variable. One such number is the *expectation* of a random variable, which is a "weighted average" of the values that X can take. Here is a more precise definition.

Definition 2.5. (Expectation of a Discrete Random Variable).
Let X be a *discrete* random variable with pdf f. The **expectation** (or
expected value) of X, denoted as $\mathbb{E}X$, is defined as

$$\mathbb{E}X = \sum_x x\,\mathbb{P}(X = x) = \sum_x x\,f(x)\,. \qquad (2.6)$$

The expectation of X is sometimes written as μ_X. It is assumed that the
sum in (2.6) is well-defined—possibly ∞ or $-\infty$. One way to interpret the
expectation is as a *long-run average payout*. Suppose in a game of dice the
payout X (dollars) is the largest of the face values of two dice. To play the
game a fee of d dollars must be paid. What would be a fair amount for d?
The answer is

$$d = \mathbb{E}X = 1 \times \mathbb{P}(X = 1) + 2 \times \mathbb{P}(X = 2) + \cdots + 6 \times \mathbb{P}(X = 6)$$
$$= 1 \times \frac{1}{36} + 2 \times \frac{3}{36} + 3 \times \frac{5}{36} + 4 \times \frac{7}{36} + 5 \times \frac{9}{36} + 6 \times \frac{11}{36} = \frac{161}{36} \approx 4.47\,.$$

Namely, if the game is played many times, the long-run fraction of tosses
where the maximum face value is $1, 2, \ldots, 6$, is $\frac{1}{36}, \frac{3}{36}, \ldots, \frac{11}{36}$, respectively.
Hence, the long-run average payout of the game is the weighted sum of
$1, 2, \ldots, 6$, where the weights are the long-run fractions (probabilities). The
game is "fair" if the long-run average profit $\mathbb{E}X - d$ is zero.

The expectation can also be interpreted as a *center of mass*. Imagine that
point masses with weights $p_1, p_2, \ldots, p_n$ are placed at positions $x_1, x_2, \ldots, x_n$
on the real line; see Fig. 2.5.

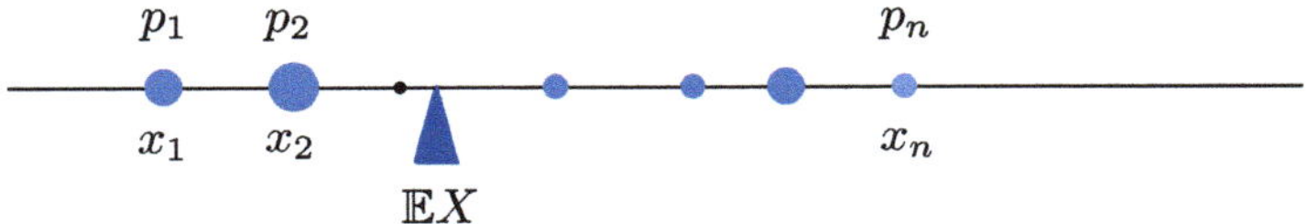

Fig. 2.5 The expectation as a center of mass

The center of mass—the place where the weights are balanced—is

$$\text{center of mass} = x_1\,p_1 + \cdots + x_n\,p_n\,,$$

which is exactly the expectation of the discrete variable X that takes values $x_1, \ldots, x_n$ with probabilities $p_1, \ldots, p_n$. An obvious consequence of this
interpretation is that for a *symmetric* pdf the expectation is equal to the
symmetry point (provided that the expectation exists). In particular, suppose that $f(c + y) = f(c - y)$ for all y. Then,

$$\mathbb{E}X = c\, f(c) + \sum_{x>c} x f(x) + \sum_{x<c} x f(x)$$

$$= c\, f(c) + \sum_{y>0} (c+y) f(c+y) + \sum_{y>0} (c-y) f(c-y)$$

$$= c\, f(c) + \sum_{y>0} c\, f(c+y) + c \sum_{y>0} f(c-y) = c \sum_{x} f(x) = c\,.$$

For continuous random variables we can define the expectation in a similar way, replacing the sum with an integral.

Definition 2.6. (Expectation of a Continuous Random Variable). Let X be a *continuous* random variable with pdf f. The **expectation** (or expected value) of X, denoted as $\mathbb{E}X$, is defined as

$$\mathbb{E}X = \int_{-\infty}^{\infty} x\, f(x)\, \mathrm{d}x\,. \tag{2.7}$$

If X is a random variable, then a function of X, such as X^2 or $\sin(X)$, is also a random variable. The following theorem simply states that the expected value of a function of X is the weighted average of the values that this function can take.

Theorem 2.2. (Expectation of a Function of a Random Variable). If X is *discrete* with pdf f, then for any real-valued function g

$$\mathbb{E}\, g(X) = \sum_{x} g(x)\, f(x)\,.$$

Similarly, if X is *continuous* with pdf f, then

$$\mathbb{E}\, g(X) = \int_{-\infty}^{\infty} g(x)\, f(x)\, \mathrm{d}x\,.$$

Proof. The proof is given for the discrete case only, as the continuous case can be proven in a similar way. Let $Y = g(X)$, where X is a discrete random variable with pdf f_X and g is a function. Let f_Y be the (discrete) pdf of the random variable Y. It can be expressed in terms of f_X in the following way:

$$f_Y(y) = \mathbb{P}(Y = y) = \mathbb{P}(g(X) = y) = \sum_{x:g(x)=y} \mathbb{P}(X = x) = \sum_{x:g(x)=y} f_X(x)\,.$$

Thus, the expectation of Y is

$$\mathbb{E}Y = \sum_y y\, f_Y(y) = \sum_y y \sum_{x:g(x)=y} f_X(x) = \sum_y \sum_{x:g(x)=y} y f_X(x)$$

$$= \sum_x g(x)\, f_X(x) \,.$$

$\square$

Example 2.5 (Die Experiment and Expectation). Find $\mathbb{E}X^2$ if X is the outcome of the toss of a fair die. We have

$$\mathbb{E}X^2 = 1^2 \times \frac{1}{6} + 2^2 \times \frac{1}{6} + 3^2 \times \frac{1}{6} + \cdots + 6^2 \times \frac{1}{6} = \frac{91}{6} \,.$$

An important consequence of Theorem 2.2 is that the expectation is "linear."

Theorem 2.3. (Properties of the Expectation). For any real numbers a and b, and functions g and h,

1. $\mathbb{E}[a X + b] = a\,\mathbb{E}X + b$.
2. $\mathbb{E}[g(X) + h(X)] = \mathbb{E}g(X) + \mathbb{E}h(X)$.

Proof. Suppose X has pdf f. The first statement follows (in the discrete case) from

$$\mathbb{E}(aX + b) = \sum_x (ax + b)f(x) = a \sum_x x\, f(x) + b \sum_x f(x) = a\,\mathbb{E}X + b \,.$$

Similarly, the second statement follows from

$$\mathbb{E}(g(X) + h(X)) = \sum_x (g(x) + h(x))f(x) = \sum_x g(x)f(x) + \sum_x h(x)f(x)$$

$$= \mathbb{E}g(X) + \mathbb{E}h(X) \,.$$

The continuous case is proven analogously, simply by replacing sums with integrals. $\square$

Another useful numerical characteristic of the distribution of X is the *variance* of X. This number, sometimes written as σ_X^2, measures the *spread* or dispersion of the distribution of X.

Definition 2.7. (Variance and Standard Deviation). The **variance** of a random variable X, denoted as $\mathrm{Var}(X)$, is defined as

$$\mathrm{Var}(X) = \mathbb{E}(X - \mathbb{E}X)^2 . \tag{2.8}$$

The square root of the variance is called the **standard deviation**. The number $\mathbb{E}X^r$ is called the r-th **moment** of X.

Theorem 2.4. (Properties of the Variance). For any random variable X the following properties hold for the variance.

1. $\mathrm{Var}(X) = \mathbb{E}X^2 - (\mathbb{E}X)^2 .$
2. $\mathrm{Var}(a + bX) = b^2 \mathrm{Var}(X) .$

Proof. Write $\mathbb{E}X = \mu$, so that $\mathrm{Var}(X) = \mathbb{E}(X - \mu)^2 = \mathbb{E}(X^2 - 2\mu X + \mu^2)$. By the linearity of the expectation, the last expectation is equal to the sum $\mathbb{E}X^2 - 2\mu\,\mathbb{E}X + \mu^2 = \mathbb{E}X^2 - \mu^2$, which proves the first statement. To prove the second statement, note that the expectation of $a + bX$ is equal to $a + b\mu$. Consequently,

$$\mathrm{Var}(a + bX) = \mathbb{E}(a + bX - (a + b\mu))^2 = \mathbb{E}(b^2(X - \mu)^2) = b^2\mathrm{Var}(X) .$$

$\square$

Note that Property 1 in Theorem 2.4 implies that $\mathbb{E}X^2 \geq (\mathbb{E}X)^2$, because $\mathrm{Var}(X) \geq 0$. This is a special case of a much more general result, regarding the expectation of convex functions. A real-valued function $h(x)$ is said to be **convex** if for each x there exists a constant v (depending on x) such that

$$h(y) \geq h(x) + v(y - x) \quad \text{for all } y . \tag{2.9}$$

Examples are the functions $x \mapsto |x|$, $x \mapsto x^2$, $x \mapsto \mathrm{e}^x$, and $x \mapsto -\ln x$.

Theorem 2.5. (Jensen's Inequality). Let $h(x)$ be a convex function and X a random variable. Then,

$$\mathbb{E}h(X) \geq h(\mathbb{E}X) . \tag{2.10}$$

Proof. Replacing x with $\mathbb{E}X$ and y with X in (2.9), it holds that $h(X) \geq h(\mathbb{E}X) + v(X - \mathbb{E}X)$ for some v, because h is convex. Taking expectations yields $\mathbb{E}h(X) \geq h(\mathbb{E}X)$. $\square$

2.4 Transforms

Many probability calculations—such as the evaluation of expectations and variances—are facilitated by the use of *transforms*. We discuss here a number of such transforms.

> **Definition 2.8. (Probability Generating Function).** Let X be a *non-negative* and *integer-valued* random variable with discrete pdf f. The **probability generating function** (PGF) of X is the function G defined by
>
> $$G(z) = \mathbb{E}\, z^X = \sum_{x=0}^{\infty} z^x f(x)\,, \quad |z| < R\,,$$
>
> where $R \geq 1$ is the **radius of convergence**.

Example 2.6 (Poisson Distribution). Let X have a discrete pdf f given by

$$f(x) = \mathrm{e}^{-\lambda}\,\frac{\lambda^x}{x!}\,, \quad x = 0, 1, 2, \ldots\,.$$

X is said to have a **Poisson distribution**. The PGF of X is given by

$$G(z) = \sum_{x=0}^{\infty} z^x\, \mathrm{e}^{-\lambda}\,\frac{\lambda^x}{x!}$$

$$= \mathrm{e}^{-\lambda} \sum_{x=0}^{\infty} \frac{(z\lambda)^x}{x!}$$

$$= \mathrm{e}^{-\lambda}\mathrm{e}^{z\lambda} = \mathrm{e}^{-\lambda(1-z)}\,.$$

As this is finite for every z, the radius of convergence is here $R = \infty$.

> **Theorem 2.6. (Derivatives of a PGF).** The k-th derivative of a PGF $\mathbb{E}z^X$ can be obtained by *differentiation under the expectation sign*:
>
> $$\frac{\mathrm{d}^k}{\mathrm{d}z^k}\mathbb{E}z^X = \mathbb{E}\frac{\mathrm{d}^k}{\mathrm{d}z^k}z^X$$
>
> $$= \mathbb{E}\left[X(X-1)\cdots(X-k+1)z^{X-k}\right] \quad \text{for } |z| < R\,,$$
>
> where $R \geq 1$ is the radius of convergence of the PGF.

☞ 477   *Proof.* The proof is deferred to Appendix B.2.   □

Let $G(z)$ be the PGF of a random variable X. Thus, $G(z) = z^0 \, \mathbb{P}(X = 0) + z^1 \, \mathbb{P}(X = 1) + z^2 \, \mathbb{P}(X = 2) + \cdots$. Substituting $z = 0$ gives $G(0) = \mathbb{P}(X = 0)$. By Theorem 2.6 the derivative of G is

$$G'(z) = \mathbb{P}(X = 1) + 2z \, \mathbb{P}(X = 2) + 3z^2 \, \mathbb{P}(X = 3) + \cdots .$$

In particular, $G'(0) = \mathbb{P}(X = 1)$. By differentiating $G'(z)$, we see that the second derivative of G at 0 is $G''(0) = 2 \, \mathbb{P}(X = 2)$. Repeating this procedure gives the following corollary to Theorem 2.6.

Corollary 2.1. (Probabilities from PGFs). Let X be a non-negative integer-valued random variable with PGF $G(z)$. Then,

$$\mathbb{P}(X = k) = \frac{1}{k!} \frac{\mathrm{d}^k}{\mathrm{d}z^k} G(0) .$$

The PGF thus uniquely determines the discrete pdf. Another consequence of Theorem 2.6 is that expectations, variances, and moments can be easily found from the PGF.

Corollary 2.2. (Moments from PGFs). Let X be a non-negative integer-valued random variable with PGF $G(z)$ and k-th derivative $G^{(k)}(z)$. Then,

$$\lim_{\substack{z \to 1 \\ |z| < 1}} \frac{\mathrm{d}^k}{\mathrm{d}z^k} G(z) = \mathbb{E}\left[X(X-1) \cdots (X - k + 1) \right] . \tag{2.11}$$

In particular, if the expectation and variance of X are finite, then $\mathbb{E}X = G'(1)$ and $\mathrm{Var}(X) = G''(1) + G'(1) - (G'(1))^2$.

Proof. The proof is deferred to Appendix B.2. $\qquad\square$ ☞ 477

Definition 2.9. (Moment Generating Function). The **moment generating function** (MGF) of a random variable X is the function $M : \mathbb{R} \to [0, \infty]$ given by

$$M(s) = \mathbb{E}\, \mathrm{e}^{sX} .$$

In particular, for a discrete random variable with pdf f,

$$M(s) = \sum_x \mathrm{e}^{sx} f(x) \,,$$

and for a continuous random variable with pdf f,

$$M(s) = \int_{-\infty}^{\infty} \mathrm{e}^{sx} f(x) \,\mathrm{d}x \,.$$

Note that $M(s)$ can be infinite for certain values of s. We sometimes write M_X to stress the role of X.

Similar to the PGF, the MGF has the **uniqueness property**: two MGFs are the same if and only if their corresponding cdfs are the same. In addition, the integer moments of X can be computed from the derivatives of M, as summarized in the next theorem. The proof is similar to that of Theorem 2.6 and Corollary 2.2 and is given in Appendix B.3.

☞ 478

Theorem 2.7. (Moments from MGFs). If the MGF is finite in an open interval containing 0, then all moments $\mathbb{E}X^n$, $n = 0, 1, \ldots$ are finite and satisfy

$$\mathbb{E}X^n = M^{(n)}(0) \,,$$

where $M^{(n)}(0)$ is the n-th derivative of M evaluated at 0.

Note that under the conditions of Theorem 2.7, the variance of X can be obtained from the moment generating function as

$$\mathrm{Var}(X) = M''(0) - (M'(0))^2 \,.$$

A transform with better analytical properties than the moment generating function is the *characteristic function*.

Definition 2.10. (Characteristic Function). The **characteristic generating function** of a random variable X is the function $\psi : \mathbb{R} \to \mathbb{C}$ given by

$$\psi(r) = \mathbb{E}\,\mathrm{e}^{\mathrm{i}rX} = \mathbb{E}\cos(rX) + \mathrm{i}\,\mathbb{E}\sin(rX), \quad r \in \mathbb{R} \,.$$

The characteristic function is well-defined and finite for any random variable, whereas for certain probability distributions the moment generating function may not be finite for any value of other than 0.

2.5 Common Discrete Distributions

In this section we give a number of common discrete distributions and list some of their properties. Note that the discrete pdf of each of these distributions, denoted f, depends on one or more parameters; so in fact we are dealing with *families* of distributions.

2.5.1 Bernoulli Distribution

Definition 2.11. (Bernoulli Distribution). A random variable X is said to have a **Bernoulli** distribution with success probability p if X can only assume the values 0 and 1, with probabilities

$$f(0) = \mathbb{P}(X = 0) = 1 - p \qquad \text{and} \qquad f(1) = \mathbb{P}(X = 1) = p \,.$$

We write $X \sim \mathsf{Ber}(p)$.

The Bernoulli distribution is the most fundamental of all probability distributions. It models a single coin toss experiment. Three important properties of the Bernoulli are summarized in the following theorem.

Theorem 2.8. (Properties of the Bernoulli Distribution). Let $X \sim \mathsf{Ber}(p)$. Then,

1. $\mathbb{E}X = p$.
2. $\mathrm{Var}(X) = p(1 - p)$.
3. The PGF is $G(z) = 1 - p + zp$.

Proof. The expectation and the variance of X can be obtained by direct computation:

$$\mathbb{E}X = 0 \times \mathbb{P}(X = 0) + 1 \times \mathbb{P}(X = 1) = 0 \times (1 - p) + 1 \times p = p$$

and

$$\mathrm{Var}(X) = \mathbb{E}X^2 - (\mathbb{E}X)^2 = \mathbb{E}X - (\mathbb{E}X)^2 = p - p^2 = p(1 - p) \,,$$

where we have used the fact that in this case $X^2 = X$. Finally, the PGF is given by $G(z) = z^0(1 - p) + z^1 p = 1 - p + zp$. $\qquad\qquad\square$

2.5.2 Binomial Distribution

Definition 2.12. (Binomial Distribution). A random variable X is said to have a **binomial** distribution with parameters n and p if X has pdf

$$f(x) = \mathbb{P}(X = x) = \binom{n}{x} p^x (1-p)^{n-x}, \quad x = 0, 1, \ldots, n \,. \qquad (2.12)$$

We write $X \sim \mathrm{Bin}(n, p)$.

☞ 17 From Example 2.2 we see that X can be interpreted as the total number of Heads in n successive coin flip experiments, with probability of Heads equal to p. An example of the graph of the pdf is given in Fig. 2.6. Theorem 2.9 lists some important properties of the binomial distribution.

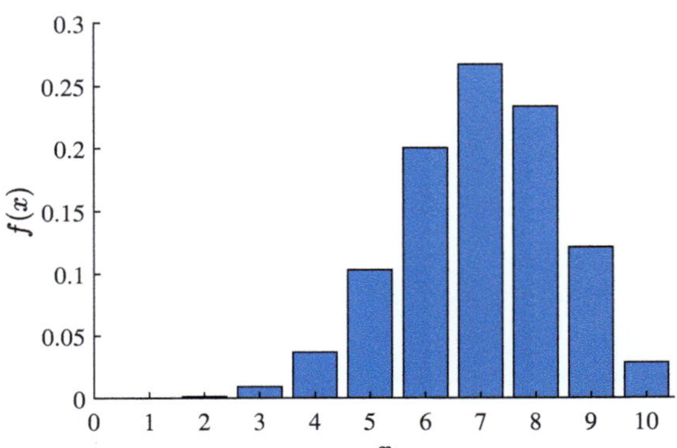

Fig. 2.6 The pdf of the Bin$(10, 0.7)$-distribution

Theorem 2.9. (Properties of the Binomial Distribution). Let $X \sim \mathrm{Bin}(n, p)$. Then,

1. $\mathbb{E}X = np$.
2. $\mathrm{Var}(X) = np(1-p)$.
3. The PGF is $G(z) = (1 - p + zp)^n$.

Proof. Using Newton's binomial formula:

$$(a + b)^n = \sum_{k=0}^{n} \binom{n}{k} a^k \, b^{n-k} \,,$$

we see that

$$G(z) = \sum_{k=0}^{n} z^k \binom{n}{k} p^k (1-p)^{n-k} = \sum_{k=0}^{n} \binom{n}{k} (z\,p)^k (1-p)^{n-k} = (1-p+zp)^n \ .$$

From Corollary 2.2 we obtain the expectation and variance via $G'(1) = np$ ☞ 35
and $G''(1) + G'(1) - (G'(1))^2 = (n-1)np^2 + np - n^2p^2 = np(1-p)$.   □

2.5.3 Geometric Distribution

Definition 2.13. (Geometric Distribution). A random variable X is said to have a **geometric** distribution with parameter p if X has pdf

$$f(x) = \mathbb{P}(X = x) = (1-p)^{x-1}p, \quad x = 1, 2, 3, \ldots. \tag{2.13}$$

We write $X \sim \mathsf{Geom}(p)$.

From Example 1.13 we see that X can be interpreted as the number of   ☞ 18
tosses needed until the first Heads occurs in a sequence of coin tosses, with the probability of Heads equal to p. An example of the graph of the pdf is given in Fig. 2.7. Theorem 2.10 summarizes some properties of the geometric distribution.

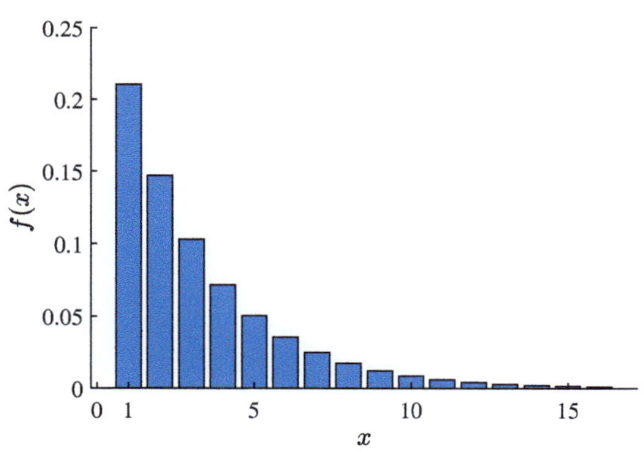

Fig. 2.7 The pdf of the Geom(0.3)-distribution

Theorem 2.10. (Properties of the Geometric Distribution). Let $X \sim \mathsf{Geom}(p)$. Then,

1. $\mathbb{E}X = 1/p$.
2. $\mathrm{Var}(X) = (1 - p)/p^2$.
3. The PGF is

$$G(z) = \frac{z\,p}{1 - z\,(1 - p)} , \quad |z| < \frac{1}{1 - p} . \tag{2.14}$$

Proof. The PGF of X follows from

$$G(z) = \sum_{x=1}^{\infty} z^x p(1 - p)^{x-1} = z\,p \sum_{k=0}^{\infty} (z(1 - p))^k = \frac{z\,p}{1 - z\,(1 - p)} ,$$

using the well-known result for *geometric sums*: $1 + a + a^2 + \cdots = (1 - a)^{-1}$, for $|a| < 1$. By Corollary 2.2 the expectation is therefore

$$\mathbb{E}X = G'(1) = \frac{1}{p} .$$

By differentiating the PGF twice we find the variance:

$$\mathrm{Var}(X) = G''(1) + G'(1) - (G''(1))^2 = \frac{2(1 - p)}{p^2} + \frac{1}{p} - \frac{1}{p^2} = \frac{1 - p}{p^2} . \qquad \square$$

One property of the geometric distribution that deserves extra attention is the **memoryless property**. Consider again the coin toss experiment. Suppose we have tossed the coin k times without a success (Heads). What is the probability that we need more than x additional tosses before getting a success? The answer is, obviously, the same as the probability that we require more than x tosses if we start from scratch, that is, $\mathbb{P}(X > x) = (1 - p)^x$, irrespective of k. The fact that we have already had k failures does not make the event of getting a success in the next trial(s) any more likely. In other words, the coin does not have a memory of what happened—hence the name memoryless property.

Theorem 2.11. (Memoryless Property). Let $X \sim \mathsf{Geom}(p)$. Then for any $x, k = 1, 2, \ldots,$

$$\mathbb{P}(X > k + x \mid X > k) = \mathbb{P}(X > x) .$$

Proof. By the definition of conditional probability,

$$\mathbb{P}(X > k + x \mid X > k) = \frac{\mathbb{P}(\{X > k + x\} \cap \{X > k\})}{\mathbb{P}(X > k)} .$$

The event $\{X > k + x\}$ is a subset of $\{X > k\}$; hence, their intersection is $\{X > k + x\}$. Moreover, the probabilities of the events $\{X > k + x\}$ and $\{X > k\}$ are $(1-p)^{k+x}$ and $(1-p)^k$, respectively. Therefore,

$$\mathbb{P}(X > k + x \mid X > k) = \frac{(1-p)^{k+x}}{(1-p)^k} = (1-p)^x = \mathbb{P}(X > x) ,$$

as required. $\qquad\square$

2.5.4 Poisson Distribution

Definition 2.14. (Poisson Distribution). A random variable X is said to have a **Poisson** distribution with **rate** parameter $\lambda > 0$ if X has pdf

$$f(x) = \mathbb{P}(X = x) = \frac{\lambda^x}{x!}\, \mathrm{e}^{-\lambda}, \quad x = 0, 1, 2, \dots . \tag{2.15}$$

We write $X \sim \mathsf{Poi}(\lambda)$.

The Poisson distribution may be viewed as the limit of the $\mathsf{Bin}(n, \lambda/n)$ distribution. Namely, if $X_n \sim \mathsf{Bin}(n, \lambda/n)$, then

$$\mathbb{P}(X_n = x) = \binom{n}{x} \left(\frac{\lambda}{n}\right)^x \left(1 - \frac{\lambda}{n}\right)^{n-x}$$

$$= \frac{\lambda^x}{x!}\, \frac{n \times (n-1) \times \cdots \times (n-x+1)}{n \times n \times \cdots \times n} \left(1 - \frac{\lambda}{n}\right)^n \left(1 - \frac{\lambda}{n}\right)^{-x} .$$

As $n \to \infty$ the second and fourth factors converge to 1, and the third factor to $\mathrm{e}^{-\lambda}$ (this is one of the defining properties of the exponential function). Hence, we have

$$\lim_{n \to \infty} \mathbb{P}(X_n = x) = \frac{\lambda^x}{x!}\, \mathrm{e}^{-\lambda}.$$

An example of the graph of the Poisson pdf is given in Fig. 2.8. Theorem 2.12 summarizes some properties of the Poisson distribution.

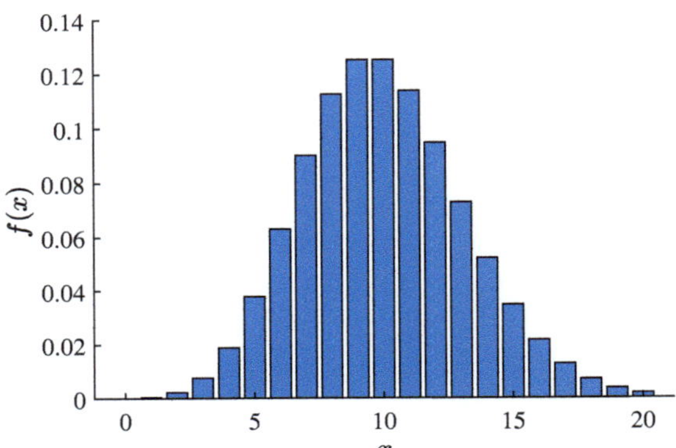

Fig. 2.8 The pdf of the Poi(10)-distribution

Theorem 2.12. (Properties of the Poisson Distribution). Let $X \sim \mathrm{Poi}(\lambda)$. Then,

1. $\mathbb{E}X = \lambda$.
2. $\mathrm{Var}(X) = \lambda$.
3. The PGF is $G(z) = \mathrm{e}^{-\lambda(1-z)}$.

☞ 34   *Proof.* The PGF was derived in Example 2.6. It follows from Corollary 2.2 that $\mathbb{E}X = G'(1) = \lambda$ and

$$\mathrm{Var}(X) = G''(1) + G'(1) - (G'(1))^2 = \lambda^2 + \lambda - \lambda^2 = \lambda \,.$$

Thus, the rate parameter λ can be interpreted as both the expectation and variance of X.   □

2.6 Common Continuous Distributions

In this section we give a number of common continuous distributions and list some of their properties. Note that the pdf of each of these distributions depends on one or more parameters; so, as in the previous section, we are dealing with *families* of distributions.

2.6.1 Uniform Distribution

Definition 2.15. (Uniform Distribution). A random variable X is said to have a **uniform** distribution on the interval $[a, b]$ if its pdf is given by

$$f(x) = \frac{1}{b-a}, \quad a \leq x \leq b.$$

We write $X \sim \mathcal{U}[a, b]$ (and $X \sim \mathcal{U}(a, b)$ for a uniform random variable on an open interval (a, b)).

The random variable $X \sim \mathcal{U}[a, b]$ can model a randomly chosen point from the interval $[a, b]$, where each choice is equally likely. A graph of the pdf is given in Fig. 2.9.

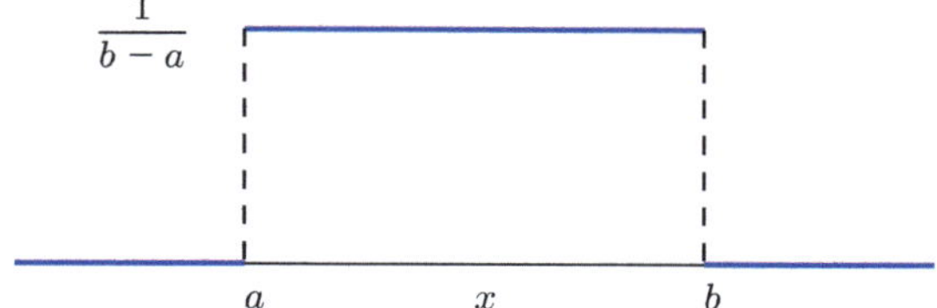

Fig. 2.9 The pdf of the uniform distribution on $[a, b]$

Theorem 2.13. (Properties of the Uniform Distribution). Let $X \sim \mathcal{U}[a, b]$. Then,

1. $\mathbb{E}X = (a + b)/2$.
2. $\mathrm{Var}(X) = (b - a)^2/12$.

Proof. We have

$$\mathbb{E}X = \int_a^b \frac{x}{b-a}\, \mathrm{d}x = \frac{1}{b-a}\left[\frac{b^2 - a^2}{2}\right] = \frac{a+b}{2}$$

and

$$\mathrm{Var}(X) = \mathbb{E}X^2 - (\mathbb{E}X)^2 = \int_a^b \frac{x^2}{b-a}\, \mathrm{d}x - \left(\frac{a+b}{2}\right)^2$$

$$= \frac{b^3 - a^3}{3(b-a)} - \left(\frac{a+b}{2}\right)^2 = \frac{(b-a)^2}{12}.$$

$\square$

2.6.2 Exponential Distribution

Definition 2.16. (Exponential Distribution). A random variable X is said to have an **exponential** distribution with **rate** parameter λ if its pdf is given by

$$f(x) = \lambda\, e^{-\lambda x}, \quad x \geq 0 . \tag{2.16}$$

We write $X \sim \mathsf{Exp}(\lambda)$.

The exponential distribution can be viewed as a continuous version of the geometric distribution. Graphs of the pdf for various values of λ are given in Fig. 2.10. Theorem 2.14 summarizes some properties of the exponential distribution.

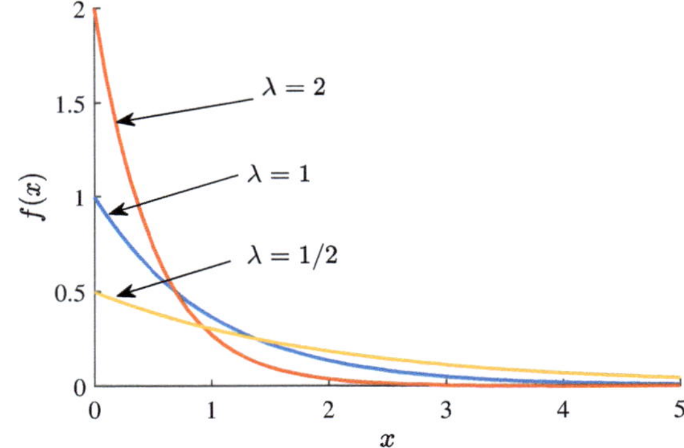

Fig. 2.10 The pdf of the Exp(λ)-distribution for various λ

Theorem 2.14. (Properties of the Exponential Distribution). Let $X \sim \mathsf{Exp}(\lambda)$. Then,

1. $\mathbb{E}X = 1/\lambda$.
2. $\mathrm{Var}(X) = 1/\lambda^2$.
3. The MGF of X is $M(s) = \lambda/(\lambda - s)$, $s < \lambda$,
4. The cdf of X is $F(x) = 1 - e^{-\lambda x}$, $x \geq 0$.
5. The **memoryless property** holds: for any $s, t > 0$,

$$\mathbb{P}(X > s + t \mid X > s) = \mathbb{P}(X > t) . \tag{2.17}$$

Proof. 3. The moment generating function is given by

$$M(s) = \int_0^\infty e^{sx} \lambda e^{-\lambda x} \mathrm{d}x = \lambda \int_0^\infty e^{-(\lambda - s)x}\, \mathrm{d}x = \lambda \left[\frac{-e^{-(\lambda - s)x}}{\lambda - s} \right]_0^\infty$$

$$= \frac{\lambda}{\lambda - s}, \quad s < \lambda \quad (\text{and } M(s) = \infty \text{ for } s \geq \lambda).$$

1. From Theorem 2.7, we obtain

$$\mathbb{E}X = M'(0) = \left.\frac{\lambda}{(\lambda - s)^2}\right|_{s=0} = \frac{1}{\lambda} \,.$$

2. Similarly, the second moment is $\mathbb{E}X^2 = M''(0) = \left.\frac{2\lambda}{(\lambda-s)^3}\right|_{s=0} = 2/\lambda^2$, so that the variance is

$$\mathrm{Var}(X) = \mathbb{E}X^2 - (\mathbb{E}X)^2 = \frac{2}{\lambda^2} - \frac{1}{\lambda^2} = \frac{1}{\lambda^2} \,.$$

4. The cdf of X is given by

$$F(x) = \mathbb{P}(X \le x) = \int_0^x \lambda e^{-\lambda u}\mathrm{d}u = \left[-e^{-\lambda u}\right]_0^x = 1 - e^{-\lambda x}, \quad x \ge 0 \,.$$

Note that the tail probability $\mathbb{P}(X > x)$ is exponentially decaying:

$$\mathbb{P}(X > x) = e^{-\lambda x}, \quad x \ge 0 \,.$$

5. Similar to the proof of the memoryless property for the geometric distribution (Theorem 2.11), we have

$$\mathbb{P}(X > s + t \mid X > s) = \frac{\mathbb{P}(X > s + t, X > s)}{\mathbb{P}(X > s)} = \frac{\mathbb{P}(X > s + t)}{\mathbb{P}(X > s)}$$
$$= \frac{e^{-\lambda(t+s)}}{e^{-\lambda s}} = e^{-\lambda t} = \mathbb{P}(X > t) \,.$$

$\square$

The memoryless property can be interpreted as a "non-aging" property. For example, when X denotes the lifetime of a machine then, given the fact that the machine is alive at time s, the remaining lifetime of the machine, $X - s$, has the same exponential distribution as a completely new machine. In other words, the machine has no memory of its age and does not deteriorate (although it will break down eventually).

2.6.3 Normal (Gaussian) Distribution

In this section we introduce the most important distribution in the study of statistics: the normal (or Gaussian) distribution. Additional properties of this distribution will be given in Sect. 3.6.

Definition 2.17. (Normal Distribution). A random variable X is said to have a **normal** or **Gaussian** distribution with parameters μ and σ^2 if its pdf is given by

$$f(x) = \frac{1}{\sigma\sqrt{2\pi}}\,\mathrm{e}^{-\frac{1}{2}\left(\frac{x-\mu}{\sigma}\right)^2}, \quad x \in \mathbb{R}\,. \tag{2.18}$$

We write $X \sim \mathcal{N}(\mu, \sigma^2)$.

The parameters μ and σ^2 turn out to be the expectation and variance of the distribution, respectively. If $\mu = 0$ and $\sigma = 1$ then

$$f(x) = \frac{1}{\sqrt{2\pi}}\,\mathrm{e}^{-x^2/2},$$

and the distribution is known as the **standard normal** distribution. The cdf of the standard normal distribution is often denoted by Φ and its pdf by φ. In Fig. 2.11 the pdf of the $\mathcal{N}(\mu, \sigma^2)$ distribution for various μ and σ is plotted.

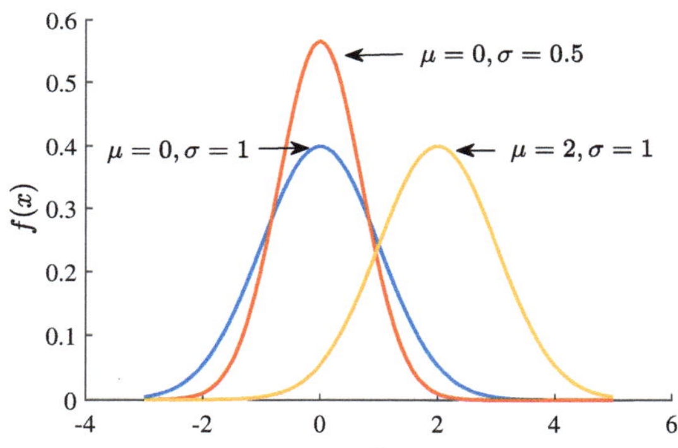

Fig. 2.11 The pdf of the $\mathcal{N}(\mu, \sigma^2)$ distribution for various μ and σ

We next consider some important properties of the normal distribution.

Theorem 2.15. (Standardization). Let $X \sim \mathcal{N}(\mu, \sigma^2)$ and define $Z = (X - \mu)/\sigma$. Then Z has a standard normal distribution.

Proof. The cdf of Z is given by

$$\mathbb{P}(Z \le z) = \mathbb{P}((X - \mu)/\sigma \le z) = \mathbb{P}(X \le \mu + \sigma z)$$

$$= \int_{-\infty}^{\mu+\sigma z} \frac{1}{\sigma\sqrt{2\pi}}\,\mathrm{e}^{-\frac{1}{2}\left(\frac{x-\mu}{\sigma}\right)^2}\,\mathrm{d}x = \int_{-\infty}^{z} \frac{1}{\sqrt{2\pi}}\,\mathrm{e}^{-y^2/2}\mathrm{d}y = \Phi(z)\,,$$

where we make a change of variable $y = (x - \mu)/\sigma$ in the fourth equation. Hence, $Z \sim \mathcal{N}(0, 1)$. $\qquad\square$

The rescaling procedure in Theorem 2.15 is called **standardization**. It follows from Theorem 2.15 that any $X \sim \mathcal{N}(\mu, \sigma^2)$ can be written as

$$X = \mu + \sigma Z, \quad \text{where } Z \sim \mathcal{N}(0, 1) \,.$$

In other words, any normal random variable can be viewed as an **affine transformation**—that is, a linear transformation plus a constant—of a standard normal random variable.

Next we prove the earlier claim that the parameters μ and σ^2 are respectively the expectation and variance of the distribution.

Theorem 2.16. (Expectation and Variance for the Normal Distribution). If $X \sim \mathcal{N}(\mu, \sigma^2)$, then $\mathbb{E}X = \mu$ and $\mathrm{Var}(X) = \sigma^2$.

Proof. Since the pdf is symmetric around μ and $\mathbb{E}X < \infty$, it follows that $\mathbb{E}X = \mu$. To show that the variance of X is σ^2, we first write $X = \mu + \sigma Z$, where $Z \sim \mathcal{N}(0, 1)$. Then, $\mathrm{Var}(X) = \mathrm{Var}(\mu + \sigma Z) = \sigma^2 \mathrm{Var}(Z)$. Hence, it suffices to show that $\mathrm{Var}(Z) = 1$. Now, since the expectation of Z is 0, we have

$$\mathrm{Var}(Z) = \mathbb{E}Z^2 = \int_{-\infty}^{\infty} z^2 \frac{1}{\sqrt{2\pi}} e^{-z^2/2} \, dz = \int_{-\infty}^{\infty} z \times \frac{z}{\sqrt{2\pi}} e^{-z^2/2} \, dz \,.$$

We apply integration by parts to the last integral to find

$$\mathbb{E}Z^2 = \left[-\frac{z}{\sqrt{2\pi}} e^{-z^2/2} \right]_{-\infty}^{\infty} + \int_{-\infty}^{\infty} \frac{1}{\sqrt{2\pi}} e^{-z^2/2} \, dz = 1 \,,$$

since the last integrand is the pdf of the standard normal distribution. $\qquad\square$

Theorem 2.17. (MGF for the Normal Distribution). The MGF of $X \sim \mathcal{N}(\mu, \sigma^2)$ is

$$\mathbb{E}e^{sX} = e^{s\mu + s^2\sigma^2/2}, \quad s \in \mathbb{R} \,. \tag{2.19}$$

Proof. Write $X = \mu + \sigma Z$, where $Z \sim \mathcal{N}(0, 1)$. We have

$$\mathbb{E}e^{sZ} = \int_{-\infty}^{\infty} e^{sz} \frac{1}{\sqrt{2\pi}} e^{-z^2/2} \, dz = e^{s^2/2} \underbrace{\int_{-\infty}^{\infty} \frac{1}{\sqrt{2\pi}} e^{-(z-s)^2/2} \, dz}_{\text{pdf of } \mathcal{N}(s,1)} = e^{s^2/2} \,,$$

so that $\mathbb{E}e^{sX} = \mathbb{E}e^{s(\mu+\sigma Z)} = e^{s\mu}\,\mathbb{E}e^{s\sigma Z} = e^{s\mu}e^{\sigma^2 s^2/2} = e^{s\mu+\sigma^2 s^2/2}$. $\square$

2.6.4 Gamma and χ^2 Distribution

Definition 2.18. (Gamma Distribution). A random variable X is said to have a **gamma** distribution with **shape** parameter $\alpha > 0$ and **rate** parameter $\lambda > 0$ if its pdf is given by

$$f(x) = \frac{\lambda^\alpha x^{\alpha-1}e^{-\lambda x}}{\Gamma(\alpha)}, \quad x \geq 0 \,, \tag{2.20}$$

where Γ is the gamma function. We write $X \sim \mathsf{Gamma}(\alpha, \lambda)$.

The **gamma function** $\Gamma(\alpha)$ is an important special function in mathematics, defined by

$$\Gamma(\alpha) = \int_0^\infty u^{\alpha-1}\,e^{-u}\,\mathrm{d}u \,. \tag{2.21}$$

We mention a few properties of the Γ function.

1. $\Gamma(\alpha + 1) = \alpha\,\Gamma(\alpha)$ for $\alpha > 0$.
2. $\Gamma(n) = (n-1)!$ for $n = 1, 2, \ldots$.
3. $\Gamma(1/2) = \sqrt{\pi}$.

Two special cases of the $\mathsf{Gamma}(\alpha, \lambda)$ distribution are worth mentioning. Firstly, the $\mathsf{Gamma}(1, \lambda)$ distribution is simply the $\mathsf{Exp}(\lambda)$ distribution. Secondly, the $\mathsf{Gamma}(n/2,\ 1/2)$ distribution, where $n \in \{1, 2, \ldots\}$, is called the **chi-squared** distribution with n **degrees of freedom**. We write $X \sim \chi_n^2$. A graph of the pdf of the χ_n^2 distribution for various n is given in Fig. 2.12.

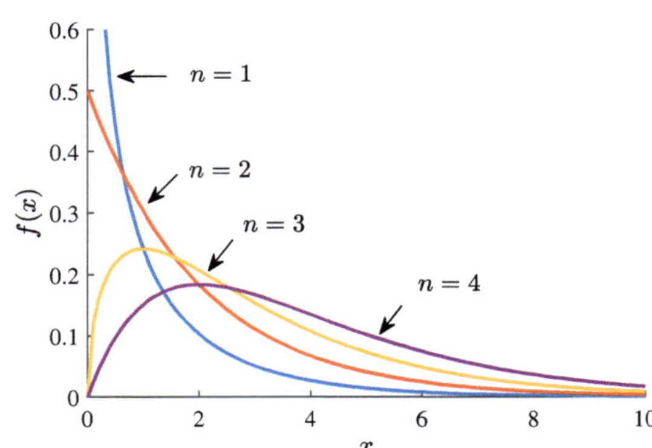

Fig. 2.12 The pdf of the χ_n^2 distribution for various degrees of freedom n

The following theorem summarizes some properties of the gamma distribution.

Theorem 2.18. (Properties of the Gamma Distribution). Let $X \sim \mathsf{Gamma}(\alpha, \lambda)$. Then,

1. $\mathbb{E}X = \alpha/\lambda$.
2. $\mathrm{Var}(X) = \alpha/\lambda^2$.
3. The MGF is $M(s) = [\lambda/(\lambda - s)]^\alpha, s < \lambda$ (and ∞ otherwise).

Proof.   3. For $s < \lambda$, the MGF of X at s is given by

$$M(s) = \mathbb{E}\,e^{sX} = \int_0^\infty \frac{e^{-\lambda x}\,\lambda^\alpha\,x^{\alpha-1}}{\Gamma(\alpha)}\,e^{sx}\,\mathrm{d}x$$

$$= \left(\frac{\lambda}{\lambda - s}\right)^\alpha \int_0^\infty \underbrace{\frac{e^{-(\lambda - s)x}\,(\lambda - s)^\alpha\,x^{\alpha-1}}{\Gamma(\alpha)}}_{\text{pdf of Gamma}(\alpha,\lambda-s)}\,\mathrm{d}x = \left(\frac{\lambda}{\lambda - s}\right)^\alpha. \qquad (2.22)$$

1. Consequently, by Theorem 2.7,

$$\mathbb{E}X = M'(0) = \frac{\alpha}{\lambda}\left(\frac{\lambda}{\lambda - s}\right)^{\alpha+1}\Bigg|_{s=0} = \frac{\alpha}{\lambda}.$$

2. Similarly, $\mathrm{Var}(X) = M''(0) - (M'(0))^2 = (\alpha + 1)\alpha/\lambda^2 - (\alpha/\lambda)^2 = \alpha/\lambda^2$.

☞ 36

2.6.5 F Distribution

Definition 2.19. (F Distribution). Let m and n be strictly positive integers. A random variable X is said to have an **F** distribution with **degrees of freedom** m and n if its pdf is given by

$$f(x) = \frac{\Gamma(\frac{m+n}{2})\,(m/n)^{m/2}x^{(m-2)/2}}{\Gamma(\frac{m}{2})\,\Gamma(\frac{n}{2})\,[1 + (m/n)x]^{(m+n)/2}}, \quad x \ge 0\,, \qquad (2.23)$$

where Γ denotes the gamma function. We write $X \sim \mathsf{F}(m, n)$.

The F distribution plays an important role in classical statistics, through Theorem 3.11. A graph of the pdf of the $\mathsf{F}(m, n)$ distribution for various m and n is given in Fig. 2.13.

☞ 88

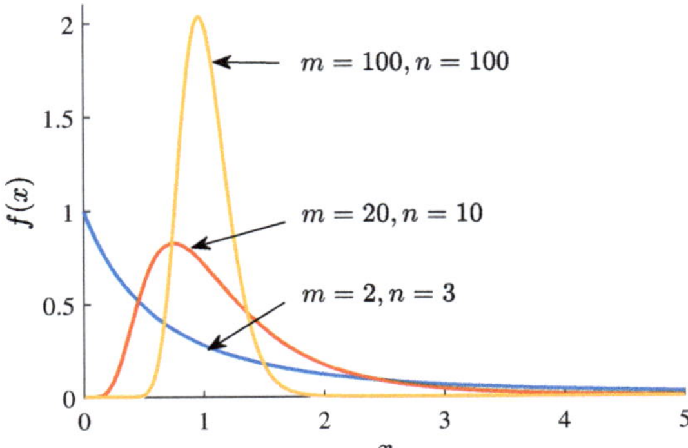

Fig. 2.13 The pdf of the $\mathsf{F}(m,n)$ distribution for various degrees of freedom m and n

2.6.6 Student's t Distribution

Definition 2.20. (Student's t Distribution). A random variable X is said to have a **Student's t** distribution with parameter $\nu > 0$ if its pdf is given by

$$f(x) = \frac{\Gamma(\frac{\nu+1}{2})}{\sqrt{\nu\pi}\,\Gamma(\frac{\nu}{2})} \left(1 + \frac{x^2}{\nu}\right)^{-(\nu+1)/2}, \quad x \in \mathbb{R}, \tag{2.24}$$

where Γ denotes the gamma function. We write $X \sim \mathsf{t}_\nu$. For integer values the parameter ν is referred to as the **degrees of freedom** of the distribution.

A graph of the pdf of the t_ν distribution for various ν is given in Fig. 2.14. Note that the pdf is symmetric. Moreover, it can be shown that the pdf of the t_ν distribution converges to the pdf of the $\mathcal{N}(0,1)$ distribution as $\nu \to \infty$. The t_1 distribution is called the **Cauchy distribution**.

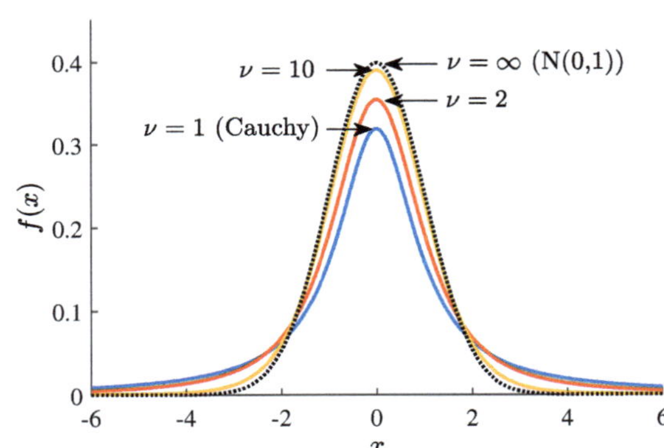

Fig. 2.14 The pdfs of t_1 (Cauchy), t_2, t_{10}, and $\mathsf{t}_\infty(\mathcal{N}(0,1))$ distributions

For completeness we mention that if $X \sim t_\nu$, then

$$\mathbb{E}X = 0 \quad (\nu > 1) \quad \text{and} \quad \mathrm{Var}(X) = \frac{\nu}{\nu - 2}, \quad (\nu > 2) \, .$$

The t and F distributions are related in the following way.

Theorem 2.19. (Relationship Between the t and F Distribution). For integer $n \geq 1$, if $X \sim t_n$, then $X^2 \sim F(1, n)$.

Proof. Let $Z = X^2$. We can express the cdf of Z in terms of the cdf of X. Namely, for every $z > 0$ we have

$$F_Z(z) = \mathbb{P}(X^2 \leq z) = \mathbb{P}(-\sqrt{z} \leq X \leq \sqrt{z}) = F_X(\sqrt{z}) - F_X(-\sqrt{z}) \, .$$

Differentiating with respect to z gives the following relation between the two pdfs:

$$f_Z(z) = f_X(\sqrt{z})\frac{1}{2\sqrt{z}} + f_X(-\sqrt{z})\frac{1}{2\sqrt{z}} = f_X(\sqrt{z})\frac{1}{\sqrt{z}} \, ,$$

using the symmetry of the t distribution. Substituting (2.24) into the last equation yields

$$f_Z(z) = c(n) \, \frac{z^{-1/2}}{(1 + z/n)^{(n+1)/2}}, \quad z > 0$$

for some constant $c(n)$. The only pdf of this form is that of the $F(1, n)$ distribution. $\qquad\qquad\square$

2.7 Generating Random Variables

This section shows how to generate random variables on a computer. We first discuss a modern uniform random generator and then introduce two general methods for drawing from an arbitrary one-dimensional distribution: the inverse-transform method and the acceptance–rejection method.

2.7.1 Generating Uniform Random Variables

The **rand** function in Julia simulates the drawing of a uniform random number on the interval $(0, 1)$ by generating *pseudo*-random numbers, that is, numbers that, although not actually random (because the computer is a deterministic device), behave for all intended purposes as truly random. The following algorithm (L'Ecuyer (1999)) uses simple recurrences to produce high-quality pseudo-random numbers, in the sense that the numbers pass all currently known statistical tests for randomness and uniformity.

Algorithm 2.1. (Combined Multiple-Recursive Generator).

1. Suppose N random numbers are required. Define $m_1 = 2^{32} - 209$ and $m_2 = 2^{32} - 22853$.
2. Initialize a vector $(X_{-2}, X_{-1}, X_0) = (12345, 12345, 12345)$ and a vector $(Y_{-2}, Y_{-1}, Y_0) = (12345, 12345, 12345)$.
3. For $t = 1$ to N let

$$X_t = (1403580\, X_{t-2} - 810728\, X_{t-3}) \bmod m_1\,,$$

$$Y_t = (527612\, Y_{t-1} - 1370589\, Y_{t-3}) \bmod m_2\,,$$

and output the t-th random number as

$$U_t = \begin{cases} \dfrac{X_t - Y_t + m_1}{m_1 + 1} & \text{if } X_t \le Y_t\,, \\[2ex] \dfrac{X_t - Y_t}{m_1 + 1} & \text{if } X_t > Y_t\,. \end{cases}$$

Here, $x \bmod m$ means the remainder of x when divided by m. The initialization in Step 2 determines the initial state—the so-called seed— of the random number stream. Restarting the stream from the same seed produces the same sequence.

The current default random number generator in Julia is Xoshiro256++ (XOR/rotate/shift/rotate). A typical usage of Julia's uniform random number generator is as follows.

```julia
using Random # Loading the Random package
Random.seed!(1234)   # set the seed to 1234
rand(1,5)    # 1x5 matrix of random numbers

Random.seed!(1234)   # reset the seed to 1234
rand(5)       # vector of random numbers
```

```
1x5 Matrix{Float64}:
0.325977  0.549051  0.218587  0.894245  0.353112

5-element Vector{Float64}:
```

```
0.32597672886359486
0.5490511363155669
0.21858665481883066
0.8942454282009883
0.35311164439921205
```

The package **Random** was loaded to set the random seed of the random number generator. This is useful for testing purposes, as always the same random sequence is generated. If the random seed is not required, one does not need to load the **Random** package to execute the **rand** function, as the latter is part of the base package of Julia.

2.7.2 Inverse-Transform Method

Once we have a method for drawing a uniform random number, we can, in principle, simulate a random variable X from *any* cdf F by using the following algorithm.

Algorithm 2.2. (Inverse-Transform Method).

1. Generate U from $\mathcal{U}(0, 1)$.
2. Return $X = F^{-1}(U)$, where F^{-1} is the inverse function of F.

Figure 2.15 illustrates the inverse-transform method. We see that the random variable $X = F^{-1}(U)$ has cdf F, since

$$\mathbb{P}(X \leq x) = \mathbb{P}(F^{-1}(U) \leq x) = \mathbb{P}(U \leq F(x)) = F(x) \ . \tag{2.25}$$

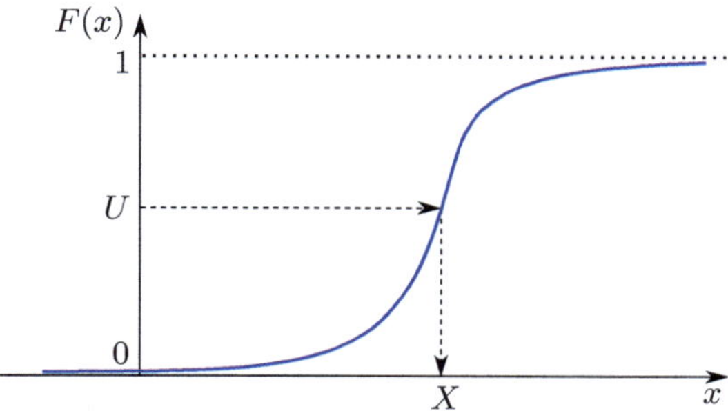

Fig. 2.15 The inverse-transform method

Example 2.7 (Generating Uniformly on a Unit Disk). Suppose we wish to draw a random point (X, Y) uniformly on the unit disk; see Fig. 2.16.

In polar coordinates we have $X = R\cos\Theta$ and $Y = R\sin\Theta$, where Θ has a $\mathcal{U}(0, 2\pi)$ distribution. The cdf of R is given by

$$F(r) = \mathbb{P}(R \leq r) = \frac{\pi r^2}{\pi} = r^2, \quad 0 < r < 1.$$

Its inverse is $F^{-1}(u) = \sqrt{u}$, $0 < u < 1$. We can thus generate R via the inverse-transform method as $R = \sqrt{U_1}$, where $U_1 \sim \mathcal{U}(0,1)$. In addition, we can simulate Θ as $\Theta = 2\pi U_2$, where $U_2 \sim \mathcal{U}(0,1)$. Note that U_1 and U_2 should be independent draws from $\mathcal{U}(0,1)$.

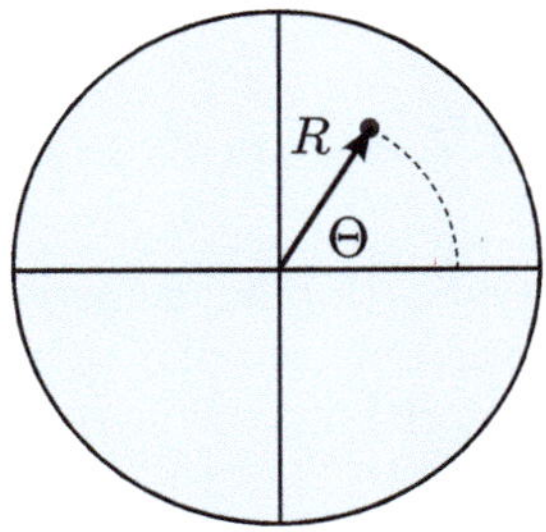

Fig. 2.16 Draw a point (X, Y) uniformly on the unit disk

The inverse-transform method holds for general cdfs F. Note that F for discrete random variables is a step function, as illustrated in Fig. 2.17. The algorithm for generating a random variable X from a discrete distribution that takes values $x_1, x_2, \ldots$ with probabilities $p_1, p_2, \ldots$ is thus as follows.

Algorithm 2.3. (Discrete Inverse-Transform Method).

1. Generate $U \sim \mathcal{U}(0,1)$.
2. Find the smallest positive integer k such that $F(x_k) \geq U$ and return $X = x_k$.

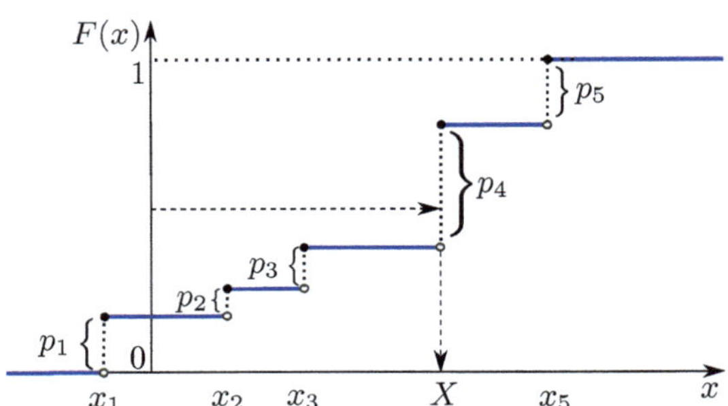

Fig. 2.17 The inverse-transform method for a discrete random variable

Drawing one of the numbers $1, \ldots, n$ according to a probability vector $[p_1, \ldots, p_n]$ can be done in one line of Julia code:

```julia
minimum(findall(cumsum(p) .> rand()))
```

Here **p** is the vector of probabilities, such as $[0.3, 0.2, 0.5]$, **cumsum** gives the cumulative vector, e.g., $[0.3, 0.5, 1]$, **findall** finds all the indices i such that the cumulative probability is greater than some random number **rand()**, and **minimum** takes the smallest of these indices.

2.7.3 Acceptance–Rejection Method

The inverse-transform method may not always be easy to implement, in particular when the inverse cdf is difficult to compute. In that case the **acceptance–rejection** method may prove to be useful. The idea of this method is depicted in Fig. 2.18. Suppose we wish to sample from a pdf f. Let g be another pdf such that for some constant $C \geq 1$ we have that $Cg(x) \geq f(x)$ for all x. It is assumed that it is easy to sample from g, for example, via the inverse-transform method.

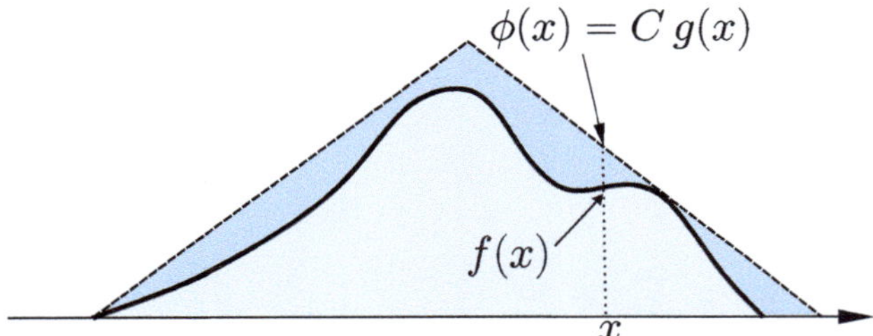

Fig. 2.18 Illustration of the acceptance–rejection method

It is intuitively clear that if a random point (X, Y) is *uniformly* distributed under the graph of f—that is, on the set $\{(x, y) : 0 \leq y \leq f(x)\}$—then X must have pdf f. To construct such a point, let us first draw a random point (Z, V) by drawing Z from g and then drawing V uniformly on $[0, Cg(Z)]$. The point (Z, V) is uniformly distributed under the graph of Cg. If we keep drawing such a point (Z, V) *until it lies under the graph of f*, then the resulting point (X, Y) must be uniformly distributed under the graph of f and hence the X coordinate must have pdf f. This leads to the following algorithm.

Algorithm 2.4. (Acceptance–Rejection Method).

1 repeat
2 | Generate $X \sim g$.
3 | Generate $Y \sim \mathcal{U}(0, C\,g(X))$.
4 until $Y \leq f(X)$
5 return X

Example 2.8 (Generating from the Standard Normal Distribution).

To sample from the standard normal pdf via the inverse-transform method requires knowledge of the inverse of the corresponding cdf, which involves numerical integration. Instead, we can use acceptance–rejection. First, observe that the standard normal pdf is symmetric around 0. Hence, if we can generate a random variable X from the **positive normal** pdf (see Fig. 2.19),

$$f(x) = \sqrt{\frac{2}{\pi}}\; \mathrm{e}^{-x^2/2}, \qquad x \geq 0 , \tag{2.26}$$

then we can generate a standard normal random variable by multiplying X with 1 or -1, each with probability $1/2$. We can bound $f(x)$ by $C\,g(x)$, where $g(x) = \mathrm{e}^{-x}$ is the pdf of the $\mathsf{Exp}(1)$ distribution. The smallest constant C such that $f(x) \leq Cg(x)$ is $\sqrt{2\mathrm{e}/\pi}$.

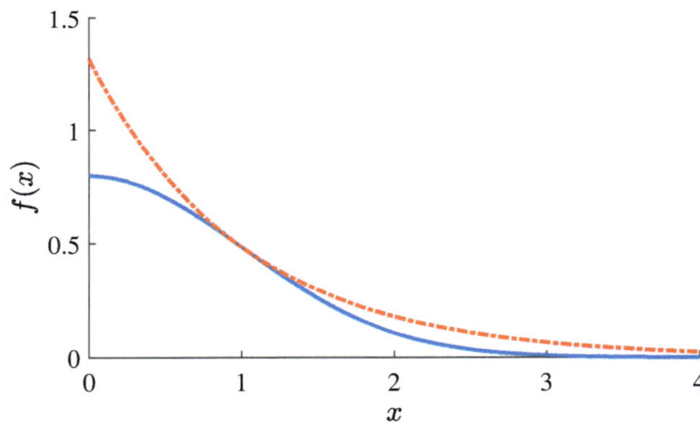

Fig. 2.19 Bounding the positive normal density (solid curve) via an $\mathsf{Exp}(1)$ pdf (times $C \approx 1.3155$)

Drawing from the $\mathsf{Exp}(1)$ distribution can be easily done via the inverse-transform method, noting that the corresponding cdf is the function $1 - \mathrm{e}^{-x}, x \geq 0$, whose inverse is the function $-\ln(1 - u)$, $u \in (0,1)$. This gives the following specification of Algorithm 2.4, where f and C are defined above.

Algorithm 2.5. ($\mathcal{N}(0, 1)$ Generator).

1 repeat
2 $\quad$ Draw $U_1 \sim \mathcal{U}(0, 1)$ and let $Z = -\ln U_1$.
3 $\quad$ Draw $U_2 \sim \mathcal{U}(0, 1)$ and let $Y = U_2\, C\, e^{-Z}$.
4 until $Y \leq f(Z)$
5 Draw $U_3 \sim \mathcal{U}(0, 1)$ and let $X = Z\left(2\, \mathbb{1}_{\{U_3 < 1/2\}} - 1\right)$
6 return X

In Step 2, we have used the fact that if $U \sim \mathcal{U}(0, 1)$ then also $1 - U \sim \mathcal{U}(0, 1)$. In Step 5, $\mathbb{1}_{\{U_3 < 1/2\}}$ denotes the **indicator** of the event $\{U_3 < 1/2\}$, which is 1 if $U_3 < 1/2$ and 0 otherwise. An alternative generation method is given in Algorithm 3.2. In Julia normal random variable generation is implemented via the **randn** function. ☞ 82

2.8 Problems

2.1. Two fair dice are thrown and the smallest of the face values, M say, is noted.

a. Give the discrete pdf of M in table form, as in Table 2.1. ☞ 28
b. What is the probability that M is at least 3?
c. Calculate the expectation and variance of M.

2.2. A continuous random variable X has cdf

$$
F(x) = \begin{cases}
0, & x < 0 \\
x^2/5, & 0 \leq x \leq 1 \\
\frac{1}{5}\left(-x^2 + 6x - 4\right), & 1 < x \leq 3 \\
1, & x > 3 .
\end{cases}
$$

a. Find the corresponding pdf and plot its graph.
b. Calculate the following probabilities:

$\quad$ i. $\mathbb{P}(X \leq 2)$
$\quad$ ii. $\mathbb{P}(1 < X \leq 2)$
$\quad$ iii. $\mathbb{P}(1 \leq X \leq 2)$.
$\quad$ iv. $\mathbb{P}(X > 1/2)$.

c. Show that $\mathbb{E}X = 22/15$.

2.3. In this book most random variables are either discrete or continuous; that is, they have either a discrete or continuous pdf. It is also possible to define random variables that have a mix of discrete and continuous characteristics. A simple example is a random variable X with cdf

$$F(x) = \begin{cases} 0, & x < 0 \\ 1 - c\,e^{-x}, & x \geq 0 \end{cases}$$

for some fixed $0 < c < 1$.

a. Sketch the cdf F.
b. Find the following probabilities:

    i. $\mathbb{P}(0 \leq X \leq x)$, $x \geq 0$.
    ii. $\mathbb{P}(0 < X \leq x)$, $x \geq 0$.
    iii. $\mathbb{P}(X = x)$, $x \geq 0$.

c. Describe how the inverse-transform method can be used to draw samples from this distribution.

2.4. Let X be a positive random variable with cdf F. Prove that

$$\mathbb{E}X = \int_0^\infty (1 - F(x))\,\mathrm{d}x \ . \tag{2.27}$$

2.5. Let X be a random variable that can possibly take values $-\infty$ and ∞ with probabilities $\mathbb{P}(X = -\infty) = a$ and $\mathbb{P}(X = \infty) = b$, respectively. Show that the corresponding cdf F satisfies $\lim_{x \to -\infty} F(x) = a$ and $\lim_{x \to \infty} F(x) = 1 - b$.

2.6. Suppose that in a large population the fraction of left-handers is 12%. We select at random 100 people from this population. Let X be the number of left-handers among the selected people. What is the distribution of X? What is the probability that at most seven of the selected people are left-handed?

2.7. Let $X \sim \mathsf{Geom}(p)$. Show that

$$\mathbb{P}(X > k) = (1 - p)^k.$$

2.8. Find the moment generating function (MGF) of $X \sim \mathcal{U}[a, b]$.

☞ 43   **2.9.** Let $X = a + (b - a)U$, where $U \sim \mathcal{U}[0, 1]$. Prove that $X \sim \mathcal{U}[a, b]$. Use this to provide a more elegant proof of Theorem 2.13.

2.10. Show that the exponential distribution is the *only* continuous (positive) distribution that possesses the memoryless property. Hint: show that the memoryless property implies that the tail probability $g(x) = \mathbb{P}(X > x)$ satisfies $g(x + y) = g(x)g(y)$.

2.11. Let $X \sim \mathsf{Exp}(2)$. Calculate the following quantities:

a. $\mathbb{P}(-1 \le X \le 1)$.
b. $\mathbb{P}(X > 4)$.
c. $\mathbb{P}(X > 4 \mid X > 2)$.
d. $\mathbb{E} X^2$.

2.12. What is the expectation of a random variable X with the following discrete pdf on the set of integer numbers, excluding 0:

$$f(x) = \frac{3}{\pi^2} \frac{1}{x^2}, \quad x \in \mathbb{Z} \setminus \{0\} \ ?$$

What is the pdf of the absolute value $|X|$ and what is its expectation?

2.13. A random variable X is said to have a **discrete uniform distribution** on the set $\{a, a+1, \ldots, b\}$ if

$$\mathbb{P}(X = x) = \frac{1}{b - a + 1}, \quad x = a, a+1, \ldots, b \ .$$

a. What is the expectation of X?
b. Show that $\mathrm{Var}(X) = (b - a)(b - a + 2)/12$.
c. Find the probability generating function (PGF) of X.
d. Describe a simple way to generate X using a uniform number generator.

2.14. Let X and Y be random variables. Prove that if $X \le Y$, then $\mathbb{E} X \le \mathbb{E} Y$.

2.15. A continuous random variable is said to have a **logistic** distribution if its pdf is given by

$$f(x) = \frac{\mathrm{e}^{-x}}{(1 + \mathrm{e}^{-x})^2}, \quad x \in \mathbb{R} \ . \tag{2.28}$$

a. Plot the graph of the pdf.
b. Show that $\mathbb{P}(X > x) = 1/(1 + \mathrm{e}^x)$ for all x.
c. Write an algorithm based on the inverse-transform method to generate random variables from this distribution.

2.16. An electrical component has a lifetime (in years) that is distributed according to an exponential distribution with expectation 3. What is the probability that the component is still functioning after 4.5 years, given that it still works after 4 years? Answer the same question for the case where the component's lifetime is normally distributed with the same expected value and variance as before.

2.17. Consider the pdf given by

$$f(x) = \begin{cases} 4\,e^{-4(x-1)}, & x \geq 1\,, \\ 0, & x < 1\,. \end{cases}$$

a. If X is distributed according to this pdf f, what is its expectation?
b. Specify how one can generate a random variable $X \sim f$ using a uniform random number generator.

2.18. Let $X \sim \mathsf{N}(4,9)$.

a. Plot the graph of the pdf.
b. Express the following probabilities in terms of the cdf Φ of the standard normal distribution:

   i. $\mathbb{P}(X \leq 3)$.
  ii. $\mathbb{P}(X > 4)$.
 iii. $\mathbb{P}(-1 \leq X \leq 5)$.

c. Find $\mathbb{E}[2X + 1]$.
d. Calculate $\mathbb{E}X^2$.

2.19. Let Φ be the cdf of $X \sim \mathsf{N}(0,1)$. The integral

$$\Phi(x) = \int_{-\infty}^{x} \frac{1}{\sqrt{2\pi}} e^{-\frac{1}{2}u^2}\, du$$

needs to be evaluated numerically. In Julia there are several ways to do this.

1. If the package `Distributions` is loaded, the cdf can be evaluated via the function `x -> cdf(Normal(0,1),x)`. The inverse cdf can be evaluated via `p -> quantile(Normal(0,1),p)`.
2. Or use the **error function** from the package `SpecialFunctions`, defined as
$$\operatorname{erf}(x) = \frac{2}{\sqrt{\pi}} \int_0^x e^{-u^2}\, du\,, \quad x \in \mathbb{R}\,.$$

   The inverse of `erf` is implemented in the same package as `erfinv`.
3. A third alternative is to use numerical integration (quadrature) via the package `QuadGK`. For example, `quadgk(f,0,x)` integrates a function `f` on the interval $[0, x]$.

a. Show that $\Phi(x) = (\operatorname{erf}(x/\sqrt{2}) + 1)/2$.
b. Evaluate $\Phi(x)$ for $x = 1, 2$, and 3 via (a) the error function and (b) numerical integration of the pdf, using the fact that $\Phi(0) = 1/2$.
c. Show that the inverse of Φ is given by

$$\Phi^{-1}(y) = \sqrt{2}\,\operatorname{erf}^{-1}(2y - 1)\,, \quad 0 < y < 1\,.$$

2.20. Based on Julia's **rand** and **randn** functions *only*, implement algorithms that generate random variables from the following distributions:

a. $\mathcal{U}[2,3]$.
b. $\mathcal{N}(3,9)$.
c. $\mathsf{Exp}(4)$.
d. $\mathsf{Bin}(10,1/2)$.
e. $\mathsf{Geom}(1/6)$.

2.21. The **Weibull** distribution $\mathsf{Weib}(\alpha,\lambda)$ has cdf

$$F(x) = 1 - \mathrm{e}^{-(\lambda x)^{\alpha}}, \quad x \geq 0. \tag{2.29}$$

It can be viewed as a generalization of the exponential distribution. Write a Julia program that draws 1000 samples from the $\mathsf{Weib}(2,1)$ distribution using the inverse-transform method. Give a histogram of the sample.

2.22. Consider the pdf

$$f(x) = c\,\mathrm{e}^{-x}x(1-x), \quad 0 \leq x \leq 1.$$

a. Show that $c = \mathrm{e}/(3-\mathrm{e})$.
b. Devise an acceptance–rejection algorithm to generate random variables that are distributed according to f.
c. Implement the algorithm in Julia.

2.23. Implement two different algorithms to draw 100 uniformly generated points on the unit disk: one based on Example 2.7 and the other using (two-dimensional) acceptance–rejection. ☞ 53

Chapter 3
Joint Distributions

Often a random experiment is described via more than one random variable. Here are some examples.

1. We randomly select $n = 10$ people and observe their heights. Let $X_1, \ldots, X_n$ be the individual heights.
2. We toss a coin repeatedly. Let $X_i = 1$ if the i-th toss is Heads and $X_i = 0$ otherwise. The experiment is thus described by the sequence $X_1, X_2, \ldots$ of Bernoulli random variables.
3. We randomly select a person from a large population and measure his/her weight X and height Y.

How can we specify the behavior of the random variables above? We should not just specify the pdf of the individual random variables, but also say something about the interaction (or lack thereof) between the random variables. For example, in the third experiment above if the height Y is large, then most likely X is large as well. In contrast, in the first two experiments it is reasonable to assume that the random variables are "independent" in some way; that is, information about one of the random variables does not give extra information about the others. What we need to specify is the **joint distribution** of the random variables. The theory below for multiple random variables follows a similar path to that of a single random variable described in Sects. 2.1–2.3.

Let $X_1, \ldots, X_n$ be random variables describing some random experiment. We can accumulate the $\{X_i\}$ into a **random vector** $\boldsymbol{X} = [X_1, \ldots, X_n]$ (row vector) or $\boldsymbol{X} = [X_1, \ldots, X_n]^\top$ (column vector). Recall that the distribution of a *single* random variable X is completely specified by its cumulative distribution function. For *multiple* random variables we have the following generalization.

☞ 23

© The Author(s), under exclusive license to Springer Science+Business Media, LLC, part of Springer Nature 2025
J. C. C. Chan, D. P. Kroese, *Statistical Modeling and Computation*,
Springer Texts in Statistics, https://doi.org/10.1007/978-1-0716-4132-3_3

Definition 3.1. (Joint Cdf). The **joint cdf** of $X_1, \ldots, X_n$ is the function $F : \mathbb{R}^n \to [0,1]$ defined by

$$F(x_1, \ldots, x_n) = \mathbb{P}(X_1 \leq x_1, \ldots, X_n \leq x_n) \,.$$

Notice that we have used the abbreviation $\mathbb{P}(\{X_1 \leq x_1\} \cap \cdots \cap \{X_n \leq x_n\}) = \mathbb{P}(X_1 \leq x_1, \ldots, X_n \leq x_n)$ to denote the probability of the intersection of events. We will use this abbreviation throughout the book.

As in the univariate (i.e., single-variable) case we distinguish between *discrete* and *continuous* distributions.

3.1 Discrete Joint Distributions

Example 3.1 (Dice Experiment). In a box there are three dice. Die 1 is an ordinary die; die 2 has no six faces, but instead two 5 faces; die 3 has no five faces, but instead two 6 faces. The experiment consists of selecting a die at random followed by a toss with that die. Let X be the die number that is selected and let Y be the face value of that die. The probabilities $\mathbb{P}(X = x, Y = y)$ in Table 3.1 specify the joint distribution of X and Y. Note that it is more convenient to specify the joint probabilities $\mathbb{P}(X = x, Y = y)$ than the joint cumulative probabilities $\mathbb{P}(X \leq x, Y \leq y)$. The latter can be found, however, from the former by applying the sum rule. For example, $\mathbb{P}(X \leq 2, Y \leq 3) = \mathbb{P}(X = 1, Y = 1) + \cdots + \mathbb{P}(X = 2, Y = 3) = 6/18 = 1/3$. Moreover, by that same sum rule, the distribution of X is found by summing the $\mathbb{P}(X = x, Y = y)$ over all values of y—giving the last column of Table 3.1. Similarly, the distribution of Y is given by the column totals in the last row of the table.

Table 3.1 The joint distribution of X (die number) and Y (face value)

		1	2	3	4	5	6	$\sum$
	1	$\frac{1}{18}$	$\frac{1}{18}$	$\frac{1}{18}$	$\frac{1}{18}$	$\frac{1}{18}$	$\frac{1}{18}$	$\frac{1}{3}$
x	2	$\frac{1}{18}$	$\frac{1}{18}$	$\frac{1}{18}$	$\frac{1}{18}$	$\frac{1}{9}$	0	$\frac{1}{3}$
	3	$\frac{1}{18}$	$\frac{1}{18}$	$\frac{1}{18}$	$\frac{1}{18}$	0	$\frac{1}{9}$	$\frac{1}{3}$
$\sum$		$\frac{1}{6}$	$\frac{1}{6}$	$\frac{1}{6}$	$\frac{1}{6}$	$\frac{1}{6}$	$\frac{1}{6}$	1

(column heading y spans columns 1–6)

In general, for discrete random variables $X_1, \ldots, X_n$ the joint distribution is easiest to specify via the joint pdf.

Definition 3.2. (Discrete Joint Pdf). The **joint pdf** f of discrete random variables $X_1, \ldots, X_n$ is given by the function

$$f(x_1, \ldots, x_n) = \mathbb{P}(X_1 = x_1, \ldots, X_n = x_n) .$$

We sometimes write $f_{X_1, \ldots, X_n}$ instead of f to show that this is the pdf of the random variables $X_1, \ldots, X_n$. Or, if $\boldsymbol{X} = [X_1, \ldots, X_n]$ is the corresponding random vector, we can write $f_{\boldsymbol{X}}$ instead.

If the joint pdf f is known, we can calculate the probability of any event $\{\boldsymbol{X} \in B\}$, B in $\mathbb{R}^n$, via the sum rule as

$$\mathbb{P}(\boldsymbol{X} \in B) = \sum_{\boldsymbol{x} \in B} f(\boldsymbol{x}) .$$

Compare this with (2.2). In particular, as explained in Example 3.1, we can find the pdf of X_i—often referred to as a **marginal** pdf, to distinguish it from the joint pdf—by summing the joint pdf over all possible values of the other variables:

$$\mathbb{P}(X_i = x) = \sum_{x_1} \cdots \sum_{x_{i-1}} \sum_{x_{i+1}} \cdots \sum_{x_n} f(x_1, \ldots, x_{i-1}, x, x_{i+1}, x_n) . \qquad (3.1)$$

The converse is not true: from the marginal distributions one cannot in general reconstruct the joint distribution. For example, in Example 3.1 we cannot reconstruct the inside of the two-dimensional table if only given the column and row totals.

However, there is one important exception, namely, when the random variables are *independent*. We have so far only defined what independence is for *events*. We can define random variables $X_1, \ldots, X_n$ to be independent if events $\{X_1 \in B_1\}, \ldots, \{X_n \in B_n\}$ are independent for any choice of sets $\{B_i\}$. Intuitively, this means that any information about one of the random variables does not affect our knowledge about the others.

Definition 3.3. (Independence). Random variables $X_1, \ldots, X_n$ are called **independent** if for all events $\{X_i \in B_i\}$ with $B_i \subseteq \mathbb{R}$, $i = 1, \ldots, n$

$$\mathbb{P}(X_1 \in B_1, \ldots, X_n \in B_n) = \mathbb{P}(X_1 \in B_1) \cdots \mathbb{P}(X_n \in B_n) . \qquad (3.2)$$

A direct consequence of the above definition is the following important theorem.

Theorem 3.1. (Independence and Product Rule). Random variables $X_1, \ldots, X_n$ with joint pdf f are independent if and only if

$$f(x_1, \ldots, x_n) = f_{X_1}(x_1) \cdots f_{X_n}(x_n) \tag{3.3}$$

for all $x_1, \ldots, x_n$, where $\{f_{X_i}\}$ are the marginal pdfs.

Proof. The theorem is true in both the discrete and continuous case. We only show the discrete case, where (3.3) is a special case of (3.2). It follows that (3.3) is a *necessary* condition for independence. To see that it is also a *sufficient* condition, let $\boldsymbol{X} = (X_1, \ldots, X_n)$ and observe that

$$\mathbb{P}(X_1 \in B_1, \ldots, X_n \in B_n) = \mathbb{P}(\boldsymbol{X} \in \underbrace{B_1 \times \cdots \times B_n}_{A}) = \sum_{\boldsymbol{x} \in A} f(\boldsymbol{x})$$

$$= \sum_{\boldsymbol{x} \in A} f_{X_1}(x_1) \cdots f_{X_n}(x_n) = \sum_{x_1 \in B_1} f_{X_1}(x_1) \cdots \sum_{x_n \in B_n} f_{X_n}(x_n)$$

$$= \mathbb{P}(X_1 \in B_1) \cdots \mathbb{P}(X_n \in B_n) .$$

Here $A = B_1 \times \cdots \times B_n$ denotes the Cartesian product of $B_1, \ldots, B_n$. $\qquad \square$

Example 3.2 (Dice Experiment Continued). We repeat the experiment in Example 3.1 with three ordinary fair dice. Since the events $\{X = x\}$ and $\{Y = y\}$ are now independent, each entry in the pdf table is $\frac{1}{3} \times \frac{1}{6}$. Clearly in the first experiment not *all* events $\{X = x\}$ and $\{Y = y\}$ are independent.

Remark 3.1. An *infinite* sequence $X_1, X_2, \ldots$ of random variables is said to be *independent* if for any finite choice of positive integers $i_1, i_2, \ldots, i_n$ (none of them the same) the random variables $X_{i_1}, \ldots, X_{i_n}$ are independent. Many statistical models involve random variables $X_1, X_2, \ldots$ that are **independent and identically distributed**, abbreviated as **iid**. We will use this abbreviation throughout this book and write the corresponding model as

$$X_1, X_2, \ldots \overset{\text{iid}}{\sim} \mathsf{Dist} \text{ (or } f \text{ or } F) ,$$

where Dist is the common distribution with pdf f and cdf F.

Example 3.3 (Bernoulli Process). Consider the experiment where we toss a biased coin n times, with probability p of Heads. We can model this experiment in the following way. For $i = 1, \ldots, n$ let X_i be the result of the i-th toss: $\{X_i = 1\}$ means Heads (or success), and $\{X_i = 0\}$ means Tails (or failure). Also, let

$$\mathbb{P}(X_i = 1) = p = 1 - \mathbb{P}(X_i = 0), \quad i = 1, 2, \ldots, n .$$

Finally, assume that $X_1, \ldots, X_n$ are *independent*. The sequence

$$X_1, X_2, \ldots \overset{\text{iid}}{\sim} \mathsf{Ber}(p)$$

is called a **Bernoulli process** with success probability p. Let $X = X_1 + \cdots + X_n$ be the total number of successes in n trials (tosses of the coin). Denote by B_k the set of all binary vectors $\boldsymbol{x} = [x_1, \ldots, x_n]$ such that $\sum_{i=1}^{n} x_i = k$. Note that B_k has $\binom{n}{k}$ elements. We have for every $k = 0, \ldots, n$,

$$
\begin{aligned}
\mathbb{P}(X = k) &= \sum_{\boldsymbol{x} \in B_k} \mathbb{P}(X_1 = x_1, \ldots, X_n = x_n) \\
&= \sum_{\boldsymbol{x} \in B_k} \mathbb{P}(X_1 = x_1) \cdots \mathbb{P}(X_n = x_n) = \sum_{\boldsymbol{x} \in B_k} p^k (1 - p)^{n-k} \\
&= \binom{n}{k} p^k (1 - p)^{n-k} .
\end{aligned}
$$

In other words, $X \sim \mathsf{Bin}(n, p)$. Compare this with Example 2.2.   ☞ 24

For the joint pdf of *dependent* discrete random variables we can write, as a consequence of the product rule (1.5),   ☞ 14

$$
\begin{aligned}
f(x_1, \ldots, x_n) &= \mathbb{P}(X_1 = x_1, \ldots, X_n = x_n) \\
&= \mathbb{P}(X_1 = x_1) \, \mathbb{P}(X_2 = x_2 \mid X_1 = x_1) \times \cdots \\
&\quad \cdots \times \mathbb{P}(X_n = x_n \mid X_1 = x_1, \ldots, X_{n-1} = x_{n-1}) ,
\end{aligned}
$$

assuming that all probabilities $\mathbb{P}(X = x_1), \ldots, \mathbb{P}(X_1 = x_1, \ldots, X_{n-1} = x_{n-1})$ are non-zero. The function which maps, *for a fixed x_1*, each variable x_2 to the conditional probability

$$\mathbb{P}(X_2 = x_2 \mid X_1 = x_1) = \frac{\mathbb{P}(X_1 = x_1, X_2 = x_2)}{\mathbb{P}(X_1 = x_1)} \tag{3.4}$$

is called the **conditional pdf** of X_2 given $X_1 = x_1$. We write it as $f_{X_2 \mid X_1}(x_2 \mid x_1)$. Similarly, the function $x_n \mapsto \mathbb{P}(X_n = x_n \mid X_1 = x_1, \ldots, X_{n-1} = x_{n-1})$ is the conditional pdf of X_n given $X_1 = x_1, \ldots, X_{n-1} = x_{n-1}$, which is written as $f_{X_n \mid X_1, \ldots, X_{n-1}}(x_n \mid x_1, \ldots, x_{n-1})$.

Example 3.4 (Generating Uniformly on a Triangle). We uniformly select a point (X, Y) from the triangle $T = \{(x, y) : x, y \in \{1, \ldots, 6\}, y \le x\}$ in Fig. 3.1.

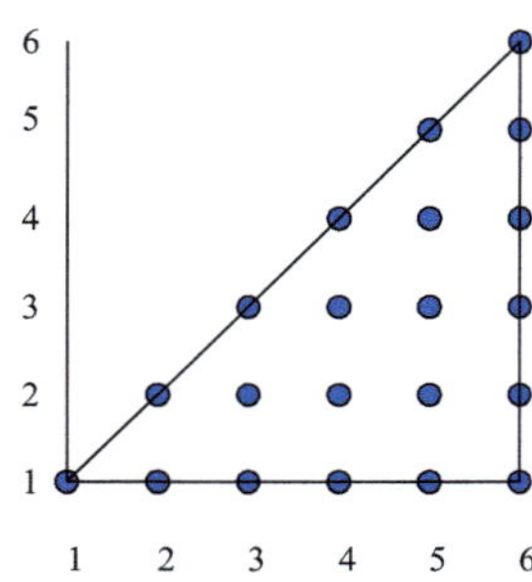

Fig. 3.1 Uniformly select
a point from the triangle

Because each of the 21 points is equally likely to be selected, the joint pdf
is constant on T:

$$f(x,y) = \frac{1}{21}, \quad (x,y) \in T \, .$$

The pdf of X is found by summing $f(x,y)$ over all y. Hence,

$$f_X(x) = \frac{x}{21}, \quad x \in \{1,\ldots,6\} \, .$$

Similarly,

$$f_Y(y) = \frac{7-y}{21}, \quad y \in \{1,\ldots,6\} \, .$$

For a fixed $x \in \{1,\ldots,6\}$ the conditional pdf of Y given $X = x$ is

$$f_{Y|X}(y\,|\,x) = \frac{f(x,y)}{f_X(x)} = \frac{1/21}{x/21} = \frac{1}{x}, \quad y \in \{1,\ldots,x\} \, ,$$

which simply means that, given $X = x$, Y has a discrete uniform distribution
on $\{1,\ldots,x\}$.

3.1.1 Multinomial Distribution

An important discrete joint distribution is the multinomial distribution. It
can be viewed as a generalization of the binomial distribution. We give the
definition and then an example of how this distribution arises in applications.

Definition 3.4. (Multinomial Distribution). A random vector $[X_1, X_2, \ldots, X_k]$ is said to have a **multinomial** distribution with parameters n and $p_1, p_2, \ldots, p_k$ (positive and summing up to 1), if

$$\mathbb{P}(X_1 = x_1, \ldots, X_k = x_k) = \frac{n!}{x_1!\, x_2! \cdots x_k!}\, p_1^{x_1} p_2^{x_2} \cdots p_k^{x_k} , \qquad (3.5)$$

for all $x_1, \ldots, x_k \in \{0, 1, \ldots, n\}$ such that $x_1 + x_2 + \cdots + x_k = n$. We write $(X_1, \ldots, X_k) \sim \mathsf{Mnom}(n, p_1, \ldots, p_k)$.

Example 3.5 (Urn Problem). We independently throw n balls into k urns, such that each ball is thrown in urn i with probability p_i, $i = 1, \ldots, k$; see Fig. 3.2.

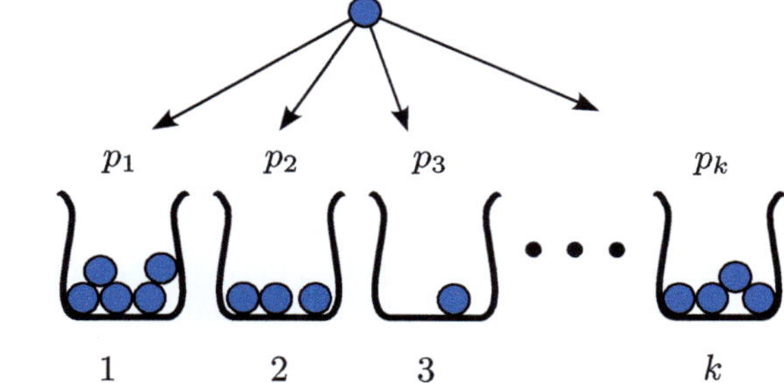

Fig. 3.2 Throwing n balls into k urns with probabilities $p_1, \ldots, p_k$. The random configuration of balls has a multinomial distribution

Let X_i be the total number of balls in urn i, $i = 1, \ldots, k$. We show that $[X_1, \ldots, X_k] \sim \mathsf{Mnom}(n, p_1, \ldots, p_k)$. Let $x_1, \ldots, x_k$ be integers between 0 and n that sum up to n. The probability that the *first* x_1 balls fall in the first urn, the *next* x_2 balls fall in the second urn, etc., is

$$p_1^{x_1} p_2^{x_2} \cdots p_k^{x_k}.$$

To find the probability that there are x_1 balls in the first urn, x_2 in the second, and so on, we have to multiply the probability above with the number of ways in which we can fill the urns with $x_1, x_2, \ldots, x_k$ balls, i.e., $n!/(x_1!\, x_2! \cdots x_k!)$. This gives (3.5).

Remark 3.2. Note that for the *binomial* distribution there are only *two* possible urns. Also, note that for each $i = 1, \ldots, k$, $X_i \sim \mathsf{Bin}(n, p_i)$.

3.2 Continuous Joint Distributions

Joint distributions for continuous random variables are usually defined via their joint pdf. The theoretical development below follows very similar lines
☞ 28   to both the univariate continuous case in Sect. 2.2.2 and the multivariate
☞ 64   discrete case in Sect. 3.1.

> **Definition 3.5. (Continuous Joint Pdf).** Continuous random variables $X_1, \ldots, X_n$ are said to have a **joint pdf** f if
>
> $$\mathbb{P}(a_1 < X_1 \le b_1, \ldots, a_n < X_n \le b_n) = \int_{a_1}^{b_1} \cdots \int_{a_n}^{b_n} f(x_1, \ldots, x_n) \, \mathrm{d}x_1 \cdots \mathrm{d}x_n$$
>
> for all $a_1, \ldots, b_n$.

☞ 28   This implies, similar to the univariate case in (2.3), that the probability of any event pertaining to $\boldsymbol{X} = [X_1, \ldots, X_n]$—say event $\{\boldsymbol{X} \in B\}$, where B is some subset of $\mathbb{R}^n$—can be found by *integration*:

$$\mathbb{P}(\boldsymbol{X} \in B) = \int_B f(x_1, \ldots, x_n) \, \mathrm{d}x_1 \ldots \mathrm{d}x_n \ . \tag{3.6}$$

☞ 29   As in (2.5) we can interpret $f(x_1, \ldots, x_n)$ as the *density* of the probability distribution at $[x_1, \ldots, x_n]$. For example, in the two-dimensional case, for small $h > 0$,

$$\mathbb{P}(x_1 \le X_1 \le x_1 + h, \, x_2 \le X_2 \le x_2 + h)$$

$$= \int_{x_1}^{x_1+h} \int_{x_2}^{x_2+h} f(u, v) \, \mathrm{d}u \, \mathrm{d}v \approx h^2 \, f(x_1, x_2) \ .$$

Similar to the discrete multivariate case in (3.1), the marginal pdfs can be recovered from the joint pdf by integrating out the other variables:

$$f_{X_i}(x) = \int_{-\infty}^{\infty} \cdots \int_{-\infty}^{\infty} f(x_1, \ldots, x_{i-1}, x, x_{i+1}, \ldots, x_n) \, \mathrm{d}x_1 \ldots \mathrm{d}x_{i-1} \, \mathrm{d}x_{i+1} \ldots \mathrm{d}x_n \ .$$

We illustrate this for the two-dimensional case. We have

$$F_{X_1}(x) = \mathbb{P}(X_1 \le x, X_2 \le \infty) = \int_{-\infty}^{x} \left(\int_{-\infty}^{\infty} f(x_1, x_2) \, \mathrm{d}x_2 \right) \mathrm{d}x_1 \ .$$

By differentiating the last integral with respect to x, we obtain

$$f_{X_1}(x) = \int_{-\infty}^{\infty} f(x, x_2) \, \mathrm{d}x_2 \ .$$

It is not possible, in general, to reconstruct the joint pdf from the marginal pdfs. An exception is when the random variables are *independent*; see Definition 3.3. By modifying the arguments in the proof of Theorem 3.3 to the continuous case—basically replacing sums with integrals—it is not difficult to see that the theorem also holds in the continuous case. In particular, continuous random variables $X_1, \ldots, X_n$ are independent if and only if their joint pdf, f say, is the product of the marginal pdfs:

$$f(x_1, \ldots, x_n) = f_{X_1}(x_1) \cdots f_{X_n}(x_n) \tag{3.7}$$

for all $x_1, \ldots, x_n$. Independence for an infinite sequence of random variables is discussed in Remark 3.1.

☞ 66

Example 3.6 (Generating a General iid Sample). Consider the sequence of numbers produced by a uniform random number generator such as Julia's **rand** function. A mathematical model for the output stream is: $U_1, U_2, \ldots$, are independent and $\mathcal{U}(0, 1)$-distributed; that is,

$$U_1, U_2, \ldots \overset{\text{iid}}{\sim} \mathcal{U}(0, 1) \ .$$

Using the inverse-transform method it follows that for any cdf F,

☞ 53

$$F^{-1}(U_1), F^{-1}(U_2), \ldots \overset{\text{iid}}{\sim} F \ .$$

Example 3.7 (Quotient of Two Independent Random Variables). Let X and Y be independent continuous random variables, with $Y > 0$. What is the pdf of the quotient $U = X/Y$ in terms of the pdfs of X and Y? Consider first the cdf of U. We have

$$F_U(u) = \mathbb{P}(U \le u) = \mathbb{P}(X/Y \le u) = \mathbb{P}(X \le Yu)$$

$$= \int_0^\infty \int_{-\infty}^{yu} f_X(x) f_Y(y) \, \mathrm{d}x \, \mathrm{d}y = \int_{-\infty}^u \int_0^\infty y f_X(yz) f_Y(y) \, \mathrm{d}y \, \mathrm{d}z \ ,$$

where we have used the change of variable $z = x/y$ and changed the order of integration in the last equation. It follows that the pdf is given by

$$f_U(u) = \frac{\mathrm{d}}{\mathrm{d}u} F_U(u) = \int_0^\infty y f_X(yu) f_Y(y) \, \mathrm{d}y \ . \tag{3.8}$$

As a particular example, suppose that X and V both have a standard normal distribution. Note that X/V has the same distribution as $U = X/Y$, where $Y = |V| > 0$ has a *positive normal* distribution. It follows from (3.8) that

☞ 56

$$f_U(u) = \int_0^\infty y \frac{1}{\sqrt{2\pi}} e^{-\frac{1}{2}y^2 u^2} \frac{2}{\sqrt{2\pi}} e^{-\frac{1}{2}y^2} \mathrm{d}y$$

$$= \int_0^\infty y \frac{1}{\pi} e^{-\frac{1}{2}y^2(1+u^2)} \, \mathrm{d}y = \frac{1}{\pi} \frac{1}{1+u^2}, \quad u \in \mathbb{R} \ .$$

☞ 50   This is the pdf of the *Cauchy* distribution.

Definition 3.6. (Conditional Pdf). Let X and Y have joint pdf f and suppose $f_X(x) > 0$. The **conditional pdf** of Y given $X = x$ is defined as

$$f_{Y|X}(y \mid x) = \frac{f(x, y)}{f_X(x)} \quad \text{for all } y \,. \tag{3.9}$$

For the discrete case, this is just a rewrite of (3.4). For the continuous case, the interpretation is that $f_{Y|X}(y \mid x)$ is the density corresponding to the cdf $F_{Y|X}(y \mid x)$ defined by the limit

$$F_{Y|X}(y \mid x) = \lim_{h \downarrow 0} \mathbb{P}(Y \le y \mid x \le X \le x{+}h) = \lim_{h \downarrow 0} \frac{\mathbb{P}(Y \le y, \, x \le X \le x + h)}{\mathbb{P}(x \le X \le x + h)} \,.$$

In many statistical situations, the conditional and marginal pdfs are known and (3.9) is used to find the joint pdf via

$$f(x, y) = f_X(x) \, f_{Y|X}(y \mid x) \,,$$

or, more generally for the n-dimensional case:

$$\begin{aligned} f(x_1, \ldots, x_n) = \\ f_{X_1}(x_1) \, f_{X_2|X_1}(x_2 \mid x_1) \cdots f_{X_n|X_1,\ldots,X_{n-1}}(x_n \mid x_1, \ldots, x_{n-1}) \,, \end{aligned} \tag{3.10}$$

☞ 14   which in the discrete case is just a rephrasing of the *product rule* in terms of probability densities. For independent random variables (3.10) reduces to (3.7). Equation (3.10) also shows how one could sequentially generate a random vector $\boldsymbol{X} = [X_1, \ldots, X_n]$ according to a pdf f, provided that it is possible to generate random variables from the successive conditional distributions, as summarized in the following algorithm.

Algorithm 3.1. (Dependent Random Variable Generation).

1 Draw X_1 from pdf f_{X_1}.
2 **for** $t = 2$ **to** n **do**
3   $\quad$ Given $X_1 = x_1, \ldots, X_t = x_t$, generate X_{t+1} from the
$\quad\quad$ conditional pdf $f_{X_{t+1}|X_1,\ldots,X_t}(x_{t+1} \mid x_1, \ldots, x_t)$.
4 **return** $\boldsymbol{X} = [X_1, \ldots, X_n]$

Example 3.8 (Non-uniform Distribution on Triangle). We select a point (X, Y) from the triangle $(0,0)$–$(1,0)$–$(1,1)$ in such a way that X has a uniform distribution on $(0, 1)$ and the conditional distribution of Y given $X =$

x is uniform on $(0, x)$. Figure 3.3 shows the result of 1000 independent draws from the joint pdf $f(x, y) = f_X(x)\, f_{Y|X}(y\,|\,x)$, generated via Algorithm 3.1. It is clear that the points are not uniformly distributed over the triangle.

```
using Plots
N = 1000
x = rand(N)
y = rand(N).*x
scatter(x,y)
```

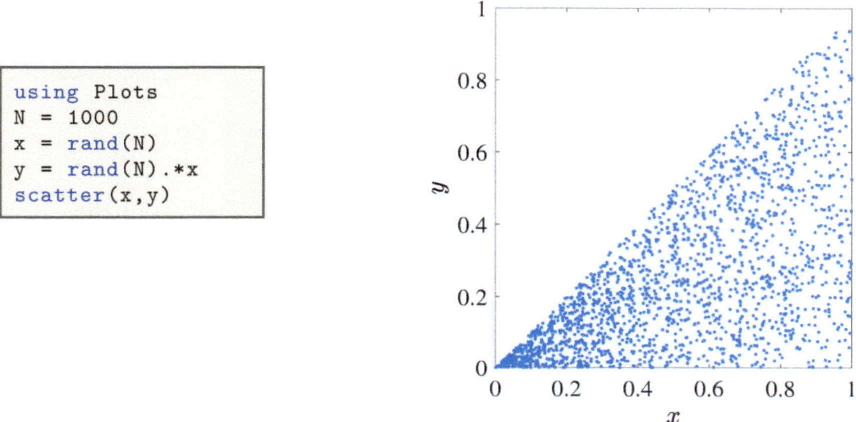

Fig. 3.3 1000 realizations from the joint density $f(x, y)$, generated using the Julia program on the left, which implements Algorithm 3.1

Random variable X has a uniform distribution on $(0, 1)$; hence, its pdf is $f_X(x) = 1$ on $x \in (0, 1)$. For any fixed $x \in (0, 1)$, the conditional distribution of Y given $X = x$ is uniform on the interval $(0, x)$, which means that

$$f_{Y|X}(y\,|\,x) = \frac{1}{x}, \quad 0 < y < x \,.$$

It follows that the joint pdf is given by

$$f(x, y) = f_X(x)\, f_{Y|X}(y\,|\,x) = \frac{1}{x}, \quad 0 < x < 1, \quad 0 < y < x \,.$$

From the joint pdf we can obtain the pdf of Y as

$$f_Y(y) = \int_{-\infty}^{\infty} f(x, y)\, \mathrm{d}x = \int_{y}^{1} \frac{1}{x}\, \mathrm{d}x = -\ln y, \quad 0 < y < 1 \,.$$

Finally, for any fixed $y \in (0, 1)$ the conditional pdf of X given $Y = y$ is

$$f_{X|Y}(x\,|\,y) = \frac{f(x, y)}{f_Y(y)} = \frac{-1}{x \ln y}, \quad y < x < 1 \,.$$

3.3 Mixed Joint Distributions

So far we have only considered joint distributions in which the random variables are all discrete or all continuous. The theory can be extended to mixed cases in a straightforward way. For example, the joint pdf of a discrete variable X and a continuous variable Y is defined as the function $f(x, y)$ such that for all events $\{(X, Y) \in A\}$, where $A \subseteq \mathbb{R}^2$,

$$\mathbb{P}((X, Y) \in A) = \sum_x \int \mathbb{1}_{\{(x,y) \in A\}}\, f(x, y)\, \mathrm{d}y \, ,$$

where $\mathbb{1}$ denotes the indicator. The pdf is often specified via (3.10).

Example 3.9 (Beta Distribution). Let $\Theta \sim \mathcal{U}(0, 1)$ and $(X \mid \Theta = \theta) \sim \mathrm{Bin}(n, \theta)$. Using (3.10), the joint pdf of X and Θ is given by

$$f(x, \theta) = \binom{n}{x} \theta^x (1 - \theta)^{n-x}, \quad \theta \in (0, 1), \; x = 0, 1, \ldots, n \, .$$

By integrating out θ, we find the pdf of X:

$$f_X(x) = \int_0^1 \binom{n}{x} \theta^x (1 - \theta)^{n-x} \mathrm{d}\theta = \binom{n}{x} B(x + 1, n - x + 1) \, ,$$

where B is the **beta function**, defined as

$$B(\alpha, \beta) = \int_0^1 t^{\alpha-1} (1 - t)^{\beta-1} \mathrm{d}t = \frac{\Gamma(\alpha)\Gamma(\beta)}{\Gamma(\alpha + \beta)} \, , \tag{3.11}$$

☞ 48 and Γ is the gamma function in (2.21). The conditional pdf of Θ given $X = x$, where $x \in \{0, \ldots, n\}$, is

$$f_{\Theta \mid X}(\theta \mid x) = \frac{f(\theta, x)}{f_X(x)} = \frac{\theta^x (1 - \theta)^{n-x}}{B(x + 1, n - x + 1)}, \quad \theta \in (0, 1) \, .$$

The continuous distribution with pdf

$$f(x; \alpha, \beta) = \frac{x^{\alpha-1}(1 - x)^{\beta-1}}{B(\alpha, \beta)}, \quad x \in (0, 1) \tag{3.12}$$

is called the **beta distribution** with parameters α and β. Both parameters are assumed to be strictly positive. We write $\mathrm{Beta}(\alpha, \beta)$ for this distribution. For this example we have thus $(\Theta \mid X = x) \sim \mathrm{Beta}(x + 1, n - x + 1)$.

3.4 Expectations for Joint Distributions

Similar to the univariate case in Theorem 2.2, the expected value of a real-valued function h of $(X_1, \ldots, X_n) \sim f$ is a weighted average of all values that $h(X_1, \ldots, X_n)$ can take. Specifically, in the continuous case, ☞ 31

$$\mathbb{E}h(X_1, \ldots, X_n) = \int \cdots \int h(x_1, \ldots, x_n)\, f(x_1, \ldots, x_n)\, \mathrm{d}x_1 \ldots \mathrm{d}x_n . \quad (3.13)$$

In the discrete case replace the integrals above with sums.

Two important special cases are the expectation of the *sum* (or more generally affine transformations) of random variables and the *product* of random variables.

> **Theorem 3.2. (Properties of the Expectation).** Let $X_1, \ldots, X_n$ be random variables with expectations $\mu_1, \ldots, \mu_n$. Then,
>
> $$\mathbb{E}[a + b_1 X_1 + b_2 X_2 + \cdots + b_n X_n] = a + b_1 \mu_1 + \cdots + b_n \mu_n \quad (3.14)$$
>
> for all constants $a, b_1, \ldots, b_n$. Also, for *independent* random variables,
>
> $$\mathbb{E}[X_1 X_2 \cdots X_n] = \mu_1 \mu_2 \cdots \mu_n . \quad (3.15)$$

Proof. We show it for the continuous case with two variables only. The general case follows by analogy and, for the discrete case, by replacing integrals with sums. Let X_1 and X_2 be continuous random variables with joint pdf f. Then, by (3.13),

$$\mathbb{E}[a + b_1 X_1 + b_2 X_2] = \iint (a + b_1 x_1 + b_2 x_2)\, f(x_1, x_2)\, \mathrm{d}x_1\, \mathrm{d}x_2$$

$$= a + b_1 \iint x_1 f(x_1, x_2)\, \mathrm{d}x_1\, \mathrm{d}x_2 + b_2 \iint x_2 f(x_1, x_2)\, \mathrm{d}x_1\, \mathrm{d}x_2$$

$$= a + b_1 \int x_1 \left(\int f(x_1, x_2)\, \mathrm{d}x_2 \right) \mathrm{d}x_1 + b_2 \int x_2 \left(\int f(x_1, x_2)\, \mathrm{d}x_1 \right) \mathrm{d}x_2$$

$$= a + b_1 \int x_1 f_{X_1}(x_1)\, \mathrm{d}x_1 + b_2 \int x_2 f_{X_2}(x_2)\, \mathrm{d}x_2 = a + b_1 \mu_1 + b_2 \mu_2 .$$

Next, assume that X_1 and X_2 are independent, so that $f(x_1, x_2) = f_{X_1}(x_1) \times f_{X_2}(x_2)$. Then,

$$\mathbb{E}[X_1 X_2] = \iint x_1 x_2 f_{X_1}(x_1) f_{X_2}(x_2)\, \mathrm{d}x_1\, \mathrm{d}x_2$$

$$= \int x_1 f_{X_1}(x_1)\, \mathrm{d}x_1 \times \int x_2 f_{X_2}(x_2)\, \mathrm{d}x_2 = \mu_1 \mu_2 .$$

$\square$

Definition 3.7. (Covariance). The **covariance** of two random variables X and Y with expectations $\mathbb{E}X = \mu_X$ and $\mathbb{E}Y = \mu_Y$ is defined as

$$\mathrm{Cov}(X, Y) = \mathbb{E}[(X - \mu_X)(Y - \mu_Y)] \,.$$

The covariance is a measure of the amount of linear dependency between two random variables. A scaled version of the covariance is given by the **correlation coefficient**:

$$\varrho(X, Y) = \frac{\mathrm{Cov}(X, Y)}{\sigma_X \, \sigma_Y} \,, \tag{3.16}$$

where $\sigma_X^2 = \mathrm{Var}(X)$ and $\sigma_Y^2 = \mathrm{Var}(Y)$. The correlation coefficient always lies between -1 and 1; see Problem 3.16.

For easy reference Theorem 3.3 lists some important properties of the variance and covariance.

Theorem 3.3. (Properties of the Variance and Covariance). For random variables X, Y, and Z and constants a and b, we have

1. $\mathrm{Var}(X) = \mathbb{E}X^2 - (\mathbb{E}X)^2$.
2. $\mathrm{Var}(a + bX) = b^2 \mathrm{Var}(X)$.
3. $\mathrm{Cov}(X, Y) = \mathbb{E}XY - \mathbb{E}X \, \mathbb{E}Y$.
4. $\mathrm{Cov}(X, Y) = \mathrm{Cov}(Y, X)$.
5. $\mathrm{Cov}(aX + bY, Z) = a \, \mathrm{Cov}(X, Z) + b \, \mathrm{Cov}(Y, Z)$.
6. $\mathrm{Cov}(X, X) = \mathrm{Var}(X)$.
7. $\mathrm{Var}(X + Y) = \mathrm{Var}(X) + \mathrm{Var}(Y) + 2 \, \mathrm{Cov}(X, Y)$.
8. If X and Y are independent, then $\mathrm{Cov}(X, Y) = 0$.

Proof. For simplicity of notation we write $\mathbb{E}Z = \mu_Z$ for a generic random variable Z. Properties 1 and 2 were already shown in Theorem 2.4.

3. $\mathrm{Cov}(X, Y) = \mathbb{E}[(X - \mu_X)(Y - \mu_Y)] = \mathbb{E}[XY - X\mu_Y - Y\mu_X + \mu_X\mu_Y] = \mathbb{E}[XY] - \mu_X\mu_Y$.
4. $\mathrm{Cov}(X, Y) = \mathbb{E}[(X - \mu_X)(Y - \mu_Y)] = \mathbb{E}[(Y - \mu_Y)(X - \mu_X)] = \mathrm{Cov}(Y, X)$.
5. $\mathrm{Cov}(aX + bY, Z) = \mathbb{E}[(aX + bY)Z] - \mathbb{E}[aX + bY]\mathbb{E}Z = a\,\mathbb{E}[XZ] - a\,\mathbb{E}X\mathbb{E}Z + b\,\mathbb{E}[YZ] - b\,\mathbb{E}Y\mathbb{E}Z = a\,\mathrm{Cov}(X, Z) + b\,\mathrm{Cov}(Y, Z)$.
6. $\mathrm{Cov}(X, X) = \mathbb{E}[(X - \mu_X)(X - \mu_X)] = \mathbb{E}[(X - \mu_X)^2] = \mathrm{Var}(X)$.
7. By Property 6, $\mathrm{Var}(X+Y) = \mathrm{Cov}(X+Y, X+Y)$. By Property 5, $\mathrm{Cov}(X+Y, X+Y) = \mathrm{Cov}(X, X) + \mathrm{Cov}(Y, Y) + \mathrm{Cov}(X, Y) + \mathrm{Cov}(Y, X) = \mathrm{Var}(X) + \mathrm{Var}(Y) + 2\,\mathrm{Cov}(X, Y)$, where in the last equation Properties 4 and 6 are used.

8. If X and Y are independent, then $\mathbb{E}[X\,Y] = \mu_X\,\mu_Y$. Therefore, $\mathrm{Cov}(X, Y)$ $= 0$ follows immediately from Property 3.

As a consequence of Properties 2 and 7, we have the following general result for the variance of affine transformations of random variables.

Corollary 3.1. (Variance of an Affine Transformation). Let $X_1, \ldots, X_n$ be random variables with variances $\sigma_1^2, \ldots, \sigma_n^2$. Then,

$$\mathrm{Var}\left(a + \sum_{i=1}^{n} b_i X_i\right) = \sum_{i=1}^{n} b_i^2\,\sigma_i^2 + 2\sum_{i<j} b_i b_j \mathrm{Cov}(X_i, X_j) \qquad (3.17)$$

for any choice of constants a and $b_1, \ldots, b_n$. In particular, for *independent* random variables $X_1, \ldots, X_n$,

$$\mathrm{Var}(a + b_1 X_1 + \cdots + b_n X_n) = b_1^2 \sigma_1^2 + \cdots + b_n^2 \sigma_n^2 . \qquad (3.18)$$

Let $\boldsymbol{X} = [X_1, \ldots, X_n]^\top$ be a random column vector. Sometimes it is convenient to write the expectations and covariances in vector notation.

Definition 3.8. (Expectation Vector and Covariance Matrix). For any random column vector $\boldsymbol{X}$ we define the **expectation vector** as the vector of expectations

$$\boldsymbol{\mu} = [\mu_1, \ldots, \mu_n]^\top = [\mathbb{E}X_1, \ldots, \mathbb{E}X_n]^\top .$$

The **covariance matrix** $\boldsymbol{\Sigma}$ is defined as the matrix whose (i, j)-th element is

$$\mathrm{Cov}(X_i, X_j) = \mathbb{E}[(X_i - \mu_i)(X_j - \mu_j)] .$$

If we define the expectation of a matrix to be the matrix of expectations, then we can write the covariance matrix succinctly as

$$\boldsymbol{\Sigma} = \mathbb{E}\left[(\boldsymbol{X} - \boldsymbol{\mu})(\boldsymbol{X} - \boldsymbol{\mu})^\top\right] .$$

Note that any covariance matrix $\boldsymbol{\Sigma}$ is symmetric and **positive semidefinite**; that is, for any (column) vector $\boldsymbol{u}$,

$$\boldsymbol{u}^\top \boldsymbol{\Sigma}\, \boldsymbol{u} \geq 0 . \qquad (3.19)$$

To see this, let $\boldsymbol{Y} = \boldsymbol{X} - \boldsymbol{\mu}$. Then,

$$\boldsymbol{u}^\top \boldsymbol{\Sigma} \boldsymbol{u} = \boldsymbol{u}^\top \mathbb{E}\left[\boldsymbol{Y}\boldsymbol{Y}^\top\right] \boldsymbol{u} = \mathbb{E}\left[\boldsymbol{u}^\top \boldsymbol{Y}\boldsymbol{Y}^\top \boldsymbol{u}\right]$$
$$= \mathbb{E}\left[(\boldsymbol{Y}^\top \boldsymbol{u})^\top \boldsymbol{Y}^\top \boldsymbol{u}\right] = \mathbb{E}(\boldsymbol{Y}^\top \boldsymbol{u})^2 \geq 0.$$

Definition 3.9. (Conditional Expectation). The **conditional expectation** of Y given $X = x$, denoted $\mathbb{E}[Y \mid X = x]$, is the expectation corresponding to the conditional pdf $f_{Y\mid X}(y \mid x)$. That is, in the continuous case,

$$\mathbb{E}[Y \mid X = x] = \int y\, f_{Y\mid X}(y \mid x)\, \mathrm{d}y \; .$$

In the discrete case replace the integral with a sum.

Note that $\mathbb{E}[Y \mid X = x]$ is a function of x, say $h(x)$. The corresponding random variable $h(X)$ is written as $\mathbb{E}[Y \mid X]$. The expectation of $\mathbb{E}[Y \mid X]$ is, in the continuous case,

$$\mathbb{E}\mathbb{E}[Y \mid X] = \int \mathbb{E}[Y \mid X = x] f_X(x)\, \mathrm{d}x = \int \int y\, \frac{f(x,y)}{f_X(x)} f_X(x)\, \mathrm{d}y\, \mathrm{d}x$$
$$= \int y\, f_Y(y)\, \mathrm{d}y = \mathbb{E}Y \; . \tag{3.20}$$

This "stacking" of (conditional) expectations is referred to as **repeated conditioning**.

Example 3.10 (Non-uniform Distribution on Triangle Continued). In Example 3.8 the conditional expectation of Y given $X = x$, with $0 < x < 1$, is

$$\mathbb{E}[Y \mid X = x] = \frac{1}{2}x \; ,$$

because conditioned on $X = x$, Y is uniformly distributed on the interval $(0, x)$. Using the repeated conditioning rule we find

$$\mathbb{E}Y = \frac{1}{2}\mathbb{E}X = \frac{1}{4} \; .$$

3.5 Functions of Random Variables

Suppose $X_1, \ldots, X_n$ are measurements of a random experiment. What can be said about the distribution of a *function* of the data, say $Z = g(X_1, \ldots, X_n)$, when the joint distribution of $X_1, \ldots, X_n$ is known?

Example 3.11 (Pdf of an Affine Transformation). Let X be a continuous random variable with pdf f_X and let $Z = a + bX$, where $b \neq 0$. We wish to determine the pdf f_Z of Z. Suppose that $b > 0$. We have for any z

$$F_Z(z) = \mathbb{P}(Z \leq z) = \mathbb{P}(X \leq (z-a)/b) = F_X\big((z-a)/b\big) \, .$$

Differentiating this with respect to z gives $f_Z(z) = f_X\big((z-a)/b\big)/b$. For $b < 0$ we similarly obtain $f_Z(z) = f_X\big((z-a)/b\big)/(-b)$. Thus, in general,

$$f_Z(z) = \frac{1}{|b|} f_X\left(\frac{z-a}{b}\right) \, . \tag{3.21}$$

Example 3.12 (Pdf of a Monotone Transformation). Generalizing the previous example, suppose that $Z = g(X)$ for some strictly increasing function g. To find the pdf of Z from that of X we first write

$$F_Z(z) = \mathbb{P}(Z \leq z) = \mathbb{P}\left(X \leq g^{-1}(z)\right) = F_X\left(g^{-1}(z)\right) \, ,$$

where g^{-1} is the inverse of g. Differentiating with respect to z now gives

$$f_Z(z) = f_X(g^{-1}(z)) \frac{\mathrm{d}}{\mathrm{d}z} g^{-1}(z) = \frac{f_X(g^{-1}(z))}{g'(g^{-1}(z))} \, . \tag{3.22}$$

For strictly decreasing functions, g' needs to be replaced with its negative value.

3.5.1 Linear Transformations

Let $\boldsymbol{x} = [x_1, \ldots, x_n]^{\top}$ be a column vector in $\mathbb{R}^n$ and $\mathbf{B}$ an $m \times n$ matrix. The mapping $\boldsymbol{x} \mapsto \boldsymbol{z}$, with $\boldsymbol{z} = \mathbf{B}\boldsymbol{x}$, is called a **linear transformation**. Now consider a *random* vector $\boldsymbol{X} = [X_1, \ldots, X_n]^{\top}$, and let

$$\boldsymbol{Z} = \mathbf{B}\boldsymbol{X} \, .$$

Then $\boldsymbol{Z}$ is a random vector in $\mathbb{R}^m$. In principle, if we know the joint distribution of $\boldsymbol{X}$, then we can derive the joint distribution of $\boldsymbol{Z}$. Let us first see how the expectation vector and covariance matrix are transformed.

Theorem 3.4. (Expectation and Covariance Under a Linear Transformation). If $\boldsymbol{X}$ has expectation vector $\boldsymbol{\mu}_{\boldsymbol{X}}$ and covariance matrix $\boldsymbol{\Sigma}_{\boldsymbol{X}}$, then the expectation vector and covariance matrix of $\boldsymbol{Z} = \mathbf{B}\boldsymbol{X}$ are given by

$$\boldsymbol{\mu}_{\boldsymbol{Z}} = \mathbf{B}\boldsymbol{\mu}_{\boldsymbol{X}} \tag{3.23}$$

and

$$\boldsymbol{\Sigma}_{\boldsymbol{Z}} = \mathbf{B}\,\boldsymbol{\Sigma}_{\boldsymbol{X}}\,\mathbf{B}^{\top}\,. \tag{3.24}$$

Proof. We have $\boldsymbol{\mu}_{\boldsymbol{Z}} = \mathbb{E}\boldsymbol{Z} = \mathbb{E}\mathbf{B}\boldsymbol{X} = \mathbf{B}\,\mathbb{E}\boldsymbol{X} = \mathbf{B}\boldsymbol{\mu}_{\boldsymbol{X}}$ and

$$\begin{aligned}
\boldsymbol{\Sigma}_{\boldsymbol{Z}} &= \mathbb{E}[(\boldsymbol{Z} - \boldsymbol{\mu}_{\boldsymbol{Z}})(\boldsymbol{Z} - \boldsymbol{\mu}_{\boldsymbol{Z}})^{\top}] = \mathbb{E}[\mathbf{B}(\boldsymbol{X} - \boldsymbol{\mu}_{\boldsymbol{X}})(\mathbf{B}(\boldsymbol{X} - \boldsymbol{\mu}_{\boldsymbol{X}}))^{\top}] \\
&= \mathbf{B}\,\mathbb{E}[(\boldsymbol{X} - \boldsymbol{\mu}_{\boldsymbol{X}})(\boldsymbol{X} - \boldsymbol{\mu}_{\boldsymbol{X}})^{\top}]\mathbf{B}^{\top} \\
&= \mathbf{B}\,\boldsymbol{\Sigma}_{\boldsymbol{X}}\,\mathbf{B}^{\top}\,.
\end{aligned}$$

$\square$

Suppose that $\mathbf{B}$ is an *invertible* $n \times n$ matrix. If $\boldsymbol{X}$ has a joint pdf $f_{\boldsymbol{X}}$, what is the joint density $f_{\boldsymbol{Z}}$ of $\boldsymbol{Z}$? Let us consider the continuous case. For any fixed $\boldsymbol{x}$, let $\boldsymbol{z} = \mathbf{B}\boldsymbol{x}$. Hence, $\boldsymbol{x} = \mathbf{B}^{-1}\boldsymbol{z}$. Consider the n-dimensional cube $C = [z_1, z_1 + h] \times \cdots \times [z_n, z_n + h]$. Then, by definition of the joint density for $\boldsymbol{Z}$, we have

$$\mathbb{P}(\boldsymbol{Z} \in C) \approx h^n\, f_{\boldsymbol{Z}}(\boldsymbol{z})\,.$$

Let D be the image of C under $\mathbf{B}^{-1}$—that is, the parallelepiped of all points $\boldsymbol{x}$ such that $\mathbf{B}\boldsymbol{x} \in C$; see Fig. 3.4.

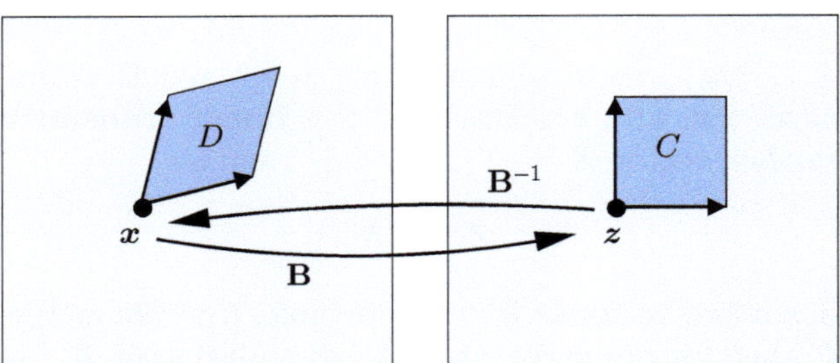

Fig. 3.4 Linear transformation

A basic result from linear algebra is that any matrix $\mathbf{B}$ linearly transforms an n-dimensional rectangle with volume V into an n-dimensional parallelepiped with volume $V\,|\mathbf{B}|$, where $|\mathbf{B}| = |\det(\mathbf{B})|$. Thus, in addition to the above expression for $\mathbb{P}(\boldsymbol{Z} \in C)$ we also have

$$\mathbb{P}(\boldsymbol{Z} \in C) = \mathbb{P}(\boldsymbol{X} \in D) \approx h^n |\mathbf{B}^{-1}| \, f_{\boldsymbol{X}}(\boldsymbol{x}) = h^n |\mathbf{B}|^{-1} \, f_{\boldsymbol{X}}(\boldsymbol{x}) \,.$$

Equating these two expressions for $\mathbb{P}(\boldsymbol{Z} \in C)$ and letting h go to 0, we obtain

$$f_{\boldsymbol{Z}}(\boldsymbol{z}) = \frac{f_{\boldsymbol{X}}(\mathbf{B}^{-1}\boldsymbol{z})}{|\mathbf{B}|}, \quad \boldsymbol{z} \in \mathbb{R}^n. \tag{3.25}$$

3.5.2 General Transformations

We can apply similar reasoning as in the previous subsection to deal with general transformations $\boldsymbol{x} \mapsto \boldsymbol{g}(\boldsymbol{x})$, written out as

$$\begin{bmatrix} x_1 \\ x_2 \\ \vdots \\ x_n \end{bmatrix} \mapsto \begin{bmatrix} g_1(\boldsymbol{x}) \\ g_2(\boldsymbol{x}) \\ \vdots \\ g_n(\boldsymbol{x}) \end{bmatrix}.$$

For a fixed $\boldsymbol{x}$, let $\boldsymbol{z} = \boldsymbol{g}(\boldsymbol{x})$. Suppose $\boldsymbol{g}$ is invertible; hence, $\boldsymbol{x} = \boldsymbol{g}^{-1}(\boldsymbol{z})$. Any infinitesimal n-dimensional rectangle at $\boldsymbol{x}$ with volume V is transformed into an n-dimensional parallelepiped at $\boldsymbol{z}$ with volume $V\,|\mathbf{J}_{\boldsymbol{g}}(\boldsymbol{x})|$, where $\mathbf{J}_{\boldsymbol{g}}(\boldsymbol{x})$ is the *matrix of Jacobi* at $\boldsymbol{x}$ of the transformation $\boldsymbol{g}$; that is, ☞ 47

$$\mathbf{J}_{\boldsymbol{g}}(\boldsymbol{x}) = \begin{bmatrix} \frac{\partial g_1}{\partial x_1} & \cdots & \frac{\partial g_1}{\partial x_n} \\ \vdots & \ddots & \vdots \\ \frac{\partial g_n}{\partial x_1} & \cdots & \frac{\partial g_n}{\partial x_n} \end{bmatrix}.$$

Now consider a random column vector $\boldsymbol{Z} = \boldsymbol{g}(\boldsymbol{X})$. Let C be a small cube around $\boldsymbol{z}$ with volume h^n. Let D be the image of C under $\boldsymbol{g}^{-1}$. Then, as in the linear case,

$$h^n \, f_{\boldsymbol{Z}}(\boldsymbol{z}) \approx \mathbb{P}(\boldsymbol{Z} \in C) \approx h^n |\mathbf{J}_{\boldsymbol{g}^{-1}}(\boldsymbol{z})| \, f_{\boldsymbol{X}}(\boldsymbol{x}) \,.$$

Hence, we have the following result.

Theorem 3.5. (Transformation Rule). Let $\boldsymbol{X}$ be a continuous n-dimensional random vector with pdf $f_{\boldsymbol{X}}$ and $\boldsymbol{g}$ a function from $\mathbb{R}^n$ to $\mathbb{R}^n$ with inverse $\boldsymbol{g}^{-1}$. Then, $\boldsymbol{Z} = \boldsymbol{g}(\boldsymbol{X})$ has pdf

$$f_{\boldsymbol{Z}}(\boldsymbol{z}) = f_{\boldsymbol{X}}(\boldsymbol{g}^{-1}(\boldsymbol{z}))\,|\mathbf{J}_{\boldsymbol{g}^{-1}}(\boldsymbol{z})|, \quad \boldsymbol{z} \in \mathbb{R}^n. \tag{3.26}$$

Remark 3.3. Note that $|\mathbf{J}_{\boldsymbol{g}^{-1}}(\boldsymbol{z})| = 1/|\mathbf{J}_{\boldsymbol{g}}(\boldsymbol{x})|$.

Example 3.13 (Box–Muller Method). The joint distribution of $X, Y \overset{\text{iid}}{\sim} \mathcal{N}(0, 1)$ is

$$f_{X,Y}(x, y) = \frac{1}{2\pi} e^{-\frac{1}{2}(x^2 + y^2)}, \quad (x, y) \in \mathbb{R}^2 .$$

In polar coordinates we have

$$X = R \cos \Theta \quad \text{and} \quad Y = R \sin \Theta , \tag{3.27}$$

where $R \geq 0$ and $\Theta \in (0, 2\pi)$. What is the joint pdf of R and Θ? Consider the inverse-transformation $\boldsymbol{g}^{-1}$, defined by

$$\begin{bmatrix} r \\ \theta \end{bmatrix} \overset{\boldsymbol{g}^{-1}}{\longmapsto} \begin{bmatrix} r \cos \theta \\ r \sin \theta \end{bmatrix} = \begin{bmatrix} x \\ y \end{bmatrix} .$$

The corresponding matrix of Jacobi is

$$\mathbf{J}_{\boldsymbol{g}^{-1}}(r, \theta) = \begin{bmatrix} \cos \theta & -r \sin \theta \\ \sin \theta & r \cos \theta \end{bmatrix} ,$$

which has determinant r. Since $x^2 + y^2 = r^2(\cos^2 \theta + \sin^2 \theta) = r^2$, it follows that

$$f_{R,\Theta}(r, \theta) = f_{X,Y}(x, y) \, r = \frac{1}{2\pi} e^{-\frac{1}{2} r^2} r, \quad \theta \in (0, 2\pi), \quad r \geq 0 .$$

By integrating out θ and r, respectively, we find $f_R(r) = r \, e^{-r^2/2}$ and $f_\Theta(\theta) = 1/(2\pi)$. Since $f_{R,\Theta}$ is the product of f_R and f_Θ, the random variables R and Θ are independent. This shows how X and Y could be generated: independently generate $R \sim f_R$ and $\Theta \sim \mathcal{U}(0, 2\pi)$ and return X and Y via (3.27). Generation ☞ 53 from f_R can be done via the inverse-transform method. In particular, R has the same distribution as $\sqrt{-2 \ln U}$ with $U \sim \mathcal{U}(0, 1)$. This leads to the following method for generating standard normal random variables.

Algorithm 3.2. (Box–Muller Method).

1. Generate $U_1, U_2 \overset{\text{iid}}{\sim} \mathcal{U}(0, 1)$.
2. Return two independent standard normal variables, X and Y, via

$$X = \sqrt{-2 \ln U_1} \, \cos(2\pi U_2) ,$$
$$Y = \sqrt{-2 \ln U_1} \, \sin(2\pi U_2) . \tag{3.28}$$

3.6 Multivariate Normal Distribution

It is helpful to view a normally distributed random variable as an affine transformation of a standard normal random variable. In particular, if Z has a standard normal distribution, then $X = \mu + \sigma Z$ has a $\mathcal{N}(\mu, \sigma^2)$ distribution; see Theorem 2.15.

   ☞ 46

We now generalize this to n dimensions. Let $Z_1, \ldots, Z_n$ be independent and standard normal random variables. The joint pdf of $\boldsymbol{Z} = [Z_1, \ldots, Z_n]^\top$ is given by

$$f_{\boldsymbol{Z}}(\boldsymbol{z}) = \prod_{i=1}^{n} \frac{1}{\sqrt{2\pi}} \, \mathrm{e}^{-\frac{1}{2}z_i^2} = (2\pi)^{-\frac{n}{2}} \, \mathrm{e}^{-\frac{1}{2}\boldsymbol{z}^\top \boldsymbol{z}}, \quad \boldsymbol{z} \in \mathbb{R}^n. \tag{3.29}$$

We write $\boldsymbol{Z} \sim \mathcal{N}(\boldsymbol{0}, \mathbb{I}_n)$, where $\mathbb{I}_n$ is the identity matrix. Consider the affine transformation (i.e., a linear transformation plus a constant vector)

$$\boldsymbol{X} = \boldsymbol{\mu} + \mathbf{B}\,\boldsymbol{Z} \tag{3.30}$$

for some $m \times n$ matrix $\mathbf{B}$ and m-dimensional vector $\boldsymbol{\mu}$. Note that, by Theorem 3.4, $\boldsymbol{X}$ has expectation vector $\boldsymbol{\mu}$ and covariance matrix $\boldsymbol{\Sigma} = \mathbf{B}\mathbf{B}^\top$.

> **Definition 3.10. (Multivariate Normal Distribution).** A random vector $\boldsymbol{X}$ of dimension m is said to have a **multivariate normal** or **multivariate Gaussian** distribution with mean vector $\boldsymbol{\mu}$ and covariance matrix $\boldsymbol{\Sigma}$ if it can be written as $\boldsymbol{X} = \boldsymbol{\mu} + \mathbf{B}\,\boldsymbol{Z}$, where $\boldsymbol{Z} \sim \mathcal{N}(\boldsymbol{0}, \mathbb{I}_n)$ and $\mathbf{B}\mathbf{B}^\top = \boldsymbol{\Sigma}$. We write $\boldsymbol{X} \sim \mathcal{N}(\boldsymbol{\mu}, \boldsymbol{\Sigma})$.

Suppose that $\mathbf{B}$ is an invertible $n \times n$ matrix. Then, by (3.25), the density of $\boldsymbol{Y} = \boldsymbol{X} - \boldsymbol{\mu}$ is given by

$$f_{\boldsymbol{Y}}(\boldsymbol{y}) = \frac{1}{|\mathbf{B}|\sqrt{(2\pi)^n}} \, \mathrm{e}^{-\frac{1}{2}(\mathbf{B}^{-1}\boldsymbol{y})^\top \mathbf{B}^{-1}\boldsymbol{y}} = \frac{1}{|\mathbf{B}|\sqrt{(2\pi)^n}} \, \mathrm{e}^{-\frac{1}{2}\boldsymbol{y}^\top (\mathbf{B}^{-1})^\top \mathbf{B}^{-1}\boldsymbol{y}}.$$

We have $|\mathbf{B}| = \sqrt{|\boldsymbol{\Sigma}|}$ and $(\mathbf{B}^{-1})^\top \mathbf{B}^{-1} = (\mathbf{B}^\top)^{-1}\mathbf{B}^{-1} = (\mathbf{B}\mathbf{B}^\top)^{-1} = \boldsymbol{\Sigma}^{-1}$, so that

$$f_{\boldsymbol{Y}}(\boldsymbol{y}) = \frac{1}{\sqrt{(2\pi)^n \, |\boldsymbol{\Sigma}|}} \, \mathrm{e}^{-\frac{1}{2}\boldsymbol{y}^\top \boldsymbol{\Sigma}^{-1}\boldsymbol{y}}.$$

Because $\boldsymbol{X}$ is obtained from $\boldsymbol{Y}$ by simply adding a constant vector $\boldsymbol{\mu}$, we have $f_{\boldsymbol{X}}(\boldsymbol{x}) = f_{\boldsymbol{Y}}(\boldsymbol{x} - \boldsymbol{\mu})$ and therefore

$$f_{\boldsymbol{X}}(\boldsymbol{x}) = \frac{1}{\sqrt{(2\pi)^n \, |\boldsymbol{\Sigma}|}} \, \mathrm{e}^{-\frac{1}{2}(\boldsymbol{x}-\boldsymbol{\mu})^\top \boldsymbol{\Sigma}^{-1}(\boldsymbol{x}-\boldsymbol{\mu})}, \quad \boldsymbol{x} \in \mathbb{R}^n. \tag{3.31}$$

Figure 3.5 shows the pdfs of two bivariate (i.e., two-dimensional) normal distributions. In both cases the mean vector is $\boldsymbol{\mu} = [0, 0]^\top$ and the variances (the diagonal elements of $\boldsymbol{\Sigma}$) are 1. The correlation coefficients (or, equivalently here, the covariances) are respectively $\varrho = 0$ and $\varrho = 0.8$.

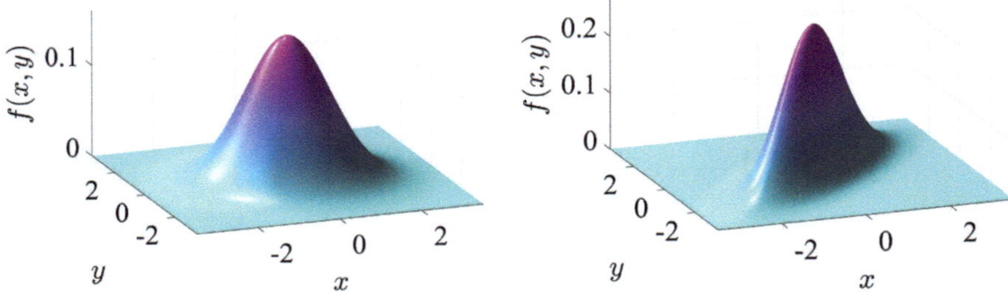

Fig. 3.5 Pdfs of bivariate normal distributions with means zero, variances 1, and correlation coefficients 0 (left) and 0.8 (right)

Conversely, given a positive-definite[1] covariance matrix $\boldsymbol{\Sigma} = [\sigma_{ij}]$, there exists a unique lower triangular matrix $\mathbf{B}$ such that $\boldsymbol{\Sigma} = \mathbf{B}\mathbf{B}^\top$. In Julia, the function **cholesky** from the **LinearAlgebra** package accomplishes this matrix factorization. Note that the function returns a Julia **struct** object, from which the matrix needs to be extracted using the field name L; see the code in Example 3.3. Once the Cholesky factorization is determined, it is easy to sample from a multivariate normal distribution.

☞ 444

> **Algorithm 3.3. (Normal Random Vector Generation).** To generate N independent draws from a $\mathcal{N}(\boldsymbol{\mu}, \boldsymbol{\Sigma})$ distribution of dimension n carry out the following steps:
>
> 1. Determine the lower Cholesky factorization $\boldsymbol{\Sigma} = \mathbf{B}\mathbf{B}^\top$.
> 2. Generate $\boldsymbol{Z} = [Z_1, \ldots, Z_n]^\top$ by drawing $Z_1, \ldots, Z_n \sim_{\text{iid}} \mathcal{N}(0, 1)$.
> 3. Output $\boldsymbol{X} = \boldsymbol{\mu} + \mathbf{B}\boldsymbol{Z}$.
> 4. Repeat Steps 2 and 3 independently N times.

Example 3.14 (Generating from a Bivariate Normal Distribution). The Julia code below draws 1000 samples from the two pdfs in Fig. 3.5. The resulting point clouds are given in Fig. 3.6.

---

[1] A positive-definite matrix satisfies (3.19) with strict inequality.

```julia
using Plots, LinearAlgebra, Random
N = 1000; rho = 0.8;
Sigma = [1 rho; rho 1];
B = cholesky(Sigma).L;    # lower-triangular Cholesky matrix
x = B*randn(2,N);
scatter(x[1,:],x[2,:],ms=2,msw=0,legend=false)
```

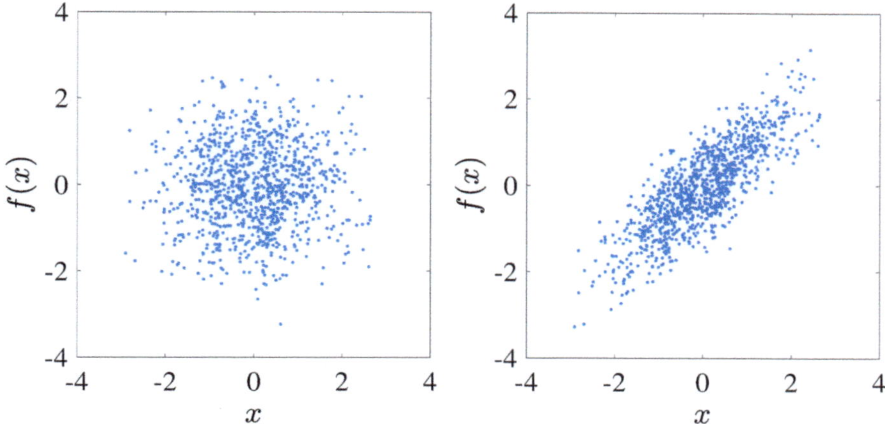

Fig. 3.6 1000 realizations of bivariate normal distributions with means zero, variances 1, and correlation coefficients 0 (left) and 0.8 (right)

The following theorem states that any affine combination of independent multivariate normal random variables is again multivariate normal.

Theorem 3.6. (Affine Transformation of Normal Random Vectors). Let $\boldsymbol{X}_1, \boldsymbol{X}_2, \ldots, \boldsymbol{X}_r$ be independent m_i-dimensional normal random vectors, with $\boldsymbol{X}_i \sim \mathcal{N}(\boldsymbol{\mu}_i, \boldsymbol{\Sigma}_i)$, $i = 1, \ldots, r$. Then, for any $n \times 1$ vector $\boldsymbol{a}$ and $n \times m_i$ matrices $\mathbf{B}_1, \ldots, \mathbf{B}_r$,

$$\boldsymbol{a} + \sum_{i=1}^{r} \mathbf{B}_i \, \boldsymbol{X}_i \sim \mathcal{N}\left(\boldsymbol{a} + \sum_{i=1}^{r} \mathbf{B}_i \, \boldsymbol{\mu}_i, \ \sum_{i=1}^{r} \mathbf{B}_i \, \boldsymbol{\Sigma}_i \, \mathbf{B}_i^{\top}\right). \tag{3.32}$$

Proof. Denote the n-dimensional random vector in the left-hand side of (3.32) by $\boldsymbol{Y}$. By Definition 3.10, each $\boldsymbol{X}_i$ can be written as $\boldsymbol{\mu}_i + \mathbf{A}_i \boldsymbol{Z}_i$, where the $\{\boldsymbol{Z}_i\}$ are independent (because the $\{\boldsymbol{X}_i\}$ are independent), so that

$$\boldsymbol{Y} = \boldsymbol{a} + \sum_{i=1}^{r} \mathbf{B}_i \, (\boldsymbol{\mu}_i + \mathbf{A}_i \boldsymbol{Z}_i) = \boldsymbol{a} + \sum_{i=1}^{r} \mathbf{B}_i \, \boldsymbol{\mu}_i + \sum_{i=1}^{r} \mathbf{B}_i \mathbf{A}_i \boldsymbol{Z}_i \, ,$$

which is an affine combination of independent standard normal random vectors. Hence, $\boldsymbol{Y}$ is multivariate normal. Its expectation vector and covariance matrix can be found easily from Theorem 3.4. $\qquad\square$

The next theorem shows that the distribution of a subvector of a multivariate normal random vector is again normal.

Theorem 3.7. (Marginal Distributions of Normal Random Vectors). Let $\boldsymbol{X} \sim \mathcal{N}(\boldsymbol{\mu}, \boldsymbol{\Sigma})$ be an n-dimensional normal random vector. Decompose $\boldsymbol{X}$, $\boldsymbol{\mu}$, and $\boldsymbol{\Sigma}$ as

$$\boldsymbol{X} = \begin{bmatrix} \boldsymbol{X}_p \\ \boldsymbol{X}_q \end{bmatrix}, \quad \boldsymbol{\mu} = \begin{bmatrix} \boldsymbol{\mu}_p \\ \boldsymbol{\mu}_q \end{bmatrix}, \quad \boldsymbol{\Sigma} = \begin{bmatrix} \boldsymbol{\Sigma}_p & \boldsymbol{\Sigma}_r \\ \boldsymbol{\Sigma}_r^\top & \boldsymbol{\Sigma}_q \end{bmatrix}, \qquad (3.33)$$

where $\boldsymbol{\Sigma}_p$ is the upper left $p \times p$ corner of $\boldsymbol{\Sigma}$ and $\boldsymbol{\Sigma}_q$ is the lower right $q \times q$ corner of $\boldsymbol{\Sigma}$. Then, $\boldsymbol{X}_p \sim \mathcal{N}(\boldsymbol{\mu}_p, \boldsymbol{\Sigma}_p)$.

Proof. Let $\mathbf{B}\mathbf{B}^\top$ be the lower Cholesky factorization of $\boldsymbol{\Sigma}$. We can write

$$\begin{bmatrix} \boldsymbol{X}_p \\ \boldsymbol{X}_q \end{bmatrix} = \begin{bmatrix} \boldsymbol{\mu}_p \\ \boldsymbol{\mu}_q \end{bmatrix} + \underbrace{\begin{bmatrix} \mathbf{B}_p & \mathbf{O} \\ \mathbf{C}_r & \mathbf{C}_q \end{bmatrix}}_{\mathbf{B}} \begin{bmatrix} \boldsymbol{Z}_p \\ \boldsymbol{Z}_q \end{bmatrix}, \qquad (3.34)$$

where $\boldsymbol{Z}_p$ and $\boldsymbol{Z}_q$ are independent p- and q-dimensional standard normal random vectors. In particular, $\boldsymbol{X}_p = \boldsymbol{\mu}_p + \mathbf{B}_p\boldsymbol{Z}_p$, which means that $\boldsymbol{X}_p \sim \mathcal{N}(\boldsymbol{\mu}_p, \boldsymbol{\Sigma}_p)$, since $\mathbf{B}_p\mathbf{B}_p^\top = \boldsymbol{\Sigma}_p$. $\qquad\square$

By relabeling the elements of $\boldsymbol{X}$ we see that Theorem 3.7 implies that *any* subvector of $\boldsymbol{X}$ has a multivariate normal distribution. For example, $\boldsymbol{X}_q \sim \mathcal{N}(\boldsymbol{\mu}_q, \boldsymbol{\Sigma}_q)$.

Not only the marginal distributions of a normal random vector are normal but also its *conditional distributions*.

Theorem 3.8. (Conditional Distributions of Normal Random Vectors). Let $\boldsymbol{X} \sim \mathcal{N}(\boldsymbol{\mu}, \boldsymbol{\Sigma})$ be an n-dimensional normal random vector with $\det(\boldsymbol{\Sigma}) > 0$. If $\boldsymbol{X}$ is decomposed as in (3.33), then

$$(\boldsymbol{X}_q \mid \boldsymbol{X}_p = \boldsymbol{x}_p) \sim \mathcal{N}(\boldsymbol{\mu}_q + \boldsymbol{\Sigma}_r^\top \boldsymbol{\Sigma}_p^{-1}(\boldsymbol{x}_p - \boldsymbol{\mu}_p), \boldsymbol{\Sigma}_q - \boldsymbol{\Sigma}_r^\top \boldsymbol{\Sigma}_p^{-1}\boldsymbol{\Sigma}_r). \quad (3.35)$$

As a consequence, $\boldsymbol{X}_p$ and $\boldsymbol{X}_q$ are *independent* if and only if they are *uncorrelated*, that is, if $\boldsymbol{\Sigma}_r = \mathbf{O}$ (zero matrix).

Proof. From (3.34) we see that

$$(\boldsymbol{X}_q \mid \boldsymbol{X}_p = \boldsymbol{x}_p) = \boldsymbol{\mu}_q + \mathbf{C}_r\,\mathbf{B}_p^{-1}(\boldsymbol{x}_p - \boldsymbol{\mu}_p) + \mathbf{C}_q \boldsymbol{Z}_q \;,$$

where $\boldsymbol{Z}_q$ is a q-dimensional multivariate standard normal random vector. It follows that $\boldsymbol{X}_q$ conditional on $\boldsymbol{X}_p = \boldsymbol{x}_p$ has a $\mathcal{N}(\boldsymbol{\mu}_q + \mathbf{C}_r\,\mathbf{B}_p^{-1}(\boldsymbol{x}_p - \boldsymbol{\mu}_p), \mathbf{C}_q\mathbf{C}_q^\top)$ distribution. The proof of (3.35) is completed by observing that $\boldsymbol{\Sigma}_r^\top \boldsymbol{\Sigma}_p^{-1} = \mathbf{C}_r\mathbf{B}_p^\top (\mathbf{B}_p^\top)^{-1}\mathbf{B}_p^{-1} = \mathbf{C}_r\,\mathbf{B}_p^{-1}$, and

$$\boldsymbol{\Sigma}_q - \boldsymbol{\Sigma}_r^\top \boldsymbol{\Sigma}_p^{-1}\boldsymbol{\Sigma}_r = \mathbf{C}_r\mathbf{C}_r^\top + \mathbf{C}_q\mathbf{C}_q^\top - \mathbf{C}_r\mathbf{B}_p^{-1}\underbrace{\boldsymbol{\Sigma}_r}_{\mathbf{B}_p\mathbf{C}_r^\top} = \mathbf{C}_q\mathbf{C}_q^\top \;.$$

If $\boldsymbol{X}_p$ and $\boldsymbol{X}_q$ are independent, then they are obviously uncorrelated, as $\boldsymbol{\Sigma}_r = \mathbb{E}[(\boldsymbol{X}_p - \boldsymbol{\mu}_p)(\boldsymbol{X}_q - \boldsymbol{\mu}_q)^\top] = \mathbb{E}(\boldsymbol{X}_p - \boldsymbol{\mu}_p)\,\mathbb{E}(\boldsymbol{X}_q - \boldsymbol{\mu}_q)^\top = \mathbf{O}$. Conversely, if $\boldsymbol{\Sigma}_r = \mathbf{O}$, then by (3.35) the conditional distribution of $\boldsymbol{X}_q$ given $\boldsymbol{X}_p$ is the same as the unconditional distribution of $\boldsymbol{X}_q$, that is, $\mathcal{N}(\boldsymbol{\mu}_q, \boldsymbol{\Sigma}_q)$. In other words, $\boldsymbol{X}_q$ is independent of $\boldsymbol{X}_p$. $\qquad\square$

Theorem 3.9. (Relationship Between Normal and χ^2 Distributions). If $\boldsymbol{X} \sim \mathcal{N}(\boldsymbol{\mu}, \boldsymbol{\Sigma})$ is an n-dimensional normal random vector with $\det(\boldsymbol{\Sigma}) > 0$, then

$$(\boldsymbol{X} - \boldsymbol{\mu})^\top \boldsymbol{\Sigma}^{-1}(\boldsymbol{X} - \boldsymbol{\mu}) \sim \chi_n^2 \;. \tag{3.36}$$

Proof. Let $\mathbf{B}\mathbf{B}^\top$ be the Cholesky factorization of $\boldsymbol{\Sigma}$, where $\mathbf{B}$ is invertible. Since $\boldsymbol{X}$ can be written as $\boldsymbol{\mu} + \mathbf{B}\boldsymbol{Z}$, where $\boldsymbol{Z} = [Z_1, \ldots, Z_n]^\top$ is a vector of independent standard normal random variables, we have

$$(\boldsymbol{X} - \boldsymbol{\mu})^\top \boldsymbol{\Sigma}^{-1}(\boldsymbol{X} - \boldsymbol{\mu}) = (\boldsymbol{X} - \boldsymbol{\mu})^\top (\mathbf{B}\mathbf{B}^\top)^{-1}(\boldsymbol{X} - \boldsymbol{\mu}) = \boldsymbol{Z}^\top \boldsymbol{Z} = \sum_{i=1}^{n} Z_i^2 \;.$$

The moment generating function of $Y = \sum_{i=1}^{n} Z_i^2$ is given by

$$\mathbb{E}\,\mathrm{e}^{tY} = \mathbb{E}\,\mathrm{e}^{t(Z_1^2 + \cdots + Z_n^2)} = \mathbb{E}\left[\mathrm{e}^{tZ_1^2} \cdots \mathrm{e}^{tZ_n^2}\right] = \left(\mathbb{E}\,\mathrm{e}^{tZ^2}\right)^n \;,$$

where $Z \sim \mathcal{N}(0, 1)$. The moment generating function of Z^2 is

$$\mathbb{E}\,\mathrm{e}^{tZ^2} = \int_{-\infty}^{\infty} \mathrm{e}^{tz^2}\frac{1}{\sqrt{2\pi}}\mathrm{e}^{-z^2/2}\mathrm{d}z = \frac{1}{\sqrt{2\pi}}\int_{-\infty}^{\infty}\mathrm{e}^{-\frac{1}{2}(1-2t)z^2}\mathrm{d}z = \frac{1}{\sqrt{1-2t}} \;,$$

so that

$$\mathbb{E}e^{tY} = \left(\frac{\frac{1}{2}}{\frac{1}{2} - t}\right)^{\frac{n}{2}}, \quad t < \frac{1}{2},$$

which is the moment generating function of the $\mathsf{Gamma}(n/2, 1/2)$ distribution, that is, the χ_n^2 distribution—see Theorem 2.18. $\qquad\square$

A consequence of Theorem 3.9 is that if $\boldsymbol{X} = [X_1, \ldots, X_n]^\top$ is n-dimensional standard normal, then the squared length $\|\boldsymbol{X}\|^2 = X_1^2 + \cdots + X_n^2$ has a χ_n^2 distribution. If instead $X_i \sim \mathcal{N}(\mu_i, 1)$, $i = 1, \ldots$, then $\|\boldsymbol{X}\|^2$ is said to have a **noncentral χ_n^2 distribution**. This distribution depends on the $\{\mu_i\}$ only through the norm $\|\boldsymbol{\mu}\|$; see Problem 3.22. We write $\|\boldsymbol{X}\|^2 \sim \chi_n^2(\theta)$, where $\theta = \|\boldsymbol{\mu}\|$ is the **noncentrality parameter**.

Such distributions frequently occur in statistics when considering *projections* of multivariate normal random variables. The proof of the following theorem can be found in Appendix B.4.

Theorem 3.10. (Relationship Between Normal and Noncentral χ^2 Distributions). Let $\boldsymbol{X} \sim \mathcal{N}(\boldsymbol{\mu}, \mathbb{I}_n)$ be an n-dimensional normal random vector and let $\mathcal{V}_k$ and $\mathcal{V}_m$ be linear subspaces of dimensions k and m, respectively, with $k < m \le n$. Let $\boldsymbol{X}_k$ and $\boldsymbol{X}_m$ be orthogonal projections of $\boldsymbol{X}$ onto $\mathcal{V}_k$ and $\mathcal{V}_m$, and let $\boldsymbol{\mu}_k$ and $\boldsymbol{\mu}_m$ be the corresponding projections of $\boldsymbol{\mu}$. Then, the following holds:

1. The random vectors $\boldsymbol{X}_k$, $\boldsymbol{X}_m - \boldsymbol{X}_k$, and $\boldsymbol{X} - \boldsymbol{X}_m$ are independent.

2. $\|\boldsymbol{X}_k\|^2 \sim \chi_k^2(\|\boldsymbol{\mu}_k\|)$, $\|\boldsymbol{X}_m - \boldsymbol{X}_k\|^2 \sim \chi_{m-k}^2(\|\boldsymbol{\mu}_m - \boldsymbol{\mu}_k\|)$, and $\|\boldsymbol{X} - \boldsymbol{X}_m\|^2 \sim \chi_{n-m}^2(\|\boldsymbol{\mu} - \boldsymbol{\mu}_m\|)$.

Theorem 3.10 is frequently used in the statistical analysis of *normal linear models*; see Sect. 5.3.1. In typical situations $\boldsymbol{\mu}$ lies in the subspace $\mathcal{V}_m$ or even $\mathcal{V}_k$—in which case $\|\boldsymbol{X}_m - \boldsymbol{X}_k\|^2 \sim \chi_{m-k}^2$ and $\|\boldsymbol{X} - \boldsymbol{X}_m\|^2 \sim \chi_{n-m}^2$, independently. The (scaled) quotient then turns out to have an F distribution—a consequence of the following theorem.

Theorem 3.11. (Relationship Between χ^2 and F Distributions). Let $U \sim \chi_m^2$ and $V \sim \chi_n^2$ be independent. Then,

$$\frac{U/m}{V/n} \sim \mathsf{F}(m, n).$$

Proof. For notational simplicity, let $c = m/2$ and $d = n/2$. It follows from Example 3.7 that the pdf of $W = U/V$ is given by

☞ 71

$$
\begin{aligned}
f_W(w) &= \int_0^\infty f_U(wv)\, v\, f_V(v)\, \mathrm{d}v \\[2mm]
&= \int_0^\infty \frac{(wv)^{c-1}\, \mathrm{e}^{-wv/2}}{\Gamma(c)\, 2^c}\, v\, \frac{v^{d-1} \mathrm{e}^{-v/2}}{\Gamma(d)\, 2^d}\, \mathrm{d}v \\[2mm]
&= \frac{w^{c-1}}{\Gamma(c)\, \Gamma(d)\, 2^{c+d}} \int_0^\infty v^{c+d-1}\, \mathrm{e}^{-(1+w)v/2}\, \mathrm{d}v \\[2mm]
&= \frac{\Gamma(c+d)}{\Gamma(c)\, \Gamma(d)}\, \frac{w^{c-1}}{(1+w)^{c+d}}\, ,
\end{aligned}
$$

where the last equality follows from the fact that the integrand is equal to $\Gamma(\alpha)\lambda^\alpha$ times the density of the $\mathsf{Gamma}(\alpha, \lambda)$ distribution with $\alpha = c + d$ and $\lambda = (1 + w)/2$. The proof is completed by observing that the density of $Z = \frac{n}{m}\frac{U}{V}$ is given by

$$
f_Z(z) = f_W(z\, m/n)\, m/n\, .
$$

$\square$

Corollary 3.2. (Relationship Between Normal, χ^2, and t Distributions). Let $Z \sim \mathsf{N}(0, 1)$ and $V \sim \chi_n^2$ be independent. Then,

$$
\frac{Z}{\sqrt{V/n}} \sim \mathsf{t}_n\, .
$$

Proof. Let $T = Z/\sqrt{V/n}$. Because $Z^2 \sim \chi_1^2$, we have by Theorem 3.11 that $T^2 \sim \mathsf{F}(1, n)$. The result follows now from Theorem 2.19 and the symmetry around 0 of the pdf of T.

☞ 51

$\square$

3.7 Limit Theorems

Two main results in probability are the *law of large numbers* and *the central limit theorem*. Both are limit theorems involving sums of independent random variables. In particular, consider a sequence $X_1, X_2, \ldots$ of iid random variables with finite expectation μ and finite variance σ^2. For each n define $S_n = X_1 + \cdots + X_n$. What can we say about the (random) sequence of sums $S_1, S_2, \ldots$ or averages $S_1, S_2/2, S_3/3, \ldots$? By (3.14) and (3.18) we

☞ 75

have $\mathbb{E}[S_n/n] = \mu$ and $\mathrm{Var}(S_n/n) = \sigma^2/n$. Hence, as n increases the variance of the (random) average S_n/n goes to 0. Informally, this means that (S_n/n) tends to the constant μ, as $n \to \infty$. This makes intuitive sense, but the important point is that the mathematical theory *confirms* our intuition in this respect. Here is a more precise statement.

Theorem 3.12. (Weak Law of Large Numbers). If $X_1, \ldots, X_n$ are iid with finite expectation μ and finite variance σ^2, then for all $\varepsilon > 0$

$$\lim_{n \to \infty} \mathbb{P}\left(|S_n/n - \mu| > \varepsilon\right) = 0 \,.$$

Proof. Let $Y = (S_n/n - \mu)^2$ and $\delta = \varepsilon^2$. We have

$$\mathrm{Var}(S_n/n) = \mathbb{E}Y = \mathbb{E}[Y\mathbb{1}_{\{Y>\delta\}}] + \mathbb{E}[Y\mathbb{1}_{\{Y\leq\delta\}}] \geq \mathbb{E}[\delta\,\mathbb{1}_{\{Y>\delta\}}] + 0$$
$$= \delta\,\mathbb{P}(Y > \delta) = \varepsilon^2\,\mathbb{P}(|S_n/n - \mu| > \varepsilon) \,.$$

Rearranging gives

$$\mathbb{P}(|S_n/n - \mu| > \varepsilon) \leq \frac{\mathrm{Var}(S_n/n)}{\varepsilon^2} = \frac{\sigma^2}{n\,\varepsilon^2} \,.$$

The proof is concluded by observing that $\sigma^2/(n\varepsilon^2)$ goes to 0 as $n \to \infty$. $\square$

Remark 3.4. In Theorem 3.12 the qualifier "weak" is used to distinguish the result from the *strong* law of large numbers, which states that

$$\mathbb{P}(\lim_{n \to \infty} S_n/n = \mu) = 1 \,.$$

In terms of a computer simulation this means that the probability of drawing a sequence for which the sequence of averages fails to converge to μ is zero. The strong law implies the weak law, but is more difficult to prove in its full generality; see, for example, Feller (1970).

The central limit theorem describes the approximate distribution of S_n (or S_n/n), and it applies to both continuous and discrete random variables. Loosely, it states that

> *the sum of a large number of iid random variables*
> *approximately has a normal distribution.*

Specifically, the random variable S_n has a distribution that is approximately normal, with expectation $n\mu$ and variance $n\sigma^2$. A more precise statement is given next.

Theorem 3.13. (Central Limit Theorem). If $X_1, \ldots, X_n$ are iid with finite expectation μ and finite variance σ^2, then for all $x \in \mathbb{R}$,

$$\lim_{n \to \infty} \mathbb{P}\left(\frac{S_n - n\mu}{\sigma\sqrt{n}} \leq x \right) = \Phi(x) \, ,$$

where Φ is the cdf of the standard normal distribution.

Proof. (Sketch) A full proof is out of the scope of this book. However, the main ideas are not difficult. Without loss of generality assume $\mu = 0$ and $\sigma = 1$. This amounts to replacing X_n by $(X_n - \mu)/\sigma$. We also assume, for simplicity, that the moment generating function of X_i is finite in an open interval containing 0, so that we can use Theorem 2.7. We wish to show ☞ 36 that the cdf of $S_n/\sqrt{n}$ converges to that of the standard normal distribution. It can be proved (and makes intuitive sense) that this is equivalent (up to some technical conditions) to demonstrating that the corresponding moment generating functions converge. That is, we wish to show that

$$\lim_{n \to \infty} \mathbb{E}\exp\left(t\frac{S_n}{\sqrt{n}} \right) = e^{\frac{1}{2}t^2}, \ \ t \in \mathbb{R} \, ,$$

where the right-hand side is the moment generating function of the standard normal distribution. Because $\mathbb{E}X_1 = 0$ and $\mathbb{E}X_1^2 = \mathrm{Var}(X_1) = 1$, we have by Theorem 2.7 that the moment generation function of X_1 has the following Taylor expansion: ☞ 47

$$M(t) \stackrel{\mathrm{def}}{=} \mathbb{E}\,e^{tX_1} = 1 + t\,\mathbb{E}X_1 + \frac{1}{2}t^2\,\mathbb{E}X_1^2 + o(t^2) = 1 + \frac{1}{2}\,t^2 + o(t^2) \, ,$$

where $o(t^2)$ is a function for which $\lim_{t\downarrow 0} o(t^2)/t^2 = 0$. Because the $\{X_i\}$ are iid, it follows that the moment generating function of $S_n/\sqrt{n}$ satisfies

$$\mathbb{E}\exp\left(t\frac{S_n}{\sqrt{n}} \right) = \mathbb{E}\exp\left(\frac{t}{\sqrt{n}}(X_1 + \cdots + X_n) \right) = \prod_{i=1}^{n} \mathbb{E}\exp\left(\frac{t}{\sqrt{n}}X_i \right)$$

$$= M^n\left(\frac{t}{\sqrt{n}} \right) = \left[1 + \frac{t^2}{2n} + o(t^2/n) \right]^n \longrightarrow e^{\frac{1}{2}t^2}$$

as $n \to \infty$. $\qquad\qquad\square$

Figure 3.7 shows central limit theorem in action. The left part shows the pdfs of $S_1, \ldots, S_4$ for the case where the $\{X_i\}$ have a $\mathcal{U}[0,1]$ distribution. The right part shows the same for the $\mathsf{Exp}(1)$ distribution. We clearly see convergence to a bell-shaped curve, characteristic of the normal distribution.

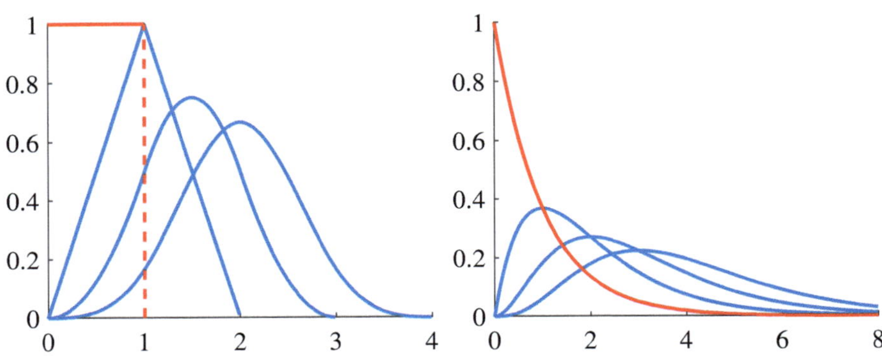

Fig. 3.7 Illustration of the central limit theorem for (left) the uniform distribution and (right) the exponential distribution

Recall that a binomial random variable $X \sim \mathsf{Bin}(n, p)$ can be viewed as the sum of n iid $\mathsf{Ber}(p)$ random variables: $X = X_1 + \cdots + X_n$. As a direct consequence of the central limit theorem it follows that for large n $\mathbb{P}(X \leq k) \approx \mathbb{P}(Y \leq k)$, where $Y \sim \mathcal{N}(np, np(1-p))$. As a rule of thumb, this normal approximation to the binomial distribution is accurate if both np and $n(1-p)$ are larger than 5.

There is also a central limit theorem for random vectors. The multidimensional version is as follows.

Theorem 3.14. (Multivariate Central Limit Theorem). Let $\boldsymbol{X}_1, \ldots, \boldsymbol{X}_n$ be iid random vectors with expectation vector $\boldsymbol{\mu}$ and covariance matrix $\boldsymbol{\Sigma}$. For large n the random vector $\boldsymbol{X}_1 + \cdots + \boldsymbol{X}_n$ approximately has a $\mathcal{N}(n\boldsymbol{\mu}, n\boldsymbol{\Sigma})$ distribution.

A more precise formulation of the above theorem is that the average random vector $\boldsymbol{Z}_n = (\boldsymbol{X}_1 + \cdots + \boldsymbol{X}_n)/n$, when rescaled via $\sqrt{n}(\boldsymbol{Z}_n - \boldsymbol{\mu})$, converges in distribution to a random vector $\boldsymbol{K} \sim \mathcal{N}(\mathbf{0}, \boldsymbol{\Sigma})$ as $n \to \infty$. A useful consequence of this is given next.

Theorem 3.15. (Delta Method). Let $\boldsymbol{Z}_1, \boldsymbol{Z}_2, \ldots$ be a sequence of random vectors such that $\sqrt{n}(\boldsymbol{Z}_n - \boldsymbol{\mu}) \to \boldsymbol{K} \sim \mathcal{N}(\mathbf{0}, \boldsymbol{\Sigma})$ as $n \to \infty$. Then, for any continuously differentiable function $\boldsymbol{g}$ of $\boldsymbol{Z}_n$,

$$\sqrt{n}(\boldsymbol{g}(\boldsymbol{Z}_n) - \boldsymbol{g}(\boldsymbol{\mu})) \to \boldsymbol{R} \sim \mathcal{N}(\mathbf{0}, \mathbf{J}\boldsymbol{\Sigma}\mathbf{J}^{\top}), \tag{3.37}$$

where $\mathbf{J} = \mathbf{J}(\boldsymbol{\mu}) = (\partial g_i(\boldsymbol{\mu})/\partial x_j)$ is the Jacobian matrix of $\boldsymbol{g}$ evaluated at $\boldsymbol{\mu}$.

Proof. (Sketch) A formal proof requires some deeper knowledge of statistical convergence, but the idea of the proof is quite straightforward. The key step is to construct the first-order Taylor expansion (see Theorem B.1) of $\boldsymbol{g}$ around ☞ 47 $\boldsymbol{\mu}$, which yields

$$\boldsymbol{g}(\boldsymbol{Z}_n) = \boldsymbol{g}(\boldsymbol{\mu}) + \mathbf{J}(\boldsymbol{\mu})(\boldsymbol{Z}_n - \boldsymbol{\mu}) + \mathcal{O}(\|\boldsymbol{Z}_n - \boldsymbol{\mu}\|^2) \ .$$

As $n \to \infty$, the remainder term goes to 0, because $\boldsymbol{Z}_n \to \boldsymbol{\mu}$. Hence, the left-hand side of (3.37) is approximately $\mathbf{J}\sqrt{n}(\boldsymbol{Z}_n - \boldsymbol{\mu})$. For large n this converges to a random vector $\boldsymbol{R} = \mathbf{J}\boldsymbol{K}$, where $\boldsymbol{K} \sim \mathcal{N}(\mathbf{0}, \boldsymbol{\Sigma})$. Finally, by Theorem 3.4 ☞ 80 we have $\boldsymbol{R} \sim \mathcal{N}(\mathbf{0}, \mathbf{J}\boldsymbol{\Sigma}\mathbf{J}^{\top})$. □

Example 3.15 (Ratio Estimator). Let $[X_1, Y_1]^{\top}, \ldots, [X_n, Y_n]^{\top}$ be iid copies of a random (column) vector $[X, Y]^{\top}$ with mean vector $[\mu_X, \mu_Y]^{\top}$ and covariance matrix $\boldsymbol{\Sigma}$. Denoting the average of the $\{X_i\}$ and $\{Y_i\}$ by $\overline{X}$ and $\overline{Y}$, respectively, what can we say about the distribution of $\overline{X}/\overline{Y}$ for large n?

Let $\boldsymbol{Z}_n = [\overline{X}, \overline{Y}]^{\top}$ and $\boldsymbol{\mu} = [\mu_X, \mu_Y]^{\top}$. By the multivariate central limit theorem, $\boldsymbol{Z}_n$ has approximately a $\mathcal{N}(\boldsymbol{\mu}, \boldsymbol{\Sigma}/n)$ distribution. More precisely, $\sqrt{n}(\boldsymbol{Z}_n - \boldsymbol{\mu})$ converges to a $\mathcal{N}(\mathbf{0}, \boldsymbol{\Sigma})$-distributed random vector.

We apply the delta method using the function $g : \mathbb{R}^2 \to \mathbb{R}$ defined by $g(x, y) = x/y$, whose Jacobian matrix is

$$\mathbf{J}(x, y) = \left[\frac{\partial g(x, y)}{\partial x}, \quad \frac{\partial g(x, y)}{\partial y} \right] = \left[\frac{1}{y}, \quad \frac{-x}{y^2} \right] \ .$$

It follows from (3.37) that $g(\overline{X}, \overline{Y}) = \overline{X}/\overline{Y}$ has approximately a normal distribution with expectation $g(\boldsymbol{\mu}) = \mu_X/\mu_Y$ and variance σ^2/n, where

$$\sigma^2 = \mathbf{J}(\boldsymbol{\mu})\,\boldsymbol{\Sigma}\,\mathbf{J}^{\top}(\boldsymbol{\mu}) = \left[\frac{1}{\mu_Y}, \quad \frac{-\mu_X}{\mu_Y^2} \right] \begin{bmatrix} \mathrm{Var}(X) & \mathrm{Cov}(X, Y) \\ \mathrm{Cov}(X, Y) & \mathrm{Var}(Y) \end{bmatrix} \begin{bmatrix} \frac{1}{\mu_Y} \\ \frac{-\mu_X}{\mu_Y^2} \end{bmatrix}$$

$$= \left(\frac{\mu_X}{\mu_Y} \right)^2 \left(\frac{\mathrm{Var}(X)}{\mu_X^2} + \frac{\mathrm{Var}(Y)}{\mu_Y^2} - 2\frac{\mathrm{Cov}(X, Y)}{\mu_X\,\mu_Y} \right) \ .$$

$$(3.38)$$

3.8 Problems

3.1. Let U and V be independent random variables with $\mathbb{P}(U = 1) = \mathbb{P}(V = 1) = 1/4$ and $\mathbb{P}(U = -1) = \mathbb{P}(V = -1) = 3/4$. Define $X = U/V$ and $Y = U + V$. Give the joint discrete pdf of X and Y in table form, as in Table 3.1. Are X and Y independent? ☞ 64

3.2. Let $X_1, \ldots, X_4 \sim_{\text{iid}} \mathsf{Ber}(p)$.

a. Give the joint discrete pdf of $X_1, \ldots, X_4$.
b. Give the joint discrete pdf of $X_1, \ldots, X_4$ given $X_1 + \cdots + X_4 = 2$.

3.3. Three identical-looking urns each have four balls. Urn 1 has one red and three white balls, Urn 2 has two red and two white balls, and Urn 3 has three red and one white ball. We randomly select an urn with equal probability. Let X be the number of the urn. We then draw two balls from the selected urn. Let Y be the number of red balls drawn. Find the following discrete pdfs:

a. The pdf of X.
b. The conditional pdf of Y given $X = x$ for $x = 1, 2, 3$.
c. The joint pdf of X and Y.
d. The pdf of Y.
e. The conditional pdf of X given $Y = y$ for $y = 0, 1, 2$.

☞ 68   **3.4.** We randomly select a point $[X, Y]$ from the triangle $\{[x, y] : x, y \in \{1, \ldots, 6\}, y \le x\}$ (see Fig. 3.1) in the following *non-uniform* way. First, select X discrete uniformly from $\{1, \ldots, 6\}$. Then, given $X = x$, select Y discrete uniformly from $\{1, \ldots, x\}$. Find the conditional distribution of X given $Y = 1$ and its corresponding conditional expectation.

☞ 72   **3.5.** We randomly and uniformly select a continuous random point (X, Y) in the triangle $(0, 0)$–$(1, 0)$–$(1, 1)$—the same triangle as in Example 3.8.

a. Give the joint pdf of X and Y.
b. Calculate the pdf of Y and sketch its graph.
c. Specify the conditional pdf of Y given $X = x$ for any fixed $x \in (0, 1)$.
d. Determine $\mathbb{E}[Y \mid X = 1/2]$.

3.6. Let $X \sim \mathcal{U}[0, 1]$ and $Y \sim \mathsf{Exp}(1)$ be independent.

a. Determine the joint pdf of X and Y and sketch its graph.
b. Calculate $\mathbb{P}((X, Y) \in [0, 1] \times [0, 1])$.
c. Calculate $\mathbb{P}(X + Y < 1)$.

3.7. Let $X \sim \mathsf{Exp}(\lambda)$ and $Y \sim \mathsf{Exp}(\mu)$ be independent.

a. Show that $\min(X, Y)$ also has an exponential distribution, and determine its corresponding parameter.
b. Show that
$$\mathbb{P}(X < Y) = \frac{\lambda}{\lambda + \mu} \, .$$

3.8. Let $X \sim \mathsf{Exp}(1)$ and $(Y \mid X = x) \sim \mathsf{Exp}(x)$.

a. What is the joint pdf of X and Y?
b. What is the marginal pdf of Y?

☞ 72   **3.9.** Let $X \sim \mathcal{U}(-\pi/2, \pi/2)$. Show that $Y = \tan(X)$ has a Cauchy distribution.

3.10. Let $X \sim \mathsf{Exp}(3)$ and $Y = \ln(X)$. What is the pdf of Y?

3.11. We draw n numbers independently and uniformly from the interval $[0,1]$ and denote their sum S_n.

a. Determine the pdf of S_2 and sketch its graph.
b. What is approximately the distribution of S_{20}?
c. Approximate the probability that the average of the 20 numbers is greater than 0.6.

3.12. A certain type of electrical component has an exponential lifetime distribution with an expected lifetime of $1/2$ year. When the component fails it is immediately replaced by a second (new) component; when the second component fails, it is replaced by a third, etc. Suppose there are ten such identical components. Let T be the time that the last of the components fails.

a. What is the expectation and variance of T?
b. Approximate, using the central limit theorem, the probability that T exceeds 6 years.
c. What is the exact distribution of T?

3.13. Let $\mathbf{A}$ be an invertible $n \times n$ matrix and let $X_1, \ldots, X_n \sim_{\text{iid}} \mathcal{N}(0, 1)$. Define $\mathbf{X} = [X_1, \ldots, X_n]^\top$ and let $[Z_1, \ldots, Z_n]^\top = \mathbf{A}\mathbf{X}$. Show that $Z_1, \ldots, Z_n$ are iid standard normal only if $\mathbf{A}\mathbf{A}^\top = \mathbb{I}_n$ (identity matrix), in other words, only if $\mathbf{A}$ is an *orthogonal* matrix. Can you find a geometric interpretation of this?

3.14. Let $X_1, \ldots, X_n$ be independent and identically distributed random variables with mean μ and variance σ^2. Let $\overline{X} = (X_1 + \cdots + X_n)/n$. Calculate the correlation coefficient of X_1 and $\overline{X}$.

3.15. Suppose that $X_1, \ldots, X_6$ are iid with pdf

$$f(x) = \begin{cases} 3x^2, & 0 \leq x \leq 1, \\ 0, & \text{elsewhere.} \end{cases}$$

a. What is the probability that all $\{X_i\}$ are greater than $1/2$?
b. Find the probability that at least one of the $\{X_i\}$ is less than $1/2$.

3.16. Let X and Y be random variables.

a. Express $\mathrm{Var}(-aX + Y)$, where a is a constant, in terms of $\mathrm{Var}(X), \mathrm{Var}(Y)$, and $\mathrm{Cov}(X, Y)$.
b. Take $a = \mathrm{Cov}(X, Y)/\mathrm{Var}(X)$. Using the fact that the variance in (a) is always non-negative, prove the following **Cauchy–Schwartz inequality**:

$$(\mathrm{Cov}(X, Y))^2 \leq \mathrm{Var}(X)\,\mathrm{Var}(Y).$$

c. Show that, as a consequence, the correlation coefficient of X and Y must lie between -1 and 1.

3.17. Suppose X and Y are independent uniform random variables on $[0,1]$. Let $U = X/Y$ and $V = XY$, which means $X = \sqrt{UV}$ and $Y = \sqrt{V/U}$.

a. Sketch the two-dimensional region where the density of $[U, V]$ is non-zero.
b. Find the matrix of Jacobi for the transformation $[x, y]^\top \mapsto [u, v]^\top$.
c. Show that its determinant is $2x/y = 2u$.
d. What is the joint pdf of U and V?
e. Show that the marginal pdf of U is

$$f_U(u) = \begin{cases} \frac{1}{2}, & 0 < u < 1 \\ \frac{1}{2u^2}, & u \geq 1 \end{cases} . \tag{3.39}$$

3.18. Let $X_1, \ldots, X_n$ be iid with mean μ and variance σ^2. Let $\overline{X} = \frac{1}{n} \sum_{i=1}^n X_i$ and $Y = \frac{1}{n} \sum_{i=1}^n (X_i - \overline{X})^2$.

a. Show that

$$Y = \frac{1}{n} \sum_{i=1}^n X_i^2 - \overline{X}^2 .$$

b. Calculate $\mathbb{E}Y$.
c. Show that $\mathbb{E}Y \to \sigma^2$ as $n \to \infty$.

3.19. Let $\boldsymbol{X} = [X_1, \ldots, X_n]^\top$, with $\{X_i\} \sim_{\text{iid}} \mathcal{N}(\mu, 1)$. Consider the orthogonal projection, denoted $\boldsymbol{X}_1$, of $\boldsymbol{X}$ onto the subspace spanned by $\boldsymbol{1} = [1, \ldots, 1]^\top$.

a. Show that $\boldsymbol{X}_1 = \overline{X}\boldsymbol{1}$.
b. Show that $\boldsymbol{X}_1$ and $\boldsymbol{X} - \boldsymbol{X}_1$ are independent.
c. Show that $\|\boldsymbol{X} - \boldsymbol{X}_1\|^2 = \sum_{i=1}^n (X_i - \overline{X})^2$ has a χ_{n-1}^2 distribution.

Hint: apply Theorem 3.10.

3.20. Let $X_1, \ldots, X_6$ be the weights of six randomly chosen people. Assume each weight is $\mathcal{N}(75, 100)$ distributed (in kg). Let $W = X_1 + \cdots + X_6$ be the total weight of the group. Explain why the distribution of W is equal or not equal to $6X_1$.

3.21. Let $X \sim \chi_m^2$ and $Y \sim \chi_n^2$ be independent. Show that $X + Y \sim \chi_{m+n}^2$. Hint: use moment generating functions.

3.22. Let $X \sim \mathcal{N}(\mu, 1)$. Show that the moment generation function of X^2 is

$$M(t) = \frac{e^{\mu^2 t/(1-2t)}}{\sqrt{1 - 2t}} \quad t < 1/2 .$$

Next, consider independent random variables $X_i \sim \mathcal{N}(\mu_i, 1)$, $i = 1, \ldots, n$. Use the result above to show that the distribution of $\|\boldsymbol{X}\|^2$ only depends on n and $\|\boldsymbol{\mu}\|$. Can you find a symmetry argument why this must be so?

3.23. A machine produces cylinders with a diameter which is normally distributed with mean 3.97 cm and standard deviation 0.03 cm. Another machine produces (independently of the first machine) shafts with a diameter which is normally distributed with mean 4.05 cm and standard deviation 0.02 cm. What is the probability that a randomly chosen cylinder fits into a randomly chosen shaft?

3.24. A sieve with diameter d is used to separate a large number of blueberries into two classes: small and large. Suppose that the diameters of the blueberries are normally distributed with an expectation $\mu = 1$ (cm) and a standard deviation $\sigma = 0.1$ (cm).

a. Find the diameter of the sieve such that the proportion of large blueberries is 30%.
b. Suppose that the diameter is chosen such as in (a). What is the probability that out of 1000 blueberries, fewer than 280 end up in the "large" class?

3.25. Suppose X, Y, and Z are independent $\mathcal{N}(1, 2)$-distributed random variables. Let $U = X - 2Y + 3Z$ and $V = 2X - Y + Z$. Give the joint distribution of U and V.

3.26. For many of the above problems it is instructive to simulate the corresponding model on a computer in order to better understand the theory.

a. Generate 10^5 points (X, Y) from the model in Problem 3.6.
b. Compare the fraction of points falling in the unit square $[0, 1] \times [0, 1]$ with the theoretical probability in Problem 3.6 (b).
c. Do the same for the probability $\mathbb{P}(X + Y < 1)$.

3.27. Simulate 10^5 draws from $\mathcal{U}(-\pi/2, \pi/2)$ and transform these using the tangent function, as in Problem 3.9. Compare the histogram of the transformed values with the theoretical (Cauchy) pdf.

3.28. Simulate 10^5 independent draws of $[U, V]$ in Problem 3.17. Verify with a histogram of the U-values that the pdf of U is of the form (3.39).

3.29. Consider the Julia experiments in Example 3.14.

a. Carry out the experiments with $\varrho = 0.4, 0.7, 0.9, 0.99$, and -0.8, and observe how the outcomes change. ☞ 84
b. Plot the corresponding pdfs, as in Fig. 3.6.
c. Give also the contour plots of the pdfs, for $\varrho = 0$ and $\varrho = 0.8$. Observe that the contours are *ellipses*.
d. Show that these ellipses are of the form

$$x_1^2 + 2\varrho\, x_1 x_2 + x_2^2 = \text{constant} .$$

Part II

Statistical Modeling and Frequentist and Bayesian Inference

In Part II of the book, we consider the modeling and analysis of random data. We describe various common models for data and discuss the mathematical tools of statistical inference. Both the classical (frequentist) and Bayesian viewpoints of statistics are covered. Frequentist statistics' main focus is the *likelihood* concept, whereas Bayesian statistics deals primarily with the *posterior distribution* of the model parameters. Both frequentist and Bayesian methods often involve *Monte Carlo sampling* techniques. It is assumed that the reader is familiar with the probability topics discussed in Part I.

Chapter 4
Common Statistical Models

The conceptual framework for statistical modeling and analysis is sketched in Fig. 4.1. The starting point is some real-life problem (*reality*) and a corresponding set of *data*. On the basis of the data we wish to say something about the real-life problem. The second step consists of finding a probabilistic *model* for the data. This model contains what we know about the reality and how the data were obtained. Within the model we carry out our calculations and analysis. This leads to conclusions about the model. Finally, the conclusions about the model are translated into conclusions about the reality.

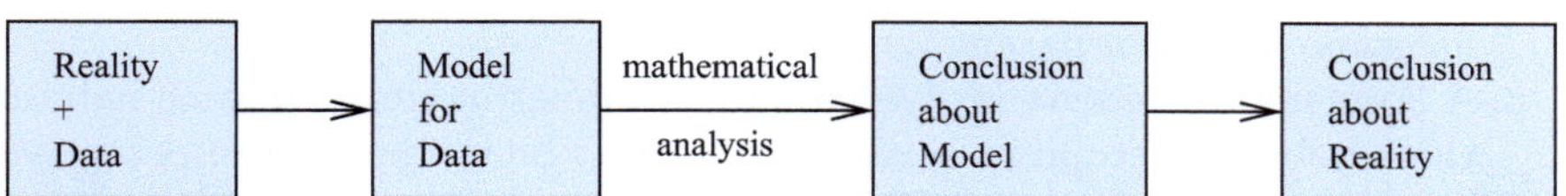

Fig. 4.1 Statistical modeling and analysis

Mathematical statistics uses probability theory and other branches of mathematics to study data. In particular, the data are viewed as realizations of random variables whose joint distribution is specified in advance, possibly up to some unknown parameter(s). The mathematical analysis is then purely about the model and its parameters. ☞ 63

4.1 Independent Sampling from a Fixed Distribution

One of the simplest statistical models is the one where the data $X_1, \ldots, X_n$ are assumed to be independent and identically distributed (iid). We write ☞ 66

© The Author(s), under exclusive license to Springer Science+Business Media, LLC, part of Springer Nature 2025   101
J. C. C. Chan, D. P. Kroese, *Statistical Modeling and Computation*,
Springer Texts in Statistics, https://doi.org/10.1007/978-1-0716-4132-3_4

$$X_1, \ldots, X_n \overset{\text{iid}}{\sim} \mathring{f} \quad \text{or} \quad X_1, \ldots, X_n \overset{\text{iid}}{\sim} \text{Dist} ,$$

to indicate that the random variables form an iid sample from a sampling pdf $\mathring{f}$ or sampling distribution Dist. Let f denote the joint pdf of $X_1, \ldots, X_n$. Then, by Theorem 3.1,

$$f(x_1, \ldots, x_n) = \mathring{f}(x_1) \cdots \mathring{f}(x_n) .$$

Example 4.1 (Experiments with Iid Samples). Each of the following scenarios can be modeled via an iid sample.

1. We roll a die 100 times, and record at each throw whether a 6 appears or not. Let $X_i = 1$ if the i-th throw yields a 6 and $X_i = 0$ otherwise, for $i = 1, \ldots, 100$. Then,

$$X_1, \ldots, X_{100} \overset{\text{iid}}{\sim} \text{Ber}(p)$$

for some known or unknown p. For example, if the die is known to be fair, then $p = 1/6$.
2. From a large population we select 300 men between 40 and 50 years of age and measure their heights. Let X_i be the height of the i-th selected person, $i = 1, \ldots, 300$. Then,

$$X_1, \ldots, X_{300} \overset{\text{iid}}{\sim} \mathcal{N}(\mu, \sigma^2)$$

for some unknown parameters μ and σ^2.
3. A large marine reserve is divided into 20 similar habitats. In each habitat the number of octopuses is recorded. Let X_i be the number of octopuses in habitat i, $i = 1, \ldots, 20$. Then,

$$X_1, \ldots, X_{20} \overset{\text{iid}}{\sim} \text{Poi}(\mu)$$

for some unknown parameter $\mu > 0$.
4. We run a simulation program for a production system for cars and record the total production in a day. We repeat this 10 times, each time starting the simulation with a different seed. Let X_i be the production per day in the i-th simulation, $i = 1, \ldots, 10$. Then,

$$X_1, \ldots, X_{10} \overset{\text{iid}}{\sim} \text{Dist}$$

for some unknown distribution Dist.

Remark 4.1 (About Statistical Modeling). At this point it is good to emphasize a few points about modeling.

- *Any* model for data is likely to be *wrong*. For example, in Scenario 2 above the height would normally be recorded on a discrete scale, say 1000–2200 (mm). However, samples from a $\mathcal{N}(\mu, \sigma^2)$ can take any real value, including negative values. Nevertheless, the normal distribution could be a reasonable approximation to the real sampling distribution. An important advantage of using a normal distribution is that it has many nice mathematical properties, as described in Sect. 3.6.

☞ 83

- Most statistical models depend on a number of *unknown* parameters. One of the main objectives of *statistical inference*—to be discussed in subsequent chapters—is to gain knowledge of the unknown parameters on the basis of the observed data. Even in Scenario 4 of Example 4.1 the model depends on underlying simulation parameters, although the distribution Dist may not be explicitly known.
- Any model for data needs to be checked for suitability. An important criterion is that data simulated from the model should resemble the observed data—at least for a certain choice of model parameters. This is automatically satisfied for Scenario 4 but should be verified for Scenarios 2 and 3. Model checking and selection is discussed in Sects. 5.3.1, 5.4, 8.6, and 12.1.1.

☞ 147

☞ 257

☞ 352

4.2 Multiple Independent Samples

The single iid sample in Sect. 4.1 is easily generalized to multiple iid samples. The most common models involve Bernoulli and normal random variables.

Example 4.2 (Two-Sample Binomial Model). To assess whether there is a difference between boys and girls in their preference for two brands of cola, say *Sweet* and *Ultra* cola, we select at random 100 boys and 100 girls and ask whether they prefer *Sweet* or *Ultra*. We could model this via two independent Bernoulli samples. That is, for each $i = 1, \ldots, 100$ let $X_i = 1$ if the i-th boy prefers *Sweet* and let $X_i = 0$ otherwise. Similarly, let $Y_i = 1$ if the i-th girl prefers *Sweet* over *Ultra*. We thus have the model:

$$X_1, \ldots, X_{100} \overset{\text{iid}}{\sim} \mathsf{Ber}(p_1) \, ,$$

$$Y_1, \ldots, Y_{100} \overset{\text{iid}}{\sim} \mathsf{Ber}(p_2) \, ,$$

$$X_1, \ldots, X_{100}, Y_1, \ldots, Y_{100} \ \text{independent, with } p_1 \text{ and } p_2 \text{ unknown.}$$

The objective is to assess the difference $p_1 - p_2$ on the basis of the observed values for $X_1, \ldots, X_{100}, Y_1, \ldots, Y_{100}$. Note that it suffices to only record the total number of boys or girls who prefer *Sweet* cola in each group; that is, $X = \sum_{i=1}^{100} X_i$ and $Y = \sum_{i=1}^{100} Y_i$. This gives the **two-sample binomial model**:

$$X \sim \mathsf{Bin}(100, p_1) \, ,$$

$$Y \sim \mathsf{Bin}(100, p_2) \, ,$$

$$X, Y \ \text{independent, with } p_1 \text{ and } p_2 \text{ unknown.}$$

Example 4.3 (Two-Sample Normal Model).   From a large population we select 200 men between 25 and 30 years of age and measure their heights. For each person we also record whether the mother smoked during pregnancy or not. Suppose that 60 mothers smoked during pregnancy.

Let $X_1, \ldots, X_{60}$ be the heights of the men whose mothers smoked, and let $Y_1, \ldots, Y_{140}$ be the heights of the men whose mothers did not smoke. Then, a possible model is the **two-sample normal model**:

$$X_1, \ldots, X_{60} \overset{\text{iid}}{\sim} \mathcal{N}(\mu_1, \sigma_1^2) \,,$$

$$Y_1, \ldots, Y_{140} \overset{\text{iid}}{\sim} \mathcal{N}(\mu_2, \sigma_2^2) \,,$$

$$X_1, \ldots, X_{60}, Y_1, \ldots, Y_{140} \quad \text{independent},$$

where the model parameters μ_1, μ_2, σ_1^2, and σ_2^2 are unknown. One would typically like to assess the difference $\mu_1 - \mu_2$. That is, does smoking during pregnancy affect the (expected) height of the child? A typical simulation outcome of the model is given in Fig. 4.2, using parameters $\mu_1 = 170, \mu_2 = 175, \sigma_1^2 = 36$, and $\sigma_2^2 = 64$.

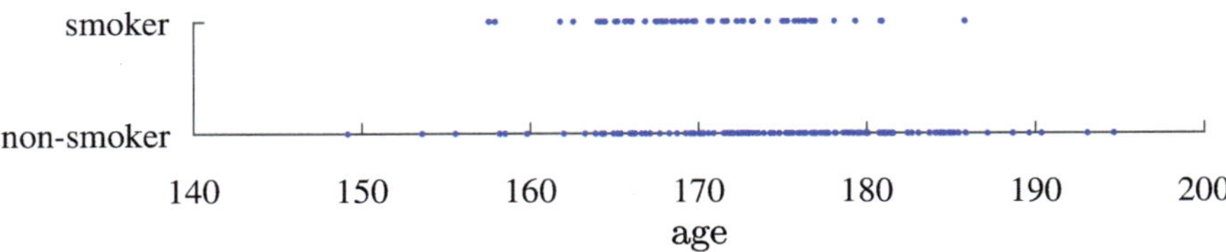

Fig. 4.2 Simulated height data from a two-sample normal model

Instead of dividing the data into two groups, one could further divide the "smoking mother" group into several subgroups according to the intensity of smoking, e.g., rarely, moderately, and heavily, so that in this case the data could be modeled via four independent samples from a normal distribution. This model would, in general, depend on eight unknown parameters—four expectations and four variances.

4.3 Regression Models

Francis Galton observed in an article in 1889 that the heights of adult offspring are, on the whole, more "average" than the heights of their parents. Galton interpreted this as a degenerative phenomenon, using the term *regression* to indicate this "return to mediocrity." Karl Pearson continued Galton's original work and conducted comprehensive studies comparing various relationships between members of the same family. Figure 4.3 depicts the measurements of the heights of 1078 fathers and their adult sons (one son per father).

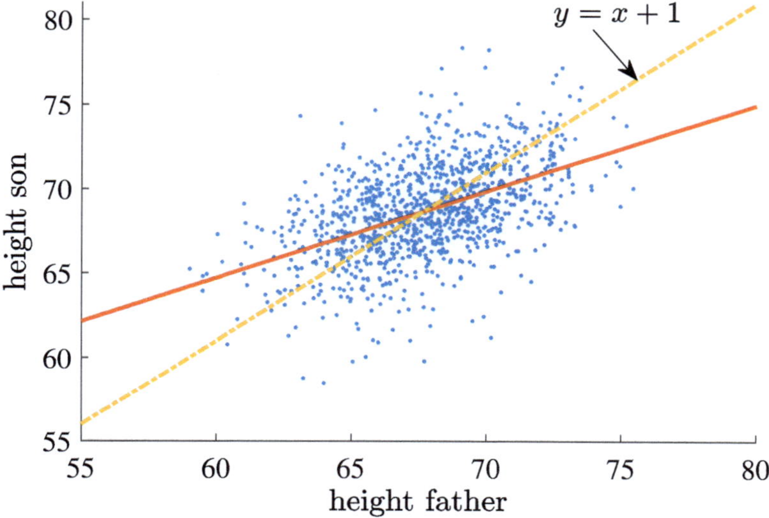

Fig. 4.3 A scatter plot of heights from Pearson's data

The average height of the fathers was 67 inches and of the sons 68 inches. Because sons are on average 1 inch taller than the fathers, we could try to "explain" the height of the son by taking the height of his father and adding 1 inch. However, the line $y = x + 1$ (dashed) does not seem to predict the height of the sons as accurately as the solid line in Fig. 4.3. This line has a slope less than 1 and demonstrates Galton's "regression" effect. For example, if a father is 5% taller than average, then his son will be on the whole *less* than 5% taller than average.

In general, regression analysis is about finding relationships between a number of variables. In particular, there is a **response** variable which we would like to "explain" via one or more **explanatory** variables. Explanatory variables are also called **predictors, covariates,** and **independent variables.** In the latter case the response variable is called the **dependent variable.** Regression is usually seen as a functional relationship between *continuous* variables.

4.3.1 Simple Linear Regression

The most basic regression model involves a linear relationship between the response and a single explanatory variable. As in Pearson's height data, we have measurements $(x_1, y_1), \ldots, (x_n, y_n)$ that lie approximately on a straight line. It is assumed that these measurements are outcomes of pairs $(x_1, Y_1), \ldots, (x_n, Y_n)$, where, for each *deterministic* explanatory variable x_i, the response variable Y_i is a *random* variable with

$$\mathbb{E}Y_i = \beta_0 + \beta_1\, x_i, \quad i = 1, \ldots, n \tag{4.1}$$

for certain *unknown* parameters β_0 and β_1. The (unknown) line

$$y = \beta_0 + \beta_1\, x \tag{4.2}$$

is called the **regression line**. To completely specify the model, we need to designate the joint distribution of $Y_1, \ldots, Y_n$. The most common linear regression model is given next. The adjective "simple" refers to the fact that a *single* explanatory variable is used to explain the response.

Definition 4.1. (Simple Linear Regression Model). In a **simple linear regression model** the response data $Y_1, \ldots, Y_n$ depend on explanatory variables $x_1, \ldots, x_n$ via the linear relationship

$$Y_i = \beta_0 + \beta_1\, x_i + \varepsilon_i, \quad i = 1, \ldots, n, \tag{4.3}$$

where $\varepsilon_1, \ldots, \varepsilon_n \overset{\text{iid}}{\sim} \mathcal{N}(0, \sigma^2)$.

This formulation makes it even more obvious that we view the responses as random variables which would lie exactly on the regression line, were it not for some "disturbance" or "error" term (represented by the $\{\varepsilon_i\}$).

Note that the simple linear regression model (4.3) is a *Gaussian* model; that is, $\boldsymbol{Y} = [Y_1, \ldots, Y_n]^\top$ has a multivariate normal distribution. Namely,

$$\boldsymbol{Y} \sim \mathcal{N}(\beta_0 \mathbf{1} + \beta_1 \boldsymbol{x}, \ \sigma^2\, \mathbb{I}_n), \tag{4.4}$$

where $\boldsymbol{x} = [x_1, \ldots, x_n]^\top$, $\mathbf{1}$ is the n-dimensional column vector of 1s, and $\mathbb{I}_n$ is the n-dimensional identity matrix.

4.3.2 Multiple Linear Regression

A linear regression model that contains more than one explanatory variable is called a **multiple linear regression model**.

Definition 4.2. (Multiple Linear Regression Model). In a (Gaussian) **multiple linear regression model** the response data $Y_1, \ldots, Y_n$ depend on d-dimensional explanatory variables $\boldsymbol{x}_1, \ldots, \boldsymbol{x}_n$, with $\boldsymbol{x}_i = [x_{i1}, \ldots, x_{id}]^\top$, via the linear relationship

$$Y_i = \beta_0 + \beta_1 x_{i1} + \cdots + \beta_d x_{id} + \varepsilon_i , \quad i = 1, \ldots, n , \qquad (4.5)$$

where $\varepsilon_1, \ldots, \varepsilon_n \overset{\text{iid}}{\sim} \mathcal{N}(0, \sigma^2)$.

We can write (4.5) as $Y_i = \beta_0 + \boldsymbol{x}_i^\top \boldsymbol{\beta} + \varepsilon_i$, where $\boldsymbol{\beta} = [\beta_1, \ldots, \beta_d]^\top$. In other words, the data $(\boldsymbol{x}_i, Y_i)$—where the $\{Y_i\}$ are random—lie approximately on the plane $y = \beta_0 + \boldsymbol{x}^\top \boldsymbol{\beta}$ for some (typically unknown) constant β_0 and vector $\boldsymbol{\beta}$. Defining $\boldsymbol{Y} = [Y_1, \ldots, Y_n]^\top$ and $\mathbf{A}$ as the matrix

$$\mathbf{A} = \begin{bmatrix} \boldsymbol{x}_1^\top \\ \boldsymbol{x}_2^\top \\ \vdots \\ \boldsymbol{x}_n^\top \end{bmatrix},$$

we can reformulate (4.5) as the Gaussian model

$$\boldsymbol{Y} \sim \mathcal{N}(\beta_0 \mathbf{1} + \mathbf{A}\boldsymbol{\beta}, \, \sigma^2 \, \mathbb{I}_n) , \qquad (4.6)$$

where $\mathbf{1}$ is the n-dimensional column vector of 1s and $\mathbb{I}_n$ is the n-dimensional identity matrix.

Example 4.4 (Multiple Linear Regression Model). Figure 4.4 gives a realization of the multiple linear regression model

$$Y_i = x_{i1} + x_{i2} + \varepsilon_i , \quad i = 1, \ldots, 100 ,$$

where $\varepsilon_1, \ldots, \varepsilon_{100} \sim_{\text{iid}} \mathcal{N}(0, 1/16)$. The fixed vectors $[x_{i1}, x_{i2}], i = 1, \ldots, 100$ of explanatory variables lie in the unit square.

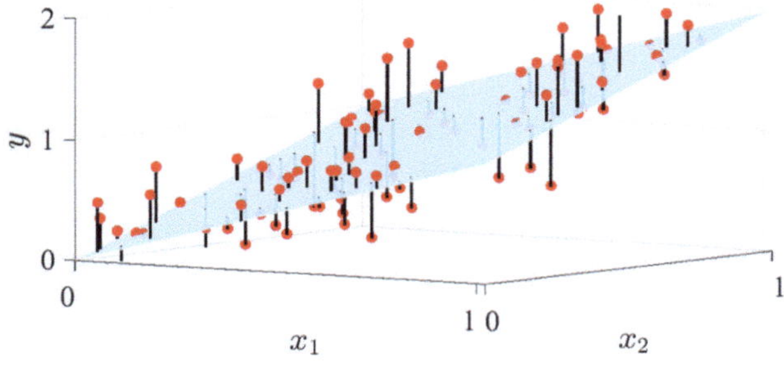

Fig. 4.4 Multiple linear regression

The multiple linear regression model can be viewed as a first-order approximation of the general model

$$Y_i = b(\boldsymbol{x}_i) + \varepsilon_i , \quad i = 1, \ldots, n , \tag{4.7}$$

where $\varepsilon_1, \ldots, \varepsilon_n \overset{\text{iid}}{\sim} \mathcal{N}(0, \sigma^2)$ and $b(\boldsymbol{x})$ is some known or unknown function of a d-dimensional vector $\boldsymbol{x}$ of explanatory variables. To see this, replace $b(\boldsymbol{x})$ with its first-order Taylor approximation around some point $\boldsymbol{x}_0$:

$$
\begin{aligned}
b(\boldsymbol{x}) &\approx b(\boldsymbol{x}_0) + (\boldsymbol{x} - \boldsymbol{x}_0)^\top \nabla b(\boldsymbol{x}_0) \\
&= \underbrace{b(\boldsymbol{x}_0) - \boldsymbol{x}_0^\top \nabla b(\boldsymbol{x}_0)}_{\beta_0} + \boldsymbol{x}^\top \underbrace{\nabla b(\boldsymbol{x}_0)}_{\boldsymbol{\beta}} = \beta_0 + \boldsymbol{x}^\top \boldsymbol{\beta} .
\end{aligned}
\tag{4.8}
$$

4.3.3 Regression in General

General regression models not only deal with multiple explanatory variables but also with *nonlinear* relationships between the response and explanatory variables. A broad class of regression models is (similar to (4.7)) of the form

$$Y_i = g(\boldsymbol{x}_i; \boldsymbol{\beta}) + \varepsilon_i, \quad i = 1, \ldots, n , \tag{4.9}$$

where $\varepsilon_1, \ldots, \varepsilon_n \sim_{\text{iid}} \mathcal{N}(0, \sigma^2)$ and $g(\boldsymbol{x}; \boldsymbol{\beta})$ is a known function of the explanatory vector $\boldsymbol{x}$ and the parameter vector $\boldsymbol{\beta}$. Both σ^2 and $\boldsymbol{\beta}$ are assumed to be unknown.

To specify regression models of this form, it suffices to report only the functional relationship between the expected response $y = \mathbb{E}Y$ and the explanatory variable (x or $\boldsymbol{x}$). For the generic model in (4.9) this corresponds to reporting only $y = g(\boldsymbol{x}; \boldsymbol{\beta})$. We will do this from now on in this section, keeping in mind the general formulation where there are n independent response variables, each with its own explanatory variable and error term.

When $g(\boldsymbol{x}; \boldsymbol{\beta})$ is a *linear* function, i.e., of the form $\boldsymbol{x} \mapsto \boldsymbol{x}^\top \boldsymbol{\beta}$, the model is said to be a **linear regression model**. The obvious examples are the simple linear regression and multiple linear regression models (note that we need to include the constant term as an explanatory variable). The following example gives another important class of linear regression models.

Example 4.5 (Polynomial Regression Models). Suppose the expected response y depends on a single explanatory variable u via a polynomial relationship

$$y = \beta_0 + \beta_1 u + \beta_2 u^2 + \cdots + \beta_d u^d . \tag{4.10}$$

This is an example of a **polynomial regression model**. If we define $\boldsymbol{x} = [1, u, u^2, \ldots, u^d]^\top$ and $\boldsymbol{\beta} = [\beta_0, \ldots, \beta_d]^\top$, then we can write

$$y = \boldsymbol{x}^\top \boldsymbol{\beta},$$

and so the model is linear with respect to the explanatory variable $\boldsymbol{x}$. In a similar way one can consider polynomial regression models with multiple explanatory variables, as in

$$y = \beta_0 + \beta_1 \, x_1 + \beta_2 \, x_2 + \beta_{11} \, x_1^2 + \beta_{22} \, x_2^2 + \beta_{12} \, x_1 \, x_2 \, , \tag{4.11}$$

which defines a second-order polynomial regression model with two explanatory variables. Similar to (4.8), this model can be viewed as a second-order approximation to a general regression model of the form

$$y = b(x_1, x_2)$$

for some known or unknown function b. Polynomial regression models are also called **response surface models**.

Common examples of *nonlinear* regression models are the following:

- **Exponential Model** with parameters a and b:

$$y = a \, \mathrm{e}^{bx} \, .$$

- **Power Law Model** with parameters a and b:

$$y = a \, x^b \, .$$

- **Logistic Model** with parameters a and b and fixed L:

$$y = \frac{L}{1 + \mathrm{e}^{a+bx}} \, .$$

- **Weibull Model** with parameters a and b:

$$y = 1 - \mathrm{e}^{-\frac{x^b}{a}} \, .$$

Example 4.6 (Exponential Model). Table 4.1 lists the free chlorine concentration (in mg per liter) in a swimming pool, recorded every 8 hours for 4 days.

Table 4.1 Chlorine concentration (in mg/L) as a function of time (hours)

Hours	Concentration	Hours	Concentration
0	1.0056	56	0.3293
8	0.8497	64	0.2617
16	0.6682	72	0.2460
24	0.6056	80	0.1839
32	0.4735	88	0.1867
40	0.4745	96	0.1688
48	0.3563		

A simple chemistry-based model for the chlorine concentration y as a function of time t is

$$y = a\,\mathrm{e}^{-b\,t}\,,$$

where a is the initial concentration and $b > 0$ is the *reaction rate*. Figure 4.5 shows that the data closely follow the curve $y = \mathrm{e}^{-0.02t}$. A common method for fitting regression curves to data is the *least-squares* method, which will be discussed in Sect. 5.1.2.

☞ 129

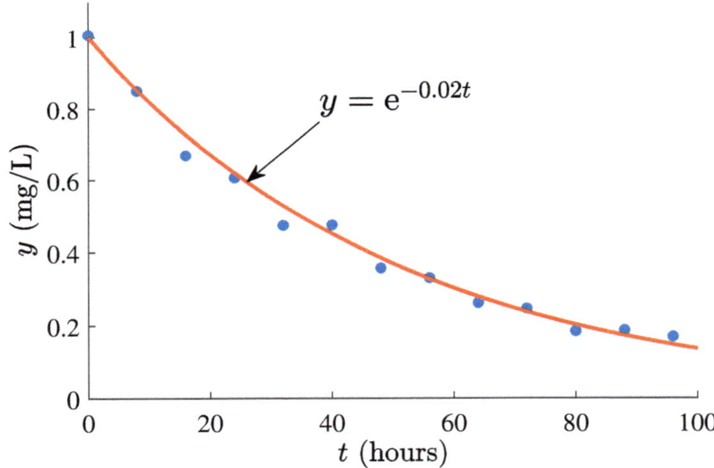

Fig. 4.5 The chlorine concentration seems to have an exponential decay

Another way to deal with nonlinearities in the data is to *transform* the data in order to achieve a linear relationship.

Example 4.7 (Log-Linear Model). Suppose that the expected chlorine concentration in Example 4.6 satisfies $y = a\,\mathrm{e}^{-bt}$ for some unknown a and $b > 0$. Then, $\ln y = \ln a - b\,t$. Hence, there is a *linear* relationship between t and $\ln y$. Thus, if for some given data $(t_1, y_1), \ldots, (t_n, y_n)$ we plot

$(t_1, \ln y_1), \ldots, (t_n, \ln y_n)$, these points should approximately lie on a straight line, and hence the simple linear regression model applies. Figure 4.6 illustrates that the transformed data indeed lie approximately on a straight line.

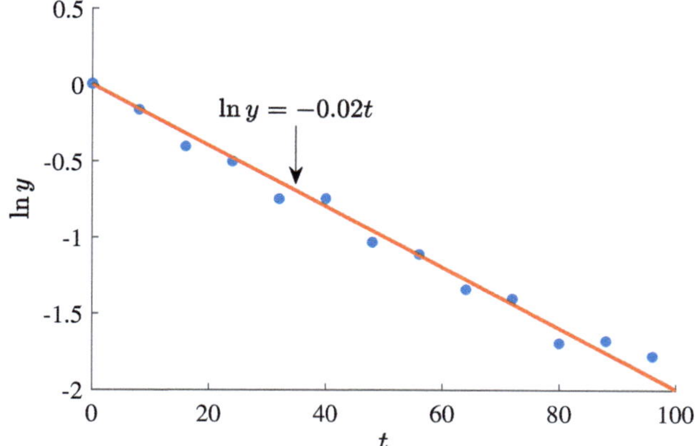

Fig. 4.6 The log-transform of the chlorine concentration can be modeled via a simple linear regression

4.4 Analysis of Variance (ANOVA) Models

In this section we discuss models that describe functional relationships between *continuous* response variables and explanatory variables that take values in a *discrete* number of categories, such as yes/no, green/blue/brown, and male/female. Such variables are often called **categorical**. By assigning numerical values to the categories, such as 0/1 and 1/2/3, one can treat them as discrete variables. Models with continuous responses and categorical explanatory variables often arise in **factorial experiments**. These are controlled statistical experiments in which the aim is to assess how a response variable is affected by one or more **factors** tested at several **levels**. A typical example is an agricultural experiment where one wishes to investigate how the yield of a food crop depends on two factors: (1) pesticide, at two levels (yes and no), and (2) fertilizer, at three levels (low, medium, and high). In factorial experiments one usually wishes to collect one or more responses from each of the different combinations of levels. A fictitious data set for the above agricultural experiment with three responses (crop yield) per level pair is given in Table 4.2.

Table 4.2 Crop yield

| | Fertilizer | | |
Pesticide	Low	Medium	High
No	3.23, 3.20, 3.16	2.99, 2.85, 2.77	5.72, 5.77, 5.62
Yes	6.78, 6.73, 6.79	9.07, 9.09, 8.86	8.12, 8.04, 8.31

☞ 147 The main statistical tool to analyze such data is **analysis of variance** (ANOVA), which will be discussed in Sect. 5.3.1. We describe next two common models that are used in such situations.

4.4.1 Single-Factor ANOVA

Consider a response variable which depends on a single factor with d levels. Within each level i there are n_i independent measurements of the response variable. The data thus consist of d independent samples with sizes $n_1, \ldots, n_d$:

$$\underbrace{Y_1, \ldots, Y_{n_1}}_{\text{level 1}}, \underbrace{Y_{n_1+1}, \ldots, Y_{n_1+n_2}}_{\text{level 2}}, \ldots, \underbrace{Y_{n-n_d+1}, \ldots, Y_n}_{\text{level } d} , \qquad (4.12)$$

☞ 104 where $n = n_1 + \cdots + n_d$. An obvious model for the data is that the $\{Y_i\}$ are assumed to be independent and normally distributed with a mean and variance which depend only on the level. Such a model is simply a d-sample generalization of the two-sample normal model in Example 4.3. To be able to analyze the model via ANOVA, one needs however the additional model assumption that the *variances are all equal*; that is, they are the same for each level. Writing Y_{ik} as the response for the k-th replication at level i, we can define the model as follows.

Definition 4.3.   (Single-Factor ANOVA Model). In a **single-factor ANOVA model**, let Y_{ik} be the response for the k-th replication at level i. Then,

$$Y_{ik} = \mu_i + \varepsilon_{ik} , \quad k = 1, \ldots, n_i , \; i = 1, \ldots, d , \qquad (4.13)$$

where $\{\varepsilon_{ik}\} \stackrel{\text{iid}}{\sim} \mathcal{N}(0, \sigma^2)$.

Instead of (4.13) one often sees the "factor effects" formulation

$$Y_{ik} = \mu + \alpha_i + \varepsilon_{ik} , \quad k = 1, \ldots, n_i , \; i = 1, \ldots, d , \qquad (4.14)$$

where μ is interpreted as the *overall* effect, common to all levels, and $\alpha_i = \mu_i - \mu$ is the *incremental effect* of level i. Although μ can be defined in several ways, it is customary to define it as the expected average response:

$$\mu = \mathbb{E}\left[\frac{Y_1 + \cdots + Y_n}{n}\right] = \frac{\sum_{i=1}^{d} n_i \, \mu_i}{n} \, ,$$

in which case the $\{\alpha_i\}$ must satisfy the relation

$$\sum_{i=1}^{d} \frac{n_i}{n} \alpha_i = 0 \, . \tag{4.15}$$

In particular, for **balanced** designs— where the sample sizes in each group are equal—we have $\sum_{i=1}^{d} \alpha_i = 0$.

Returning to the sequence of response variables $Y_1, \ldots, Y_n$ in (4.12), suppose that for each Y_k we denote the corresponding level by u_k, $k = 1, \ldots, n$. We can then write the model in a form closely resembling a multiple linear regression model, namely,

$$Y_k = \mu_1 \, \mathbb{1}_{\{u_k = 1\}} + \cdots + \mu_d \, \mathbb{1}_{\{u_k = d\}} + \varepsilon_k \, , \quad k = 1, \ldots, n \, , \tag{4.16}$$

where $\{\varepsilon_k\} \sim_{\text{iid}} \mathcal{N}(0, \sigma^2)$ and $\mathbb{1}_{\{u=a\}} = 1$ if $u = a$ and 0 otherwise. It follows that the vector $\boldsymbol{Y} = [Y_1, \ldots, Y_n]^\top$ has a multivariate normal distribution with a mean vector whose k-th component is $\mu_1 \, \mathbb{1}_{\{u_k = 1\}} + \cdots + \mu_d \, \mathbb{1}_{\{u_k = d\}}$, and with covariance matrix $\sigma^2 \, \mathbb{I}_n$, where $\mathbb{I}_n$ is the n-dimensional identity matrix.

4.4.2 Two-Factor ANOVA

Many designed experiments deal with responses that depend on more than one factor. We consider for simplicity only the two-factor ANOVA model. Models with more than two factors can be formulated analogously.

Suppose Factor 1 has d_1 levels and Factor 2 has d_2 levels. Within each pair of levels (i, j) we assume that there are n_{ij} replications. Let Y_{ijk} be the k-th observation at level (i, j). A direct generalization of (4.13) gives the following model.

Definition 4.4. (Two-Factor ANOVA Model). In a **two-factor ANOVA model** let Y_{ijk} be the response for the k-th replication at level (i, j). Then,

$$Y_{ijk} = \mu_{ij} + \varepsilon_{ijk} \, , \quad k = 1, \ldots, n_{ij} \, , i = 1, \ldots, d_1, j = 1, \ldots, d_2 \, , \tag{4.17}$$

where $\{\varepsilon_{ijk}\} \sim_{\text{iid}} \mathcal{N}(0, \sigma^2)$.

Note that the variances of the responses are assumed to be equal σ^2. To obtain a "factor effects" representation, we can reparameterize model (4.17) as follows:

$$Y_{ijk} = \mu + \alpha_i + \beta_j + \gamma_{ij} + \varepsilon_{ijk} \,,$$
$$k = 1, \ldots, n_{ij} \,,\ i = 1, \ldots, d_1 \,, j = 1, \ldots, d_2 \,. \tag{4.18}$$

The parameter μ can be interpreted as the overall mean response, α_i as the incremental effect due to Factor 1 at level i, and β_j as the incremental effect of Factor 2 at level j. The $\{\gamma_{ij}\}$ represent the interaction effects of the two factors. As in the one-factor model, the parameters can be defined in several ways. For the most important *balanced* case (all the n_{ij} are the same), the default choice for the parameters is as follows:

$$\mu = \mathbb{E}\overline{Y}_{\bullet\bullet} = \frac{\sum_i \sum_j \mu_{ij}}{d_1 d_2} \,. \tag{4.19}$$

$$\alpha_i = \mathbb{E}[\overline{Y}_{i\bullet} - \overline{Y}_{\bullet\bullet}] = \frac{\sum_j \mu_{ij}}{d_2} - \mu \,. \tag{4.20}$$

$$\beta_j = \mathbb{E}[\overline{Y}_{\bullet j} - \overline{Y}_{\bullet\bullet}] = \frac{\sum_i \mu_{ij}}{d_1} - \mu \,. \tag{4.21}$$

$$\gamma_{ij} = \mathbb{E}[Y_{ij} - \overline{Y}_{i\bullet} - \overline{Y}_{\bullet j} + \overline{Y}_{\bullet\bullet}] = \mu_{ij} - \mu - \alpha_i - \beta_j \,. \tag{4.22}$$

Here, $\overline{Y}_{\bullet\bullet}$ indicates the average of all the $\{Y_{ijk}\}$. Similarly, $\overline{Y}_{i\bullet}$ is the average of all the $\{Y_{ijk}\}$ within level i of Factor 1, and $\overline{Y}_{\bullet j}$ denotes the average of all the $\{Y_{ijk}\}$ within level j of Factor 2. For this case it is easy to see that $\sum_i \alpha_i = \sum_j \beta_j = 0$ and $\sum_i \gamma_{ij} = \sum_j \gamma_{ij} = 0$ for all i and j. Note that under these restrictions model (4.18) has the same number of parameters as model (4.17); see Problem 4.5.

One objective of ANOVA is to assess whether the data are best described by a "saturated" model such as (4.18) or if simpler models, with fewer parameters, suffice. For example, a model without interaction terms is

$$Y_{ijk} = \mu + \alpha_i + \beta_j + \varepsilon_{ijk} \,.$$

A model where Factor 2 is irrelevant is

$$Y_{ijk} = \mu + \alpha_i + \varepsilon_{ijk} \,.$$

If neither Factor 1 or Factor 2 have an influence on the response, then the appropriate model would simply be

$$Y_{ijk} = \mu + \varepsilon_{ijk} \,,$$

that is, $Y_{ijk} \sim_{\text{iid}} \mathcal{N}(\mu, \sigma^2)$.

Remark 4.2 (Blocking). Not all of the factors in an ANOVA model need to be of primary interest to the researcher. Some of the factors are included in the experiment to reduce the variability of the measurements. Such factors are called **nuisance** factors. An example of a nuisance factor in the crop data in Table 4.2 is the *plant location* of the crop. Suppose the data were gathered from three different locations. Different soil conditions in these locations could greatly influence the crop yield and hence the findings of the research. To reduce the effect of plant location, one could take one measurement for each (pesticide, fertilizer, location) triplet. The data in Table 4.2 could represent this situation, where the three measurements for each (pesticide, fertilizer) pair correspond to location 1, 2, and 3. The idea of grouping data into levels of a nuisance factor in order to reduce the experimental error is called **blocking** and is important in the design of controlled experiments.

4.5 Normal Linear Model

The regression model in Sect. 4.3 and the ANOVA models in Sects. 4.4.1 and 4.4.2 are both examples of *normal (or Gaussian) linear models*.

Definition 4.5. (Normal Linear Model). In a **normal linear model** the response Y depends on a p-dimensional explanatory variable $\boldsymbol{x} = [x_1, \ldots, x_p]^\top$, via the linear relationship

$$Y = \boldsymbol{x}^\top \boldsymbol{\beta} + \varepsilon, \tag{4.23}$$

where $\varepsilon \sim \mathcal{N}(0, \sigma^2)$.

Note that (4.23) is a model for a single pair $(\boldsymbol{x}, Y)$. The model for multiple data $\{(\boldsymbol{x}_i, Y_i)\}$ is simply that each Y_i satisfies (4.23) (with $\boldsymbol{x} = \boldsymbol{x}_i$) and that the $\{Y_i\}$ are independent. Gathering all responses in the vector $\boldsymbol{Y} = [Y_1, \ldots, Y_n]^\top$, we can write

$$\boldsymbol{Y} = \mathbf{X}\boldsymbol{\beta} + \boldsymbol{\varepsilon}, \tag{4.24}$$

where $\boldsymbol{\varepsilon} = [\varepsilon_1, \ldots, \varepsilon_n]^\top$ is a vector of iid copies of ε and $\mathbf{X}$ is the so-called model matrix or design matrix with rows $\boldsymbol{x}_1^\top, \ldots, \boldsymbol{x}_n^\top$. Consequently, $\boldsymbol{Y}$ has a multivariate normal distribution with mean vector $\mathbf{X}\boldsymbol{\beta}$ and covariance matrix $\sigma^2 \mathbb{I}_n$, where $\mathbb{I}_n$ is the identity matrix of dimension n. From (3.31) it follows that the joint density of $\boldsymbol{Y}$ at $\boldsymbol{y}$ is given by

☞ 83

$$f_{\boldsymbol{Y}}(\boldsymbol{y}) = (2\pi\sigma^2)^{-\frac{n}{2}} \, \mathrm{e}^{-\frac{1}{2\sigma^2}(\boldsymbol{y}-\mathbf{X}\boldsymbol{\beta})^\top(\boldsymbol{y}-\mathbf{X}\boldsymbol{\beta})} = (2\pi\sigma^2)^{-\frac{n}{2}} \, \mathrm{e}^{-\frac{1}{2\sigma^2}\|\boldsymbol{y}-\mathbf{X}\boldsymbol{\beta}\|^2}.$$

The situation is graphically depicted in Fig. 4.7. Imagine drawing multiple realizations of the random vector $\mathbf{Y}$. These would form a spherically symmetric cloud of points centered around $\mathbf{X}\boldsymbol{\beta}$.

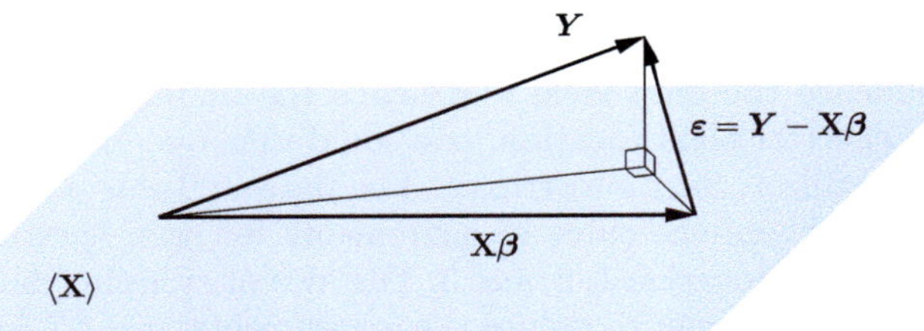

Fig. 4.7 Normal linear model. $\langle \mathbf{X} \rangle$ is the subspace of $\mathbb{R}^n$ spanned by the columns of $\mathbf{X}$

☞ 106   To see that the simple linear regression model (4.3) is of the form (4.23), take

$$\mathbf{X} = \begin{bmatrix} 1 & x_1 \\ 1 & x_2 \\ \vdots & \vdots \\ 1 & x_n \end{bmatrix} \qquad \text{and} \qquad \boldsymbol{\beta} = \begin{bmatrix} \beta_0 \\ \beta_1 \end{bmatrix}.$$

An equivalent formulation is given in (4.4). Similarly, for the multiple linear
☞ 107   regression model (4.5) we have, in view of (4.6),

$$\mathbf{Y} = \underbrace{\begin{bmatrix} 1 & \boldsymbol{x}_1^\top \\ 1 & \boldsymbol{x}_2^\top \\ \vdots & \vdots \\ 1 & \boldsymbol{x}_n^\top \end{bmatrix}}_{\mathbf{X}} \underbrace{\begin{bmatrix} \beta_0 \\ \boldsymbol{\beta} \end{bmatrix}}_{\tilde{\boldsymbol{\beta}}} + \boldsymbol{\varepsilon} .$$

To see that the one-factor ANOVA model is also of the form (4.3), let us define $\mathbf{1}_m$ as the m-dimensional column vector of 1s and $\mathbf{0}_m$ as the vector of 0s. Using the "regression" form (4.16) we can now write the vector $\mathbf{Y}$ as $\mathbf{X}\boldsymbol{\beta} + \boldsymbol{\varepsilon}$ with

$$\mathbf{X} = \begin{bmatrix} \mathbf{1}_{n_1} & \mathbf{0}_{n_1} & \cdots & \mathbf{0}_{n_1} \\ \mathbf{0}_{n_2} & \mathbf{1}_{n_2} & \cdots & \mathbf{0}_{n_2} \\ \vdots & \vdots & \ddots & \vdots \\ \mathbf{0}_{n_d} & \mathbf{0}_{n_d} & \cdots & \mathbf{1}_{n_d} \end{bmatrix} \qquad \text{and} \qquad \boldsymbol{\beta} = \begin{bmatrix} \mu_1 \\ \vdots \\ \mu_d \end{bmatrix}.$$

A similar formulation can be given for the multifactor ANOVA case, as illustrated in the following example.

Example 4.8 (ANOVA as a Normal Linear Model). Regression and ANOVA data are often represented in the form of a **spreadsheet**, where each row corresponds to a single measurement, and the columns correspond to the response variable and the various factors. Table 4.3 gives such a spreadsheet for the crop yield data in Table 4.2.

Table 4.3 Crop yield data as a spreadsheet

Crop yield	Pesticide	Fertilizer
3.23	No	Low
3.20	No	Low
3.16	No	Low
2.99	No	Medium
2.85	No	Medium
2.77	No	Medium
5.72	No	High
5.77	No	High
5.62	No	High
6.78	Yes	Low
6.73	Yes	Low
6.79	Yes	Low
9.07	Yes	Medium
9.09	Yes	Medium
8.86	Yes	Medium
8.12	Yes	High
8.04	Yes	High
8.31	Yes	High

The design matrix can be directly constructed from this table. For example, consider the representation (4.17) and define $\boldsymbol{\beta} = [\mu_{11}, \mu_{12}, \mu_{13}, \mu_{21}, \mu_{22}, \mu_{23}]^\top$. With the responses $\{Y_{ijk}\}$ ordered as $[Y_1, \ldots, Y_{18}]^\top$ as in Table 4.3, the 18×6 design matrix is given by

$$\mathbf{X} = \begin{bmatrix} \mathbf{1} & \mathbf{0} & \cdots & \mathbf{0} \\ \mathbf{0} & \mathbf{1} & \cdots & \mathbf{0} \\ \vdots & \ddots & \ddots & \vdots \\ \mathbf{0} & \mathbf{0} & \cdots & \mathbf{1} \end{bmatrix},$$

where $\mathbf{1} = [1, 1, 1]^\top$ and $\mathbf{0} = [0, 0, 0]^\top$. This may be written in compact notation as $\mathbf{X} = \mathbb{I}_6 \otimes \mathbf{1}$, where $\mathbf{A} \otimes \mathbf{B}$ indicates the **Kronecker product** of $\mathbf{A} = (a_{ij})$ and $\mathbf{B}$, that is, the block matrix with (i, j)-th block $a_{ij}\mathbf{B}$. For the "factor effects" representation (4.18), define $\boldsymbol{\beta} = [\mu, \alpha_1, \alpha_2, \beta_1, \beta_2,$

$\beta_3, \gamma_{11}, \gamma_{12}, \gamma_{13}, \gamma_{21}, \gamma_{22}, \gamma_{23}]^\top$. In this case the design matrix is an 18×12 matrix given by

$$
\mathbf{X} =
\begin{bmatrix}
1 & 1 & 0 & 1 & 0 & 0 & 1 & 0 & 0 & 0 & 0 & 0 \\
1 & 1 & 0 & 0 & 1 & 0 & 0 & 1 & 0 & 0 & 0 & 0 \\
1 & 1 & 0 & 0 & 0 & 1 & 0 & 0 & 1 & 0 & 0 & 0 \\
1 & 0 & 1 & 1 & 0 & 0 & 0 & 0 & 0 & 1 & 0 & 0 \\
1 & 0 & 1 & 0 & 1 & 0 & 0 & 0 & 0 & 0 & 1 & 0 \\
1 & 0 & 1 & 0 & 0 & 1 & 0 & 0 & 0 & 0 & 0 & 1 \\
\end{bmatrix} .
$$

Note that in this case the parameters are linearly dependent. For example, $\alpha_2 = -\alpha_1$ and $\gamma_{13} = -(\gamma_{11} + \gamma_{12})$. To retain only 6 linearly independent variables (as in the case (4.17)), one could consider the six-dimensional parameter vector $\widetilde{\boldsymbol{\beta}} = [\mu, \alpha_1, \beta_1, \beta_2, \gamma_{11}, \gamma_{12}]^\top$, which is related to the 12-dimensional parameter vector $\boldsymbol{\beta}$ via the transformation

$$
\underbrace{
\begin{bmatrix}
1 & 0 & 0 & 0 & 0 & 0 \\
0 & 1 & 0 & 0 & 0 & 0 \\
0 & -1 & 0 & 0 & 0 & 0 \\
0 & 0 & 1 & 0 & 0 & 0 \\
0 & 0 & 0 & 1 & 0 & 0 \\
0 & 0 & -1 & -1 & 0 & 0 \\
0 & 0 & 0 & 0 & 1 & 0 \\
0 & 0 & 0 & 0 & 0 & 1 \\
0 & 0 & 0 & 0 & -1 & -1 \\
0 & 0 & 0 & 0 & -1 & 0 \\
0 & 0 & 0 & 0 & 0 & -1 \\
0 & 0 & 0 & 0 & 1 & 1 \\
\end{bmatrix}
}_{\mathbf{M}}
\underbrace{
\begin{bmatrix}
\mu \\ \alpha_1 \\ \beta_1 \\ \beta_2 \\ \gamma_{11} \\ \gamma_{12}
\end{bmatrix}
}_{\widetilde{\boldsymbol{\beta}}}
=
\underbrace{
\begin{bmatrix}
\mu \\ \alpha_1 \\ \alpha_2 \\ \beta_1 \\ \beta_2 \\ \beta_3 \\ \gamma_{11} \\ \gamma_{12} \\ \gamma_{13} \\ \gamma_{21} \\ \gamma_{22} \\ \gamma_{23}
\end{bmatrix}
}_{\boldsymbol{\beta}}
=
\begin{bmatrix}
\mu \\ \alpha_1 \\ -\alpha_1 \\ \beta_1 \\ \beta_2 \\ -\beta_1 - \beta_2 \\ \gamma_{11} \\ \gamma_{12} \\ -\gamma_{11} - \gamma_{12} \\ -\gamma_{11} \\ -\gamma_{12} \\ \gamma_{11} + \gamma_{12}
\end{bmatrix} .
$$

The design matrix corresponding to $\widetilde{\boldsymbol{\beta}}$ is simply $\widetilde{\mathbf{X}} = \mathbf{X}\mathbf{M}$; see also Problem 4.10.

4.6 Statistical Learning

It is useful to view the modeling of data in the wider framework of **statistical learning**. Here the goal is to accurately predict some future quantity of interest, given some observed data, or to discover unusual or interesting patterns in the data. In the first case we speak of **supervised** learning and in the second case of **unsupervised** learning. In both supervised and unsupervised learning the modeling of the data goes hand in hand with the selection of a suitable "learning" function. In particular, in supervised learning the goal is to find a **prediction function** g which takes as input a vector $\boldsymbol{x}$ of explanatory variables (features) and outputs a **g**uess $g(\boldsymbol{x})$ for the response variable y. This is the basic paradigm for regression.

We can measure the closeness of a prediction $\widehat{y} = g(\boldsymbol{x})$ to a response y by using some **loss function** $\mathrm{Loss}(y, \widehat{y})$. In a regression setting the usual choice is the **squared-error loss** $(y - \widehat{y})^2$. However, there are many other loss functions possible. Probability enters the scene by viewing each pair $(\boldsymbol{x}, y)$ as the outcome of a random pair $(\boldsymbol{X}, Y)$ with some (unknown) probability density $f(\boldsymbol{x}, y)$. A good prediction function g is one that gives a small loss for any random pair $(\boldsymbol{X}, Y)$ drawn from f. More precisely, we seek a g that minimizes the **risk**, defined as the expected loss

$$r(g) = \mathbb{E}\,\mathrm{Loss}(Y, g(\boldsymbol{X})), \tag{4.25}$$

where $(Y, \boldsymbol{X}) \sim f$.

For the squared-error loss $\mathrm{Loss}(y, \widehat{y}) = (y - \widehat{y})^2$, the optimal prediction function g^* is equal to the conditional expectation of Y given $\boldsymbol{X} = \boldsymbol{x}$:

$$g^*(\boldsymbol{x}) = \mathbb{E}[Y \mid \boldsymbol{X} = \boldsymbol{x}].$$

To see this, let $g^*(\boldsymbol{x}) = \mathbb{E}[Y \mid \boldsymbol{X} = \boldsymbol{x}]$ and define $U = Y - g^*(\boldsymbol{X})$ and $V = g^*(\boldsymbol{X}) - g(\boldsymbol{X})$. Note that,

$$\mathbb{E}UV = \mathbb{E}\mathbb{E}[UV \mid \boldsymbol{X}] = \mathbb{E}[V\mathbb{E}[U \mid \boldsymbol{X}]] = \mathbb{E}[V(\mathbb{E}[Y \mid \boldsymbol{X}] - \mathbb{E}[Y \mid \boldsymbol{X}])] = 0,$$

using repeated conditioning (see (3.20)). Then, for any function g, we have

$$\begin{aligned}
r(g) = \mathbb{E}(Y - g(\boldsymbol{X}))^2 &= \mathbb{E}(Y - g^*(\boldsymbol{X}) + g^*(\boldsymbol{X}) - g(\boldsymbol{X}))^2 \\
&= \mathbb{E}U^2 + 2\mathbb{E}UV + \mathbb{E}V^2 \\
&\geq \mathbb{E}U^2 = \mathbb{E}(Y - g^*(\boldsymbol{X}))^2 = r(g^*),
\end{aligned}$$

showing that g^* yields the smallest squared-error risk.

In contrast, **unsupervised learning** makes no distinction between response and explanatory variables, and the objective is simply to learn the unknown pdf f from data $\boldsymbol{x}_1, \ldots, \boldsymbol{x}_n$ drawn from f. In this case the guess $g(\boldsymbol{x})$ is an approximation of $f(\boldsymbol{x})$ and the risk is of the form

$$r(g) = \mathbb{E}\,\mathrm{Loss}(f(\boldsymbol{X}), g(\boldsymbol{X})). \tag{4.26}$$

A convenient loss function is

$$\mathrm{Loss}(f(\boldsymbol{x}), g(\boldsymbol{x})) = \ln \frac{f(\boldsymbol{x})}{g(\boldsymbol{x})} = \ln f(\boldsymbol{x}) - \ln g(\boldsymbol{x}).$$

The expected value of this loss (i.e., the risk) is thus

$$r(g) = \mathbb{E}\ln \frac{f(\boldsymbol{X})}{g(\boldsymbol{X})} = \int f(\boldsymbol{x}) \ln \frac{f(\boldsymbol{x})}{g(\boldsymbol{x})} \,\mathrm{d}\boldsymbol{x}. \tag{4.27}$$

The integral in (4.27) provides a fundamental way to measure the distance between two densities and is called the **Kullback–Leibler (KL) divergence** between f and g. Note that the KL divergence is not symmetric in f and g. Moreover, it is always greater than or equal to 0 and equal to 0 when $f = g$.

4.6.1 Training and Test Loss

Returning to the supervised case, it is typically not possible to compute the risk $r(g)$ in (4.25), let alone find the optimal prediction function g^*, as we do not know the underlying pdf f. However, we can approximate $r(g)$ from a **training set** $\mathcal{T} = \{(\boldsymbol{X}_1, Y_1), \ldots, (\boldsymbol{X}_n, Y_n)\}$ consisting of independent copies of $(\boldsymbol{X}, Y)$; we denote its (deterministic) outcome by $\tau = \{(\boldsymbol{x}_1, y_1), \ldots, (\boldsymbol{x}_n, y_n)\}$. This approximation of $r(g)$ is simply the average loss:

$$r_\tau(g) = \frac{1}{n} \sum_{i=1}^{n} \mathrm{Loss}(y_i, g(\boldsymbol{x}_i)), \tag{4.28}$$

which is called the **training loss**. We then choose g in some class $\mathcal{G}$ of functions that minimizes the training loss. A similar results hold for the unsupervised case.

Example 4.9 (Linear Model). The simplest and most important model for supervised learning is where we choose $\mathcal{G}$ to be the class of *linear* prediction functions and assume that it is rich enough to contain the true g^*. In particular, letting $\boldsymbol{X} = [X_1, \ldots, X_p]^\top$ be the p-dimensional explanatory variable and Y the response variable, the model assumption is that, conditional on $\boldsymbol{X} = \boldsymbol{x}$, the response Y depends on $\boldsymbol{x}$ via the linear relationship

$$Y = \boldsymbol{x}^\top \boldsymbol{\beta} + \varepsilon, \tag{4.29}$$

where $\mathbb{E}\,\varepsilon = 0$ and $\mathrm{Var}\,\varepsilon = \sigma^2$. Thus, a normal linear model (in the sense of Definition 4.5) is a linear model with normal error terms. Similar to (4.24) the model for multiple data $\{(\boldsymbol{x}_i, Y_i)\}$ is

$$\boldsymbol{Y} = \mathbf{X}\boldsymbol{\beta} + \boldsymbol{\varepsilon}, \tag{4.30}$$

where $\boldsymbol{\varepsilon}$ is a zero-mean vector with independent components, and $\mathbf{X}$ is the model matrix with rows $\boldsymbol{x}_1^\top, \ldots, \boldsymbol{x}_n^\top$. If we view $\tau = \{(\boldsymbol{x}_i, y_i)\}$ as the training data, then the squared-error training loss of a prediction function $g : \boldsymbol{x} \mapsto \boldsymbol{x}^\top \boldsymbol{\beta}$ is given by

$$r_\tau(g) = \frac{1}{n} \sum_{i=1}^{n} (y_i - \boldsymbol{x}_i^\top \boldsymbol{\beta})^2 = \frac{1}{n} \|\boldsymbol{y} - \mathbf{X}\boldsymbol{\beta}\|^2.$$

The optimal prediction function, or **learner**, $g_\mathcal{T}$ in this class $\mathcal{G}$ of linear functions is the function $x \mapsto x^\top \beta^*$ for some β^* which minimizes $\|y - X\beta\|$.

Once a class $\mathcal{G}$ of functions has been chosen and a training set τ is available, an approximation of the optimal prediction function g^* (the minimizer of the risk $r(g)$) is given by

$$g_\mathcal{T}^\mathcal{G} = \underset{g \in \mathcal{G}}{\operatorname{argmin}}\, r_\mathcal{T}(g)\,. \tag{4.31}$$

Note that minimizing the training loss over all possible functions g (rather than over all $g \in \mathcal{G}$) does not lead to a meaningful optimization problem, as any function g for which $g(x_i) = y_i$ for all i gives minimal training loss. In particular, for a squared-error loss, the training loss will be 0. Unfortunately, such functions have a poor ability to predict new (i.e., independent from $\mathcal{T}$) pairs of data. This poor generalization performance is called **overfitting**.

The prediction accuracy of new pairs of data is measured by the **generalization risk** of the learner. For a *fixed* training set τ it is defined as

$$r(g_\mathcal{T}^\mathcal{G}) = \mathbb{E}\,\mathrm{Loss}(Y, g_\mathcal{T}^\mathcal{G}(X))\,, \tag{4.32}$$

where (X, Y) is distributed according to $f(x, y)$. We can approximate the generalization risk via the **test loss**:

$$r_{\mathcal{T}'}(g_\mathcal{T}^\mathcal{G}) = \frac{1}{n'} \sum_{i=1}^{n'} \mathrm{Loss}(Y_i', g_\mathcal{T}^\mathcal{G}(X_i'))\,, \tag{4.33}$$

where $\mathcal{T}' = \{(X_1', Y_1'), \ldots, (X_{n'}', Y_{n'}')\}$ is a so-called test sample. The test sample is completely separate from the training set, but is drawn in the same way, that is, via independent draws from $f(x, y)$, for some sample size n'.

4.6.2 Trade-Offs in Statistical Learning

Choosing a suitable class $\mathcal{G}$ of prediction functions involves the balancing of various competing demands. For example, $\mathcal{G}$ should be rich enough to adequately approximate, or even contain, the optimal predication function g^*, but also be simple enough to allow fast computations to determine the learner.

To better understand the relation between model complexity, computational simplicity, and estimation accuracy, it is useful to decompose the generalization risk into several parts, so that the trade-offs between these parts can be studied. For example, we can decompose the generalization risk (4.32) into the following three components:

$$r(g_\mathcal{T}^\mathcal{G}) = \underbrace{r^*}_{\text{irreducible risk}} + \underbrace{r(g^\mathcal{G}) - r^*}_{\text{approximation error}} + \underbrace{r(g_\mathcal{T}^\mathcal{G}) - r(g^\mathcal{G})}_{\text{statistical error}}\,, \tag{4.34}$$

where $r^* = r(g^*)$ is the **irreducible risk** and $g^{\mathcal{G}} = \text{argmin}_{g \in \mathcal{G}} r(g)$ is the best learner within class $\mathcal{G}$. No learner can predict a new response with a smaller risk than r^*.

The second component is the **approximation error**; it measures the difference between the irreducible risk and the best possible risk that can be obtained by selecting the best prediction function in the selected class of functions $\mathcal{G}$. Determining a suitable class $\mathcal{G}$ and minimizing $r(g)$ over this class is purely a problem of numerical and functional analysis, as the training data τ are not present. For a fixed $\mathcal{G}$ that does not contain the optimal g^*, the approximation error cannot be made arbitrarily small and may be the dominant component in the generalization risk. The only way to reduce the approximation error is by expanding the class $\mathcal{G}$ to include a larger set of possible functions.

The third component is the **statistical (estimation) error**. It depends on the training set τ and, in particular, on how well the learner $g_\tau^{\mathcal{G}}$ estimates the best possible prediction function, $g^{\mathcal{G}}$, within class $\mathcal{G}$. For any sensible estimator this error should decay to zero as the training size tends to infinity.

We thus have two competing demands pitted against each other. The first is that the class $\mathcal{G}$ has to be simple enough so that the statistical error is not too large. The second is that the class $\mathcal{G}$ has to be rich enough to ensure a small approximation error. Thus, there is a trade-off between the approximation and estimation errors.

4.7 Problems

4.1. Formulate a statistical model for each of the situations below, in terms of one or more iid samples. If a model has more than one parameter, specify which parameter is of primary interest.

a. A ship builder buys each week hundreds of tins of paint, labeled as containing 20 liters. The builder suspects that the tins contain, on average, less than 20 liters, and decides to determine the volume of paint in 9 randomly chosen tins.
b. An electronics company wishes to examine if the rate of productivity differs significantly between male and female employees involved in assembly work. The time of completion of a certain component is observed for 12 men and 12 women.
c. The head of a mathematics department suspects that lecturers A and B differ significantly in the way they assess student work. To test this, 12 exams are both assessed by lecturer A and B.
d. We wish to investigate if a certain coin is fair. We toss the coin 500 times and examine the results.
e. We investigate the effectiveness of a new teaching method, by dividing 20 students into 2 groups of 10, where the first group is taught by the old

method and the second group is taught by the new method. Each student is asked to complete an exam before and after the teaching period.

f. We wish to assess which of two scales is the more sensitive. We measure, for each scale, 10 times a standard weight of 1kg.

g. To investigate if the support for the *Honest* party is the same in two different cities, one hundred voters in each city are asked if they would vote for the *Honest* party or not.

h. In a study on the effectiveness of an advertising campaign, a survey was conducted among 15 retail outlets. For each outlet the sales on a typical Saturday was recorded 1 month before and 1 month after the advertising campaign.

i. To focus their marketing of remote-controlled cars, an electronics company wishes to investigate who in the end decides to buy: the child or the father. It records who decides in 400 transactions involving a father and a son.

4.2. Formulate appropriate statistical models for the data occurring in the following quality control processes.

a. Consider a packaging line for 500 gm packets of *Yummy* breakfast cereal. The process is monitored by recording each hour the average weight of five randomly selected packets.

b. A mail-order company selects each day at random 50 invoices from the many invoices it receives on a day and has these examined for errors. The number of invoices with errors is recorded.

4.3. An alternative approach to model the height data in Fig. 4.3 is to assume that the observations are outcomes of iid random vectors $[X_1, Y_1], \ldots,$ $[X_n, Y_n]$. What would be a suitable two-dimensional distribution?

4.4. Consider a Gaussian model $\boldsymbol{Y} \sim \mathcal{N}(\boldsymbol{\mu}, \Sigma)$, where $\boldsymbol{Y}$ is of dimension n. Show that the maximum number of model parameters is $n(n+3)/2$.

4.5. Show that under the restrictions $\sum_i \alpha_i = \sum_j \beta_j = 0$ and $\sum_i \gamma_{ij} = \sum_j \gamma_{ij} = 0$ the factor effects ANOVA model in (4.18) has $d_1 d_2 + 1$ free parameters. ☞ 114

4.6. Verify the relation (4.15). ☞ 113

4.7. For each of the following situations, formulate a regression or ANOVA model.

a. In a study of shipping costs, a company controller has randomly selected 9 air freight invoices from current shippers in order to assess the relationship between shipping costs and distance, for a given volume of goods.

b. We wish to test if three different brands of compact cars have the same average fuel consumption. The fuel consumption for a traveled distance of 100 km is measured for 20 cars of each brand.

c. Heart rates were monitored for 20 laboratory rats during 3 different stages of sleep.
d. For the last t10 years a peace organization has been keeping record of the yearly military expenditure and gross national product of a country, which appear to be related linearly.
e. We investigate the effectiveness of a new fertilizer, by dividing a large patch of land into 20 test plots, each of which is divided into 3 small subplots. In each of the 3 subplots a different concentration of fertilizer is tested: *weak*, *moderate*, and *strong*. The product yield for each subplot is recorded.
f. One hundred adults are randomly selected from a large population. The height and weight of each person is recorded, along with their body mass index (i.e., the weight in kilogram divided by the square of the height in meters).

4.8. Let $Y_1, \ldots, Y_n$ be data from the polynomial regression model (4.10), with corresponding explanatory variables $x_1, \ldots, x_n$. Write the model as a Gaussian linear model of the form (4.23).

4.9. Specify the design matrix for the multiple polynomial regression model (4.11), based on n explanatory variable pairs $(x_{11}, x_{21}), \ldots, (x_{1n}, x_{2n})$.

4.10. Give the 18×6 design matrix corresponding to the parameter vector $\widetilde{\boldsymbol{\beta}}$ for the two-factor ANOVA model in Example 4.8. Verify that the first column, consisting of only 1s, is orthogonal (perpendicular) to all the other columns.

4.11. Table 4.2 was produced using the ANOVA model (4.18), with the following parameters: $\mu = 6$, $\sigma = 0.1$, $(\alpha_1, \alpha_2) = (-2, 2)$, $(\beta_1, \beta_2, \beta_3) = (-1, 0, 1)$, and

$$\begin{bmatrix} \gamma_{11} & \gamma_{12} & \gamma_{13} \\ \gamma_{21} & \gamma_{22} & \gamma_{23} \end{bmatrix} = \begin{bmatrix} 0.2 & -1 & 0.8 \\ -0.2 & 1 & -0.8 \end{bmatrix} .$$

Implement a Julia program to draw realizations from this model, producing data similar to that in Table 4.2.

4.12. The data in Table 4.1 was computer generated from the nonlinear regression model

$$Y_i = e^{-0.02\, t_i} + \varepsilon_i \,,$$

where $t_i = (i - 1)8, i = 1, \ldots, 13$ and $\{\varepsilon_i\} \sim_{\text{iid}} \mathcal{N}(0, (0.03)^2)$. Implement a Julia program that generates (new) data from the model. Plot the data and the regression curve as in Fig. 4.5.

Chapter 5
Statistical Inference

Recall the conceptual framework for Statistics in Fig. 4.1. *Statistical infer-* ☞ 10
ence deals with the middle part of this framework. That is, how to obtain
conclusions about the model on the basis of the observed data. The two main
approaches to statistical inference are:

- Frequentist statistics
- Bayesian statistics

In *frequentist statistics* the data vector x is viewed as the outcome of a
random vector X described by a probabilistic model—usually the model is
specified up to a (multidimensional) parameter θ; that is, $X \sim f(\cdot; \theta)$. The
statistical inference is then purely concerned with the model and in particular
with the parameter θ. For example, on the basis of the data one may wish to

1. Estimate the parameter
2. Perform statistical tests on the parameter

A main difference between the frequentist and the *Bayesian* approach is that
in the latter case *prior information* on the parameter vector θ is used, most
often represented by a probability density for θ. Thus, for the purpose of
computations, we can view θ as as a *random* vector. Inference about θ is
carried out by analyzing the conditional pdf $f(\theta \,|\, x)$—the so-called *posterior*
pdf. Bayesian inference is discussed in Chap. 8. For the remainder of this ☞ 23
chapter we will explain the main ingredients of the classical (frequentist)
approach to statistical inference, starting with a simple motivating example.

Example 5.1 (Biased Coin). We throw a coin 1000 times and observe 570
Heads. Using this information, what can we say about the "fairness" of the
coin? The data (or better, *datum*) here is the number $x = 570$. Suppose we

© The Author(s), under exclusive license to Springer Science+Business   125
Media, LLC, part of Springer Nature 2025
J. C. C. Chan, D. P. Kroese, *Statistical Modeling and Computation*,
Springer Texts in Statistics, https://doi.org/10.1007/978-1-0716-4132-3_5

view x as the outcome of a random variable X which describes the number of Heads in 1000 tosses. Our statistical model is then:

$$X \sim \text{Bin}(1000, p) \,,$$

where $p \in [0, 1]$ is unknown. Any statement about the fairness of the coin is expressed in terms of p and is assessed via this model. It is important to understand that p will *never be known*. The best we can do is to provide an *estimate* of p. A common-sense estimate of p is simply the proportion of Heads $x/1000 = 0.570$. But how accurate is this estimate? Is it possible that the unknown p could in fact be 0.5? One can make sense of these questions through detailed analysis of the statistical model.

5.1 Estimation

Suppose the distribution of the data $\boldsymbol{X}$ is completely specified up to an unknown parameter vector $\boldsymbol{\theta}$. The aim is to estimate $\boldsymbol{\theta}$ on the basis of the observed data $\boldsymbol{x}$ only. Mathematically, the goal is to find function $\boldsymbol{T} = \boldsymbol{T}(\boldsymbol{X})$ of the data $\boldsymbol{X}$ such that the random vector $\boldsymbol{T}$ is close to $\boldsymbol{\theta}$. The random variable $\boldsymbol{T}$ is called an **estimator** of $\boldsymbol{\theta}$. The corresponding outcome $\boldsymbol{t} = \boldsymbol{T}(\boldsymbol{x})$ is the **estimate** of $\boldsymbol{\theta}$. The **bias** of an estimator $\boldsymbol{T}$ is defined as $\mathbb{E}\boldsymbol{T} - \boldsymbol{\theta}$. $\boldsymbol{T}$ is said to be **unbiased** if $\mathbb{E}\boldsymbol{T} = \boldsymbol{\theta}$. It is important to note that $\boldsymbol{T}$ is a function of the data only and not of the parameter. Such a function is called a **statistic**.

Example 5.2 (Iid Sample from a Normal Distribution). Consider the
standard model for data (see Sect. 4.1):

$$X_1, \ldots, X_n \sim \mathcal{N}(\mu, \sigma^2) \,,$$

where μ and σ^2 are unknown. The random measurements $\{X_i\}$ could represent the weights of randomly selected teenagers, the heights of the dorsal fin of sharks, the dioxin concentrations in hamburgers, and so on. Suppose, for example, that with $n = 10$, the observed measurements $x_1, \ldots, x_n$ are:
$$77.01,\ 71.37,\ 77.15,\ 79.89,\ 76.46,\ 78.10,\ 77.18,\ 74.08,\ 75.88,\ 72.63.$$

A common-sense *estimate* (a number) for μ is the **sample mean**

$$\overline{X} = \frac{x_1 + \cdots + x_n}{n} = 75.975 \,. \tag{5.1}$$

Note that the estimate $\overline{X}$ is a function of the data $\boldsymbol{x} = [x_1, \ldots, x_n]$ only. The corresponding *estimator* (a random variable) is

$$\overline{X} = \frac{X_1 + \cdots + X_n}{n} \,.$$

To justify why $\overline{X}$ is a good estimate of μ, imagine that we carry out the experiment and the estimation *tomorrow*, obtaining the (random) sample mean $\overline{X}$ as our guess for μ. From the affine transformation property of the normal distribution (see Theorem 3.6), we see that $\overline{X} \sim \mathcal{N}(\mu, \sigma^2/n)$. Hence, $\overline{X}$ is an unbiased estimator for μ—it is in expectation equal to the unknown μ. Moreover, for large n, the variance of $\overline{X}$ tends to zero, implying that $\overline{X}$ gets closer to μ as the sample size n is increased. To specify exactly how close $\overline{X}$ is to μ one needs to estimate also σ^2, which is discussed in the next section.

☞ 85

Remark 5.1 (Notation). It is customary in statistics to denote the estimate of a parameter $\boldsymbol{\theta}$ by $\widehat{\boldsymbol{\theta}}$; for example, $\widehat{\mu} = \overline{X}$, in the example above. The *same* notation, $\widehat{\boldsymbol{\theta}}$, is often also used for the corresponding (random) *estimator*. It should be clear from the context which meaning is used.

Three systematic approaches to constructing good estimators are the *maximum likelihood method*, the *method of moments*, and *least-squares minimization*. Maximum likelihood estimation is the most powerful of the three and is based on the concept of the *likelihood function*, which plays a central role in statistics. The whole of Chap. 6 is devoted to likelihood methods. In particular, Sect. 6.3 deals with maximum likelihood estimation. The other two estimation procedures are described next.

☞ 17?

5.1.1 Method of Moments

Suppose $x_1, \ldots, x_n$ are outcomes from an iid sample $X_1, \ldots, X_n \sim_{\text{iid}} f(x; \boldsymbol{\theta})$, where $\boldsymbol{\theta} = [\theta_1, \ldots, \theta_k]$ is unknown. The *moments* of the sampling distribution can be easily estimated. Namely, if $X \sim f(x; \boldsymbol{\theta})$, then the r-th moment of X, that is, $\mu_r(\boldsymbol{\theta}) = \mathbb{E}_{\boldsymbol{\theta}} X^r$ (assuming it exists), can be estimated through the **sample r-th moment**

☞ 32

$$m_r = \frac{1}{n} \sum_{i=1}^{n} x_i^r \ .$$

The **method of moments** involves choosing the estimate $\widehat{\boldsymbol{\theta}}$ of $\boldsymbol{\theta}$ such that each of the first k sample moments is matched with the true moments; that is,

$$m_r = \mu_r(\widehat{\boldsymbol{\theta}}), \quad r = 1, 2, \ldots, k \ .$$

In general, this gives a set of nonlinear equations, and so its solution often has to be found numerically. In the following examples, however, the solution can be obtained analytically.

Example 5.3 (Sample Mean and Sample Variance). Suppose that the data are given by $\boldsymbol{X} = [X_1, \ldots, X_n]^\top$, where the $\{X_i\}$ form an iid sample from a general distribution with mean μ and variance $\sigma^2 < \infty$. Matching the first moment gives the equation

$$\frac{1}{n}\sum_{i=1}^{n} x_i = \widehat{\mu} \,, \tag{5.2}$$

which yields the *sample mean* $\widehat{\mu} = \overline{X}$ (already introduced in Example 5.2) as the method of moments estimate for μ. Matching the second moment, $\mathbb{E}X^2 = (\mathbb{E}X)^2 + \mathrm{Var}(X)$, gives the equation

$$\frac{1}{n}\sum_{i=1}^{n} x_i^2 = (\widehat{\mu})^2 + \widehat{\sigma^2} \,. \tag{5.3}$$

The method of moments estimate for σ^2 is therefore

$$\widehat{\sigma^2} = \frac{1}{n}\sum_{i=1}^{n} x_i^2 - (\overline{X})^2 = \frac{1}{n}\sum_{i=1}^{n}(x_i - \overline{X})^2 \,. \tag{5.4}$$

The corresponding estimator turns out to be biased:

$$\mathbb{E}\widehat{\sigma^2} = \mathbb{E}X^2 - \mathbb{E}(\overline{X})^2 = \mathrm{Var}(X) + (\mathbb{E}X)^2 - (\mathrm{Var}(\overline{X}) + (\mathbb{E}\overline{X})^2)$$
$$= \sigma^2 + \mu^2 - \sigma^2/n - \mu^2 = \frac{n-1}{n}\,\sigma^2 \,.$$

By multiplying $\widehat{\sigma^2}$ with $n/(n-1)$ we obtain an *unbiased* estimator of σ^2, called the **sample variance**, often denoted by S^2:

$$S^2 = \widehat{\sigma^2}\,\frac{n}{n-1} = \frac{1}{n-1}\sum_{i=1}^{n}(X_i - \overline{X})^2 \,. \tag{5.5}$$

The square root of the sample variance $S = \sqrt{S^2}$ is called the **sample standard deviation**.

The method of moments can also be used to estimate parameters of iid random vectors, as illustrated in the following example.

Example 5.4 (Sample Correlation Coefficient).   Let $(X_1, Y_1), \ldots,$ (X_n, Y_n) be independent copies of a pair (X, Y) of random variables with unknown correlation coefficient $\varrho = \varrho(X, Y)$. Think of iid samples from a bivariate normal distribution. We can estimate ϱ by using the same "moment matching" ideas as in the one-dimensional case. In particular, write

$$\varrho = \frac{\mathbb{E}[XY] - \mu_X\,\mu_Y}{\sigma_X\,\sigma_Y} \,, \tag{5.6}$$

where μ_X and μ_Y are the expectations of X and Y, respectively, and σ_X and σ_Y are the standard deviations of X and Y, respectively. We can estimate these parameters via the corresponding moment estimators, as discussed above. Moreover, we can estimate $\mathbb{E}[XY]$ via the moment estimator

$$\frac{1}{n}\sum_{i=1}^{n}X_iY_i\,.$$

Hence, we can estimate the numerator of (5.6) as

$$\frac{1}{n}\sum_{i=1}^{n}X_iY_i-\overline{X}\,\overline{Y}=\frac{1}{n}\sum_{i=1}^{n}(X_i-\overline{X})(Y_i-\overline{Y})\,.$$

This leads to the following estimator of ϱ:

$$\frac{\sum_{i=1}^{n}(X_i-\overline{X})(Y_i-\overline{Y})}{\sqrt{\sum_{i=1}^{n}(X_i-\overline{X})^2}\,\sqrt{\sum_{i=1}^{n}(Y_i-\overline{Y})^2}}\,,\tag{5.7}$$

which is called the **sample correlation coefficient**.

5.1.2 Least-Squares Estimation

Least-squares estimation is a simple estimation technique that is particularly useful in regression analysis. In particular, consider the normal linear model (4.23)

$$\boldsymbol{Y}=\mathbf{X}\boldsymbol{\beta}+\boldsymbol{\varepsilon}\,,\quad \boldsymbol{\varepsilon}\sim\mathcal{N}(\mathbf{0},\sigma^2\,\mathbb{I}_n)\,,$$

where the $n\times m$ design matrix $\mathbf{X}=[x_{ij}]$ is known, but the parameters $\boldsymbol{\beta}=[\beta_1,\ldots,\beta_m]^{\top}$ and σ^2 need to be estimated from an outcome $\boldsymbol{y}=[y_1,\ldots,y_n]^{\top}$ of $\boldsymbol{Y}$. We assume that $n>m$; that is, there are at least as many observations as model parameters. The main idea is illustrated in Fig. 5.1: choose estimate $\widehat{\boldsymbol{\beta}}$ of $\boldsymbol{\beta}$ such that the (Euclidean) distance between $\mathbf{X}\widehat{\boldsymbol{\beta}}$ and the observed data $\boldsymbol{y}$ is as small as possible.

In other words, we seek to minimize $\|\boldsymbol{y}-\mathbf{X}\boldsymbol{\beta}\|$ with respect to $\boldsymbol{\beta}$. This is equivalent to minimizing the squared distance

$$\|\boldsymbol{y}-\mathbf{X}\boldsymbol{\beta}\|^2=\sum_{i=1}^{n}\Big(y_i-\sum_{j=1}^{m}x_{ij}\beta_j\Big)^2\,.\tag{5.8}$$

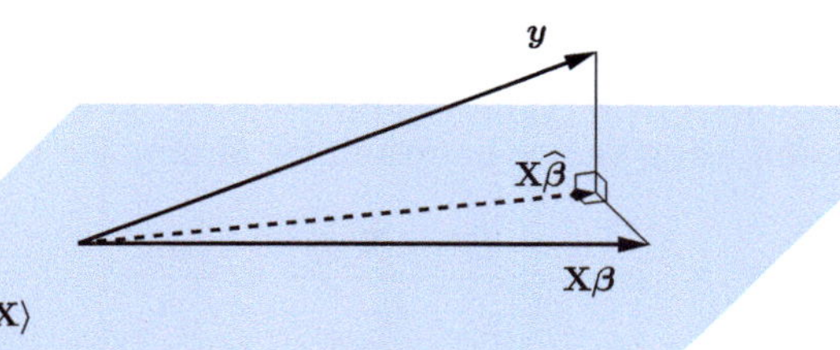

Fig. 5.1 $\mathbf{X}\widehat{\boldsymbol{\beta}}$ is the orthogonal projection of $\boldsymbol{y}$ onto the linear space spanned by the columns of the design matrix $\mathbf{X}$

To find the optimal $\beta_1, \ldots, \beta_m$ we take the derivative of (5.8) with respect to each $\beta_k, k = 1, \ldots, m$ and set it equal to 0. This leads to the set of linear equations

$$\frac{\partial \sum_{i=1}^n (y_i - \sum_{j=1}^m x_{ij}\beta_j)^2}{\partial \beta_k} = -\sum_{i=1}^n \left\{ 2(y_i - \sum_{j=1}^m x_{ij}\beta_j)x_{ik} \right\} = 0 \,, k = 1, \ldots, m \,,$$

which can be written in matrix notation as

$$\mathbf{X}^\top \mathbf{X} \boldsymbol{\beta} = \mathbf{X}^\top \boldsymbol{y} \,. \tag{5.9}$$

These are the so-called normal equations. The **rank** of $\mathbf{X}$ is the number of linearly independent columns (recall that we assume that the number of columns is less than the number of rows). If $\mathbf{X}$ is of *full rank* (i.e., none of the columns can be expressed as a linear combination of the other columns), then $\mathbf{X}^\top \mathbf{X}$ is *invertible*. In that case,

$$\widehat{\boldsymbol{\beta}} = (\mathbf{X}^\top \mathbf{X})^{-1} \mathbf{X}^\top \boldsymbol{y} \,. \tag{5.10}$$

Note that the matrix $\mathbf{P} = \mathbf{X}(\mathbf{X}^\top \mathbf{X})^{-1} \mathbf{X}^\top$ is the *projection matrix* onto the subspace $\langle \mathbf{X} \rangle$ spanned by the columns of $\mathbf{X}$—and hence $\mathbf{X}\widehat{\boldsymbol{\beta}} = \mathbf{P}\boldsymbol{y}$. Namely, $\mathbf{P}$ maps each vector in $\langle \mathbf{X} \rangle$ to itself, because $\mathbf{PX} = \mathbf{X}$, and $\mathbf{P}$ maps any vector $\boldsymbol{v}$ perpendicular to $\langle \mathbf{X} \rangle$ to $\mathbf{0}$, because $\mathbf{X}^\top \boldsymbol{v} = \mathbf{0}$. The $m \times n$ matrix

$$\mathbf{X}^+ = (\mathbf{X}^\top \mathbf{X})^{-1} \mathbf{X}^\top \tag{5.11}$$

is called the (right) **pseudo-inverse** of $\mathbf{X}$, because $\mathbf{X}^+ \mathbf{X} = \mathbb{I}_m$—the m-dimensional identity matrix. We thus have

$$\widehat{\boldsymbol{\beta}} = \mathbf{X}^+ \boldsymbol{y} \,. \tag{5.12}$$

Let $\varepsilon_i = Y_i - (\mathbf{X}\boldsymbol{\beta})_i$ be the i-th component of $\boldsymbol{\varepsilon}$. Note that the $\{\varepsilon_i\}$ form an iid sample from the $\mathcal{N}(0, \sigma^2)$ distribution. To obtain the method-of-moment estimate of σ^2, we match the second moment of $\varepsilon \sim \mathcal{N}(0, \sigma^2)$ to its sample average

$$\frac{1}{n} \sum_{i=1}^n (Y_i - (\mathbf{X}\widehat{\boldsymbol{\beta}})_i)^2 \,,$$

where we have plugged in the least-squares estimate $\widehat{\boldsymbol{\beta}}$ for $\boldsymbol{\beta}$. The estimated errors $u_i = Y_i - [\mathbf{X}\widehat{\boldsymbol{\beta}}]_i, i = 1, \ldots, n$ are called the **residuals**. Simplifying the above expression using vector notation, we obtain the estimator

$$\widehat{\sigma^2} = \frac{\|\boldsymbol{Y} - \mathbf{X}\widehat{\boldsymbol{\beta}}\|^2}{n} = \frac{\|\boldsymbol{u}\|^2}{n} \,, \tag{5.13}$$

where $\boldsymbol{u} = [u_1, \ldots, u_n]^\top$ is the vector of residuals.

Example 5.5 (Simple Linear Regression). For the simple linear regression case we have a design matrix

$$\mathbf{X} = [\mathbf{1}\ \boldsymbol{x}] = \begin{bmatrix} 1 & x_1 \\ 1 & x_2 \\ \vdots & \vdots \\ 1 & x_n \end{bmatrix},$$

and a parameter vector $\boldsymbol{\beta} = [\beta_0, \beta_1]^\top$. The least-squares estimator of $\boldsymbol{\beta}$ is given by

$$\widehat{\boldsymbol{\beta}} = (\mathbf{X}^\top \mathbf{X})^{-1} \mathbf{X}^\top \boldsymbol{Y} = \begin{bmatrix} n & \sum_{i=1}^{n} x_i \\ \sum_{i=1}^{n} x_i & \sum_{i=1}^{n} x_i^2 \end{bmatrix}^{-1} \begin{bmatrix} \sum_{i=1}^{n} Y_i \\ \sum_{i=1}^{n} x_i Y_i \end{bmatrix}.$$

It is straightforward to write this out to obtain explicit expressions for $\widehat{\beta}_0$ and $\widehat{\beta}_1$ (see Problem 5.10), but in practice it is easier to simply solve the normal equations (5.10) numerically. The estimator for σ^2 is

$$\widehat{\sigma^2} = \frac{1}{n} \|\boldsymbol{Y} - \mathbf{X}\widehat{\boldsymbol{\beta}}\|^2 = \frac{1}{n} \sum_{i=1}^{n} (Y_i - \widehat{\beta}_0 - \widehat{\beta}_1\, x_i)^2 .$$

By taking the square root of the above expression, one obtains a natural estimator for σ.

The following Julia program draws $N = 100$ samples from a simple linear regression model with parameters $\boldsymbol{\beta} = [6, 13]^\top$ and $\sigma = 2$, where the x-coordinates are evenly spaced on the interval $[0, 1]$. The parameters are estimated in the last two lines of the program. An important thing to keep in mind when solving linear equations is that one should avoid computing costly inverses. In particular, an equation such as $\mathbf{A}\boldsymbol{x} = \boldsymbol{b}$ should never be solved numerically via $\boldsymbol{x} = \mathbf{A}^{-1}\boldsymbol{b}$. Instead, use Julia's syntax $\boldsymbol{x} = \mathbf{A} \setminus \boldsymbol{b}$, as in the second-last line of code below. Typical estimates for $\boldsymbol{\beta}$ and σ are $\widehat{\boldsymbol{\beta}} = [6.3, 12.2]^\top$ and $\widehat{\sigma} = 1.86$.

```julia
linregest.jl

using LinearAlgebra, Plots
N = 100; x = collect(1:N)/N ;
beta = [6; 13]; sigma = 2;              # parameters
X = [ones(N,1) x];                      # design matrix
y = X*beta + sigma*randn(N);            # draw the y-data
scatter(x,y)                            # plot the data
betahat = X'*X(X'*y)         # solve the normal equations
sigmahat = norm(y - X*betahat)/sqrt(N) # estimate for sigma
```

5.2 Confidence Intervals

An essential part of any estimation procedure is to provide an assessment
of the *accuracy* of the estimate. Indeed, without information on its accuracy
the estimate itself would be meaningless. Confidence intervals (sometimes
called **interval estimates**) provide a precise way of describing the uncertainty in the estimate. In Sect. 6.3.1 we will discuss a systematic approach
for constructing (approximate) confidence intervals, based on the *likelihood*
concept. The *bootstrap method,* see Sect. 7.3, provides another useful way
to construct confidence intervals. The analogue of a confidence interval in
Bayesian statistics is the **credible interval**; see Example 8.1.

> **Definition 5.1. (Confidence Interval).** Let $X_1, \ldots, X_n$ be random
> variables with a joint distribution depending on a parameter $\theta \in \Theta$.
> Let $T_1 < T_2$ be functions of the data but not of θ. The random in-
> terval (T_1, T_2) is called a **stochastic confidence interval** for θ with
> confidence $1 - \alpha$ if
>
> $$\mathbb{P}_\theta(T_1 < \theta < T_2) \geq 1 - \alpha \quad \text{for all } \theta \in \Theta. \tag{5.14}$$
>
> If t_1 and t_2 are the observed values of T_1 and T_2, then the interval (t_1, t_2)
> is called the **numerical confidence interval** for θ with confidence
> $1 - \alpha$.

If (5.14) only holds approximately, the interval is called an **approximate
confidence interval**. The probability $\mathbb{P}_\theta(T_1 < \theta < T_2)$ is called the **coverage probability**. The subscript θ in $\mathbb{P}_\theta$ indicates that the joint distribution
of $X_1, \ldots, X_n$ depends on θ. The coverage probability for an exact $1 - \alpha$ confidence interval is, by definition, at least $1 - \alpha$ for every θ. For approximate
$1 - \alpha$ confidence intervals the actual coverage probability could well be less
than $1 - \alpha$ for certain choices of θ. An example is given in Problem 5.22.

Remark 5.2. Reducing α widens the confidence interval. A very large confidence interval is not very useful. Common choices for α are $0.01, 0.05$, and
0.1.

We next describe a simple approach to constructing exact or approximate
confidence intervals that uses a so-called **pivot** variable $T = T(\boldsymbol{X}, \theta)$, which
is a function of the data $\boldsymbol{X}$ *and* of the parameter of interest θ, and for
which the distribution is known (sometimes only approximately) and does
not depend on θ. The construction depends on specific *quantiles* of the pivot
distribution. For $\gamma \in (0, 1)$, the γ-**quantile** of a distribution with cdf F is
a number z_γ for which $F(z_\gamma) = \gamma$ or, equivalently, $z_\gamma = F^{-1}(\gamma)$. Numerical
values for quantiles of various distributions can be obtained in Julia via the
`quantile` function from the `Distributions` package; see Sect. A.9.

In general, constructing a confidence interval using a pivot variable involves the following steps.

Steps in the Pivot Method

1. Formulate a statistical model for the data $\boldsymbol{X}$.
2. Choose an appropriate pivot variable $T(\boldsymbol{X}, \theta)$.
3. Determine the (approximate) distribution of the pivot.
4. Calculate quantiles q_1 and q_2 for the (approximate) pivot distribution such that $\mathbb{P}(q_1 < T(\boldsymbol{X}, \theta) < q_2) = 1 - \alpha$.
5. Rearrange the event $\{q_1 < T(\boldsymbol{X}, \theta) < q_2\}$ into $\{T_1 < \theta < T_2\}$ and return (T_1, T_2) as an (approximate) stochastic $1 - \alpha$ confidence interval for θ.

Remark 5.3. For a one-sided confidence interval, such as (T, ∞) or (c, T), where c is fixed, only a single quantile needs to be calculated in Step 4.

Example 5.6 (Confidence Interval for Iid Normal Data). Suppose $X_1, \ldots, X_n \sim_{\text{iid}} \mathcal{N}(\mu, 1)$. We have seen that we can estimate μ with the sample mean $\overline{X}$. Here, $\overline{X} \sim \mathcal{N}(\mu, 1/n)$, so $T = (\overline{X} - \mu)n^{1/2} \sim \mathcal{N}(0, 1)$. Since T depends only on μ and the data and has a distribution which does not depend on μ, we can use it as a pivot variable. To construct a 95% confidence interval (hence $\alpha = 0.05$) we consider the $1 - \alpha/2 = 0.975$- and $\alpha/2 = 0.025$-quantiles of the $\mathcal{N}(0, 1)$ distribution, which are 1.96 and -1.96, respectively. Hence, $\mathbb{P}(-1.96 < T < 1.96) = 0.95$. Rearranging $\{-1.96 < (\overline{X} - \mu)n^{1/2} < 1.96\}$ into $\{\overline{X} - 1.96\, n^{-1/2} < \mu < \overline{X} + 1.96\, n^{-1/2}\}$ gives the 0.95 stochastic confidence interval $(\overline{X} - 1.96\, n^{-1/2}, \overline{X} + 1.96\, n^{-1/2})$, sometimes written as $\overline{X} \pm 1.96\, n^{-1/2}$. Thus, if we would repeat the experiment many times, and get many outcomes of the interval $\overline{X} \pm 1.96\, n^{-1/2}$, the true μ would be contained in these intervals in 95% of the cases.

The remainder of this section is about the construction of (approximate) confidence intervals for a number of standard situations, using appropriate pivots.

5.2.1 Iid Data: Approximate Confidence Interval for μ

Let $X_1, \ldots, X_n$ be an iid sample from a distribution with mean μ and variance $\sigma^2 < \infty$ (both assumed to be unknown). By the central limit theorem the sample mean $\overline{X}$ has approximately a $\mathcal{N}(\mu, \sigma^2/n)$ distribution, so $(\overline{X} - \mu)/(\sigma/\sqrt{n})$ has approximately a standard normal distribution. However, this is not yet a pivot variable for μ, because it still depends on the

☞ 90

unknown standard deviation σ. This can be remedied by substituting σ with the sample standard deviation S_X, which, by the law of large numbers, will be close to σ for large n. This gives the pivot variable

$$T = \frac{\overline{X} - \mu}{S_X/\sqrt{n}} \overset{\text{approx.}}{\sim} \mathcal{N}(0,1) . \tag{5.15}$$

For $\gamma \in (0,1)$, let z_γ denote the γ-quantile of the standard normal distribution. Rearranging the approximate equality $\mathbb{P}(|T| \le z_{1-\alpha/2}) \approx 1 - \alpha$ yields

$$\mathbb{P}\left(\overline{X} - z_{1-\alpha/2}\frac{S_X}{\sqrt{n}} \le \mu \le \overline{X} + z_{1-\alpha/2}\frac{S_X}{\sqrt{n}}\right) \approx 1 - \alpha ,$$

so that

$$\left(\overline{X} - z_{1-\alpha/2}\frac{S_X}{\sqrt{n}},\ \overline{X} + z_{1-\alpha/2}\frac{S_X}{\sqrt{n}}\right) , \tag{5.16}$$

abbreviated as $\overline{X} \pm z_{1-\alpha/2}S_X/\sqrt{n}$, is an approximate stochastic $1 - \alpha$ confidence interval for μ.

Since (5.16) is only an asymptotic result, care should be taken when applying it to cases where the sample size is small or moderate and the sampling distribution is heavily skewed.

Example 5.7 (Monte Carlo Integration). In **Monte Carlo integration**, random sampling is used to evaluate complicated integrals. Consider, for example, the integral

$$\mu = \int_{-\infty}^{\infty} \int_{-\infty}^{\infty} \int_{-\infty}^{\infty} \sqrt{|z_1 + z_2 + z_3|}\, e^{-(z_1^2 + z_2^2 + z_3^2)/2}\, dz_1\, dz_2\, dz_3 .$$

Defining $X = |Z_1 + Z_2 + Z_3|^{1/2}(2\pi)^{3/2}$, with $Z_1, Z_2, Z_3 \overset{\text{iid}}{\sim} \mathcal{N}(0,1)$, we can write $\mu = \mathbb{E}X$. In the following Julia program we generate an iid sample of $N = 10^6$ copies of X and estimate μ via the corresponding sample mean. A typical outcome is given in the output.

`mcint.jl`

```julia
using Statistics, Printf
c = (2*pi)^(3/2); N = 10^8;
H =  z -> c*sqrt.(abs.(sum(z,dims=2)))
Z = randn(N,3); X = H(Z);
mX = mean(X); sX = std(X);
R = 1.96*sX/sqrt(N);
LCI = mX - R; UCI = mX + R;
@printf("Estimate = %.3f, CI = (%.3f,%.3f)",mX,LCI,UCI)
```

```
Estimate = 17.053, CI = (17.039,17.067)
```

5.2.2 Normal Data: Confidence Intervals for μ and σ^2

For the standard model $X_1, \ldots, X_n \sim_{\text{iid}} \mathcal{N}(\mu, \sigma^2)$ it is possible to construct *exact* confidence intervals for both μ and σ^2, based on the following result.

> **Theorem 5.1. (Student t and χ^2 Statistics for Normal Data).**
> Let $Y_1, \ldots, Y_n \sim_{\text{iid}} \mathcal{N}(0, 1)$ and let $\overline{Y}$ and S_Y^2 be the sample mean and sample variance. Then, $\overline{Y}\sqrt{n} \sim \mathcal{N}(0, 1)$ and $(n-1)S_Y^2 \sim \chi^2_{n-1}$, independently. Moreover,
>
> $$T = \frac{\overline{Y}\sqrt{n}}{S_Y} \sim t_{n-1} \; . \qquad (5.17)$$

Proof. By the linearity property of the normal distribution (see Theorem 3.6), we have $\overline{Y}\sqrt{n} \sim \mathcal{N}(0, 1)$. Let $\boldsymbol{Y} = [Y_1, \ldots, Y_n]^\top$, and let $\boldsymbol{Y}_1 = \overline{Y}\mathbf{1}$ be the orthogonal projection of $\boldsymbol{Y}$ onto $\mathbf{1} = [1, \ldots, 1]^\top$. By Theorem 3.10, $\|\boldsymbol{Y}_1\|^2 = n\overline{Y}^2$ is independent of $\|\boldsymbol{Y} - \boldsymbol{Y}_1\|^2 = (n-1)S_Y^2$, and $\|\boldsymbol{Y} - \boldsymbol{Y}_1\|^2 \sim \chi^2_{n-1}$. The result now follows from Corollary 3.2. $\qquad\Box$ ☞ 85 ☞ 88 ☞ 89

To obtain a stochastic confidence for μ we take the same pivot as in (5.15). Defining $Y_i = (X_i - \mu)/\sigma$, $i = 1, \ldots, n$, we can write

$$T = \frac{\overline{X} - \mu}{S_X/\sqrt{n}} = \frac{\overline{Y}\sqrt{n}}{S_Y} \; , \qquad (5.18)$$

where the $\{Y_i\}$ form an iid sample from the standard normal distribution. By Theorem 5.1, T has a Student's t distribution with $n - 1$ degrees of freedom. We now rearrange, similar to what was done in Sect. 5.2.1, the equality $\mathbb{P}(|T| \leq t_{n-1;1-\alpha/2}) = 1 - \alpha$, where $t_{n-1;1-\alpha/2}$ is the $1 - \alpha/2$ quantile of the t_{n-1} distribution, to find an exact confidence interval for μ:

$$\overline{X} \pm t_{n-1;1-\alpha/2}\frac{S_X}{\sqrt{n}} \; . \qquad (5.19)$$

To obtain an exact confidence interval for σ^2, we can use the pivot

$$\frac{(n-1)S_X^2}{\sigma^2} = (n-1)S_Y^2 \; ,$$

which by Theorem 5.1 has a χ^2_{n-1} distribution. Note that the corresponding pdf is not symmetric. Let $\chi^2_{n;\gamma}$ be γ-quantile of the χ^2_n distribution. Then,   ☞ 48

$$\mathbb{P}\left(\chi^2_{n-1;\alpha/2} < \frac{(n-1)S_X^2}{\sigma^2} < \chi^2_{n-1;1-\alpha/2}\right) = 1 - \alpha \; .$$

Rearranging gives:

$$\mathbb{P}\left(\frac{(n-1)S_X^2}{\chi_{n-1;1-\alpha/2}^2} < \sigma^2 < \frac{(n-1)S_X^2}{\chi_{n-1;\alpha/2}^2}\right) = 1-\alpha\,.$$

Hence, a $(1-\alpha)$ stochastic confidence interval for σ^2 is

$$\left(\frac{(n-1)S_X^2}{\chi_{n-1;1-\alpha/2}^2},\ \frac{(n-1)S_X^2}{\chi_{n-1;\alpha/2}^2}\right).\tag{5.20}$$

Example 5.8 (Monte Carlo Experiment for Confidence Intervals).
The following Julia program draws an iid sample of size $n = 10$ from the
$\mathcal{N}(3, 0.25)$ distribution. It then determines 95% confidence intervals for μ
and σ^2 and checks if the true values are contained in the intervals or not.
This is repeated independently 100 times and the total number of times that
μ and σ^2 are contained in the confidence intervals is reported. The quantiles
for the t and χ^2 distributions are determined by using the `Distributions`
package. The values are `tq` $= 2.2622$, `cq1` $= 19.0228$, and `cq2` $= 2.7004$. A
typical estimate of μ is $\widehat{\mu} = 3.22$, with a 95% confidence interval $(3.02, 3.41)$.
For σ^2 a typical estimate is $\widehat{\sigma^2} = 0.0761$, with a 95% confidence interval
$(0.0360, 0.2535)$. In this case only the second confidence interval contains the
true parameter. However, out of the 100 confidence intervals typically only
95 contain the true parameter. The output shows that in this particular case
92 confidence intervals for μ contained the true value, and the true σ^2 was
contained in 97 cases.

```
confintnorm.jl

using Distributions, Random, Statistics
mu = 3; sig = 0.5
# true parameters
alpha = 0.05; n = 10; mu_count = 0; sig_count = 0
for k in 1:100
    x = randn(n)*sig .+ mu   # draw the iid sample
    mu_est = mean(x)   # estimate mu
    sig_est = std(x)   # estimate sigma
    tq = quantile(TDist(n-1),1-alpha/2)
    mu_lo = mu_est - tq*sig_est/sqrt(n)   # low bound CI for mu
    mu_hi = mu_est + tq*sig_est/sqrt(n)   # upper bound
    cq1 = quantile(Chisq(n-1),1-alpha/2)
    cq2 = quantile(Chisq(n-1),alpha/2)
    sig_lo = (n-1)*sig_est^2/cq1; # lower bound CI for sigma
    sig_hi = (n-1)*sig_est^2/cq2;   # upper bound
    global mu_count = mu_count + (mu_lo < mu < mu_hi)
```

```
    global sig_count = sig_count + (sig_lo < sig^2 < sig_hi)
end
println(mu_count, "    ", sig_count)
```
```
92    97
```

5.2.3 Two Normal Samples: Confidence Intervals for $\mu_X - \mu_Y$ and σ_X^2/σ_Y^2

Suppose we have two independent samples $X_1, \ldots, X_m$ and $Y_1, \ldots, Y_n$ from respectively a $\mathcal{N}(\mu_X, \sigma_X^2)$ and $\mathcal{N}(\mu_Y, \sigma_Y^2)$ distribution. We wish to make confidence intervals for $\mu_X - \mu_Y$ and σ_X^2/σ_Y^2. The difference $\mu_X - \mu_Y$ tells us how the two *means* relate to each other, and σ_X^2/σ_Y^2 gives an indication how the *variances* relate to each other.

Constructing a confidence interval for $\mu_X - \mu_Y$ is very similar to the one-sample case *provided* that we make the *extra model assumption* that *the variances of the two samples are the same*. That is, we assume that $\sigma_X^2 = \sigma_Y^2 = \sigma^2$ for some unknown σ^2. The analysis now proceeds as follows. The natural estimator for $\mu_X - \mu_Y$ is $\overline{X} - \overline{Y}$. Next, observe that

$$\frac{(\overline{X} - \overline{Y}) - (\mu_X - \mu_Y)}{\sigma\sqrt{1/m + 1/n}} \sim \mathcal{N}(0, 1) \ .$$

If σ^2 is unknown, we must replace it with an appropriate estimator in order to obtain a pivot variable for μ. For this we will use the **pooled sample variance**, S_p^2, which is defined as

$$S_p^2 = \frac{(m-1)S_X^2 + (n-1)S_Y^2}{m + n - 2} \ , \tag{5.21}$$

where S_X^2 and S_Y^2 are the sample variances for the $\{X_i\}$ and $\{Y_i\}$, respectively. It is not difficult to show that S_p^2 is an unbiased estimator of σ^2; see Problem 5.9. The following result is the analogue of Theorem 5.1 and is proved in Appendix B.5.

☞ 47

Theorem 5.2. (t Statistic for Two Normal Samples). Let the random variables $X_1, \ldots, X_n, Y_1, \ldots, Y_m$ be defined as above, then

$$T = \frac{(\overline{X} - \overline{Y}) - (\mu_X - \mu_Y)}{S_p\sqrt{\frac{1}{m} + \frac{1}{n}}} \sim t_{m+n-2} \ .$$

Using the pivot T, we find (completely analogously to the one-sample case) the following $1 - \alpha$ stochastic confidence interval for $\mu_X - \mu_Y$:

$$\overline{X} - \overline{Y} \pm t_{m+n-2;1-\alpha/2}\, S_p \sqrt{\frac{1}{m} + \frac{1}{n}} \,. \tag{5.22}$$

If the assumption $\sigma_X^2 = \sigma_Y^2$ is dropped, the pivot method no longer provides the means to obtain an exact confidence interval for $\mu_X - \mu_Y$, although it is easy to construct approximate confidence intervals for large sample sizes; see Problem 5.15.

Next, we turn our attention to a confidence interval for σ_X^2/σ_Y^2. Here, we can employ the pivot

$$\frac{S_X^2/\sigma_X^2}{S_Y^2/\sigma_Y^2} \sim \mathsf{F}(m - 1, n - 1) \,.$$

To see that this pivot has the mentioned F distribution, first observe that, by Theorem 5.1, $(m - 1)S_X^2/\sigma_X^2 \sim \chi_{m-1}^2$ and $(n - 1)S_Y^2/\sigma_Y^2 \sim \chi_{n-1}^2$, and then apply Theorem 3.11.

☞ 88

Let $F_{m,n;\gamma}$ denote the γ quantile of the $\mathsf{F}(m, n)$ distribution. Then,

$$\mathbb{P}\left(F_{m-1,n-1;\alpha/2} < \frac{S_X^2/\sigma_X^2}{S_Y^2/\sigma_Y^2} < F_{m-1,n-1;1-\alpha/2} \right) = 1 - \alpha \,.$$

Rearranging gives the following $(1 - \alpha)$ stochastic confidence interval for σ_X^2/σ_Y^2:

$$\left(\frac{1}{F_{m-1,n-1;1-\alpha/2}}\, \frac{S_X^2}{S_Y^2}, \; \frac{1}{F_{m-1,n-1;\alpha/2}}\, \frac{S_X^2}{S_Y^2} \right) \,. \tag{5.23}$$

Example 5.9 (Comparing Two Means). A study of iron deficiency among infants compared breast-fed with formula-fed babies. A sample of 25 breast-fed infants gave a mean blood hemoglobin level of 13.3 and a standard deviation of 1.4, while a sample of 21 formula-fed infants gave a mean and standard deviation of 12.4 and 2.0, respectively. Assuming the hemoglobin levels are normally distributed, is there statistical evidence that the mean hemoglobin levels of the two groups are different?

Let the hemoglobin levels for the breast-fed and formula-fed babies be $X_1, \ldots, X_{25} \sim_{\text{iid}} \mathcal{N}(\mu_X, \sigma_X^2)$ and $Y_1, \ldots, Y_{21} \sim_{\text{iid}} \mathcal{N}(\mu_Y, \sigma_Y^2)$, respectively. The samples are assumed to be independent of each other. A 95% numerical confidence interval for σ_X^2/σ_Y^2 is

$$\left(\frac{1}{2.40756}\, \frac{1.4^2}{2.0^2}, \; \frac{1}{0.42969}\, \frac{1.4^2}{2.0^2} \right) = (0.2035, \, 1.1404) \,.$$

Because 1 is an element of this interval, there is no reason to believe that σ_X^2 is different from σ_Y^2. We thus assume that the two variances are equal, which allows us to apply (5.22). The pooled sample variance is $s_p^2 = (24(1.4)^2 + 20(2.0)^2)/44 = 2.8873$, and the 0.975 quantile of the t_{44} distribution is 2.0154, so that a 95% confidence interval for $\mu_X - \mu_Y$ is

$$13.3 - 12.4 \pm 2.0154\,\sqrt{2.8873}\,\sqrt{1/25 + 1/21} = (-0.11,\ 1.91)\,,$$

which contains 0. Hence, on the basis of these data and the assumptions of normality, there is no ground to believe that the expected hemoglobin levels are different for the two groups.

5.2.4 Binomial Data: Approximate Confidence Intervals for Proportions

Suppose we have an outcome x of a random variable X with a $\mathrm{Bin}(n,p)$ distribution. We wish to construct a confidence interval for p. In fact, it is not so easy to find an *exact* confidence interval for p, so we settle for an approximate one. For large n, X has approximately a $\mathcal{N}(np, np(1-p))$ distribution; see (3.7). The natural estimator for p, that is, $\widehat{p} = X/n$, has therefore approximately a $\mathcal{N}(p, p(1-p)/n)$ distribution. Thus, using the pivot $(\widehat{p} - p)/\sqrt{p(1-p)/n}$, we have

☞ 92

$$\mathbb{P}\left(-z_{1-\alpha/2} < \frac{\widehat{p} - p}{\sqrt{p(1-p)/n}} < z_{1-\alpha/2}\right) \approx 1 - \alpha\,,$$

where $z_{1-\alpha/2}$ is the $1 - \alpha/2$ quantile of the standard normal distribution. Rearranging gives:

$$\mathbb{P}\left(\widehat{p} - z_{1-\alpha/2}\sqrt{\frac{p(1-p)}{n}} < p < \widehat{p} + z_{1-\alpha/2}\sqrt{\frac{p(1-p)}{n}}\right) \approx 1 - \alpha\,.$$

This would suggest that we take $\widehat{p} \pm z_{1-\alpha/2}\sqrt{\frac{p(1-p)}{n}}$ as an approximate $1 - \alpha$ confidence interval for p, were it not for the fact that the bounds still contain the unknown p. However, for large n the estimator $\widehat{p}$ is close to the real p, so that we may replace p with $\widehat{p}$ under the square roots in the expression above. Hence, an approximate $1 - \alpha$ confidence interval for p is

$$\widehat{p} \pm z_{1-\alpha/2}\sqrt{\frac{\widehat{p}(1-\widehat{p})}{n}}\,. \tag{5.24}$$

Example 5.10 (Approximate Confidence Interval for Proportion).
In an opinion poll of 1000 registered voters, 227 voters say they will vote for
the *Honest* party. We wish to find a 95% approximate confidence interval for
the proportion p of *Honest* voters of the total population. We hereto view
the datum, 227, as the outcome of a random variable X (the number of
Honest voters out of 1000 registered voters) with a $\mathsf{Bin}(1000, p)$ distribution.
We have $\widehat{p} = 227/1000 = 0.227$, and $z_{0.975} = 1.96$, so that an approximate
95% numerical confidence interval for p is

$$0.227 \pm 1.96 \times 0.0132 = (0.20,\ 0.25)\,.$$

The same methodology can be used to construct approximate confidence
intervals for the difference between two proportions. In particular, consider
outcomes x and y of two independent random variables $X \sim \mathsf{Bin}(m, p_X)$ and
$Y \sim \mathsf{Bin}(n, p_Y)$. We wish to construct an approximate confidence interval for
$p_X - p_Y$. The corresponding estimator is $\widehat{p}_X - \widehat{p}_Y = X/m - Y/n$. As in the
one-sample case, for m and n sufficiently large,

$$\mathbb{P}\left(-z_{1-\alpha/2} \le \frac{\widehat{p}_X - \widehat{p}_Y - (p_X - p_Y)}{\sqrt{\frac{p_X(1-p_X)}{m} + \frac{p_Y(1-p_Y)}{n}}} \le z_{1-\alpha/2}\right) \approx 1 - \alpha\,.$$

Rewriting this gives

$$\mathbb{P}\left(\widehat{p}_X - \widehat{p}_Y - z_{1-\alpha/2}\sqrt{\frac{p_X(1-p_X)}{m} + \frac{p_Y(1-p_Y)}{n}} \le p_X - p_Y\right.$$
$$\left.\le \widehat{p}_X - \widehat{p}_Y + z_{1-\alpha/2}\sqrt{\frac{p_X(1-p_X)}{m} + \frac{p_Y(1-p_Y)}{n}}\right) \approx 1 - \alpha\,.$$

By substituting p_X and p_Y with their estimators, we obtain the following
approximate $1 - \alpha$ confidence interval for $p_X - p_Y$:

$$\widehat{p}_X - \widehat{p}_Y \pm z_{1-\alpha/2}\sqrt{\frac{\widehat{p}_X(1-\widehat{p}_X)}{m} + \frac{\widehat{p}_Y(1-\widehat{p}_Y)}{n}}\,. \tag{5.25}$$

**Example 5.11 (Approximate Confidence Interval for the Difference
of Two Proportions).** Two groups of men and women are asked whether
they would buy *Happy* or *Fun* cola, if they were forced to choose between the
two. The results are given in Table 5.1.

Table 5.1 Counts of men and women preferring *Happy* or *Fun* cola

	Men	Women
Happy	55	60
Fun	105	132

The observed proportions of *Happy* cola drinkers among the men and women are $55/160 = 34.4\%$ and $60/192 = 31.3\%$, respectively. Is this difference statistically significant or due to chance?

We view the data as outcomes of a two-sample binomial model. Specifically, let X be the number of *Happy* cola drinkers among 160 men, and Y the number of *Happy* cola drinkers among 192 women. We assume that $X \sim \mathsf{Bin}(160, p_X)$ and $Y \sim \mathsf{Bin}(192, p_Y)$ are independent. To assess the difference between the true proportions p_X and p_Y, we simply evaluate the numerical confidence interval of the form (5.25). We have $\widehat{p}_X = 0.344$, $\widehat{p}_Y = 0.313$, and $z_{0.975} = 1.96$, so that a 95% numerical confidence interval for $p_X - p_Y$ is

$$0.031 \pm 0.099 = (-0.07,\ 0.13)\,.$$

This interval contains 0, so there is no evidence that men and women differ in their preference for the two brands of cola.

5.2.5 Confidence Intervals for the Normal Linear Model

Consider the normal linear model

$$\boldsymbol{Y} = \mathbf{X}\boldsymbol{\beta} + \boldsymbol{\varepsilon}, \quad \boldsymbol{\varepsilon} \sim \mathcal{N}(\mathbf{0}, \sigma^2\,\mathbb{I}_n)\,,$$

where $\mathbf{X}$ is an $n \times m$ matrix $(m < n)$ of full rank m—thus, the columns of $\mathbf{X}$ are linearly independent, and, as a consequence, the matrix $\mathbf{X}^\top\mathbf{X}$ has an inverse.

We saw in Sect. 5.1.2 that the parameter vector $\boldsymbol{\beta}$ can be estimated via the estimator

$$\widehat{\boldsymbol{\beta}} = \mathbf{X}^+\boldsymbol{Y} = (\mathbf{X}^\top\mathbf{X})^{-1}\mathbf{X}^\top\boldsymbol{Y}\,.$$

☞ 12

Since the random vector $\widehat{\boldsymbol{\beta}}$ is a linear transformation of a normal random vector, it has a multivariate normal distribution. The mean vector and covariance matrix follow from Theorem 3.4:

☞ 80

$$\mathbb{E}\widehat{\boldsymbol{\beta}} = (\mathbf{X}^\top\mathbf{X})^{-1}\mathbf{X}^\top\mathbb{E}\boldsymbol{Y} = (\mathbf{X}^\top\mathbf{X})^{-1}\mathbf{X}^\top\mathbf{X}\boldsymbol{\beta} = \boldsymbol{\beta}$$

and

$$\boldsymbol{\Sigma}_{\widehat{\boldsymbol{\beta}}} = (\mathbf{X}^\top\mathbf{X})^{-1}\mathbf{X}^\top\sigma^2\mathbb{I}_n\left((\mathbf{X}^\top\mathbf{X})^{-1}\mathbf{X}^\top\right)^\top = \sigma^2(\mathbf{X}^\top\mathbf{X})^{-1}\,.$$

Let $\boldsymbol{a}$ be any m-dimensional vector. A natural estimator for $\theta = \boldsymbol{a}^\top \boldsymbol{\beta}$ is $\widehat{\theta} = \boldsymbol{a}^\top \widehat{\boldsymbol{\beta}}$. The following theorem gives an exact confidence interval for θ.

Theorem 5.3. (Confidence Interval for the Normal Linear Model). A $1 - \alpha$ stochastic confidence interval for $\theta = \boldsymbol{a}^\top \boldsymbol{\beta}$ is

$$\widehat{\theta} \pm t_{n-m;1-\alpha/2}\, \frac{\|\boldsymbol{Y} - \mathbf{X}\widehat{\boldsymbol{\beta}}\|\, \sqrt{\boldsymbol{a}^\top (\mathbf{X}^\top \mathbf{X})^{-1} \boldsymbol{a}}}{\sqrt{n - m}}\,, \qquad (5.26)$$

where $t_{n-m;1-\alpha/2}$ is the $1 - \alpha/2$ quantile of the t_{n-m} distribution.

Proof. Being linear in the components of $\boldsymbol{\beta}$, the random variable $\widehat{\theta} = \boldsymbol{a}^\top \widehat{\boldsymbol{\beta}}$ has a normal distribution, with expectation $\boldsymbol{a}^\top \boldsymbol{\beta} = \theta$ and variance $\sigma^2 \boldsymbol{a}^\top (\mathbf{X}^\top \mathbf{X})^{-1} \boldsymbol{a}$. Let

$$\widehat{\sigma^2} = \frac{\|\boldsymbol{Y} - \boldsymbol{Y}_m\|^2}{n}\,,$$

with $\boldsymbol{Y}_m = \mathbf{X}\widehat{\boldsymbol{\beta}}$, be the least-squares estimator of σ^2. The random variable
☞ 88 　$\|\boldsymbol{Y} - \boldsymbol{Y}_m\|^2/\sigma^2$ has, by Theorem 3.10, a χ^2_{n-m} distribution and is independent of $\boldsymbol{Y}_m$. Since $\widehat{\boldsymbol{\beta}} = \mathbf{X}^+ \mathbf{X}\widehat{\boldsymbol{\beta}} = \mathbf{X}^+ \boldsymbol{Y}_m$, we have that $\|\boldsymbol{Y} - \boldsymbol{Y}_m\|^2$ is independent
☞ 89 　of $\widehat{\boldsymbol{\beta}}$. Using Corollary 3.2, we see that the pivot

$$T = \frac{(\widehat{\theta} - \theta)/\sqrt{\boldsymbol{a}^\top (\mathbf{X}^\top \mathbf{X})^{-1} \boldsymbol{a}}}{\sqrt{\|\boldsymbol{Y} - \mathbf{X}\widehat{\boldsymbol{\beta}}\|^2/(n - m)}}$$

has a t_{n-m} distribution. By rearranging the identity $\mathbb{P}(|T| \le t_{n-m;1-\alpha/2}) = 1 - \alpha$ in the usual way, we arrive at the confidence interval (5.26). $\qquad\square$

Example 5.12 (Confidence Limits in Simple Linear Regression).
☞ 131 　We continue Example 5.5 by including confidence intervals, $(l(x), u(x))$ say, of the parameter $\theta(x) = \beta_0 + \beta_1 x$, for various x. The points $u(x), x \in [0, 1]$ form an upper confidence curve for the regression line $y = \beta_0 + \beta_1 x$; and $l(x)$ gives the lower confidence curve. The following Julia code, to be appended to the code in Example 5.5, implements (5.26) and yields a plot of the true regression line and confidence curves similar to Fig. 5.2.

linregestconf.jl

```julia
tquant = quantile(TDist(N-2),0.975) # 0.975 quantile
ucl = zeros(N); lcl = zeros(N); # upper/lower conf. limits
rl = zeros(N)   # (true) regression line
u=0
```

```
for i in 1:N
   global u = u + 1/N
   a = [1;u]
   rl[i] = a'*beta;
   ucl[i] = dot(a,betahat) .+ tquant*norm(y - X*betahat)*sqrt(
       a'*inv(X'*X)*a)/sqrt(N-2)
   lcl[i] = dot(a,betahat) .- tquant*norm(y - X*betahat)*sqrt(
       a'*inv(X'*X)*a)/sqrt(N-2)
end
plot!(x,rl,legend=false); plot!(x,ucl,legend=false);
plot!(x,lcl,legend=false); scatter!(x,y,legend=false)
```

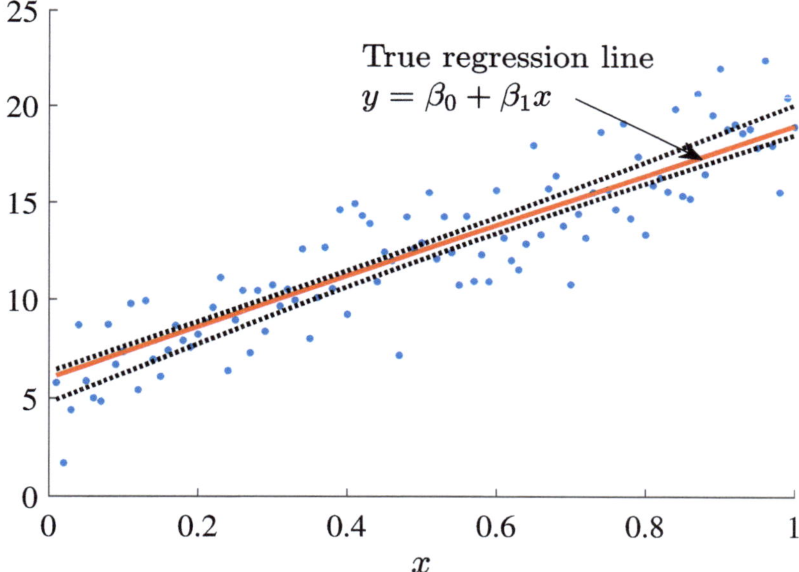

Fig. 5.2 The true regression line (solid) and the upper and lower 95% confidence curves (dashed)

5.3 Hypothesis Testing

Hypothesis testing involves making *decisions* about certain hypotheses on the basis of the observed data. In many cases we have to decide whether the observations are due to "chance" or due to an "effect." Hypothesis testing has traditionally played a prominent role in statistics, and many introductory books still are predominantly about hypothesis testing. Modern statistical analyses however, especially those based on computer intensive methods, do not so heavily rely on hypothesis testing any more, preferring, for example, inference via confidence intervals to inference based on hypothesis tests. In Bayesian statistics hypothesis testing is done in a different way, via *Bayes factors*. We will address the main ideas of frequentist hypothesis testing in this section.

☞ 257

Suppose the model for the data X is described by a family of probability distributions that depend on a parameter $\theta \in \Theta$. The aim of **hypothesis testing** is to decide, on the basis of the observed data x, which of two competing hypotheses, $H_0 : \theta \in \Theta_0$ (the **null hypothesis**) and $H_1 : \theta \in \Theta_1$ (the **alternative hypothesis**), holds true, where Θ_0 and Θ_1 are subsets of the parameter space Θ. Traditionally, the null hypothesis and alternative hypothesis do not play equivalent roles. H_0 contains the "status quo" statement and is only rejected if the observed data are very unlikely to have happened under H_0.

The decision whether to reject H_0 or not is dependent on the outcome of a **test statistic $T = T(X)$**. For simplicity, we discuss only the one-dimensional case $T \equiv T$.

The **p-value** is the probability that under H_0 the (random) test statistic takes a value as extreme as or more extreme than the one observed. Let t be the observed outcome of the test statistic T. We consider three types of tests:

- **Left one-sided test.** Here H_0 is rejected for small values of t, and the p-value is defined as $p = \mathbb{P}_{H_0}(T \leq t)$.
- **Right one-sided test:** Here H_0 is rejected for large values of t, and the p-value is defined as $p = \mathbb{P}_{H_0}(T \geq t)$,
- **Two-sided test:** In this test H_0 is rejected for small or large values of t, and the p-value is defined as $p = \min\{2\mathbb{P}_{H_0}(T \leq t),\ 2\mathbb{P}_{H_0}(T \geq t)\}$.

The smaller the p-value, the greater the strength of the evidence against H_0 provided by the data. As a rule of thumb:

$$p < 0.10 \text{ suggestive evidence,}$$
$$p < 0.05 \text{ reasonable evidence,}$$
$$p < 0.01 \text{ strong evidence.}$$

The following decision rule is generally used to decide between H_0 and H_1:

Decision rule : *Reject H_0 if the p-value is smaller than some* **significance level** α.

In general, a statistical test involves the following steps.

Steps for a Statistical Test

1. Formulate a statistical model for the data.
2. Give the null and alternative hypotheses (H_0 and H_1).
3. Choose an appropriate test statistic.
4. Determine the distribution of the test statistic under H_0.
5. Evaluate the outcome of the test statistic.
6. Calculate the p-value.
7. Accept or reject H_0 based on the p-value.

Choosing an appropriate test statistic is akin to selecting a good estimator for the unknown parameter $\boldsymbol{\theta}$. The test statistic should summarize the information about $\boldsymbol{\theta}$ and make it possible to distinguish between the alternative hypotheses. The *likelihood ratio test* provides a systematic approach to constructing powerful test statistics; see Sect. 6.4.

☞ 18

Example 5.13 (Blood Pressure). Suppose the systolic blood pressure for white males aged 35–44 is known to be normally distributed with expectation 127 and standard deviation 7. A paper in a public health journal considers a sample of 101 diabetic males and reports a sample mean of 130. Is this good evidence that diabetics have on average a higher blood pressure than the general population?

To assess this, we could ask the question how likely it would be, *if diabetics were similar to the general population*, that a sample of 101 diabetics would have a mean blood pressure this far from 127.

Let us perform the seven steps of a statistical test. A reasonable model for the data is $X_1, \ldots, X_{101} \sim_{\text{iid}} \mathcal{N}(\mu, 49)$. Alternatively, the model could simply be $\overline{X} \sim \mathcal{N}(\mu, 49/101)$, since we only have an outcome of the sample mean of the blood pressures. The null hypothesis (the status quo) is $H_0 : \mu = 127$; the alternative hypothesis is $H_1 : \mu > 127$. We take $\overline{X}$ as the test statistic. Note that we have a right one-sided test here, because we would reject H_0 for high values of $\overline{X}$. Under H_0 we have $\overline{X} \sim \mathcal{N}(127, 49/101)$. The outcome of $\overline{X}$ is 130, so that the p-value is given by

$$\mathbb{P}(\overline{X} \geq 130) = \mathbb{P}\left(\frac{\overline{X} - 127}{\sqrt{49/101}} > \frac{130 - 127}{\sqrt{49/101}} \right) = \mathbb{P}(Z > 4.31) = 8.16 \cdot 10^{-6},$$

where $Z \sim \mathcal{N}(0, 1)$. So it is extremely unlikely that the event $\{\overline{X} \geq 130\}$ occurs if the two groups are the same with regard to blood pressure. However, the event *has* occurred. Therefore, there is *strong* evidence that the blood pressure of diabetics differs from the general public.

Example 5.14 (Binomial Test). We suspect a certain die to be loaded. Throwing 100 times we observe 25 sixes. Is there enough evidence to justify our suspicion?

We ask ourselves the same type of question as in the previous example: Suppose that the die is fair. What is the probability that out of 100 tosses 25 or more sixes would appear? To calculate this, let X be the number of sixes out of 100. Our model is $X \sim \text{Bin}(100, p)$, with p unknown. We would like to show the hypothesis $H_1 : p > 1/6$; otherwise, we do not reject (accept) the null hypothesis $H_0 : p = 1/6$. Our test statistic is simply X. Under H_0, $X \sim \text{Bin}(100, 1/6)$, so that the p-value for this right one-sided test is

$$\mathbb{P}(X \geq 25) = \sum_{k=25}^{100} \binom{100}{k} (1/6)^k (5/6)^{100-k} \approx 0.0217 \,.$$

This is quite small. Hence, we have *reasonable* evidence that the die is loaded. Such statistical tests involving count data are often called **binomial tests**.

Example 5.15 (One-Sample t-Test). In a **one-sample t-test** the data are assumed to follow the standard model: $Z_1, \ldots, Z_n \sim_{\text{iid}} \mathcal{N}(\mu, \sigma^2)$. One typically wishes to test the null hypothesis $H_0 : \mu = 0$ against $H_1 : \mu \neq 0$ or some one-sided alternative. The test statistic in this case is

$$T = \frac{\overline{Z}\sqrt{n}}{S_Z} \,,$$

where $\overline{Z}$ and S_Z are the sample mean and sample standard deviation of the data. By Theorem 5.1 T has a t_{n-1} distribution under H_0.

☞ 135

As a specific example, consider the before and after weights (actually, masses) of 10 participants in a "miracle" weight loss program, given in Table 5.2.

Table 5.2 Weight loss data in kilograms

Before	280	140	90	128	135	98	111	97	89	156
After	240	135	89	135	120	95	99	103	87	140
Loss	40	5	1	−7	15	3	12	−6	2	16

Although the data involve *paired* observations in which the before and after weights are highly correlated, it is reasonable to assume that the weight *losses* (weight before − weight after), $Z_1, \ldots, Z_{10}$, follow the standard model above. The outcome of the test statistic is here $t = 27/\sqrt{209} \approx 1.87$. For the alternative hypothesis $H_1 : \mu > 0$ (the weight loss program works!), we obtain the p-value $\mathbb{P}(T \geq t) = 0.047$, giving modest evidence that the program is effective.

Example 5.16 (Two-Sample t-Test). We return to Example 5.9 and test whether breast-fed and formula-fed babies have the same hemoglobin levels. The null and alternative hypotheses are $H_0 : \mu_X = \mu_Y$ and $H_1 : \mu_X \neq \mu_Y$. For the test statistic we take

$$T = \frac{\overline{X} - \overline{Y}}{S_p\sqrt{\frac{1}{m} + \frac{1}{n}}} \, ,$$

which by Theorem 5.2 has a t_{44} distribution under H_0. As we have here a two-sample normal model, the resulting test is called a **two-sample t-test**.

The outcome of T is here

$$t = \frac{(\overline{X} - \overline{y})}{s_p\sqrt{\frac{1}{m} + \frac{1}{n}}} = \frac{13.3 - 12.4}{\sqrt{2.8873}\sqrt{\frac{1}{25} + \frac{1}{21}}} = 1.7894 \, .$$

The corresponding p-value for this two-sided test is 0.08, providing insufficient evidence that the expected hemoglobin levels are different and corroborating the findings in Example 5.9.

5.3.1 ANOVA for the Normal Linear Model

Hypothesis testing for the normal linear model in Sect. 4.23 is often related to *model selection*. In particular, suppose we have the following model for the data $\boldsymbol{Y} = [Y_1, \ldots, Y_n]^\top$:

$$\boldsymbol{Y} = \underbrace{\mathbf{X}_1\boldsymbol{\beta}_1 + \mathbf{X}_2\boldsymbol{\beta}_2}_{X\beta} + \boldsymbol{\varepsilon}, \quad \boldsymbol{\varepsilon} \sim \mathcal{N}(0, \sigma^2\, \mathbb{I}_n) \, , \tag{5.27}$$

where $\boldsymbol{\beta}_1$ and $\boldsymbol{\beta}_2$ are unknown vectors of dimension k and $m - k$, respectively; and $\mathbf{X}_1$ and $\mathbf{X}_2$ are full-rank design matrices of dimensions $n \times k$ and $n \times (m - k)$, respectively. Above we implicitly defined $\mathbf{X} = [\mathbf{X}_1, \mathbf{X}_2]$ and $\boldsymbol{\beta}^\top = [\boldsymbol{\beta}_1^\top, \boldsymbol{\beta}_2^\top]$.

Suppose we wish to test the hypothesis $H_0 : \boldsymbol{\beta}_2 = 0$ against $H_1 : \boldsymbol{\beta}_2 \neq 0$. We saw in Sect. 5.1.2 how to estimate the parameters via least squares. Let $\widehat{\boldsymbol{\beta}}$ be the estimate of $\boldsymbol{\beta}$ under the full model, and let $\widehat{\boldsymbol{\beta}}_1$ denote the estimate of $\boldsymbol{\beta}_1$ for the reduced model; that is, under H_0. To simplify notation, let $\boldsymbol{Y}_m = \mathbf{X}\widehat{\boldsymbol{\beta}}$ be the projection of $\boldsymbol{Y}$ onto the space $\langle \mathbf{X} \rangle$ spanned by the columns of $\mathbf{X}$; and let $\boldsymbol{Y}_k = \mathbf{X}_1\widehat{\boldsymbol{\beta}}_1$ be the projection of $\boldsymbol{Y}$ onto the space $\langle \mathbf{X}_1 \rangle$ spanned by the columns of $\mathbf{X}_1$ only.

A sensible strategy for deciding upon the reduced or full model is to compare $\|\boldsymbol{Y} - \boldsymbol{Y}_k\|$ with $\|\boldsymbol{Y} - \boldsymbol{Y}_m\|$ via the quotient of the two. The larger this quotient, the more evidence for the full model. It is more convenient to use instead the equivalent statistic

$$T = \frac{n - m}{m - k} \times \frac{\|\boldsymbol{Y} - \boldsymbol{Y}_k\|^2 - \|\boldsymbol{Y} - \boldsymbol{Y}_m\|^2}{\|\boldsymbol{Y} - \boldsymbol{Y}_m\|^2} = \frac{\|\boldsymbol{Y}_m - \boldsymbol{Y}_k\|^2/(m - k)}{\|\boldsymbol{Y} - \boldsymbol{Y}_m\|^2/(n - m)} \, , \tag{5.28}$$

☞ 118

☞ 129

where we have used Pythagoras' theorem in the second equation above, as illustrated in Fig. 5.3.

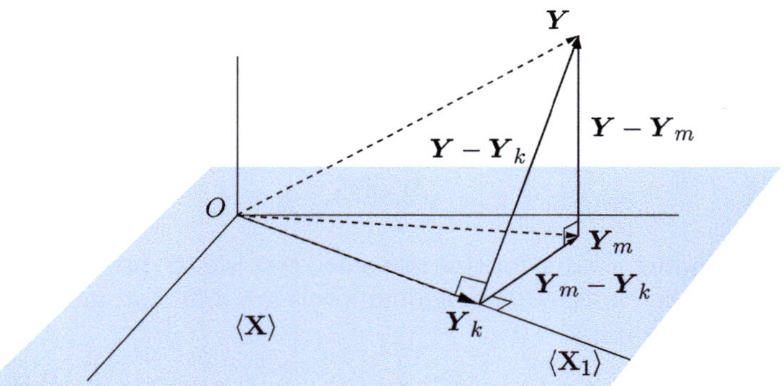

Fig. 5.3 Pythagoras' theorem

Define $X = Y/\sigma$ with expectation $\mu = X\beta/\sigma$, and $X_j = Y_j/\sigma$ with expectation μ_j, $j = k, m$. Note that $\mu = \mu_m$, and under H_0, $\mu_m = \mu_k$. We can directly apply Theorem 3.10 to find that $\|Y - Y_m\|^2/\sigma^2 = \|X - X_m\|^2 \sim \chi^2_{n-m}$, and, under H_0, $\|Y_m - Y_k\|^2/\sigma^2 \sim \chi^2_{m-k}$. Moreover, these random variables are independent of each other. It follows from Theorem 3.11 that, under H_0,

$$T \sim \mathsf{F}(m - k, n - m) \, .$$

We reject H_0 for large values of T. The above methodology is often referred to as **analysis of variance** (ANOVA).

Example 5.17 (Hypothesis Testing for Randomized Block Design). In a randomized block design the data are collected in blocks, in order to reduce variability in the experiment. Consider, for example, the data in Table 5.3, representing the crop yield using four different crop treatments (e.g., strengths of fertilizer) on four different blocks (plots).

Table 5.3 Crop yield

		Treatment		
Block	1	2	3	4
1	9.2988	9.4978	9.7604	10.1025
2	8.2111	8.3387	8.5018	8.1942
3	9.0688	9.1284	9.3484	9.5086
4	8.2552	7.8999	8.4859	8.9485

Let us consider the data first as coming from four different groups, depending only on the level of treatment. A possible model would be the single-factor ANOVA model

☞ 11

$$Y_{ik} = \mu + \alpha_i + \varepsilon_{ik}, \quad i, k = 1, \ldots, 4,$$

with $\{\varepsilon_{ik}\} \sim_{\text{iid}} \mathcal{N}(0, \sigma^2)$, and $\sum_{i=1}^{4} \alpha_i = 0$. Ordering the $\{Y_{ik}\}$ into a column vector $\boldsymbol{Y} = [Y_{11}, Y_{12}, \ldots Y_{14}, Y_{21}, \ldots, Y_{44}]^\top$, we can write $\boldsymbol{Y}$ in the form (5.27):

$$\boldsymbol{Y} = \underbrace{\begin{bmatrix} 1 \\ 1 \\ 1 \\ 1 \end{bmatrix}}_{\boldsymbol{X}_1} \mu + \underbrace{\begin{bmatrix} 1 & 0 & 0 \\ 0 & 1 & 0 \\ 0 & 0 & 1 \\ -1 & -1 & -1 \end{bmatrix}}_{\boldsymbol{X}_2} \underbrace{\begin{bmatrix} \alpha_1 \\ \alpha_2 \\ \alpha_3 \end{bmatrix}}_{\boldsymbol{\beta}_2} + \boldsymbol{\varepsilon},$$

where $\boldsymbol{1}$ and $\boldsymbol{0}$ are vectors of 1s and 0s, respectively. We wish to test whether the treatments make a difference to the crop yield or not. The null hypothesis $H_0 : \alpha_1 = \alpha_2 = \alpha_3 = 0$ is that the treatments have no effect. As a test statistic we use (5.28). For the present model we have $n = 16$, $m = 4$, and $k = 1$. The squared norm $\|\boldsymbol{Y} - \boldsymbol{Y}_m\|^2 = \|\boldsymbol{Y} - \boldsymbol{X}\widehat{\boldsymbol{\beta}}\|^2$ is often written as SS_{error}, that is, the sum of squares of the error terms. Note that $\|\boldsymbol{Y} - \boldsymbol{X}\widehat{\boldsymbol{\beta}}\|^2 / (n - m)$ is an unbiased estimator of the variance σ^2 of the model error.

Similarly, $\|\boldsymbol{Y}_m - \boldsymbol{Y}_k\|^2$ represents the sum of squares due to the treatment effect and is written as $\text{SS}_{\text{treatment}}$. Our test statistic T in (5.28) can thus be written as

$$T = \frac{\text{SS}_{\text{treatment}}/(m - k)}{\text{SS}_{\text{error}}/(n - m)} \overset{\text{def}}{=} \frac{\text{MS}_{\text{treatment}}}{\text{MS}_{\text{error}}},$$

where "MS" stands for "mean square." Under H_0 the test statistic T has an $\mathsf{F}(m - k, n - m) = \mathsf{F}(3, 12)$ distribution.

```
solvehypotcrop1.jl
```

```julia
using LinearAlgebra, Statistics, Distributions
yy = [9.2988 9.4978 9.7604 10.1025;
   8.2111 8.3387 8.5018 8.1942;
   9.0688 9.1284 9.3484 9.5086;
   8.2552 7.8999 8.4859 8.9485]
n = length(yy); (nrow,ncol) = size(yy); y = vec(yy)
X_1 = ones(n,1)
KM = kron(diagm(ones(ncol)),ones(nrow,1)); X_2 = KM[:,1:ncol
    -1]
X_2[n-nrow+1:n,:] = -ones(nrow,ncol-1)
X = [X_1 X_2]
m = size(X,2);
betahat = X'*X(X'*y)
```

```
ym = X*betahat
yk = X_1*mean(y); # omitting treatment effect
k = 1 # number of parameters in reduced model
T = (n-m)/(m-k)*(norm(ym - yk)^2)/norm(y-ym)^2
pval = 1 - cdf(FDist(m-k,n-m),T)
```

The outcome of T is found to be 0.4724, which gives a p-value of 0.7072. This suggests that the treatment does not have an effect on the crop yield. But what if the crop yield is not only determined by the treatment levels but also by the blocks? To investigate this, we could describe the data via a two-factor ANOVA model:

$$Y_{ik} = \mu + \alpha_i + \tau_k + \varepsilon_{ik}, \quad i, k = 1, \ldots, 4 \,,$$

with $\{\varepsilon_{ik}\} \sim_{\text{iid}} \mathcal{N}(0, \sigma^2)$ and $\sum_{i=1}^{4} \alpha_i = 0$ and $\sum_{i=1}^{4} \tau_i = 0$. Ordering the data in the same way as for the one-factor case, we can write

$$\boldsymbol{Y} = \mathbf{X}_1 \mu + \mathbf{X}_2 \boldsymbol{\beta}_2 + \underbrace{\begin{bmatrix} \mathbf{C} \\ \mathbf{C} \\ \mathbf{C} \\ \mathbf{C} \end{bmatrix}}_{\mathbf{X}_3} \underbrace{\begin{bmatrix} \tau_1 \\ \tau_2 \\ \tau_3 \end{bmatrix}}_{\boldsymbol{\beta}_3} + \boldsymbol{\varepsilon}, \quad \text{with} \quad \mathbf{C} = \begin{bmatrix} 1 & 0 & 0 \\ 0 & 1 & 0 \\ 0 & 0 & 1 \\ -1 & -1 & -1 \end{bmatrix},$$

and $\mathbf{X}_1$ and $\mathbf{X}_2$ are the same as in the one-factor case. We wish to test first if using such an extended model (as opposed to the previous one-factor model) is justified. In particular, we test if $\tau_1 = 0, \ldots, \tau_4 = 0$. We can use again a statistic of the form (5.28). Now the vector $\boldsymbol{Y}_m$ is the projection of $\boldsymbol{Y}$ onto the ($m = 7$)-dimensional space spanned by the columns of $\mathbf{X} = [\mathbf{X}_1, \mathbf{X}_2, \mathbf{X}_3]$; and $\boldsymbol{Y}_k$ is the projection of $\boldsymbol{Y}$ onto the ($k = 4$)-dimensional space spanned by the columns of $\mathbf{X}_{12} = [\mathbf{X}_1, \mathbf{X}_2]$. The test statistic (5.28), which we could write as

$$T_{12} = \frac{\text{MS}_{\text{blocks}}}{\text{MS}_{\text{error}}} \,,$$

has under H_0 an $\mathsf{F}(3, 9)$ distribution.

The Julia code below, which has to be appended to the first seven lines of code for the one-factor case, calculates the outcome of the test statistic T_{12} and the corresponding p-value. We find $t_{12} = 34.9998$, which gives a p-value 2.73×10^{-5}. This shows that the block effects are extremely important for explaining the data.

Using the extended model—thus with the block effects—we can again test whether the $\{\alpha_i\}$ are all 0 or not. This is done in the last six lines of the code below. The outcome of the test statistic is 4.4878, with a p-value of 0.0346. By including the block effects, we effectively reduce the uncertainty in the model and are able to more accurately assess the effects of the treatments, to conclude that the treatment *does* seem to have an effect on the crop yield. A closer look at the data shows that within each block (row) the crop yield roughly increases with the treatment level.

```julia
solvehypotcrop2.jl

C = vcat(diagm(ones(nrow-1)), -ones(1,nrow-1))
X_3 = repeat(C,ncol,1)
X = [X_1 X_2 X_3]
m = size(X,2); # number of parameters in full model
betahat = X'*X(X'*y) # estimate under the full model
ym = X*betahat
X_12 = [X_1 X_2] # omitting the block effect
k = size(X_12,2) # number of parameters in reduced model
betahat_12 = X_12'*X_12(X_12'*y)
y_12 = X_12*betahat_12;
T_12=(n-m)/(m-k)*(norm(y-y_12)^2 - norm(y-ym)^2)/norm(y-ym)^2
pval_12 = 1 - cdf(FDist(m-k,n-m),T_12)

X_13 = [X_1 X_3]; # omitting the treatment effect
k = size(X_13,2); # number of parameters in reduced model
betahat_13 = X_13'*X_13(X_13'*y)
y_13 = X_13*betahat_13
T_13=(n-m)/(m-k)*(norm(y-y_13)^2 - norm(y-ym)^2)/norm(y-ym)^2
pval_13 = 1 - cdf(FDist(m-k,n-m),T_13)
```

5.4 Cross-Validation

For experimental data it is often the case that several competing models seem equally appropriate. As a concrete example, suppose we observe n independent points in the x-y plane, as depicted in Fig. 5.4. We wish to find a suitable polynomial that fits the data well. To that end, we consider the 5-th order polynomial regression model; see (4.10):

☞ 108

$$Y_i = \beta_0 + \beta_1 x_i + \cdots + \beta_5 x_i^5 + \varepsilon_i \,,$$

where $\{\varepsilon_i\} \sim_{\text{iid}} \mathcal{N}(0, \sigma^2)$. The fitted line is also depicted in Fig. 5.4, which seems to fit the points reasonably well.

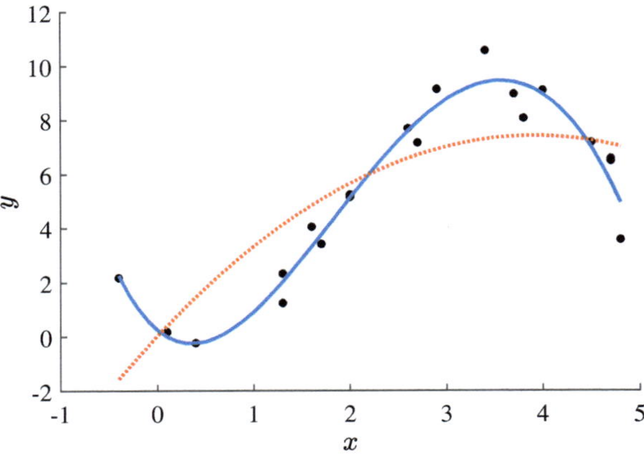

Fig. 5.4 Quadratic (dotted) and 5-th order (solid) polynomial regression lines

Since the 5-th order polynomial is adequate, we might not need to consider higher-order polynomials. However, it is plausible that a simpler model (e.g., a cubic polynomial) would fit the data almost as well, and is therefore more appropriate. One common approach is to test a sequence of hypotheses to determine the exact degree needed. That is, first we estimate the 5-th order polynomial regression model and test the null hypothesis that $\beta_5 = 0$. If the null hypothesis is rejected, we stop and use the 5-th order polynomial. Otherwise, we estimate the 4-th order polynomial regression model, and test the null hypothesis that $\beta_4 = 0$. This process is continued until a certain null hypothesis is rejected.

A more thoughtful approach is to select a model based on its predictive performance. After all, one main goal of statistical inference is to predict future observations. One way to assess the predictive ability of a model is to use it to predict a set of observations not used in the estimation. This can be done, for example, by partitioning the data into a "training set" and a "test set." Then, use the "training set" to estimate the model, and its predictive accuracy is assessed by some error measure on the "test set." This is an example of a **cross-validation**.

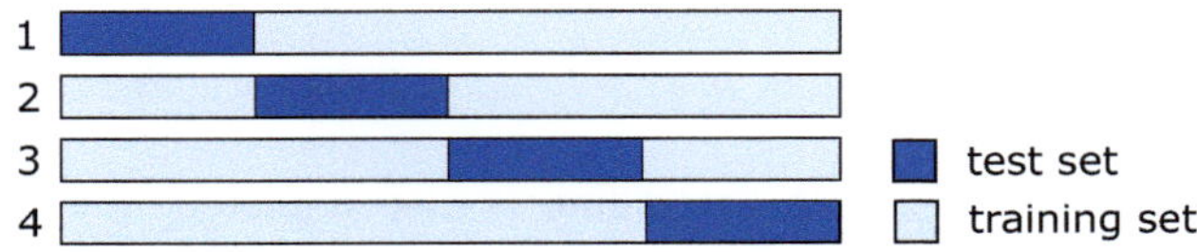

Fig. 5.5 A graphical representation of a fourfold cross-validation

More generally, a **K-fold cross-validation** is implemented as follows:

1. Partition the data into K subsamples of equal (or nearly equal) size. Number the subsamples from 1 to K.
2. For $k = 1, \ldots, K$, use all but the k-th subsample to estimate the model parameters. Compute the prediction errors for the omitted observations in the k-th subsample.
3. Summarize the predictive performance by some error measure, such as the sum of squared errors.

A graphical representation of a fourfold cross-validation is depicted in Fig. 5.5. For a sample with n observations, we can implement at most an n-fold cross-validation. In fact, this is a popular choice, and it is often called the **leave-one-out cross-validation**.

More specifically, suppose there are n independent observations $y_1, \ldots, y_n$. Let $\widehat{y}_{-k}$ denote the prediction for the k-th observation using all the data except y_k. The prediction error $y_k - \widehat{y}_{-k}$ is called a *predicted residual*—in contrast to an ordinary residual, $u_k = y_k - \widehat{y}_k$, which is the difference between an observation and its fitted value obtained using the whole sample. At the end of n iterations, we obtain the collection of predicted residuals $\{y_k - \widehat{y}_{-k}\}$. One way to summarize them is through the **predicted residual sum of squares** or **PRESS**:

$$\text{PRESS} = \sum_{k=1}^{n} (y_k - \widehat{y}_{-k})^2 \ .$$

In general, computing the PRESS is computationally intensive as it involves n separate estimations and predictions. For linear models, however, the predicted residuals can be calculated quickly using only the ordinary residuals and the projection matrix.

☞ 11

Theorem 5.4. (PRESS for Linear Models). Consider the normal linear model (4.23)

$$\boldsymbol{Y} = \mathbf{X}\boldsymbol{\beta} + \boldsymbol{\varepsilon} \ , \quad \boldsymbol{\varepsilon} \sim \mathcal{N}(\mathbf{0}, \sigma^2 \, \mathbb{I}_n) \ ,$$

where the $n \times m$ design matrix $\mathbf{X} = [x_{ij}]$ is known and is of full rank. Given an outcome $\boldsymbol{y} = [y_1, \ldots, y_n]^\top$ of $\boldsymbol{Y}$, the fitted values can be obtained as $\widehat{\boldsymbol{y}} = \mathbf{P}\boldsymbol{y}$, where $\mathbf{P} = \mathbf{X}(\mathbf{X}^\top \mathbf{X})^{-1}\mathbf{X}^\top$ is the projection matrix. Then, the predicted residual sum of squares can be written as

$$\text{PRESS} = \sum_{k=1}^{n} \left(\frac{u_k}{1 - p_k} \right)^2 ,$$

where $u_k = y_k - \widehat{y}_k = y_k - (\mathbf{X}\widehat{\boldsymbol{\beta}})_k$ is the k-th residual and p_k is the k-th diagonal element of the projection matrix $\mathbf{P}$.

Proof (Sketch). It suffices to show that the k-th predicted residual can be written as $y_k - \widehat{y}_{-k} = u_k/(1-p_k)$. Let $\mathbf{X}_{-k}$ denote the design matrix $\mathbf{X}$ with the k-th row removed, and define $\boldsymbol{y}_{-k}$ similarly. Then, the least-squares estimate for $\boldsymbol{\beta}$ using all but the k-th observation is $\widehat{\boldsymbol{\beta}}_{-k} = (\mathbf{X}_{-k}^\top \mathbf{X}_{-k})^{-1}\mathbf{X}_{-k}^\top \boldsymbol{y}_{-k}$.

☞ 162 It can be shown (see Problem 5.18) that $\widehat{\boldsymbol{\beta}}_{-k}$ is related to the full-sample least-squares estimate $\widehat{\boldsymbol{\beta}}$ via

$$\widehat{\boldsymbol{\beta}}_{-k} = \widehat{\boldsymbol{\beta}} - \frac{(\mathbf{X}^\top \mathbf{X})^{-1}\boldsymbol{x}_k u_k}{1 - p_k} \;, \tag{5.29}$$

where $\boldsymbol{x}_k^\top$ is the k-th row of the design matrix $\mathbf{X}$. It follows that the predicted value for the k-th observation is given by

$$\widehat{y}_{-k} = \boldsymbol{x}_k^\top \widehat{\boldsymbol{\beta}}_{-k} = \boldsymbol{x}_k^\top \widehat{\boldsymbol{\beta}} - \frac{\boldsymbol{x}_k^\top (\mathbf{X}^\top \mathbf{X})^{-1}\boldsymbol{x}_k u_k}{1 - p_k} = \widehat{y}_k - \frac{p_k u_k}{1 - p_k} \;,$$

where we used the fact that $p_k = \boldsymbol{x}_k^\top (\mathbf{X}^\top \mathbf{X})^{-1}\boldsymbol{x}_k$. The desired result now follows from direct calculation. $\qquad\square$

Example 5.18 (Leave-One-Out Cross-Validation for Polynomial Regressions). In this example we revisit the polynomial regression example in the beginning of this section. Specifically, given the $n = 20$ points in the x-y plane listed in Table 5.4 (see also Fig. 5.4), we wish to find the simplest polynomial that fits the points well.

Table 5.4 Polynomial regression data

x	y	x	y	x	y	x	y
4.7	6.57	3.7	8.95	4.8	3.56	0.4	−0.23
2.0	5.15	2.0	5.24	1.7	3.40	2.6	7.68
2.7	7.15	3.4	10.54	−0.4	2.18	4.0	9.09
0.1	0.18	1.3	1.24	4.5	7.16	2.9	9.13
4.7	6.48	3.8	8.05	1.3	2.32	1.6	4.04

For this purpose, we consider five different polynomial regression models:

$$Y_i = \beta_0 + \beta_1 x_i + \cdots + \beta_k x_i^k + \varepsilon_i$$

for $k = 1, \ldots, 5$, where $\{\varepsilon_i\} \sim_{\mathrm{iid}} \mathcal{N}(0, \sigma^2)$. Since they can all be written as normal linear models, we can use Theorem 5.4 to compute their predicted residual sums of squares. For each of these models, we compute the least-squares estimate and the corresponding PRESS using the Julia script below.

```
polyreg.jl
```

```julia
using LinearAlgebra
x = [4.7 2 2.7 0.1 4.7 3.7 2 3.4 1.3 3.8 4.8 1.7 -0.4 4.5 1.3
    0.4 2.6 4 2.9 1.6]'
y = [6.57 5.15 7.15 0.18 6.48 8.95 5.24 10.54 1.24 8.05 3.56
    3.4 2.18 7.16 2.32 -0.23 7.68 9.09 9.13 4.04]'
n = length(x);
press = zeros(5)
X = ones(n,1)
for k=1:5
    global X = [X x.^k]
    # construct the design matrix
    P = X*((X'*X)\X')
    e = y - P*y
    press[k] = sum((e./(1 .-diag(P))).^2)
    println(press[k])
end
```

The PRESS values for the linear, quadratic, cubic, 4-th, and 5-th order
polynomial regression models are, respectively, 117.388, 130.781, 16.0532,
16.3167, and 25.727. Hence, the cubic polynomial regression has the lowest
PRESS, indicating that it has the best predictive performance. It illustrates
that complex models do not necessarily have better predictive accuracy than
simpler models.

5.5 Sufficiency and Exponential Families

A statistic—that is, a function of the data only—is said to be **sufficient** for
a parameter (vector) $\boldsymbol{\theta}$ if it captures all the information about $\boldsymbol{\theta}$ contained in
the data. Sufficient statistics can be used to *summarize* data, often giving a
tremendous reduction in size. To formalize this concept, suppose that $\boldsymbol{T}(\boldsymbol{X})$
is a (possibly multidimensional) statistic for $\boldsymbol{\theta}$ such that any inference about
$\boldsymbol{\theta}$ depends on the data $\boldsymbol{X} = [X_1, \ldots, X_n]^\top$ only through the value $\boldsymbol{T}(\boldsymbol{X})$.
That is, if $\boldsymbol{x}$ and $\boldsymbol{y}$ are outcomes such that $\boldsymbol{T}(\boldsymbol{x}) = \boldsymbol{T}(\boldsymbol{y})$, then the inference
about $\boldsymbol{\theta}$ should be the same whether $\boldsymbol{X} = \boldsymbol{x}$ or $\boldsymbol{X} = \boldsymbol{y}$ is observed. This
observation leads to the following definition.

Definition 5.2. (Sufficient Statistic). A statistic $\boldsymbol{T}(\boldsymbol{X})$ is a **sufficient statistic** for $\boldsymbol{\theta}$ if the conditional distribution of $\boldsymbol{X}$ given $\boldsymbol{T}(\boldsymbol{X})$
does not depend on $\boldsymbol{\theta}$.

The workhorse for establishing sufficiency is the following theorem.

Theorem 5.5. (Factorization Theorem). Let $f(\boldsymbol{x}; \boldsymbol{\theta})$ denote the pdf of the data $\boldsymbol{X} = [X_1, \ldots, X_n]^\top$. A statistic $\boldsymbol{T}(\boldsymbol{X})$ is sufficient for $\boldsymbol{\theta}$ if and only if there exist functions $g(\boldsymbol{t}, \boldsymbol{\theta})$ and $h(\boldsymbol{x})$ such that, for all $\boldsymbol{x}$ and $\boldsymbol{\theta}$,

$$f(\boldsymbol{x}; \boldsymbol{\theta}) = g(\boldsymbol{T}(\boldsymbol{x}), \boldsymbol{\theta})\, h(\boldsymbol{x}) . \tag{5.30}$$

Proof. We give the proof only for the case where $\boldsymbol{X}$ is a discrete random vector. For this case we can write $f(\boldsymbol{x}; \boldsymbol{\theta})$ as

$$
\begin{aligned}
f(\boldsymbol{x}; \boldsymbol{\theta}) &= \mathbb{P}_{\boldsymbol{\theta}}(\boldsymbol{X} = \boldsymbol{x}) \\
&= \mathbb{P}_{\boldsymbol{\theta}}(\boldsymbol{X} = \boldsymbol{x}, \boldsymbol{T}(\boldsymbol{X}) = \boldsymbol{T}(\boldsymbol{x})) \\
&= \mathbb{P}_{\boldsymbol{\theta}}(\boldsymbol{T}(\boldsymbol{X}) = \boldsymbol{T}(\boldsymbol{x}))\, \mathbb{P}_{\boldsymbol{\theta}}(\boldsymbol{X} = \boldsymbol{x} \,|\, \boldsymbol{T}(\boldsymbol{X}) = \boldsymbol{T}(\boldsymbol{x})) .
\end{aligned}
$$

If $\boldsymbol{T}(\boldsymbol{X})$ is a sufficient statistic, then $\mathbb{P}_{\boldsymbol{\theta}}(\boldsymbol{X} = \boldsymbol{x} \,|\, \boldsymbol{T}(\boldsymbol{X}) = \boldsymbol{T}(\boldsymbol{x}))$ does not depend on $\boldsymbol{\theta}$. Consequently, (5.30) holds with $g(\boldsymbol{t}, \boldsymbol{\theta}) = \mathbb{P}_{\boldsymbol{\theta}}(\boldsymbol{T}(\boldsymbol{X}) = \boldsymbol{t})$ and $h(\boldsymbol{x}) = \mathbb{P}_{\boldsymbol{\theta}}(\boldsymbol{X} = \boldsymbol{x} \,|\, \boldsymbol{T}(\boldsymbol{X}) = \boldsymbol{T}(\boldsymbol{x}))$.

Conversely, suppose that (5.30) holds. We need to show that the conditional probability

$$\mathbb{P}_{\boldsymbol{\theta}}(\boldsymbol{X} = \boldsymbol{x} \,|\, \boldsymbol{T}(\boldsymbol{X}) = \boldsymbol{t}) = \frac{\mathbb{P}_{\boldsymbol{\theta}}(\boldsymbol{X} = \boldsymbol{x}, \boldsymbol{T}(\boldsymbol{X}) = \boldsymbol{t})}{\mathbb{P}_{\boldsymbol{\theta}}(\boldsymbol{T}(\boldsymbol{X}) = \boldsymbol{t})}$$

does not depend on $\boldsymbol{\theta}$. If $\boldsymbol{x}$ is a data point such that $\boldsymbol{T}(\boldsymbol{x}) \neq \boldsymbol{t}$, then clearly $\mathbb{P}_{\boldsymbol{\theta}}(\boldsymbol{X} = \boldsymbol{x} \,|\, \boldsymbol{T}(\boldsymbol{X}) = \boldsymbol{t}) = 0$. If $\boldsymbol{T}(\boldsymbol{x}) = \boldsymbol{t}$, then

$$
\begin{aligned}
\mathbb{P}_{\boldsymbol{\theta}}(\boldsymbol{X} = \boldsymbol{x} \,|\, \boldsymbol{T}(\boldsymbol{X}) = \boldsymbol{t}) &= \frac{\mathbb{P}_{\boldsymbol{\theta}}(\boldsymbol{X} = \boldsymbol{x})}{\mathbb{P}_{\boldsymbol{\theta}}(\boldsymbol{T}(\boldsymbol{X}) = \boldsymbol{t})} = \frac{f(\boldsymbol{x}; \boldsymbol{\theta})}{\sum_{\boldsymbol{y}:\boldsymbol{T}(\boldsymbol{y})=\boldsymbol{t}} f(\boldsymbol{y}; \boldsymbol{\theta})} \\[2mm]
&= \frac{g(\boldsymbol{T}(\boldsymbol{x}), \boldsymbol{\theta})\, h(\boldsymbol{x})}{\sum_{\boldsymbol{y}:\boldsymbol{T}(\boldsymbol{y})=\boldsymbol{t}} g(\boldsymbol{T}(\boldsymbol{y}), \boldsymbol{\theta})\, h(\boldsymbol{y})} = \frac{g(\boldsymbol{t}, \boldsymbol{\theta})\, h(\boldsymbol{x})}{g(\boldsymbol{t}, \boldsymbol{\theta}) \sum_{\boldsymbol{y}:\boldsymbol{T}(\boldsymbol{y})=\boldsymbol{t}} h(\boldsymbol{y})} \\[2mm]
&= \frac{h(\boldsymbol{x})}{\sum_{\boldsymbol{y}:\boldsymbol{T}(\boldsymbol{y})=\boldsymbol{t}} h(\boldsymbol{y})} ,
\end{aligned}
$$

which does not depend on $\boldsymbol{\theta}$. Hence $\boldsymbol{T}(\boldsymbol{X})$ is a sufficient statistic. $\square$

Example 5.19 (Sufficient Statistic for Iid Uniform Data). Let $\boldsymbol{X} = [X_1, \ldots, X_n]^\top$ be an iid sample from $\mathcal{U}(0, \theta)$. The pdf of $\boldsymbol{X}$ is given by

$$
f(\boldsymbol{x}; \theta) = \begin{cases} \left(\frac{1}{\theta}\right)^n & \text{for } \max\{x_1, \ldots, x_n\} \leq \theta \ \text{ and } x_i \geq 0, \ i = 1, \ldots, n \\ 0 & \text{otherwise} . \end{cases}
$$

It follows that $T(\boldsymbol{X}) = \max(X_1, \ldots, X_n)$ is a sufficient statistic for θ.

Example 5.20 (Sufficient Statistic for Iid Normal Data). Let $\boldsymbol{X} = [X_1, \ldots, X_n]^\top$ be an iid sample from $\mathcal{N}(\mu, 1)$. We show that the sample mean $T(\boldsymbol{X}) = \overline{X}$ is a sufficient statistic for μ. Namely, the pdf is

$$
f(\boldsymbol{x}; \mu) = \left(\frac{1}{\sqrt{2\pi}}\right)^n \exp\left(-\frac{1}{2}\sum_{i=1}^n (x_i - \mu)^2\right)
$$
$$
= h(\boldsymbol{x}) \underbrace{\exp\left(\mu\, n\, \overline{X} - n\,\mu^2/2\right)}_{g(T(\boldsymbol{x}),\mu)},
$$

for some function h, so that the required factorization holds.

The following general class of distributions plays an important role in statistics.

Definition 5.3. (Exponential Family). Let $\boldsymbol{X} = [X_1, \ldots, X_n]^\top$ be a random vector with pdf $f(\boldsymbol{x}; \boldsymbol{\theta})$, where $\boldsymbol{\theta} = [\theta_1, \ldots, \theta_d]^\top$ is a parameter vector. $\boldsymbol{X}$ is said to belong to an m-dimensional **exponential family** if there exist real-valued functions $t_i(\boldsymbol{x})$, $\eta_i(\boldsymbol{\theta})$, $i = 1, \ldots, m \leq n$ and $h(\boldsymbol{x}) > 0$, and a (normalizing) function $c(\boldsymbol{\theta}) > 0$, such that

$$
f(\boldsymbol{x}; \boldsymbol{\theta}) = c(\boldsymbol{\theta})\, \exp\left(\sum_{i=1}^m \eta_i(\boldsymbol{\theta}) t_i(\boldsymbol{x})\right) h(\boldsymbol{x})\,. \tag{5.31}
$$

The representation of an exponential family is in general not unique. It is often convenient to reparameterize exponential families via the $\{\eta_i\}$, that is, to take $\boldsymbol{\eta} = [\eta_1(\boldsymbol{\theta}), \ldots, \eta_m(\boldsymbol{\theta})]^\top$ as the parameter vector rather than $\boldsymbol{\theta}$. The reparameterized pdf is then

$$
\widetilde{f}(\boldsymbol{x}; \boldsymbol{\eta}) = \widetilde{c}(\boldsymbol{\eta})\, \mathrm{e}^{\boldsymbol{\eta}^\top \boldsymbol{t}(\boldsymbol{x})}\, h(\boldsymbol{x})\,, \tag{5.32}
$$

where $\widetilde{c}(\boldsymbol{\eta})$ is the normalization constant and $\boldsymbol{t}(\boldsymbol{x}) = [t_1(\boldsymbol{x}), \ldots, t_m(\boldsymbol{x})]$. Such an exponential family is said to be in **canonical form** or is said to be a **natural exponential family**.

Example 5.21 (Normal Distribution as a Two-Dimensional Exponential Family). The normal distributions $\mathcal{N}(\mu, \sigma^2)$, $\mu \in \mathbb{R}$, $\sigma^2 > 0$ form a two-dimensional exponential family with parameter $\boldsymbol{\theta} = (\mu, \sigma^2)$. To see this, write the logarithm of the pdf of the $\mathcal{N}(\mu, \sigma^2)$ distribution as

$$\ln f(x; \boldsymbol{\theta}) = \ln(1/\sqrt{2\pi\sigma^2}) - \frac{1}{2}\frac{(x-\mu)^2}{\sigma^2}$$

$$= \ln(1/\sqrt{2\pi\sigma^2}) - \frac{\mu^2}{2\sigma^2} + x\frac{\mu}{\sigma^2} - x^2\frac{1}{2\sigma^2}\,,$$

which shows that we can take $t_1(x) = x$, $t_2(x) = x^2$, $\eta_1(\boldsymbol{\theta}) = \mu/\sigma^2$, and $\eta_2(\boldsymbol{\theta}) = -1/(2\sigma^2)$, with $h(x) = 1$ and $c(\boldsymbol{\theta}) = \exp(-\mu^2/(2\sigma^2))/\sqrt{2\pi\sigma^2}$.

Many other families of distributions are of this type, such as the binomial, gamma, beta, geometric, and Poisson distributions, as summarized in Table 5.5.

Table 5.5 Various univariate exponential families

Distr.	$\boldsymbol{\theta}$	$t_1(x),\ t_2(x)$	$c(\boldsymbol{\theta})$	$\eta_1(\boldsymbol{\theta}),\ \eta_2(\boldsymbol{\theta})$	$h(x)$
$\mathsf{Beta}(\alpha,\beta)$	(α,β)	$\ln x,\ \ln(1-x)$	$1/B(\alpha,\beta)$	$\alpha-1,\ \ \beta-1$	1
$\mathsf{Bin}(n,p)$	p	$x,\ \ -$	$(1-p)^n$	$\ln\left(\frac{p}{1-p}\right),\ \ -$	$\binom{n}{x}$
$\mathsf{Gamma}(\alpha,\lambda)$	(α,λ)	$x,\ \ \ln x$	$\dfrac{\lambda^\alpha}{\Gamma(\alpha)}$	$-\lambda,\ \ \alpha-1$	1
$\mathsf{Geom}(p)$	p	$x-1,\ \ -$	p	$\ln(1-p),\ \ -$	1
$\mathcal{N}(\mu,\sigma^2)$	(μ,σ^2)	$x,\ \ x^2$	$\dfrac{e^{-\mu^2/(2\sigma^2)}}{\sqrt{2\pi\sigma^2}}$	$\dfrac{\mu}{\sigma^2},\ \ -\dfrac{1}{2\sigma^2}$	1
$\mathsf{Poi}(\lambda)$	λ	$x,\ \ -$	$e^{-\lambda}$	$\ln\lambda,\ \ -$	$\dfrac{1}{x!}$

Sufficiency (and therefore data summarization) is particularly easy to establish for exponential families of distributions. In particular, suppose that $\boldsymbol{X} = [X_1,\ldots,X_n]^\top$ is an iid sample from the exponential family with pdf

$$\mathring{f}(x; \boldsymbol{\theta}) = c(\boldsymbol{\theta})\, e^{\sum_{i=1}^m \eta_i(\boldsymbol{\theta})\, t_i(x)}\, \mathring{h}(x)\,.$$

For simplicity suppose that x is one-dimensional. By taking the product of the marginal pdfs we obtain the pdf of $\boldsymbol{X}$:

$$f(\boldsymbol{x}; \boldsymbol{\theta}) = \underbrace{c(\boldsymbol{\theta})^n\, e^{\sum_{i=1}^m \eta_i(\boldsymbol{\theta}) \sum_{k=1}^n t_i(x_k)}}_{g(\boldsymbol{T}(\boldsymbol{x}),\boldsymbol{\theta})} \underbrace{\prod_{k=1}^n \mathring{h}(x_k)}_{h(\boldsymbol{x})}\,.$$

A direct consequence of the factorization theorem is that

$$\boldsymbol{T}(\boldsymbol{X}) = \left[\sum_{k=1}^n t_1(X_k),\ldots,\sum_{k=1}^n t_m(X_k)\right]^\top \tag{5.33}$$

is a sufficient statistic for $\boldsymbol{\theta}$.

Example 5.22 (Sufficient Statistics for Iid Normal Data). As a particular instance of the previous setting, consider the case $X_1, \ldots, X_n \sim_{\mathrm{iid}} \mathcal{N}(\mu, \sigma^2)$. It follows from (5.33) and Example 5.21 that $\boldsymbol{T}(\boldsymbol{X}) = [T_1(\boldsymbol{X}), T_2(\boldsymbol{X})]^\top$, with $T_1(\boldsymbol{X}) = \sum_{k=1}^n X_k$ and $T_2(\boldsymbol{X}) = \sum_{k=1}^n X_k^2$, is a sufficient statistic for $\boldsymbol{\theta} = (\mu, \sigma^2)$. This means that for this standard data model, the data can be summarized via only T_1 and T_2.

It is not difficult to see that any one-to-one function of a sufficient statistic yields again a sufficient statistic. To see this, suppose that $\boldsymbol{T}(\boldsymbol{X})$ is a sufficient statistic and $\widetilde{\boldsymbol{T}}(\boldsymbol{X}) = \boldsymbol{r}(\boldsymbol{T}(\boldsymbol{X}))$ is another statistic, with $\boldsymbol{r}$ being invertible with inverse $\boldsymbol{r}^{-1}$. By the factorization theorem

$$f(\boldsymbol{x}; \boldsymbol{\theta}) = g(\boldsymbol{T}(\boldsymbol{x}), \boldsymbol{\theta})\, h(\boldsymbol{x}) = g(\boldsymbol{r}^{-1}(\widetilde{\boldsymbol{T}}(\boldsymbol{x})), \boldsymbol{\theta})\, h(\boldsymbol{x}) = \widetilde{g}(\widetilde{\boldsymbol{T}}(\boldsymbol{x}), \boldsymbol{\theta})\, h(\boldsymbol{x})$$

for some function $\widetilde{g}$. Thus, the factorization theorem also holds for $\widetilde{\boldsymbol{T}}$, and therefore the latter is also a sufficient statistic for $\boldsymbol{\theta}$.

Example 5.23 (Sufficient Statistics for Iid Normal Data Continued). We have seen that $T_1(\boldsymbol{X}) = \sum_{k=1}^n X_k$ and $T_2(\boldsymbol{X}) = \sum_{k=1}^n X_k^2$ are sufficient statistics for $\boldsymbol{\theta} = (\mu, \sigma^2)$ in the standard model for data. The sample mean $\widetilde{T}_1 = \overline{X}$ and the sample variance

$$\widetilde{T}_2 = \frac{1}{n-1} \sum_{k=1}^n (X_k - \overline{X})^2 = \frac{1}{n-1} \left(\sum_{k=1}^n X_k^2 - n\overline{X}^2 \right).$$

also form a pair of sufficient statistics, because the mapping

$$\widetilde{T}_1 = \frac{T_1}{n}, \qquad \widetilde{T}_2 = \frac{1}{n-1}\left(T_2 - T_1^2/n\right)$$

is invertible.

5.6 Problems

5.1. Find the method of moments estimators for the parameters of the $\mathsf{Geom}(p)$, $\mathsf{Poi}(\lambda)$, and $\mathsf{Gamma}(\alpha, \lambda)$ distributions.

5.2. The **mean square error** (MSE) of a real-valued estimator T is defined as $\mathrm{MSE} = \mathbb{E}_\theta (T - \theta)^2$. It can be used to assess the quality of an estimator: the smaller the MSE, the more efficient the estimator. Show that the MSE can be written as the sum

$$\mathrm{MSE} = \left(\mathbb{E}_\theta T - \theta\right)^2 + \mathrm{Var}_\theta(T).$$

In particular, for an *unbiased* estimator the MSE is simply equal to its variance.

5.3. The normal equations (5.10) can be derived more directly by solving $\nabla_{\beta}\|\boldsymbol{y} - \mathbf{X}\boldsymbol{\beta}\|^2 = \mathbf{0}$, where ∇_{β} indicates the gradient with respect to β. ☞ 475 Show, using Sect. B.1, that

$$\nabla_{\beta}\|\boldsymbol{y} - \mathbf{X}\boldsymbol{\beta}\|^2 = 2\mathbf{X}^{\top}(\boldsymbol{y} - \mathbf{X}\boldsymbol{\beta}) .$$

5.4. We wish to estimate the area $a = \mu_1\mu_2$ of a rectangular plot of land, with length μ_1 and width μ_2. We thus measure the length and the width twice. There are two natural ways to estimate the unknown constant a. We can either multiply the average width and length, or we can take the average of the two estimated areas. Suppose the measurements are outcomes of independent random variables $X_1, X_2 \sim \mathcal{N}(\mu_1, \sigma^2)$ and $Y_1, Y_2 \sim \mathcal{N}(\mu_2, \sigma^2)$. Here σ describes the accuracy of our measuring instrument. Let

$$T_1 = \frac{X_1 + X_2}{2} \times \frac{Y_1 + Y_2}{2} \quad \text{and} \quad T_2 = \frac{X_1 \times Y_1 + X_2 \times Y_2}{2} .$$

a. Show that T_1 and T_2 are *unbiased* estimators of a.
b. Show that $\mathrm{Var}(X_1 Y_1) = \sigma^2(\sigma^2 + \mu_1^2 + \mu_2^2)$.
c. Derive the variance of T_1 and the variance of T_2 and infer from this which estimator is preferred.

5.5. Let $X_1, \ldots, X_n \sim_{\mathrm{iid}} \mathsf{Exp}(\lambda)$ for some unknown $\lambda > 0$.

a. Show that the method of moments estimator of λ is $1/\overline{X}$.
b. Construct an approximate $1 - \alpha$ stochastic confidence interval for λ, by applying the central limit theorem to $\overline{X}$.

5.6. Let $X_1, \ldots, X_n \sim_{\mathrm{iid}} \mathcal{N}(1, \sigma^2)$, for some unknown $\sigma^2 > 0$.

a. Show that $T = \sum_{i=1}^{n}(X_i - 1)^2/\sigma^2 \sim \chi_n^2$.
b. Construct a $1 - \alpha$ stochastic confidence interval for σ^2 using the pivot T.

5.7. A *buret* is a glass tube with scales that can be used to add a specified volume of a fluid to a receiving vessel. Determine a 95% confidence interval for the expected volume of *one* drop of water that leaves the buret, if the initial volume in the buret is 25.35 (ml), the volume after 50 drops is 22.84, and the volume after 100 drops is 20.36.

5.8. On the label of a certain packet of aspirin it is written that the standard deviation of the amount of aspirin per tablet is 1.0 mg, but we suspect this is not true. To investigate this we take a sample of 25 tablets and find that the sample standard deviation of the amount of aspirin is 1.3 mg. Determine a 95% numerical confidence interval for σ. Is our suspicion justified?

5.9. Show that S_p in (5.21) is an unbiased estimator of σ^2.

5.10. Show that for the simple linear regression model in Example 5.5 we have $\widehat{\beta}_0 = \overline{Y} - \widehat{\beta}_1 \overline{X}$ and $\widehat{\beta}_1 = S_{xY}/S_{xx}$, where $\quad$ ☞ 13

$$S_{xx} = \sum_{i=1}^{n}(x_i - \overline{X})^2 \quad \text{and} \quad S_{xY} = \sum_{i=1}^{n}(x_i - \overline{X})(Y_i - \overline{Y}) .$$

5.11. Consider the model selection for the normal linear model in Sect. 5.3.1. $\quad$ ☞ 14
We wish to assess how the extended model $\boldsymbol{Y} = \mathbf{X}\boldsymbol{\beta} + \boldsymbol{\varepsilon}$, where $\boldsymbol{\varepsilon} \sim \mathcal{N}(\mathbf{0}, \sigma^2\,\mathbb{I}_n)$, fits the data, compared to the default model $\boldsymbol{Y} = \mu\mathbf{1} + \boldsymbol{\varepsilon}$ (i.e., the $\{Y_i\}$ are independent and $\mathcal{N}(\mu, \sigma^2)$ distributed). To do this we can compare the variance of the original data, estimated via $\sum_i(Y_i - \overline{Y})^2/n = \|\boldsymbol{Y} - \overline{Y}\mathbf{1}\|^2/n$, with the variance of the fitted data, estimated via $\sum_i(\widehat{Y}_i - \overline{Y})^2/n = \|\widehat{\boldsymbol{Y}} - \overline{Y}\mathbf{1}\|^2/n$, where $\widehat{\boldsymbol{Y}} = \mathbf{X}\widehat{\boldsymbol{\beta}}$. Note that, in the notation of Fig. 5.3, $\widehat{\boldsymbol{Y}} = \boldsymbol{Y}_m$ and $\overline{Y}\mathbf{1} = \boldsymbol{Y}_k$. The quantity

$$R^2 = \frac{\|\widehat{\boldsymbol{Y}} - \overline{Y}\mathbf{1}\|^2}{\|\boldsymbol{Y} - \overline{Y}\mathbf{1}\|^2} \tag{5.34}$$

is called the **coefficient of determination** of the linear model. Note that R^2 lies between 0 and 1. An R^2 value close to 1 indicates that a large proportion of the variance in the data has been explained by the model.

a. Show that

$$R^2 = 1 - \frac{\text{SS}_{\text{error}}}{\text{SS}_{\text{total}}} \stackrel{\text{def}}{=} 1 - \frac{\sum_i(Y_i - \widehat{Y}_i)^2}{\sum_i(Y_i - \overline{Y})^2} .$$

Hint: use Pythagoras' theorem, as in Fig. 5.3.
b. For the simple linear regression model in Problem 5.10 show that $R = \sqrt{R^2}$ is equal to the sample correlation coefficient (5.7) —where each X_i is replaced with x_i. Hint: write out $\widehat{Y}_i = \widehat{\beta}_0 + \widehat{\beta}_1 x_i$, using the explicit expressions for $\widehat{\beta}_0$ and $\widehat{\beta}_1$ in Problem 5.10. $\quad$ ☞ 12

5.12. A small lead ball is dropped onto a floor from different heights (measured in meters). The times (in seconds) when the ball hits the floor are given in the following table.

height	1	2	3	4
time	0.38	0.67	0.76	0.94

From physics we expect that, ignoring air resistance and the diameter of the ball, the relationship between the time y and the height h is $y = a\sqrt{h}$ for some unknown parameter a. Formulate a plausible statistical model for the data and fit a curve of the form $y = a\sqrt{h}$ to the data using the method of least squares.

5.13. In the past a milk vendor found that 30% of his milk sales were of a low fat variety. Recently, of his 1500 milk sales, 400 were low fat. Is there any indication of a move toward low fat milk? Give the p-value associated with the test.

5.14. Two lakes are being analyzed with respect to their PCB concentration in fish. The PCB concentration from 10 fish from lake A is given by

11.5 10.8 11.6 9.4 12.4 11.4 12.2 11.0 10.6 10.8

The concentration from 8 fish from lake B is given by

11.8 12.6 12.2 12.5 11.7 12.1 10.4 12.6

a. Assess whether the true variances are the same.
b. Assuming equality of variances, infer whether there is any difference in PCB concentration between the fish from the two lakes.

5.15. Let $X_1, \ldots, X_m \sim_{\text{iid}} \mathcal{N}(\mu_X, \sigma_X^2)$ and $Y_1, \ldots, Y_n \sim_{\text{iid}} \mathcal{N}(\mu_Y, \sigma_Y^2)$ be two independent normal samples with $\sigma_X^2 \neq \sigma_Y^2$. Find a pivot variable of the form

$$T = \frac{(\overline{X} - \overline{Y}) - (\mu_X - \mu_Y)}{V(X_1, \ldots, X_m, Y_1, \ldots, Y_n)}$$

that has approximately (for large m and n) a standard normal distribution and use this pivot to construct an approximate $1 - \alpha$ confidence interval for $\mu_X - \mu_Y$.

5.16. The Australian Bureau of Statistics reports that during 2003, 48,300 babies were born in the state of Queensland. Of these, 24,800 were boys and 23,500 were girls. Does this suggest that the probability of a male birth is more likely than that of a female birth? Conduct a suitable statistical analysis to find this out.

5.17. Gerrit from Gouda is an exporter of cheese. Gerrit requires that his suppliers produce cheese with an expected percentage fat content (PFC) of 40. From past experience it is known that the PFC has a normal distribution with standard deviation 4. Gerrit selects from each new batch of cheese n cheeses at random and measures their fat content. If the average PFC is less than 39 Gerrit rejects the entire batch.

a. Suppose $n = 5$. Give the distribution of the average PFC of the five cheeses.
b. Calculate the probability that Gerrit will reject the batch if the expected PFC is in fact 38.5.
c. Suppose the expected PFC is 38. How large should Gerrit choose n such that the test rejects the batch with a probability of at least 90%?

☞ 154   **5.18.** In this problem we prove the identity (5.29).

a. Suppose $\mathbf{A}$ is an $m \times m$ invertible matrix and $\boldsymbol{b}$ is an $m \times 1$ vector. Show that

$$(\mathbf{A} - \boldsymbol{b}\boldsymbol{b}^\top)^{-1} = \mathbf{A}^{-1} + \frac{\mathbf{A}^{-1}\boldsymbol{b}\boldsymbol{b}^\top\mathbf{A}^{-1}}{1 - \boldsymbol{b}^\top\mathbf{A}^{-1}\boldsymbol{b}} . \tag{5.35}$$

Hint: by direct computation, show that the right-hand side of (5.35) is indeed the inverse of $\mathbf{A} - \boldsymbol{b}\boldsymbol{b}^\top$.

b. Using (5.35), show that

$$(\mathbf{X}_{-k}^\top\mathbf{X}_{-k})^{-1} = (\mathbf{X}^\top\mathbf{X})^{-1} + \frac{(\mathbf{X}^\top\mathbf{X})^{-1}\boldsymbol{x}_k\boldsymbol{x}_k^\top(\mathbf{X}^\top\mathbf{X})^{-1}}{1 - p_k} , \tag{5.36}$$

where $\mathbf{X}_{-k}$ is the design matrix $\mathbf{X}$ with the k-th row removed, $\boldsymbol{x}_k^\top$ is the k-th row of $\mathbf{X}$, and p_k is the k-th diagonal element of the projection matrix $\mathbf{P} = \mathbf{X}(\mathbf{X}^\top\mathbf{X})^{-1}\mathbf{X}^\top$.

c. Use (5.36) to show (5.29).

5.19. Let $X_1, \ldots, X_n$ be an iid sample from the pdf

$$f(x; \theta) = \frac{\theta}{1 - \theta}\, x^{(2\theta-1)/(1-\theta)}, \quad x \in (0, 1), \quad \theta \in (\tfrac{1}{2}, 1) .$$

Show that $\{f(x; \theta)\}$ forms a one-dimensional exponential family. Show that the joint pdf of $X_1, \ldots, X_n$ forms again a one-dimensional exponential family. Show that $T = \sum_{i=1}^n \ln X_i$ is a sufficient statistic for θ.

5.20. Implement a Julia program to estimate

$$\ell = \int_0^1 \int_0^1 \frac{\sin(x)\, \mathrm{e}^{-(x+y)}}{\ln(1 + x)}\, \mathrm{d}x\, \mathrm{d}y$$

via Monte Carlo integration and give a 95% confidence interval.

5.21. Implement a Julia program to estimate

$$\ell = \int_{-2}^2 \mathrm{e}^{-x^2/2}\, \mathrm{d}x = \int H(x) f(x)\, \mathrm{d}x$$

via Monte Carlo integration using two different approaches: (1) by taking $H(x) = 4\,\mathrm{e}^{-x^2/2}$ and f the pdf of the $\mathcal{U}[-2, 2]$ distribution and (2) by taking $H(x) = \sqrt{2\pi}\, \mathbb{1}_{\{-2 \leq x \leq 2\}}$ and f the pdf of the $\mathcal{N}(0, 1)$ distribution.

a. For both cases estimate ℓ via the estimator $\widehat{\ell} = N^{-1}\sum_{i=1}^N H(X_i)$. Use a sample size of $N = 1000$.

b. Give an approximate 95% confidence interval for ℓ for both cases.

c. Using (b.), assess how large N should be such that the width of the confidence interval is less than 0.01, and carry out the simulation with this N. Compare the result with the true (numerical) value of ℓ.

5.22. Consider the approximate confidence interval (5.24) for binomial data.
☞ 139   It is possible to calculate the exact coverage probability via total enumeration. Specifically, define

$$T_1(x) = x/n - z_{1-\alpha/2}\sqrt{(x/n) \times (1 - x/n)/n}$$

and

$$T_2(x) = x/n + z_{1-\alpha/2}\sqrt{(x/n) \times (1 - x/n)/n}\,.$$

Then, the coverage probability as a function of p is

$$\mathbb{P}_p(T_1(X) < p < T_2(X)) = \sum_{x=0}^{n} \mathbb{1}_{\{T_1(x)<p<T_2(x)\}} \binom{n}{x} p^x (1-p)^{n-x}\,.$$

For various n and $\alpha = 0.05$ (so that $z_{1-\alpha/2} = 1.96$) draw the graph of the
coverage probability as a function of p and comment on the quality of the
coverage (which is aimed to be 95%).

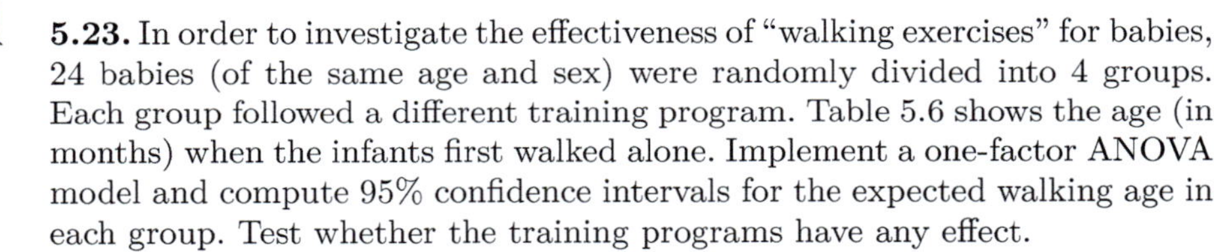

5.23. In order to investigate the effectiveness of "walking exercises" for babies,
24 babies (of the same age and sex) were randomly divided into 4 groups.
Each group followed a different training program. Table 5.6 shows the age (in
months) when the infants first walked alone. Implement a one-factor ANOVA
model and compute 95% confidence intervals for the expected walking age in
each group. Test whether the training programs have any effect.

Table 5.6 Walking age of babies (in months)

	Group		
A	B	C	D
9	11	11.5	13.25
9.5	10	12	11.5
9.75	10	9	12
10	11.75	11.5	13.5
13	10.5	13.25	11.5
9.5	15	13	11.5

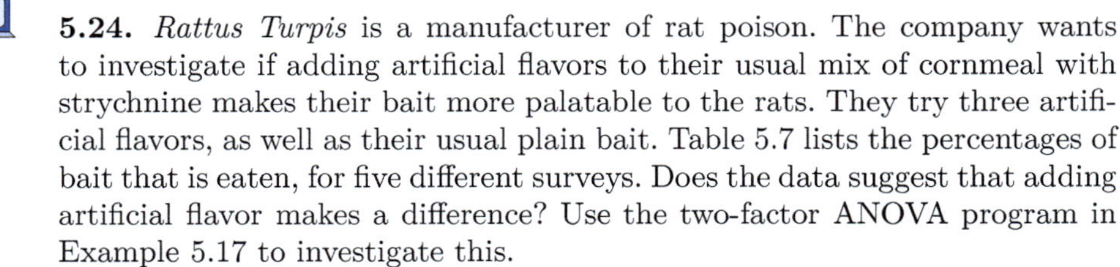

5.24. *Rattus Turpis* is a manufacturer of rat poison. The company wants
to investigate if adding artificial flavors to their usual mix of cornmeal with
strychnine makes their bait more palatable to the rats. They try three artificial flavors, as well as their usual plain bait. Table 5.7 lists the percentages of
bait that is eaten, for five different surveys. Does the data suggest that adding
artificial flavor makes a difference? Use the two-factor ANOVA program in
Example 5.17 to investigate this.

Table 5.7 Percentage of bait eaten

Survey	Flavor			
	Plain	Butter	Beef	Bread
1	13.8	11.7	14.0	12.6
2	12.9	16.7	15.5	13.8
3	25.9	29.8	27.8	25.0
4	18.0	23.1	23.0	16.9
5	15.2	20.2	19.9	13.7

Chapter 6
Likelihood

The concept of *likelihood* is central in Statistics. It describes in a precise manner the information about the parameters of the model given the observed data.

> **Definition 6.1. (Likelihood Function).** Let $\boldsymbol{X}$ be a random vector with pdf $f(\cdot\,; \boldsymbol{\theta})$ (discrete or continuous) with parameter vector $\boldsymbol{\theta} \in \Theta$. For a given outcome $\boldsymbol{x}$ of $\boldsymbol{X}$, the function
>
> $$L(\boldsymbol{\theta}; \boldsymbol{x}) = f(\boldsymbol{x}; \boldsymbol{\theta})$$
>
> is called the **likelihood function** of $\boldsymbol{\theta}$ based on $\boldsymbol{x}$.

Note that L is a function of $\boldsymbol{\theta}$ for fixed $\boldsymbol{x}$, whereas f is a function of $\boldsymbol{x}$ for fixed $\boldsymbol{\theta}$.

Example 6.1 (Binomial Likelihood). Let $X \sim \mathsf{Bin}(n, p)$. For a given observation x, the likelihood of x under p is given by

$$L(p; x) = f(x; p) = \binom{n}{x} p^x (1 - p)^{n-x}, \quad 0 < p < 1 . \tag{6.1}$$

As a particular example, consider the experiment where we flip 100 times a biased coin with success probability p. We know that the total number of successes (say Heads) in 100 tosses, X, has a $\mathsf{Bin}(100, p)$ distribution. Suppose that $x = 43$ successes were observed. Thus, the likelihood of the observed data as a function of p is

© The Author(s), under exclusive license to Springer Science+Business Media, LLC, part of Springer Nature 2025
J. C. C. Chan, D. P. Kroese, *Statistical Modeling and Computation*, Springer Texts in Statistics, https://doi.org/10.1007/978-1-0716-4132-3_6

$$L(p; 43) = \binom{100}{43} p^{43} (1-p)^{57}, \quad 0 < p < 1,$$

the graph of which is plotted in Fig. 6.1.

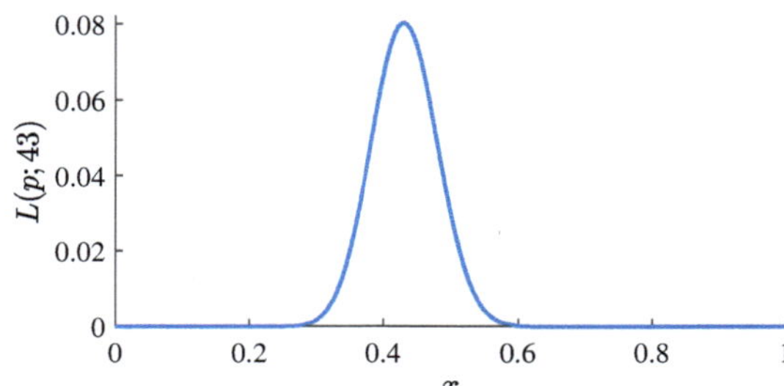

Fig. 6.1 The likelihood function for the $\mathsf{Bin}(100, p)$ distribution, with 43 observed successes

We see that the likelihood is largest for values of p that lie between 0.25 and 0.6. It is very implausible that the current datum was obtained from a p outside this interval. In this sense the likelihood is used to compare the plausibilities of various parameter values.

Example 6.2 (Normal Likelihood). Suppose we are given data $x_1, \ldots, x_n$ from an iid sample $\boldsymbol{X} = [X_1, \ldots, X_n]^\top$ of the $\mathcal{N}(\mu, \sigma^2)$ distribution, with μ and σ^2 unknown—in this case $\boldsymbol{\theta} = [\mu, \sigma^2]^\top$. The pdf of $\boldsymbol{X}$ (i.e., the joint pdf of $X_1, \ldots, X_n$) is given by the product of the marginal pdfs; see (3.7). Consequently, the likelihood of the data as a function of the parameters is

$$L(\mu, \sigma^2; \boldsymbol{x}) = \prod_{i=1}^{n} f_{X_i}(x_i; \mu, \sigma^2) = \left(\frac{1}{\sqrt{2\pi\sigma^2}}\right)^n \exp\left\{-\frac{1}{2}\sum_{i=1}^{n}\frac{(x_i - \mu)^2}{\sigma^2}\right\}$$

for $\mu \in \mathbb{R}$, $\sigma > 0$. As a particular example, suppose $n = 10$ and that the data (computer-generated from some $\mathcal{N}(\mu, \sigma^2)$ distribution) are

$$2.39876, \quad -0.149451, \quad -0.770132, \quad 0.87627, \quad -0.0852696,$$
$$1.58494, \quad 1.32772 \quad 1.35611, \quad -0.206479, \quad 0.83773 \ .$$

Figure 6.2 gives the three-dimensional graph and the corresponding contour plot of the likelihood function. Note that the values for $\boldsymbol{\theta}$ for which the likelihood of the data is largest are restricted to an ellipse-like region. The *actual* parameter values for the data were $\mu = 1$ and $\sigma^2 = 1$ in this case.

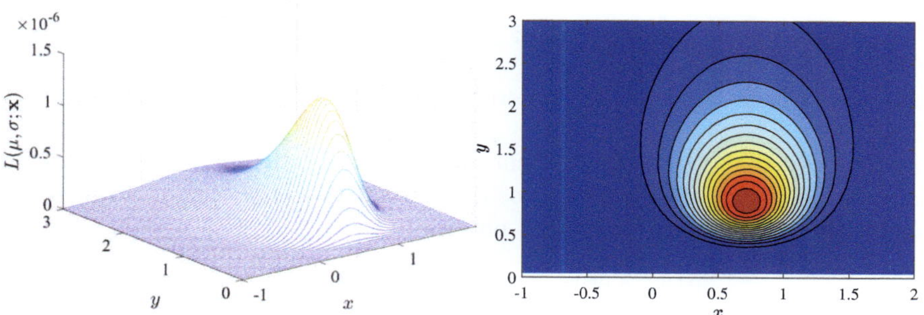

Fig. 6.2 The graph and contour plot of the likelihood function for the $\mathcal{N}(\mu, \sigma^2)$ distribution, for the given data

In general, if $X_1, \ldots, X_n$ is an iid sample from $\mathring{f}(\cdot\,; \boldsymbol{\theta})$, then the likelihood of the data $\boldsymbol{x} = [x_1, \ldots, x_n]$ under $\boldsymbol{\theta}$ is the product:

$$L(\boldsymbol{\theta}; \boldsymbol{x}) = \prod_{i=1}^{n} \mathring{f}(x_i; \boldsymbol{\theta}) \ . \tag{6.2}$$

Example 6.3 (Radioactive Source Detection). Suppose a low-intensity radioactive source is emitting particles (in pairs). A screen registers the impact of one particle from each pair. Suppose the position of the source is (a, b), and X is the x-coordinate of the location where a random particle will hit the screen, and let $Y \in (-\pi/2, \pi/2)$ be the angle between the line segments (a, b)-$(a, 0)$ and (a, b)-$(X, 0)$; see Fig. 6.3.

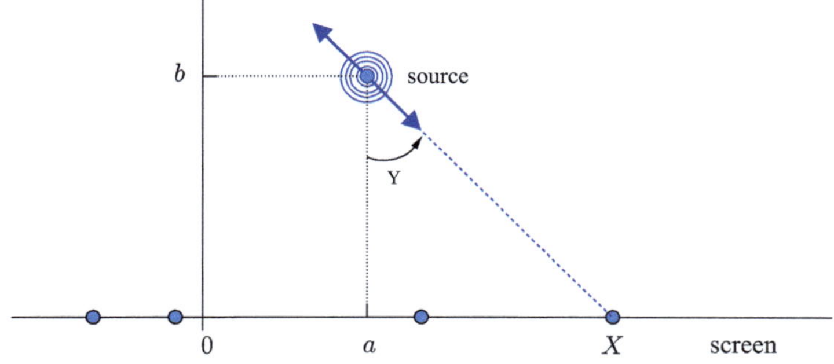

Fig. 6.3 A radioactive source at position (a, b) emits particles in a random direction

Since all angles are equally likely, Y is uniformly distributed in $(-\pi/2, \pi/2)$. Moreover, X and Y are related via $\tan(Y) = \frac{X-a}{b}$. It follows from the transformation formula (3.22) that

☞ 79

$$f_X(x) = \frac{b}{\pi(b^2 + (x - a)^2)}, \quad x \in \mathbb{R}.$$

In other words, $X = a + bZ$, where Z has a Cauchy distribution; see Problem 6.8.

Suppose that we know that the source is at a distance $b = 1$ from the screen, but we do not know its position a relative to the origin. However, we know the impact positions of ten particles:

$$1.3615, \quad 3.5616, \quad -14.2411, \quad -4.4950, \quad 2.3014,$$
$$1.1066, \quad -9.3409, \quad 0.3779, \quad 0.9386, \quad -0.1838.$$

Based on these data, what can we say about a? A naive guess is to simply take the mean of the data to estimate the location, which turns out to be -1.8613. This, however, is a fundamentally flawed approach, because the expectation of the distribution of X *does not exist*; namely, $\int_0^\infty x f_X(x)\,\mathrm{d}x = \infty$ and $\int_{-\infty}^0 x f_X(x)\,\mathrm{d}x = -\infty$, and $\infty - \infty$ is not well-defined. Of course the mode of f (the point where f is maximal) is a, but here the mode is not equal to the expectation (which does not exist). A much better approach is to plot the likelihood function for a, which is

$$L(a; \boldsymbol{x}) = \left(\frac{1}{\pi}\right)^{10} \prod_{i=1}^{10} \frac{1}{1 + (x_i - a)^2}.$$

The graph of the likelihood function is given in Fig. 6.4.

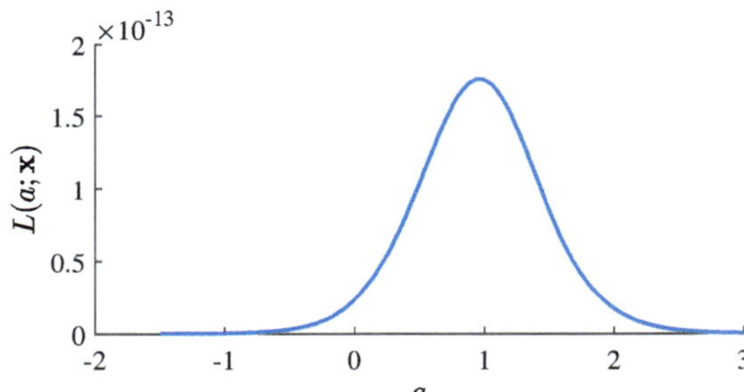

Fig. 6.4 The graph of the likelihood function for the position a of the radioactive source

We see that the most likely position is around 1 and that our initial guess of -1.8613 is extremely unlikely. We also see that the most likely positions fall between roughly -1 and 3. In fact, the actual position was $a = 1$ in this case. So we see that with relatively sparse information, we can still make well-founded decisions about a, as long as we use the likelihood.

6.1 Log-Likelihood and Score Functions

Definition 6.2. (Log-Likelihood and Score Functions). Let X be a random vector with pdf $f(\cdot; \boldsymbol{\theta})$ (discrete or continuous) with parameter vector $\boldsymbol{\theta} \in \Theta$. For a given outcome x of X, the **log-likelihood function**, denoted l, is the natural logarithm of the likelihood function:

$$l(\boldsymbol{\theta}; x) = \ln L(\boldsymbol{\theta}; x) = \ln f(x; \boldsymbol{\theta}) .$$

Its gradient, denoted S (column vector), is called the **score function**:

$$S(\boldsymbol{\theta}; x) = \nabla_{\boldsymbol{\theta}} l(\boldsymbol{\theta}; x) = \frac{\nabla_{\boldsymbol{\theta}} f(x; \boldsymbol{\theta})}{f(x; \boldsymbol{\theta})} . \tag{6.3}$$

Example 6.4 (Binomial Log-Likelihood and Score Functions). For the $\mathsf{Bin}(n, p)$ distribution with observed datum x, the log-likelihood is

$$l(p; x) = \ln\left(\binom{n}{x}\right) + x \ln(p) + (n - x) \ln(1 - p) .$$

Differentiating $l(p; x)$ with respect to p gives the score function:

$$S(p; x) = \frac{x}{p} - \frac{n - x}{1 - p} . \tag{6.4}$$

Theorem 6.1. (Log-Likelihood and Score Functions for Iid Data). Let $X = [X_1, \ldots, X_n]^\top$ be an iid sample from $\mathring{f}(\cdot; \boldsymbol{\theta})$, and let $\mathring{l}$ and $\mathring{S}$ be respectively the log-likelihood and the score function corresponding to $\mathring{f}$. Then the log-likelihood and score functions of $\boldsymbol{\theta}$ based on an outcome x of X are

$$l(\boldsymbol{\theta}; x) = \sum_{i=1}^{n} \mathring{l}(\boldsymbol{\theta}; x_i) \quad \text{and} \quad S(\boldsymbol{\theta}; x) = \sum_{i=1}^{n} \mathring{S}(\boldsymbol{\theta}; x_i) .$$

Proof. The pdf of X is $f(x; \boldsymbol{\theta}) = \prod_{i=1}^{n} \mathring{f}(x_i; \boldsymbol{\theta})$. Taking the logarithm gives the log-likelihood as the sum of the logarithms of the pdfs. By differentiating this sum, we obtain the score function as the sum of the derivatives. $\qquad\square$

Example 6.5 (Log-Likelihood and Score Functions for Normal Iid Data). Consider the standard model for data: $X_1, \ldots, X_n \sim_{\text{iid}} \mathcal{N}(\mu, \sigma^2)$. The log-likelihood function of (μ, σ^2) for a single outcome x is given by the logarithm of the pdf of the $\mathcal{N}(\mu, \sigma^2)$ distribution:

$$\mathring{l}(\mu, \sigma^2; x) = -\frac{1}{2}\ln(2\pi) - \frac{1}{2}\ln(\sigma^2) - \frac{1}{2}(x - \mu)^2/\sigma^2 \,.$$

By differentiating $\mathring{l}$ with respect μ and σ^2 (note that σ^2 is viewed as a single parameter), we obtain the two components of the score function:

$$\mathring{S}_1(\mu, \sigma^2; x) = \frac{\partial \mathring{l}(\mu, \sigma^2; x)}{\partial \mu} = \frac{x - \mu}{\sigma^2} \,,$$

and

$$\mathring{S}_2(\mu, \sigma^2; x) = \frac{\partial \mathring{l}(\mu, \sigma^2; x)}{\partial \sigma^2} = -\frac{1}{2\sigma^2} + \frac{1}{2}\frac{(x - \mu)^2}{(\sigma^2)^2} \,.$$

It follows from Theorem 6.1 that the log-likelihood and score functions of (μ, σ^2) based on an outcome $\boldsymbol{x} = [x_1, \ldots, x_n]^\top$ are given by

$$l(\mu, \sigma^2; \boldsymbol{x}) = -\frac{n}{2}\ln(2\pi) - \frac{n}{2}\ln(\sigma^2) - \sum_{i=1}^{n} \frac{1}{2}(x_i - \mu)^2/\sigma^2 \,,$$

$$S_1(\mu, \sigma^2; \boldsymbol{x}) = \sum_{i=1}^{n} \frac{x_i - \mu}{\sigma^2} \,, \tag{6.5}$$

and

$$S_2(\mu, \sigma^2; \boldsymbol{x}) = -\frac{n}{2\sigma^2} + \frac{1}{2}\sum_{i=1}^{n} \frac{(x_i - \mu)^2}{(\sigma^2)^2} \,. \tag{6.6}$$

Theorem 6.2. (Score Function for an Exponential Family). The score function for a natural exponential family with pdf: $f(\boldsymbol{x}; \boldsymbol{\theta}) = c(\boldsymbol{\theta})\, e^{\boldsymbol{\theta}^\top \boldsymbol{t}(\boldsymbol{x})}\, h(\boldsymbol{x})$ is given by

$$\boldsymbol{S}(\boldsymbol{\theta}; \boldsymbol{x}) = \frac{\nabla c(\boldsymbol{\theta})}{c(\boldsymbol{\theta})} + \boldsymbol{t}(\boldsymbol{x}) \,. \tag{6.7}$$

Proof. The log-likelihood function is $l(\boldsymbol{\theta}; \boldsymbol{x}) = \ln c(\boldsymbol{\theta}) + \boldsymbol{\theta}^\top \boldsymbol{t}(\boldsymbol{x}) + \ln h(\boldsymbol{x})$. Now take the gradient with respect to $\boldsymbol{\theta}$. $\square$

Example 6.6 (Score Function for Gamma Data). The pdf of the $\mathsf{Gamma}(\alpha, \lambda)$ distribution, where $\alpha, \lambda > 0$, is

$$f(x; \alpha, \lambda) = \frac{\lambda^{\alpha} x^{\alpha-1} e^{-\lambda x}}{\Gamma(\alpha)}, \quad x > 0 \,.$$

Let us assume that α is known. After the reparameterization $\eta = -\lambda$, we obtain (see Table 5.5) the natural exponential family with pdf

$$\widetilde{f}(x; \eta) = c(\eta) \, e^{\eta t(x)} \, h(x) \,,$$

where $c(\eta) = (-\eta)^{\alpha}$ and $t(x) = x$. Here, $h(x)$ does not depend on η (but does depend on the known constant α). Since

$$\frac{c'(\eta)}{c(\eta)} = \frac{\alpha}{\eta} \,,$$

we find the score function $\widetilde{S}(\eta; x) = \frac{\alpha}{\eta} + x$. In the original parameter, we have (chain rule) $S(\lambda; x) = \widetilde{S}(\eta(\lambda); x) \times \frac{\mathrm{d}\eta}{\mathrm{d}\lambda} = - \left(\frac{\alpha}{-\lambda} + x \right) = \frac{\alpha}{\lambda} - x.$

6.2 Fisher Information and Cramér–Rao Inequality

Definition 6.3. (Efficient Score). Let $S(\boldsymbol{\theta}; \boldsymbol{x})$ be the score function corresponding to an outcome $\boldsymbol{x}$ of $\boldsymbol{X} \sim f(\cdot; \boldsymbol{\theta})$. The *random vector* $S(\boldsymbol{\theta}) = S(\boldsymbol{\theta}; \boldsymbol{X})$ is called the **efficient score** or simply **score** of $\boldsymbol{\theta}$.

The expected score under $\boldsymbol{\theta}$ is *equal to the zero vector*; namely,

$$\begin{aligned}
\mathbb{E}_{\boldsymbol{\theta}} S(\boldsymbol{\theta}) &= \int \frac{\nabla_{\boldsymbol{\theta}} f(\boldsymbol{x}; \boldsymbol{\theta})}{f(\boldsymbol{x}; \boldsymbol{\theta})} \, f(\boldsymbol{x}; \boldsymbol{\theta}) \, \mathrm{d}\boldsymbol{x} \\
&= \int \nabla_{\boldsymbol{\theta}} f(\boldsymbol{x}; \boldsymbol{\theta}) \, \mathrm{d}\boldsymbol{x} = \nabla_{\boldsymbol{\theta}} \int f(\boldsymbol{x}; \theta) \, \mathrm{d}\boldsymbol{x} = \nabla_{\boldsymbol{\theta}} 1 = \boldsymbol{0} \,,
\end{aligned} \tag{6.8}$$

provided that the interchange of differentiation and integration is justified. This is true for large classes of distributions, including natural exponential families. From now on we simply assume that such an interchange is permitted.

Definition 6.4. (Fisher Information Matrix). For the model $\boldsymbol{X} \sim f(\cdot; \boldsymbol{\theta})$, let $\boldsymbol{S}(\boldsymbol{\theta}) = \boldsymbol{S}(\boldsymbol{\theta}; \boldsymbol{X})$ be the score of $\boldsymbol{\theta}$. The covariance matrix of the random vector $\boldsymbol{S}(\boldsymbol{\theta})$, denoted by $\mathbf{I}(\boldsymbol{\theta})$, is called the **Fisher information matrix**.

Since the expected score is $\mathbf{0}$, we have:

$$\mathbf{I}(\boldsymbol{\theta}) = \mathbb{E}_{\boldsymbol{\theta}}[\boldsymbol{S}(\boldsymbol{\theta})\boldsymbol{S}(\boldsymbol{\theta})^{\top}] \tag{6.9}$$

and in the one-dimensional case, the information number is

$$I(\theta) = \mathbb{E}_{\theta}\left(\frac{\mathrm{d}\ln f(\boldsymbol{X}; \theta)}{\mathrm{d}\theta}\right)^{2}.$$

Example 6.7 (Information Number for Binomial Data). Let $X \sim \mathrm{Bin}(n, p)$. From (6.4) we see that the score is

$$S(p; X) = \frac{X}{p} - \frac{n-X}{1-p}. \tag{6.10}$$

The information number is therefore

$$\mathrm{Var}_{p}\left(\frac{X}{p} - \frac{n-X}{1-p}\right) = \mathrm{Var}_{p}\left(\frac{X}{p(1-p)}\right) = \frac{n\,p\,(1-p)}{p^{2}\,(1-p)^{2}} = \frac{n}{p(1-p)}. \tag{6.11}$$

For iid samples the score has approximately a multivariate normal distribution that is characterized by the Fisher information of the sampling distribution, as summarized in the following theorem.

Theorem 6.3. (Asymptotic Distribution of the Score). Let $\boldsymbol{X} = [X_{1}, \ldots, X_{n}]^{\top}$ be an iid sample from $\mathring{f}(x; \boldsymbol{\theta})$ and let $\boldsymbol{S}(\boldsymbol{\theta}) = \boldsymbol{S}(\boldsymbol{\theta}; \boldsymbol{X})$ be the score of $\boldsymbol{\theta}$. Then,

1. $\frac{1}{n}\boldsymbol{S}(\boldsymbol{\theta}) \to \mathbf{0}$ as $n \to \infty$, and
2. $\boldsymbol{S}(\boldsymbol{\theta}) \overset{\text{approx.}}{\sim} \mathcal{N}(\mathbf{0}, n\,\mathring{\mathbf{I}}(\boldsymbol{\theta}))$ for large n, where $\mathring{\mathbf{I}}(\boldsymbol{\theta})$ is the Fisher information matrix corresponding to $\mathring{f}$.

Proof. By Theorem 6.1, we can write $\boldsymbol{S}(\boldsymbol{\theta}) = \sum_{i=1}^{n}\mathring{\boldsymbol{S}}(\boldsymbol{\theta}; X_{i})$. Note that the random vectors $\{\mathring{\boldsymbol{S}}(\boldsymbol{\theta}; X_{i})\}$ are independent and identically distributed with mean $\mathbf{0}$ and covariance matrix $\mathring{\mathbf{I}}(\boldsymbol{\theta})$. The law of large numbers and the multivariate central limit theorem (see Theorem 3.14) now lead directly to the two properties above. $\square$

☞ 92

It is sometimes easier to compute the information number in a different way to (6.9), based on the following equality (assuming a one-dimensional parameter θ):

$$\frac{\mathrm{d}^2}{\mathrm{d}\theta^2}\ln f(\boldsymbol{x};\theta) = \frac{\frac{\mathrm{d}^2}{\mathrm{d}\theta^2}f(\boldsymbol{x};\theta)}{f(\boldsymbol{x};\theta)} - \left(\frac{\frac{\mathrm{d}}{\mathrm{d}\theta}f(\boldsymbol{x};\theta)}{f(\boldsymbol{x};\theta)}\right)^2 .$$

Multiplying both sides with $f(\boldsymbol{x};\theta)$ and integrating with respect to $\boldsymbol{x}$ gives:

$$\mathbb{E}_\theta \frac{\mathrm{d}^2 \ln f(\boldsymbol{X};\theta)}{\mathrm{d}\theta^2} = \int \frac{\mathrm{d}^2}{\mathrm{d}\theta^2}f(\boldsymbol{x};\theta)\,\mathrm{d}\boldsymbol{x} - I(\theta) .$$

Now if we may change the order of differentiation and integration in the integral (allowed for exponential families), then

$$\int \frac{\mathrm{d}^2}{\mathrm{d}\theta^2}f(\boldsymbol{x};\theta)\,\mathrm{d}\boldsymbol{x} = \frac{\mathrm{d}^2}{\mathrm{d}\theta^2}1 = 0 ,$$

so that the Fisher information number is also given by

$$I(\theta) = -\mathbb{E}_\theta \frac{\mathrm{d}^2 \ln f(\boldsymbol{X};\theta)}{\mathrm{d}\theta^2} = -\mathbb{E}_\theta \frac{\mathrm{d}S(\theta;\boldsymbol{X})}{\mathrm{d}\theta} . \qquad (6.12)$$

Example 6.8 (Information Number for Binomial Data Continued). Differentiating the score in (6.10) with respect to p gives:

$$\frac{\mathrm{d}S(p;X)}{\mathrm{d}p} = -\frac{X}{p^2} - \frac{n-X}{(1-p)^2} .$$

The expectation of this random variable (under $X \sim \mathsf{Bin}(n,p)$) is

$$-\frac{np}{p^2} - \frac{n-np}{(1-p)^2} = -\frac{n}{p(1-p)} ,$$

which is exactly the negative of the information number found in (6.11). $\square$

The multidimensional version of (6.12) is

$$\mathbf{I}(\boldsymbol{\theta}) = -\mathbb{E}_{\boldsymbol{\theta}}\,\nabla^2 \ln f(\boldsymbol{X};\boldsymbol{\theta}) = -\mathbb{E}_{\boldsymbol{\theta}}\,\nabla S(\boldsymbol{\theta}) , \qquad (6.13)$$

where $\nabla^2 \ln f(\boldsymbol{X};\boldsymbol{\theta})$ is the *Hessian* of $\ln f(\boldsymbol{X};\boldsymbol{\theta})$; that is, the (random) matrix

$$\left[\frac{\partial^2 \ln f(\boldsymbol{X};\boldsymbol{\theta})}{\partial\theta_i\partial\theta_j}\right] = \left[\frac{\partial^2 l(\boldsymbol{\theta};\boldsymbol{X})}{\partial\theta_i\partial\theta_j}\right] = \left[\frac{\partial S_i(\boldsymbol{\theta};\boldsymbol{X})}{\partial\theta_j}\right] ,$$

where S_i denotes the i-th component of the score. The following is a direct consequence of Theorem 6.1.

Theorem 6.4. (Information Matrix for Iid Data). Let $X = [X_1, \ldots, X_n]^\top$ be an iid sample from $\mathring{f}(x; \boldsymbol{\theta})$, and let $\mathring{\mathbf{I}}(\boldsymbol{\theta})$ be the information matrix corresponding to $X \sim \mathring{f}(x; \boldsymbol{\theta})$. Then, the information matrix for $\boldsymbol{X}$ is given by

$$\mathbf{I}(\boldsymbol{\theta}) = n\,\mathring{\mathbf{I}}(\boldsymbol{\theta}) \, .$$

Example 6.9 (Information Matrix for Iid Normal Data). Let $X_1, \ldots,$ X_n be an iid sample from the $\mathcal{N}(\mu, \sigma^2)$ distribution. Using Examples 6.5 and (6.13), we see that the information matrix $\mathring{\mathbf{I}}(\mu, \sigma^2)$ is the expectation of the following matrix of partial derivatives:

$$-\begin{bmatrix} \frac{\partial \mathring{S}_1(\mu,\sigma^2;X)}{\partial \mu} & \frac{\partial \mathring{S}_1(\mu,\sigma^2;X)}{\partial \sigma^2} \\ \frac{\partial \mathring{S}_2(\mu,\sigma^2;X)}{\partial \mu} & \frac{\partial \mathring{S}_2(\mu,\sigma^2;X)}{\partial \sigma^2} \end{bmatrix} = -\begin{bmatrix} -\frac{1}{\sigma^2} & -\frac{(X-\mu)}{(\sigma^2)^2} \\ -\frac{(X-\mu)}{(\sigma^2)^2} & \frac{1}{2\sigma^4} - \frac{(X-\mu)^2}{(\sigma^2)^3} \end{bmatrix} , \tag{6.14}$$

where $X \sim \mathcal{N}(\mu, \sigma^2)$. Taking expectations gives:

$$\mathring{\mathbf{I}}(\mu, \sigma^2) = \begin{bmatrix} \sigma^{-2} & 0 \\ 0 & \frac{\sigma^{-4}}{2} \end{bmatrix} . \tag{6.15}$$

By Theorem 6.4 the information matrix corresponding to the whole iid sample is simply a factor n larger: $\mathbf{I}(\mu, \sigma^2) = n\mathring{\mathbf{I}}(\mu, \sigma^2)$.

Example 6.10 (Information Matrix for Exponential Families). Consider a natural exponential family with pdf :

$$f(\boldsymbol{x}; \boldsymbol{\theta}) = e^{\boldsymbol{\theta}^\top \boldsymbol{t}(\boldsymbol{x}) - \zeta(\boldsymbol{\theta})} h(\boldsymbol{x}) . \tag{6.16}$$

Then, similar to (6.7),

$$\boldsymbol{S}(\boldsymbol{\theta}; \boldsymbol{x}) = \boldsymbol{t}(\boldsymbol{x}) - \nabla \zeta(\boldsymbol{\theta}) . \tag{6.17}$$

Since the covariance matrix of a random vector $\boldsymbol{Z}$ is the same as that of $\boldsymbol{Z} + \boldsymbol{a}$ for any constant vector $\boldsymbol{a}$, we have that the covariance matrix of $\boldsymbol{S}(\boldsymbol{\theta}; \boldsymbol{X})$, that is, the information matrix, is simply the covariance matrix of $\boldsymbol{t}(\boldsymbol{X})$.

Example 6.11 (Information Number for Location Families). For **location families** $\{f(x; \mu)\}$; that is, when $f(x; \mu) = \widetilde{f}(x - \mu)$ for some fixed pdf $\widetilde{f}$, the Fisher information *does not depend on* μ and is therefore constant. Namely, in this case the log-likelihood satisfies $l(\mu; x) = \ln \widetilde{f}(x - \mu)$, and the score function is thus a function of $\mu - x$, say $g(x - \mu)$. The variance of the score, that is, the information number, satisfies:

$$I(\mu) = \int_{-\infty}^{\infty} S^2(\mu; x) f(x; \mu) \, \mathrm{d}x = \int_{-\infty}^{\infty} g^2(x - \mu) \widetilde{f}(x - \mu) \, \mathrm{d}x$$

$$= \int_{-\infty}^{\infty} g^2(y) \widetilde{f}(y) \, \mathrm{d}y \, ,$$

which does not depend on μ.

The importance of the Fisher information in statistics is corroborated by the famous *Cramér–Rao inequality.*

Theorem 6.5. (Cramér–Rao Information Inequality). Let $X \sim f(x; \boldsymbol{\theta})$. The variance of any unbiased estimator $Z = Z(X)$ of $g(\boldsymbol{\theta})$ is bounded from below via

$$\mathrm{Var}(Z) \geq (\nabla g(\boldsymbol{\theta}))^{\top} \, \mathbf{I}^{-1}(\boldsymbol{\theta}) \, \nabla g(\boldsymbol{\theta}) \, . \tag{6.18}$$

Proof. We prove only the one-dimensional case. All expectations and variances below are taken with respect to $f(x; \theta)$. Recall that $S = S(\theta; X) = \frac{\partial}{\partial \theta} \ln f(X; \theta)$ denotes the score and that $\mathrm{Var}(S) = I(\theta)$. The key is to apply the Cauchy–Schwartz inequality:

$$\mathrm{Cov}(Z, S) \leq \sqrt{\mathrm{Var}(Z)\mathrm{Var}(S)} \, ,$$

which immediately yields

$$\mathrm{Var}(Z) \geq \frac{(\mathrm{Cov}(Z, S))^2}{I(\theta)} \, .$$

Thus, it remains to be shown that $\mathrm{Cov}(Z, S) = g'(\theta)$. This follows from $\mathrm{Cov}(Z, S) = \mathbb{E}[ZS] - \mathbb{E}Z \, \mathbb{E}S = \mathbb{E}ZS$ (because $\mathbb{E}S = 0$) and

$$\mathbb{E}[ZS] = \mathbb{E}\left[Z \, \frac{\frac{\partial}{\partial \theta} f(X; \theta)}{f(X; \theta)} \right] = \int Z(x) \frac{\partial}{\partial \theta} f(x; \theta) \, \mathrm{d}x = \frac{\mathrm{d}}{\mathrm{d}\theta} \mathbb{E}Z = g'(\theta) \, ,$$

assuming that we may change the order of integration and differentiation. $\square$

6.3 Likelihood Methods for Estimation

Suppose we are given data x from a model $f(x; \boldsymbol{\theta})$, yielding the likelihood function $L(\boldsymbol{\theta}; x) = f(x; \boldsymbol{\theta})$. Although the entire shape of the likelihood function is valuable for our inference about the unknown parameter $\boldsymbol{\theta}$, it is often desirable to summarize the information on the likelihood function into a few key numbers. One of these numbers is the **mode** of the likelihood function, that is, the parameter value $\widehat{\boldsymbol{\theta}}$ for which the function is maximal. This number (or vector of numbers, in the multiparameter case) is in a way our best estimate for $\boldsymbol{\theta}$. It is called the **maximum likelihood estimate** (MLE). Note that $\widehat{\boldsymbol{\theta}} = \widehat{\boldsymbol{\theta}}(\boldsymbol{x})$ is a function of the data $\boldsymbol{x}$. The corresponding random variable, also denoted $\widehat{\boldsymbol{\theta}}$, is the **maximum likelihood estimator** (also abbreviated as MLE).

Since the natural logarithm is an increasing function, maximization of $L(\boldsymbol{\theta}; \boldsymbol{x})$ is equivalent (in terms of finding the mode) to maximization of the log-likelihood $l(\boldsymbol{\theta}; \boldsymbol{x})$. This is often easier, especially when $\boldsymbol{X}$ is an iid sample from some sampling distribution.

Remark 6.1 (Existence and Uniqueness). Maximum likelihood estimators may not always exist (e.g., when estimating a variance with only one data point), or could be nonunique (when the likelihood function attains its maximum at more than one point).

If $l(\boldsymbol{\theta}; \boldsymbol{x})$ is a differentiable function with respect to $\boldsymbol{\theta}$ and the maximum is attained in the *interior* of Θ, *and there exists a unique maximum point*, then we can find the MLE of $\boldsymbol{\theta}$ by differentiating $l(\boldsymbol{\theta}; \boldsymbol{x})$ with respect to $\boldsymbol{\theta}$—more precisely, by solving

$$\nabla_{\boldsymbol{\theta}}\, l(\boldsymbol{\theta}; \boldsymbol{x}) = \mathbf{0}\ .$$

In other words, the MLE is obtained by solving the root of the score function, that is, by solving

$$\boldsymbol{S}(\boldsymbol{\theta}; \boldsymbol{x}) = \mathbf{0}\ . \tag{6.19}$$

In general, solving the above equation only yields a *local* maximum. If the likelihood function is multimodal, there will be more than one point $\boldsymbol{\theta}$ that satisfies (6.19). The evaluation of l at *all* of these points may then identify the *global* maximum.

Example 6.12 (MLE for Binomial Data). Suppose x is an outcome of $X \sim \mathsf{Bin}(n, p)$. By (6.4) the MLE is found by solving:

$$\frac{x}{p} - \frac{n - x}{1 - p} = 0\ ,$$

which gives the maximum likelihood estimate $\widehat{p} = x/n$ and the corresponding estimator $\widehat{p} = X/n$.

Example 6.13 (MLE for Iid Normal Data). Suppose $x_1, \ldots, x_n$ are the outcomes of $X_1, \ldots, X_n \sim_{\text{iid}} \mathcal{N}(\mu, \sigma^2)$. The MLEs follow (see (6.5) and (6.6)$||$) from solving the set of equations:

$$\sum_{i=1}^{n} \frac{(x_i - \mu)}{\sigma^2} = 0 , \tag{6.20}$$

$$-\frac{n}{2\sigma^2} + \frac{1}{2}\sum_{i=1}^{n} \frac{(x_i - \mu)^2}{(\sigma^2)^2} = 0 , \tag{6.21}$$

giving

$$\widehat{\mu} = \frac{1}{n}\sum_{i=1}^{n} x_i = \overline{x} \qquad \text{and} \qquad \widehat{\sigma^2} = \frac{1}{n}\sum_{i=1}^{n}(x_i - \overline{x})^2 . \tag{6.22}$$

We see that the maximum likelihood method and the method of moments yield exactly the same estimates in this case.

Example 6.14 (MLE for the Normal Linear Model). Consider the normal linear model:

$$\boldsymbol{Y} = \mathbf{X}\boldsymbol{\beta} + \boldsymbol{\varepsilon} , \tag{6.23}$$

where $\mathbf{X}$ is an $n \times m$ design matrix, $\boldsymbol{\beta}$ an m-dimensional vector of parameters, and $\boldsymbol{\varepsilon}$ a vector of iid $\mathcal{N}(0, \sigma^2)$ error terms. Since $\boldsymbol{Y} \sim \mathcal{N}(\mathbf{X}\boldsymbol{\beta}, \sigma^2 \, \mathbb{I}_n)$, it follows from (3.31) that the likelihood function is

$$L(\boldsymbol{\beta}, \sigma^2; \boldsymbol{y}) = \left(\frac{1}{\sqrt{2\pi\sigma^2}}\right)^n e^{-\frac{1}{2}\|\boldsymbol{y}-\mathbf{X}\boldsymbol{\beta}\|^2/\sigma^2}$$

for a given outcome $\boldsymbol{y}$ of $\boldsymbol{Y}$. Observe that for any *fixed* σ^2 the likelihood $L(\boldsymbol{\beta}, \sigma^2; \boldsymbol{y})$, as a function of $\boldsymbol{\beta}$, is maximized by choosing $\boldsymbol{\beta}$ such that $\|\boldsymbol{y} - \mathbf{X}\boldsymbol{\beta}\|^2$ is minimized. But this gives exactly the least-squares estimate of $\boldsymbol{\beta}$; see Sect. 5.1.2. To obtain the MLE for σ^2, it remains to maximize $L(\widehat{\boldsymbol{\beta}}, \sigma^2; \boldsymbol{y})$ or, equivalently, solve:

$$-\frac{n}{2\sigma^2} + \frac{1}{2}\frac{\|\boldsymbol{y} - \mathbf{X}\widehat{\boldsymbol{\beta}}\|^2}{(\sigma^2)^2} = 0 ,$$

where $\widehat{\boldsymbol{\beta}}$ is MLE of $\boldsymbol{\beta}$. This gives the same estimate $\widehat{\sigma^2} = \|\boldsymbol{y} - \mathbf{X}\widehat{\boldsymbol{\beta}}\|^2/n$ as in (5.13). For a generalization to the general regression case (possibly nonlinear), see Problem 6.3.

Example 6.15 (MLE for Exponential Families). For natural exponential families of the form (6.16) the MLE is found by solving

$$\boldsymbol{t}(\boldsymbol{x}) - \nabla\zeta(\boldsymbol{\theta}) = \boldsymbol{t}(\boldsymbol{x}) - \mathbb{E}_{\boldsymbol{\theta}}\, \boldsymbol{t}(\boldsymbol{X}) = \boldsymbol{0} , \tag{6.24}$$

where we have used the fact that $\mathbb{E}_{\boldsymbol{\theta}}[\boldsymbol{t}(\boldsymbol{X}) - \nabla\zeta(\boldsymbol{\theta})] = \mathbb{E}_{\boldsymbol{\theta}}S(\boldsymbol{\theta}; \boldsymbol{X}) = 0$; see (6.8). Thus, $\boldsymbol{\theta}$ is chosen such that the observed and expected values of $\boldsymbol{t}(\boldsymbol{X})$ are matched.

☞ 127
☞ 113
☞ 83
☞ 129
☞ 130
☞ 173

Maximum likelihood estimation arises in a natural way from the statistical learning framework in Sect. 4.6. Consider the unsupervised setting where we have a training set $\tau = \{x_1, \dots, x_n\}$ that contains the outcomes of n iid random variables $X_1, \dots, X_n$ from some unknown pdf $\mathring{f}$. The objective is to "learn" $\mathring{f}$ from the training data, using a class of probability density functions $\mathcal{G} = \{g(\cdot; \boldsymbol{\theta}), \boldsymbol{\theta} \in \boldsymbol{\Theta}\}$. In particular, we seek the best g in $\mathcal{G}$ that minimizes the Kullback–Leibler risk $r(g)$ given in (4.27); that is,

$$r(g) = \mathbb{E} \ln \frac{\mathring{f}(X)}{g(X)} ,$$

which corresponds to the loss function

$$\mathrm{Loss}(\mathring{f}(x), g(x)) = \ln \frac{\mathring{f}(x)}{g(x)} = \ln \mathring{f}(x) - \ln g(x) .$$

Using similar notation as in Sect. 4.6, define $g^{\mathcal{G}}$ as the global minimizer of the risk in the class $\mathcal{G}$; that is, $g^{\mathcal{G}} = \mathrm{argmin}_{g \in \mathcal{G}} \, r(g)$. If we define

$$\boldsymbol{\theta}^* = \underset{\boldsymbol{\theta}}{\mathrm{argmin}} \, r(g(\cdot; \boldsymbol{\theta})) = \underset{\boldsymbol{\theta}}{\mathrm{argmin}} \int \left(\ln \mathring{f}(x) - \ln g(x; \boldsymbol{\theta}) \right) \mathring{f}(x), \mathrm{d}x$$

$$= \underset{\boldsymbol{\theta}}{\mathrm{argmax}} \int \mathring{f}(x) \ln g(x; \boldsymbol{\theta}) \, \mathrm{d}x = \underset{\boldsymbol{\theta}}{\mathrm{argmax}} \, \mathbb{E} \ln g(X; \boldsymbol{\theta}),$$

then $g^{\mathcal{G}} = g(\cdot; \boldsymbol{\theta}^*)$ and learning $g^{\mathcal{G}}$ is equivalent to learning (or estimating) $\boldsymbol{\theta}^*$. To learn $\boldsymbol{\theta}^*$ from the training set τ, we then minimize the training loss:

$$\frac{1}{n} \sum_{i=1}^{n} \mathrm{Loss}(\mathring{f}(x_i), g(x_i; \boldsymbol{\theta})) = -\frac{1}{n} \sum_{i=1}^{n} \ln g(x_i; \boldsymbol{\theta}) + \frac{1}{n} \sum_{i=1}^{n} \ln \mathring{f}(x_i),$$

giving

$$\widehat{\boldsymbol{\theta}}_n \overset{\mathrm{def}}{=} \underset{\boldsymbol{\theta}}{\mathrm{argmax}} \, \frac{1}{n} \sum_{i=1}^{n} \ln g(x_i; \boldsymbol{\theta}) . \tag{6.25}$$

As the logarithm is an increasing function, this is equivalent to

$$\widehat{\boldsymbol{\theta}}_n = \underset{\boldsymbol{\theta}}{\mathrm{argmax}} \prod_{i=1}^{n} g(x_i; \boldsymbol{\theta}),$$

where $\prod_{i=1}^{n} g(x_i; \boldsymbol{\theta})$ is the likelihood of the data under the model that $X_1, \dots, X_n \sim_{\mathrm{iid}} g(\cdot; \boldsymbol{\theta})$. We therefore have recovered the maximum likelihood estimate of $\boldsymbol{\theta}^*$. Note that this reasoning still holds even if the class $\mathcal{G}$ does not contain the true $\mathring{f}$.

6.3.1 Score Intervals

The score function is not only valuable for finding point estimates, but can also be used to construct confidence intervals. The key observation here is that for large iid samples, the score is approximately normally distributed; see Theorem 6.3. Let us concentrate on the one-dimensional case; that is, θ is real-valued.

Let $\boldsymbol{X} = [X_1, \ldots, X_n]^\top \sim_{\text{iid}} \mathring{f}(\cdot\,; \theta)$ and let $S(\theta; \boldsymbol{X})$ denote the score. By Theorem 6.3, the pivot variable $S(\theta; \boldsymbol{X})(n\mathring{I}(\theta))^{-1/2}$ has approximately a standard normal distribution, and hence

$$\left\{ \theta : -z_{1-\alpha/2} < \frac{S(\theta; \boldsymbol{X})}{\sqrt{n\mathring{I}(\theta)}} < z_{1-\alpha/2} \right\}$$

is an approximate $1 - \alpha$ stochastic **confidence set**. We use here "set" instead of "interval" because this set need not be an interval in general.

Example 6.16 (Score Interval for Iid Bernoulli Data). Let $\boldsymbol{X}$ be an iid sample from $\mathsf{Ber}(p)$. Since the Bernoulli distribution is a special case of the binomial distribution, we can use (6.10) in combination with Theorem 6.1 to find the score $S(p; \boldsymbol{X}) = \sum_{i=1}^{n}(X_i - p)/(p(1-p)) = n(\overline{X} - p)/(p(1-p))$. By a similar reasoning, we find the information number $I(p) = n/(p(1-p))$. So the confidence set becomes:

$$\left\{ p : -z_{1-\alpha/2} < \frac{n(\overline{X} - p)}{p(1-p)} \times \sqrt{\frac{p(1-p)}{n}} < z_{1-\alpha/2} \right\}$$

$$= \left\{ p : -a < \frac{\overline{X} - p}{\sqrt{p(1-p)/n}} < a \right\},$$

where we have abbreviated $z_{1-\alpha/2}$ to a. By solving with respect to p the quadratic equation

$$(\overline{X} - p)^2 = a^2\, p(1-p)/n\ ,$$

this confidence set can be written as the interval $\{T_1 < p < T_2\}$ with

$$T_1 = \frac{a^2 + 2n\overline{X} - a\sqrt{a^2 - 4n(\overline{X} - 1)\overline{X}}}{2\,(a^2 + n)}$$

$$T_2 = \frac{a^2 + 2n\overline{X} + a\sqrt{a^2 - 4n(\overline{X} - 1)\overline{X}}}{2\,(a^2 + n)}\ .$$

This **score interval** has much better coverage behavior than the "standard" confidence interval (5.24) over the complete range of p.

6.3.2 Properties of the ML Estimator

An important property of the maximum likelihood estimator is that it is *invariant* under transformations.

> **Theorem 6.6. (Invariance of the MLE).** Suppose $\boldsymbol{X} \sim f(\boldsymbol{x}; \boldsymbol{\theta})$. Let $\widehat{\boldsymbol{\theta}}$ be the MLE of $\boldsymbol{\theta}$ and let $\boldsymbol{g}$ be an invertible function. Then the MLE of $\boldsymbol{\eta} = \boldsymbol{g}(\boldsymbol{\theta})$ is $\widehat{\boldsymbol{\eta}} = \boldsymbol{g}(\widehat{\boldsymbol{\theta}})$.

Proof. Let $L(\boldsymbol{\theta}) = f(\boldsymbol{x}; \boldsymbol{\theta})$ be the likelihood function, and let $\widetilde{L}(\boldsymbol{\eta}) = L(\boldsymbol{g}^{-1}(\boldsymbol{\eta}))$ be the reparameterized likelihood function. The MLE of $\boldsymbol{\eta}$ is, by definition, that number $\widehat{\boldsymbol{\eta}}$ for which $\widetilde{L}(\widehat{\boldsymbol{\eta}})$ is maximal. Since L is maximal for $\boldsymbol{\theta} = \widehat{\boldsymbol{\theta}}$, the function $L(\boldsymbol{g}^{-1}(\boldsymbol{\eta}))$ is maximal at $\widehat{\boldsymbol{\eta}}$ for which $\boldsymbol{g}^{-1}(\widehat{\boldsymbol{\eta}}) = \widehat{\boldsymbol{\theta}}$; which gives $\widehat{\boldsymbol{\eta}} = \boldsymbol{g}(\widehat{\boldsymbol{\theta}})$. $\qquad\square$

Remark 6.2. If $\boldsymbol{g}$ is not invertible, then we can still *define* the MLE of $\boldsymbol{\eta}$ as $\widehat{\boldsymbol{\eta}} = \boldsymbol{g}(\widehat{\boldsymbol{\theta}})$. In effect, this amounts to defining $\widetilde{L}(\boldsymbol{\eta}) = \max_{\boldsymbol{\theta}:\boldsymbol{g}(\boldsymbol{\theta})=\boldsymbol{\eta}} L(\boldsymbol{\theta}; \boldsymbol{x})$.

Next, we consider the case where $\boldsymbol{X} = [X_1, \ldots, X_n]^\top$ is an iid sample from some pdf $\mathring{f}(x; \boldsymbol{\theta})$. Let $\widehat{\boldsymbol{\theta}}$ be the ML estimator of $\boldsymbol{\theta}$. The random variable $\widehat{\boldsymbol{\theta}}$ has some nice asymptotic properties.

> **Theorem 6.7. (Consistency of the MLE).** The ML estimator $\widehat{\boldsymbol{\theta}}$ is **consistent**. That is, with probability tending to 1 as $n \to \infty$, the likelihood equation has a root $\widehat{\boldsymbol{\theta}}$ such that for *all* $\varepsilon > 0$
>
> $$\mathbb{P}(\|\widehat{\boldsymbol{\theta}} - \boldsymbol{\theta}\| > \varepsilon) \to 0 \,.$$

Proof. (Sketch.) Let C_a be a sphere with radius a centered at the true parameter $\boldsymbol{\theta}$. We want to show that for sufficiently small a the probability tends to 1 that
$$l(\boldsymbol{\theta}) > l(\widetilde{\boldsymbol{\theta}})$$
at all points $\widetilde{\boldsymbol{\theta}}$ on the surface of C_a. This can be established as follows. A second-order Taylor expansion of $l(\boldsymbol{\theta})$ around $\boldsymbol{\theta}$, divided by n, yields:

☞ 477

$$\frac{1}{n}(l(\widetilde{\boldsymbol{\theta}}; \boldsymbol{X}) - l(\boldsymbol{\theta}; \boldsymbol{X})) =$$
$$\frac{1}{n}\boldsymbol{S}(\boldsymbol{\theta}; \boldsymbol{X})^\top(\widetilde{\boldsymbol{\theta}} - \boldsymbol{\theta}) + \frac{1}{n}\frac{1}{2}(\widetilde{\boldsymbol{\theta}} - \boldsymbol{\theta})^\top \mathbf{H}(\boldsymbol{\theta}; \boldsymbol{X})(\widetilde{\boldsymbol{\theta}} - \boldsymbol{\theta}) + \frac{1}{n}R_n, \qquad (6.26)$$

where $S(\theta; X)$ is the gradient of l (i.e., the score), $\mathbf{H}(\theta; X)$ is the Hessian matrix of l (i.e., the matrix of partial derivatives $(\partial^2 l/\partial\theta_i\partial\theta_j)$), and R_n a random remainder term. By Theorem 6.3, $S(\theta; X)/n$ converges to the zero vector. Similarly, by Theorem 6.1, $\mathbf{H}(\theta; X)$ can be written as the iid sum $\sum_{k=1}^n \mathring{\mathbf{H}}(\theta; X_k)$, where $\mathring{\mathbf{H}}(\theta; X_k)$ denotes the matrix of partial derivatives $(\partial^2 \mathring{l}(\theta; X_k)/\partial\theta_i\partial\theta_j)$. Hence, by the law of large numbers and (6.13),

☞ 174
☞ 17

$$\frac{1}{n}\mathbf{H}(\theta; X) \to \mathbb{E}_\theta\mathring{\mathbf{H}}(\theta; X) = -\mathring{\mathbf{I}}(\theta) \tag{6.27}$$

as $n \to \infty$, where $\mathring{\mathbf{I}}$ is the information matrix corresponding to $\mathring{f}$. Thus, the first and second term in (6.26) converge to 0 and $-\frac{1}{2}(\widetilde{\theta} - \theta)^\top\mathring{\mathbf{I}}(\theta)(\widetilde{\theta} - \theta)$ respectively as $n \to \infty$. Since the information matrix is positive definite (i.e., $w^\top\mathring{\mathbf{I}}(\theta)w > 0$ for any vector w), the second term is strictly negative. If the remainder term, which depends on the third derivative of l, can be bounded in norm by a constant times a^3/n, then with probability tending to 1 the right-hand side will be less than 0 for a small enough, proving the assertion that $l(\theta) > l(\widetilde{\theta})$ on the surface of the sphere C_a. From this we can conclude that with probability tending to 1, there must be an MLE $\widehat{\theta}$ that lies inside C_a. For a sequence of $a_n \to 0$, we can thus find a sequence of $\widehat{\theta}_n \to \theta$, showing the consistency of the estimator. $\qquad\square$

Note that the above theorem only says that there *exists* a sequence of MLEs $\{\widehat{\theta}_n\}$ that converge (in probability) to the true θ. When there are multiple local maxima, a particular sequence $\widehat{\theta}_n$ may in fact converge to a local maximum.

Theorem 6.8. (Asymptotic Distribution of the MLE). Suppose that $\{\widehat{\theta}_n\}$ is a sequence of consistent ML estimators for θ. Then, $\sqrt{n}(\widehat{\theta}_n - \theta)$ converges in distribution to a $\mathcal{N}(0, \mathring{\mathbf{I}}^{-1}(\theta))$-distributed random vector as $n \to \infty$. In other words,

$$\widehat{\theta}_n \overset{\text{approx.}}{\sim} \mathcal{N}(\theta, \mathring{\mathbf{I}}^{-1}(\theta)/n) \, .$$

Proof. A sketch of the proof for the one-dimensional case (thus, $\theta = \theta$ is a scalar) is as follows. The key idea is again to take a Taylor expansion; this time a Taylor expansion of $l'(\widehat{\theta}_n)$ around θ:

$$l'(\widehat{\theta}_n) = l'(\theta) + (\widehat{\theta}_n - \theta)l''(\theta) + \frac{1}{2}(\widehat{\theta}_n - \theta)^2 l'''(\theta^*) \, ,$$

where θ^* lies between θ and $\widehat{\theta}_n$. Since, $l'(\widehat{\theta}_n) = 0$ (by definition), it follows that

$$\sqrt{n}(\widehat{\theta}_n - \theta) = \frac{l'(\theta)/\sqrt{n}}{-l''(\theta)/n - (\widehat{\theta}_n - \theta)l'''(\theta^*)/(2n)} \, . \qquad (6.28)$$

The numerator in the right-hand side of (6.28) is $S(\theta; \boldsymbol{X})/\sqrt{n}$, which by Theorem 6.3 has approximately a $\mathcal{N}(0, \mathring{I}(\theta))$ distribution for large n. The first term of the denominator is $-\frac{1}{n} \sum_{i=1}^{n} \mathring{H}(\theta; X_i)$, which by the law of large numbers converges to $\mathring{I}(\theta)$ (see (6.27)). The second term of the denominator goes to 0 by the consistency property. This shows that either side of (6.28) is approximately $\mathcal{N}(\theta, \mathring{I}^{-1}(\theta))$-distributed. $\qquad \Box$

Example 6.17 (Asymptotic Distribution of the Binomial MLE). Let us check if this theorem makes sense for the case where $X_1, \ldots, X_n$ are iid and $\mathsf{Ber}(p)$ distributed. Here the MLE is $\overline{X}$ and the information number for $\mathsf{Ber}(p)$ is $1/(p(1-p))$ (see (6.11) with $n = 1$). Theorem 6.8 states that for large n

$$\overline{X} \overset{\text{approx.}}{\sim} \mathcal{N}\left(p, \frac{p(1-p)}{n}\right),$$

which follows also directly from the normal approximation to the binomial distribution by noting that $n\overline{X} \sim \mathsf{Bin}(n, p)$.

☞ 92

6.4 Likelihood Methods in Statistical Tests

The likelihood does not only provide a systematic way of defining good estimators (via the maximum likelihood principle), it also yields a systematic way of finding test statistics.

Let $X_1, \ldots, X_n$ be an iid sample from a distribution with unknown parameter $\boldsymbol{\theta}$. Write $\boldsymbol{X}$ for the corresponding random vector, and let $L(\boldsymbol{\theta}; \boldsymbol{x})$ be the likelihood function for a given outcome $\boldsymbol{x}$ of $\boldsymbol{X}$. Let Θ be set of possible values for $\boldsymbol{\theta}$. Suppose Θ_0 and Θ_1 are two nonoverlapping subsets of Θ such that $\Theta_0 \cup \Theta_1 = \Theta$. Consider the following hypotheses:

$$H_0 : \boldsymbol{\theta} \in \Theta_0 \, ,$$
$$H_1 : \boldsymbol{\theta} \in \Theta_1 \, .$$

Definition 6.5. (Generalized Likelihood Ratio). The **generalized likelihood ratio** is defined as the number

$$\lambda = \frac{M_0(\boldsymbol{x})}{M(\boldsymbol{x})} \overset{\text{def}}{=} \frac{\max_{\boldsymbol{\theta} \in \Theta_0} L(\boldsymbol{\theta}; \boldsymbol{x})}{\max_{\boldsymbol{\theta} \in \Theta} L(\boldsymbol{\theta}; \boldsymbol{x})} \, .$$

Note that $M(\boldsymbol{x}) = L(\widehat{\boldsymbol{\theta}}; \boldsymbol{x})$, where $\widehat{\boldsymbol{\theta}}$ is the ML estimate of $\boldsymbol{\theta}$. Let Λ denote the random generalized likelihood ratio obtained by substituting $\boldsymbol{X}$ for $\boldsymbol{x}$. We can use Λ as a test statistic for testing the above hypotheses. The general principle is to *reject H_0* if Λ is *too small* (left one-sided test). To determine the corresponding p-value $\mathbb{P}(\Lambda \le \lambda)$, we need to know the distribution of Λ under H_0. This is in general a difficult task. However, it is sometimes possible to derive the distribution of a *function* of Λ under H_0, which is then taken as an equivalent test statistic. The new rejection region is no longer necessarily left one-sided.

☞ 14

Example 6.18 (Generalized Likelihood Ratio Test for Iid Normal Data). Suppose $X_1, \ldots, X_n \sim_{\text{iid}} \mathcal{N}(\mu, \sigma^2)$, with μ and σ^2 unknown. We wish to test:

$$H_0 : \mu = \mu_0 \ ,$$
$$H_1 : \mu \ne \mu_0 \ .$$

Hence, $\Theta_0 = \{(\mu_0, \sigma^2), \sigma^2 > 0\}$. The random likelihood function is given by

$$L(\mu, \sigma^2; \boldsymbol{X}) = \left(\frac{1}{2\pi\sigma^2}\right)^{n/2} \exp\left(-\frac{1}{2}\sum_{i=1}^{n}\frac{(X_i - \mu)^2}{\sigma^2}\right).$$

Maximizing L (or $\ln L$) over Θ gives the maximum likelihood estimator $(\widehat{\mu}, \widehat{\sigma^2}) = (\overline{X}, \sum_{i=1}^{n}(X_i - \overline{X})^2/n)$. Hence, $M(\boldsymbol{X}) = L(\widehat{\mu}, \widehat{\sigma^2}; \boldsymbol{X})$. Optimizing L over Θ_0 gives the estimator $(\mu_0, \widetilde{\sigma^2})$, with

$$\widetilde{\sigma^2} = \frac{1}{n}\sum_{i=1}^{n}(X_i - \mu_0)^2 \ .$$

Consequently,

$$\Lambda = \frac{L(\mu_0, \widetilde{\sigma^2}; \boldsymbol{X})}{L(\widehat{\mu}, \widehat{\sigma^2}; \boldsymbol{X})} = \left(\frac{\sum_{i=1}^{n}(X_i - \overline{X})^2}{\sum_{i=1}^{n}(X_i - \mu_0)^2}\right)^{n/2} = \left(1 + \frac{1}{n-1}T^2\right)^{-n/2},$$

where $T = \frac{\overline{X} - \mu_0}{S/\sqrt{n}}$ and S is the sample standard deviation. Rejecting H_0 for small values of Λ is equivalent to rejecting H_0 for large values of $|T|$. By (5.18), T has a t_{n-1} distribution under H_0.

☞ 13

Theorem 6.9. (Asymptotic Distribution of the Generalized Likelihood Ratio). For a k-dimensional parameter space (thus, $\boldsymbol{\theta} = [\theta_1, \ldots, \theta_k]^\top$), if the null hypothesis has only one value $H_0 : \boldsymbol{\theta} = \boldsymbol{\theta}_0$ and the alternative hypothesis is $H_1 : \boldsymbol{\theta} \neq \boldsymbol{\theta}_0$, then for large n (under some mild regularity conditions, which are satisfied for exponential families):

$$- 2\ln\Lambda \overset{\text{approx.}}{\sim} \chi^2_k \; .$$

☞ 477   *Proof.* (Sketch.) This is again an exercise in Taylor expansions. Let $\widehat{\boldsymbol{\theta}}$ be the MLE of $\boldsymbol{\theta}$ and let $l(\boldsymbol{\theta})$ be the log-likelihood function. Under H_0

$$- 2\ln\Lambda = -2(l(\boldsymbol{\theta}_0) - l(\widehat{\boldsymbol{\theta}})) \; .$$

A second-order Taylor expansion at $\boldsymbol{\theta}_0$ around $\widehat{\boldsymbol{\theta}}$ gives:

$$l(\boldsymbol{\theta}_0) = l(\widehat{\boldsymbol{\theta}}) + (\nabla l(\widehat{\boldsymbol{\theta}}))^\top (\widehat{\boldsymbol{\theta}} - \boldsymbol{\theta}_0) + \frac{1}{2}(\widehat{\boldsymbol{\theta}} - \boldsymbol{\theta}_0)^\top \nabla^2 l(\widehat{\boldsymbol{\theta}})(\widehat{\boldsymbol{\theta}} - \boldsymbol{\theta}_0) + \mathcal{O}(\|\widehat{\boldsymbol{\theta}} - \boldsymbol{\theta}_0\|^3) \; .$$

Because $\nabla l(\widehat{\boldsymbol{\theta}}) = \mathbf{0}$ and $\nabla^2 l(\widehat{\boldsymbol{\theta}}) \approx -\mathbf{I}(\boldsymbol{\theta}_0)$, where $\mathbf{I}$ is the information matrix (of dimension k), we have:

$$- 2\ln\Lambda \approx (\widehat{\boldsymbol{\theta}} - \boldsymbol{\theta}_0)^\top \mathbf{I}(\boldsymbol{\theta}_0)(\widehat{\boldsymbol{\theta}} - \boldsymbol{\theta}_0) \; .$$

By Theorem 6.8, $\widehat{\boldsymbol{\theta}} - \boldsymbol{\theta}_0$ has approximately a $\mathcal{N}(\mathbf{0}, \mathbf{I}^{-1}(\boldsymbol{\theta}_0))$ distribution. Thus, for a large sample size, we have that $-2\ln\Lambda$ is approximately distributed as

☞ 87 $\boldsymbol{X}^\top \mathbf{I}(\boldsymbol{\theta}_0)\boldsymbol{X}$ with $\boldsymbol{X} \sim \mathcal{N}(\mathbf{0}, \mathbf{I}^{-1}(\boldsymbol{\theta}_0))$. From Theorem 3.9 it follows now that $-2\ln\Lambda$ has approximately a χ^2_k distribution.   □

6.5 Newton–Raphson Method

Recall that likelihood maximization often involves solving $\boldsymbol{S}(\boldsymbol{\theta}) = \boldsymbol{S}(\boldsymbol{\theta}; \boldsymbol{x}) = \mathbf{0}$, where $\boldsymbol{S}(\boldsymbol{\theta})$ is the score function and $\boldsymbol{\theta}$ a k-dimensional parameter vector. The maximum likelihood estimate $\widehat{\boldsymbol{\theta}}$ is the solution to this equation; that is, it is the root of $\boldsymbol{S}(\boldsymbol{\theta})$. It is often not possible to find $\widehat{\boldsymbol{\theta}}$ in an explicit form. In that case one needs to solve the equation $\boldsymbol{S}(\boldsymbol{\theta}) = \mathbf{0}$ *numerically*. There exist many standard techniques for root-finding. A well-known method is the **Newton–Raphson** procedure. This is an iterative procedure where, starting from a guess $\boldsymbol{\theta}$, a "better" guess is obtained by approximating the score via a linear function. More precisely, suppose that $\boldsymbol{\theta}$ is our initial guess for $\widehat{\boldsymbol{\theta}}$ (the

root of $\boldsymbol{S}$). If $\widehat{\boldsymbol{\theta}}$ is reasonably close to $\boldsymbol{\theta}$, a first-order Taylor approximation   ☞ 47?
of $S_i = \partial l/\partial\theta_i$ around $\boldsymbol{\theta}$ gives:

$$S_i(\widehat{\boldsymbol{\theta}}) \approx S_i(\boldsymbol{\theta}) + [\nabla S_i(\boldsymbol{\theta})]^\top (\widehat{\boldsymbol{\theta}} - \boldsymbol{\theta}), \quad i = 1,\ldots,k\ ,$$

or in matrix notation:

$$\boldsymbol{S}(\widehat{\boldsymbol{\theta}}) \approx \boldsymbol{S}(\boldsymbol{\theta}) + \mathbf{H}(\boldsymbol{\theta})(\widehat{\boldsymbol{\theta}} - \boldsymbol{\theta})\ ,$$

where $\mathbf{H}$ is the Hessian of the log-likelihood, that is, the matrix of second-order partial derivatives of l. Since $\boldsymbol{S}(\widehat{\boldsymbol{\theta}}) = \mathbf{0}$ by definition, we have:

$$\widehat{\boldsymbol{\theta}} \approx \boldsymbol{\theta} - \mathbf{H}^{-1}(\boldsymbol{\theta})\,\boldsymbol{S}(\boldsymbol{\theta})\ .$$

This suggests the following **Newton–Raphson** recursion for finding successively better guesses $\boldsymbol{\theta}_1, \boldsymbol{\theta}_2, \ldots$ converging to $\widehat{\boldsymbol{\theta}}$:

$$\boldsymbol{\theta}_{t+1} = \boldsymbol{\theta}_t - \mathbf{H}^{-1}(\boldsymbol{\theta}_t)\,\boldsymbol{S}(\boldsymbol{\theta}_t)\ . \tag{6.29}$$

The sequence of successive values is guaranteed to converge to the actual root, provided the function is smooth enough (e.g., has continuous second-order derivatives) and the initial guess is close enough to the root.

Notice that $\mathbf{H}(\boldsymbol{\theta}) = \mathbf{H}(\boldsymbol{\theta}; \boldsymbol{x})$ depends on the parameter $\boldsymbol{\theta}$ and the data $\boldsymbol{x}$, and may be quite complicated. On the other hand, the expectation of $\mathbf{H}(\boldsymbol{\theta}; \boldsymbol{X})$ under $\boldsymbol{\theta}$ is simply the negative of information matrix $\mathbf{I}(\boldsymbol{\theta})$, which does not depend on the data. This suggests the alternative iterative scheme, called **Fisher's scoring method**:

$$\boldsymbol{\theta}_{t+1} = \boldsymbol{\theta}_t + \mathbf{I}^{-1}(\boldsymbol{\theta}_t)\,\boldsymbol{S}(\boldsymbol{\theta}_t)\ , \tag{6.30}$$

which may be much easier to implement if the information matrix can be readily evaluated.

Example 6.19 (MLE for Iid Normal Data). Suppose $\boldsymbol{x} = [x_1,\ldots,x_n]^\top$ is the outcome of an iid sample from the $\mathcal{N}(\mu,\sigma^2)$ distribution (both parameters unknown). The score function is given in (6.5)–(6.6). From (6.14) we   ☞ 17?
find that the Hessian matrix is given by   ☞ 17?

$$\mathbf{H}(\mu,\sigma^2;\boldsymbol{x}) = \sum_{i=1}^{n} \mathring{\mathbf{H}}(\mu,\sigma^2;x_i) = \sum_{i=1}^{n} \begin{bmatrix} -\frac{1}{\sigma^2} & -\frac{x_i-\mu}{(\sigma^2)^2} \\ -\frac{x_i-\mu}{(\sigma^2)^2} & \frac{1}{2\sigma^4} - \frac{(x_i-\mu)^2}{(\sigma^2)^3} \end{bmatrix},$$

where $\mathring{\mathbf{H}}(\mu,\sigma^2;x)$ is the Hessian for the one-dimensional case. Apart from a starting value, this is all that is required to carry out the Newton–Raphson iteration (6.29). It is easier, however, to apply the recursion (6.30), using the exact expression for the information matrix (see (6.15)):   ☞ 17?

$$\mathbf{I}^{-1}(\mu, \sigma^2) = \left(n\mathring{\mathbf{I}}(\mu, \sigma^2) \right)^{-1} = \frac{1}{n} \begin{bmatrix} \sigma^2 & 0 \\ 0 & 2\sigma^4 \end{bmatrix} .$$

It follows that the Newton–Raphson procedure (6.30) involves the following iterative steps:

$$\mu_{t+1} = \mu_t + \frac{1}{n}\sigma_t^2 \sum_{i=1}^{n} \frac{(x_i - \mu_t)}{\sigma_t^2} = \mu_t + \frac{1}{n}\sum_{i=1}^{n}(x_i - \mu_t) = \overline{x}$$

$$\sigma_{t+1}^2 = \sigma_t^2 + \frac{2}{n}\sigma_t^4 \left(\frac{-n}{2\sigma_t^2} + \frac{1}{2}\sum_{i=1}^{n} \frac{(x_i - \mu_t)^2}{\sigma_t^4} \right) = \frac{1}{n}\sum_{i=1}^{n}(x_i - \mu_t)^2 .$$

Note that, starting from any initial guess, after only two steps, we get $\mu_t = \overline{x}$ and $\sigma_t^2 = \frac{1}{n}\sum_{i=1}^{n}(x_i - \overline{x})^2$, which are the MLEs for μ and σ^2.

Example 6.20 (MLE for the Radioactive Source Detection Example). Let us return to Example 6.3. Suppose we want to find the most likely estimate for the position a of the source. The log-likelihood function is

☞ 169

$$l(a; \boldsymbol{x}) = -n \ln \pi - \sum_{i=1}^{n} \ln(1 + (x_i - a)^2) .$$

Taking the derivative with respect to a gives the score function:

$$S(a; \boldsymbol{x}) = \sum_{i=1}^{n} \frac{2(x_i - a)}{1 + (x_i - a)^2} .$$

The information number is of form $I(a) = n\mathring{I}(a)$, where $\mathring{I}$ is the information number for a single sample. Specifically,

$$\mathring{I}(a) = \mathbb{E}_a S^2(a; X) = \int_{-\infty}^{\infty} \frac{4(x - a)^2}{(1 + (x - a)^2)^2} \frac{1}{\pi(1 + (x - a)^2)} \, \mathrm{d}x$$

$$= \int_{-\infty}^{\infty} \frac{4y^2}{\pi(1 + y^2)^3} \, \mathrm{d}y \qquad \text{(change of variable } y = x - a\text{)}$$

$$= \frac{1}{2} .$$

Thus, the information number is constant; this is in agreement with the fact that we are dealing here with a location family of distributions; see Example 6.11. Now (6.30) leads to the scheme:

$$a_{t+1} = a_t + \frac{2}{n}\sum_{i=1}^{n} \frac{2(x_i - a_t)}{1 + (x_i - a_t)^2} .$$

This is implemented in the following Julia code.

```
lighthousemle.jl
```
```julia
x = [1.3615 3.5616 -14.2411 -4.4950 2.3014 1.1066 -9.3409
    0.3779 0.9386 -0.1838]; # the data
a = 2; # initial guess
n = 10;
for i=1:7
  println(a)
  global a = a + 4*sum( (x .- a)./(1 .+ (x .- a).^2) )/n
  # note the vectorization!
end
```
```
2
1.2625662007001668
0.9535905615030806
0.9653773555988199
0.9647755245520702
0.9648071279192287
0.9648054705999485
```

Thus, the MLE is $\widehat{a} = 0.9648$, which is remarkably close to the true value $a = 1$.

6.6 Expectation–Maximization (EM) Algorithm

Another useful numerical method for likelihood maximization is the **expectation–maximization** (EM) algorithm.

Suppose that, for a given vector of observations $\boldsymbol{x} = [x_1, \ldots, x_n]^\top$, we wish to compute the maximum likelihood estimate:

$$\widehat{\boldsymbol{\theta}} = \operatorname*{argmax}_{\boldsymbol{\theta}} L(\boldsymbol{\theta}; \boldsymbol{x}) , \tag{6.31}$$

where $L(\boldsymbol{\theta}; \boldsymbol{x}) = f(\boldsymbol{x}; \boldsymbol{\theta})$ is the likelihood function.

One could use a root-finding routine, such as the Newton–Raphson method described in Sect. 6.5, to obtain $\widehat{\boldsymbol{\theta}}$. However, for many problems, computing the score function and the Hessian matrix analytically—required by the Newton–Raphson method—might be difficult. Instead of maximizing the likelihood function directly, the EM algorithm augments the data $\boldsymbol{x}$ with a suitable vector of *latent* (or hidden) variables $\boldsymbol{z}$ such that

$$f(\boldsymbol{x}; \boldsymbol{\theta}) = \int \widetilde{f}(\boldsymbol{x}, \boldsymbol{z}; \boldsymbol{\theta}) \, \mathrm{d}\boldsymbol{z} .$$

The function of $\boldsymbol{\theta}$

$$\widetilde{L}(\boldsymbol{\theta}; \boldsymbol{x}, \boldsymbol{z}) = \widetilde{f}(\boldsymbol{x}, \boldsymbol{z}; \boldsymbol{\theta})$$

is usually referred to as the **complete-data likelihood** function. The main advantage of the data augmentation step is that it is often possible to introduce latent variables z in such a way that the maximization of the complete-data likelihood $\widetilde{L}(\boldsymbol{\theta}; \boldsymbol{x}, \boldsymbol{z})$ or log-likelihood $\widetilde{l}(\boldsymbol{\theta}; \boldsymbol{x}, \boldsymbol{z}) = \ln \widetilde{L}(\boldsymbol{\theta}; \boldsymbol{x}, \boldsymbol{z})$ is much easier than maximizing the original likelihood $L(\boldsymbol{\theta}; \boldsymbol{x})$ or log-likelihood $l(\boldsymbol{\theta}; \boldsymbol{x}) = \ln L(\boldsymbol{\theta}; \boldsymbol{x})$.

Of course, the latent variables z are not observed, and neither $\widetilde{L}(\boldsymbol{\theta}; \boldsymbol{x}, \boldsymbol{z})$ nor $\widetilde{l}(\boldsymbol{\theta}; \boldsymbol{x}, \boldsymbol{z})$ are available. One feasible approach is to replace it with the expectation $\mathbb{E}_g \widetilde{l}(\boldsymbol{\theta}; \boldsymbol{x}, \boldsymbol{Z})$ with respect to a suitable density $g(\boldsymbol{z})$. It can be shown (see Problem 6.20) that for all $\boldsymbol{\theta}$ and any density g,

$$\ln f(\boldsymbol{x}; \boldsymbol{\theta}) \geq \mathcal{L}(g, \boldsymbol{\theta}) \overset{\text{def}}{=} \int g(\boldsymbol{z}) \ln \left(\frac{\widetilde{f}(\boldsymbol{x}, \boldsymbol{z}; \boldsymbol{\theta})}{g(\boldsymbol{z})} \right) \mathrm{d}\boldsymbol{z} \tag{6.32}$$
$$= \mathbb{E}_g \widetilde{l}(\boldsymbol{\theta}; \boldsymbol{x}, \boldsymbol{Z}) - \mathbb{E}_g \ln g(\boldsymbol{Z}) .$$

That is, $\mathcal{L}(g, \boldsymbol{\theta})$ is a lower bound for the log-likelihood $l(\boldsymbol{\theta}; \boldsymbol{x})$. In addition, this lower bound is attained (see Problem 6.20) for

$$g(\boldsymbol{z}) = \widetilde{f}_{\boldsymbol{Z} \mid \boldsymbol{X}}(\boldsymbol{z} \mid \boldsymbol{x}; \boldsymbol{\theta}) \overset{\text{def}}{=} \frac{\widetilde{f}(\boldsymbol{x}, \boldsymbol{z}; \boldsymbol{\theta})}{\int \widetilde{f}(\boldsymbol{x}, \boldsymbol{z}; \boldsymbol{\theta}) \mathrm{d}\boldsymbol{z}} . \tag{6.33}$$

That is, the lower bound is attained when $g(\boldsymbol{z})$ is taken as the conditional pdf of the latent data $\boldsymbol{Z}$ given the observed data $\boldsymbol{X} = \boldsymbol{x}$.

Algorithm 6.1. (EM Algorithm). Suppose $\boldsymbol{\theta}_0$ is an initial guess for the maximizer. The EM algorithm consists of iterating the following steps for $t = 1, 2, \ldots$.

1. **Expectation Step (E-Step)**: Given the current vector $\boldsymbol{\theta}_{t-1}$ maximize $\mathcal{L}(g, \boldsymbol{\theta}_{t-1})$ as a function of g. It follows from (6.33) that the exact solution is

$$g_t(\boldsymbol{z}) \overset{\text{def}}{=} \widetilde{f}_{\boldsymbol{Z} \mid \boldsymbol{X}}(\boldsymbol{z} \mid \boldsymbol{x}; \boldsymbol{\theta}_{t-1}) .$$

Compute the expected log-likelihood under g_t:

$$Q_t(\boldsymbol{\theta}) \overset{\text{def}}{=} \mathbb{E}_{g_t} \widetilde{l}(\boldsymbol{\theta}; \boldsymbol{x}, \boldsymbol{Z}) . \tag{6.34}$$

2. **Maximization Step (M-Step)**: Maximize $\mathcal{L}(g_t, \boldsymbol{\theta})$ as a function of $\boldsymbol{\theta}$. Since $\mathcal{L}(g_t, \boldsymbol{\theta}) = Q_t(\boldsymbol{\theta}) - \mathbb{E}_{g_t} \ln g_t(\boldsymbol{Z})$, this is equivalent to finding
$$\boldsymbol{\theta}_t = \underset{\boldsymbol{\theta}}{\operatorname{argmax}} \, Q_t(\boldsymbol{\theta}) .$$

3. **Stopping Condition**: If, for example, $|l(\boldsymbol{\theta}_t; \boldsymbol{x}) - l(\boldsymbol{\theta}_{t-1}; \boldsymbol{x})| \leq \varepsilon$ for some small tolerance ε, terminate the algorithm.

A direct consequence of the EM algorithm is that the sequence of log-likelihood values does not decrease with each iteration. In fact, we have:

$$l(\boldsymbol{\theta}_{t-1}; \boldsymbol{x}) = \mathcal{L}(g_t, \boldsymbol{\theta}_{t-1}) \leq \mathcal{L}(g_t, \boldsymbol{\theta}_t) \leq \mathcal{L}(g_{t+1}, \boldsymbol{\theta}_t) = l(\boldsymbol{\theta}_t; \boldsymbol{x}) \,, \qquad (6.35)$$

where the first and last equalities follow from the definitions of $\mathcal{L}$, g_t, and g_{t+1}, whereas the second and third inequalities follow from the M- and E-steps, respectively. Under certain continuity conditions, the sequence $\{\boldsymbol{\theta}_t\}$ is guaranteed to converge to a local maximizer of the log-likelihood ℓ (or the likelihood L). Convergence to a global maximizer (the MLE $\widehat{\boldsymbol{\theta}}$) depends on the appropriate choice for the starting value. Typically, the algorithm is run from different random starting points. Note that (6.35) is useful for debugging computer implementations of the EM algorithm: if likelihood values are observed to decrease at any iteration, then there is an error in the program. For a further discussion of the theoretical and practical aspects of the EM algorithm, we refer to McLachlan and Krishnan (2008). We illustrate the EM algorithm via two examples.

Example 6.21 (EM for the Genetic Linkage Experiment). In a genetic linkage experiment, n animals are randomly assigned (by nature) to four categories according to the multinomial distribution with pdf:

$$f(x_1, x_2, x_3, x_4; \theta) \propto \pi_1^{x_1} \pi_2^{x_2} \pi_3^{x_3} \pi_4^{x_4} \,,$$

where $n = x_1 + x_2 + x_3 + x_4$ and the cell probabilities are $\pi_1 = 1/2 + \theta/4$, $\pi_2 = (1 - \theta)/4$, $\pi_3 = (1 - \theta)/4$, and $\pi_4 = \theta/4$. Suppose the observed data are given as $\boldsymbol{x} = [x_1, x_2, x_3, x_4] = [125, 18, 20, 34]$, and we wish to obtain the maximum likelihood estimate for θ.

It is easy to check that the log-likelihood function is given by

$$l(\theta; \boldsymbol{x}) = x_1 \ln(2 + \theta) + (x_2 + x_3) \ln(1 - \theta) + x_4 \ln \theta + \text{const} \,.$$

The graph of the log-likelihood function (apart from the constant term) is given in Fig. 6.5.

Since this is a univariate problem, the maximum likelihood estimate for θ can be obtained by the grid search or the Newton–Raphson method (see Problem 6.25). In this example we use the EM algorithm to maximize the log-likelihood.

☞ 20

To that end, we augment the observed data as follows: suppose that the first of the original four multinomial cells could be split into two subcells having probabilities $1/2$ and $\theta/4$, respectively. Let Z and $X_1 - Z$ be the corresponding split of X_1, and note that Z is not observed. Now the random vector $[Z, X_1 - Z, X_2, X_3, X_4]$ has a multinomial distribution with the following five cell probabilities:

$$\left[\frac{1}{2}, \frac{\theta}{4}, \frac{1 - \theta}{4}, \frac{1 - \theta}{4}, \frac{\theta}{4} \right] \,,$$

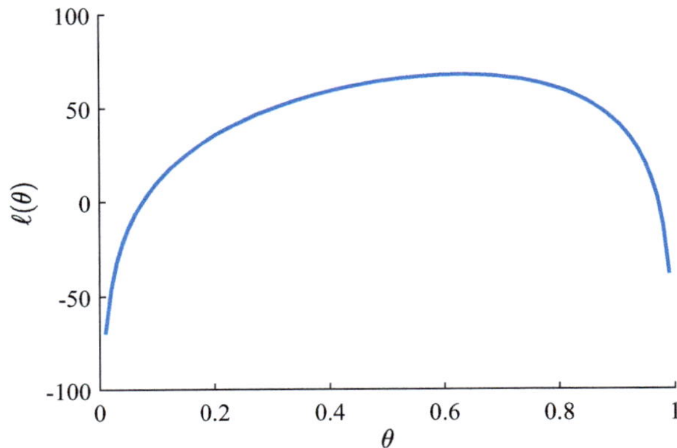

Fig. 6.5 The log-likelihood function for the genetic linkage experiment

and the complete-data log-likelihood can be written as

$$\widetilde{l}(\theta; z, \boldsymbol{x}) = (x_1 - z + x_4)\ln\theta + (x_2 + x_3)\ln(1 - \theta) + \text{const}.$$

Suppose that θ_{t-1} is the current guess for θ. To implement the E-step, we first derive the conditional density $g_t(\boldsymbol{z}) = \widetilde{f}_{\boldsymbol{Z}\mid\boldsymbol{X}}(\boldsymbol{z}\mid\boldsymbol{x};\boldsymbol{\theta}_{t-1})$. Note that given $X_1 = x_1$, Z has a $\mathsf{Bin}(x_1, p)$ distribution, with success probability

$$p = \frac{1/2}{1/2 + \theta_{t-1}/4} = \frac{2}{2 + \theta_{t-1}}.$$

Recall that for $Y \sim \mathsf{Bin}(n, p)$, we have $\mathbb{E}Y = np$. Hence, we have:

$$\mathbb{E}_{g_t} Z = \mathbb{E}[Z \mid X_1 = x_1; \theta_{t-1}] = 2x_1/(2 + \theta_{t-1}).$$

It follows that

$$Q_t(\theta) = \mathbb{E}_{g_t}\widetilde{l}(\theta; Z, \boldsymbol{x}) = \left(x_1 + x_4 - \frac{2x_1}{2 + \theta_{t-1}}\right)\ln\theta + (x_2 + x_3)\ln(1 - \theta) + \text{const}.$$

To implement the M-step, we simply solve $\frac{\mathrm{d}}{\mathrm{d}\theta}Q_t(\theta) = 0$ for θ. It is easy to check that the solution is given by

$$\theta_t = \frac{x_1 + x_4 - 2x_1/(2 + \theta_{t-1})}{n - 2x_1/(2 + \theta_{t-1})}.$$

The following Julia program implements the EM algorithm to find the maximum likelihood estimate for θ, which is estimated to be $\widehat{\theta} = 0.6268$.

```
geneticEM.jl

x = [ 125 18 20 34 ]; n = sum(x);
theta = 4*(x[1]/n-1/2);            # initial guess
err = 1;
while abs(err) > 10^(-5)           # stopping criterion
    z = 2*x[1]/(2+theta);          # E-step
    temp = (x[1]+x[4] - z)/(n-z);  # M-step
    global err = theta - temp;
    global theta = temp;
end
```

In the next example, we illustrate how one can use the EM algorithm for fitting mixture models. A **mixture pdf** is a pdf of the form:

$$f(x) = w_1 f_1(x)+\cdots+w_c\, f_c(x), \quad w_z \geq 0, z = 1,\ldots,c, \quad \sum_{z=1}^{c} w_z = 1 \,, \quad (6.36)$$

where each f_z is itself a pdf. Such a mixture pdf can be thought of in the following way. Consider two random variables, X and Z, where Z takes values $1, 2, \ldots, c$ with probabilities $w_1, \ldots, w_c$, and conditional on $Z = z$, the random variable X has pdf f_z. By the product rule (3.10), the joint pdf of X and Z is given by $f_{X,Z}(x, z) = w_z f_z(x)$, and the marginal pdf of X is found by summing the joint pdf over the values of z—this gives (6.36).   ☞ 72

Example 6.22 (EM for a Gaussian Mixture Model). Let $x_1, \ldots, x_n$ be iid observations drawn from the following *Gaussian* mixture pdf:

$$\mathring{f}(x;\boldsymbol{\theta}) = \sum_{z=1}^{c} \frac{w_z}{\sigma_z}\, \varphi\left(\frac{x - \mu_z}{\sigma_z}\right),$$

where φ is the pdf of the $\mathcal{N}(0,1)$ distribution, $\boldsymbol{\theta}^\top = [\boldsymbol{\mu}, \boldsymbol{\sigma}, \boldsymbol{w}]$ with $\boldsymbol{\mu} = [\mu_1, \ldots, \mu_c]$, $\boldsymbol{\sigma} = [\sigma_1, \ldots, \sigma_c]$, and $\boldsymbol{w} = [w_1, \ldots, w_c]$. The likelihood of $\boldsymbol{x}$ under $\boldsymbol{\theta}$ is

$$L(\boldsymbol{\theta}; \boldsymbol{x}) = f(\boldsymbol{x};\boldsymbol{\theta}) = \prod_{i=1}^{n} \mathring{f}(x_i;\boldsymbol{\theta}) = \prod_{i=1}^{n}\sum_{z=1}^{c} \frac{w_z}{\sigma_z}\, \varphi\left(\frac{x_i - \mu_z}{\sigma_z}\right). \quad (6.37)$$

Such a mixture distribution is often used for modeling unobserved heterogeneity, i.e., the presence of subpopulations that are not identified in the observed data. For example, suppose that x_i is, say, height, of the i-th student in a class. Further suppose that there are both male and female students in the class, but the genders of the students are not recorded. Then, a suitable model for the outcomes is a mixture of two Gaussian distributions.

Direct maximization of the likelihood in (6.37) could be difficult and time-consuming. To simplify the computation, introduce a vector of latent variables $\boldsymbol{Z} = [Z_1, \ldots, Z_n]^\top$, each Z_i taking values in $\{1, 2, \ldots, c\}$ and such that $(X_i \mid Z_i = z_i) \sim \mathcal{N}(\mu_{z_i}, \sigma_{z_i}^2)$. This gives the complete-data likelihood

$$\widetilde{L}(\boldsymbol{\theta}; \boldsymbol{x}, \boldsymbol{z}) = \widetilde{f}(\boldsymbol{x}, \boldsymbol{z}; \boldsymbol{\theta}) = \prod_{i=1}^{n} \frac{w_{z_i}}{\sigma_{z_i}} \, \varphi\left(\frac{x_i - \mu_{z_i}}{\sigma_{z_i}} \right). \tag{6.38}$$

Note that by summing $\widetilde{f}(\boldsymbol{x}, \boldsymbol{z}; \boldsymbol{\theta})$ over all $\boldsymbol{z}$, we obtain $f(\boldsymbol{x}; \boldsymbol{\theta})$. The discussion following (6.36) shows that the latent variable Z_i can be interpreted as the component of the mixture model from which X_i is drawn.

To implement the EM algorithm, suppose that $\boldsymbol{\theta}_{t-1}$ is the current guess for $\boldsymbol{\theta}$. In the E-step we first derive the (discrete) pdf of $\boldsymbol{Z}$ given the data $\boldsymbol{X} = \boldsymbol{x}$:

$$g_t(\boldsymbol{z}) = \widetilde{f}_{\boldsymbol{Z} \mid \boldsymbol{X}}(\boldsymbol{z} \mid \boldsymbol{x}; \boldsymbol{\theta}_{t-1}) \propto \widetilde{f}(\boldsymbol{x}, \boldsymbol{z}; \boldsymbol{\theta}_{t-1}) \,.$$

Thus, to find g_t we view the right-hand side of (6.38) as a function of $\boldsymbol{z} = [z_1, \ldots, z_n]^\top$. It follows that under g_t the components of $\boldsymbol{Z}$ are independent, and each Z_i has a (discrete) pdf

$$g_{t,i}(z) \stackrel{\text{def}}{=} \frac{w_{t-1,z}}{\sigma_{t-1,z}} \, \varphi\left(\frac{x_i - \mu_{t-1,z}}{\sigma_{t-1,z}} \right) \bigg/ \sum_{k=1}^{c} \frac{w_{t-1,k}}{\sigma_{t-1,k}} \, \varphi\left(\frac{x_i - \mu_{t-1,k}}{\sigma_{t-1,k}} \right) \tag{6.39}$$

for $i = 1, \ldots, n$ and $z = 1, \ldots, c$. The expected complete-data likelihood in the E-step is then

$$Q_t(\boldsymbol{\theta}) = \mathbb{E}_{g_t} \widetilde{l}(\boldsymbol{\theta}; \boldsymbol{x}, \boldsymbol{Z}) = \sum_{i=1}^{n} \sum_{z=1}^{c} g_{t,i}(z) \left(\ln w_z - \ln \sigma_z - \frac{(x_i - \mu_z)^2}{2\sigma_z^2} \right) + \text{const} \,.$$

Next, in the M-step, we maximize $Q_t(\boldsymbol{\theta})$ with respect to $\boldsymbol{w}$ (under the constraints $\sum_z w_z = 1$, $w_z \geq 0$ for all z), $\boldsymbol{\mu}$, and $\boldsymbol{\sigma}$. It is easy to check that for $z = 1, \ldots, c$ the solution to $\nabla Q_t(\boldsymbol{\theta}) = \boldsymbol{0}$ is

$$
\begin{aligned}
w_z &= \frac{1}{n} \sum_{i=1}^{n} g_{t,i}(z) \,, \\
\mu_z &= \frac{\sum_{i=1}^{n} g_{t,i}(z) x_i}{\sum_{i=1}^{n} g_{t,i}(z)} \,, \\
\sigma_z^2 &= \frac{\sum_{i=1}^{n} g_{t,i}(z) (x_i - \mu_z)^2}{\sum_{i=1}^{n} g_{t,i}(z)} \,.
\end{aligned}
\tag{6.40}
$$

We then set $\boldsymbol{\theta}_t$ according to the values in (6.40), and keep iterating the E-Step (6.39) and the M-Step (6.40) until convergence is reached.

6.7 Problems

6.1. In a guessing game, Albert chooses a number θ between 0 and 10, and the other people have to guess the number; the person whose guess is closest to θ wins. To facilitate the guesswork, Albert draws seven numbers uniformly from the interval $[0, \theta]$ and displays the results to the others. Suppose these seven values (the observed data) are

$$4.3180,\ 4.8007,\ 0.6730,\ 4.8409,\ 3.3515,\ 0.5170,\ 1.4760\ .$$

a. Give a model for the data $X_1, \ldots, X_7$. Show that $M = \max\{X_1, \ldots, X_7\}$ is a sufficient statistic for θ.
b. Determine the method of moments estimate of θ. Is the corresponding estimator a function of M?
c. Sketch the graph of the likelihood function, and use it to determine the maximum likelihood estimate. Is the corresponding estimator a function of M?
d. Use $T = M/\theta$ as a pivot variable to construct a 95% numerical confidence interval for θ of the form (m, a) for some $a > m$, where $m = \max\{x_1, \ldots, x_7\}$. ☞ 13⁞

6.2. Let $X_1, \ldots, X_n \sim_{\text{iid}} \mathcal{N}(\theta, \theta)$ with an unknown $\theta > 0$. Find the maximum likelihood estimator of θ.

6.3. Consider the general regression model ☞ 10⁞

$$Y_i = g(\boldsymbol{x}_i; \boldsymbol{\beta}) + \varepsilon_i, \quad i = 1, \ldots, n\ , \tag{6.41}$$

where $\varepsilon_1, \ldots, \varepsilon_n \sim_{\text{iid}} \mathcal{N}(0, \sigma^2)$ and $g(\boldsymbol{x}; \boldsymbol{\beta})$ is a known function of the explanatory vector $\boldsymbol{x}$ and the parameter vector $\boldsymbol{\beta}$. Both σ^2 and $\boldsymbol{\beta}$ are assumed to be unknown.

a. Show that the maximum likelihood estimator of $\boldsymbol{\beta}$ is found by minimizing the sum of the squared deviations between the $\{Y_i\}$ and the $\{g(\boldsymbol{x}_i; \boldsymbol{\beta})\}$; that is,

$$\widehat{\boldsymbol{\beta}} = \operatorname*{argmin}_{\boldsymbol{\beta}} \sum_{i=1}^{n} (Y_i - g(\boldsymbol{x}_i; \boldsymbol{\beta}))^2\ .$$

b. Derive the maximum likelihood estimator of σ^2.

6.4. For multidimensional parameters $\boldsymbol{\theta}$, it is sometimes useful to draw one-dimensional graphs for the likelihood function by substituting all parameters *except one* with their maximum likelihood estimates (as a function of the remaining unknown parameter). The function thus obtained is called the **profile likelihood.**

Consider the ten iid samples from the $\mathcal{N}(\mu, \sigma^2)$ distribution given in Example 6.2. ☞ 16⁞

a. Give the formula for the profile likelihood for σ^2.

b. Draw the graph of this profile likelihood. Does its mode correspond to the maximum likelihood estimate of σ^2?

6.5. Let $X_1, \ldots, X_n$ be iid random variables with pdf:

$$f(x; \theta) = (\theta + 1)\, x^\theta, \quad 0 \le x \le 1, \quad \theta > -1 .$$

a. Find the method of moments estimator of θ.

b. Find the maximum likelihood estimator of θ.

6.6. The weight X (in grams) of an egg is $\mathcal{N}(\mu, \sigma^2)$ distributed. Let $\widehat{\mu} = 56.3$ and $\widehat{\sigma} = 7.6$ be the maximum likelihood estimates of μ and σ. Give the maximum likelihood estimate of

$$\mathbb{P}(X > 68.5) .$$

6.7. For $X_1, \ldots, X_n \overset{\text{iid}}{\sim} \mathcal{N}(\mu, \sigma^2)$, let S^2 be the sample variance and let $\widehat{\sigma^2}$ be the maximum likelihood estimator of σ^2.

a. Which of the two is an unbiased estimator of σ^2?

b. Is $\sqrt{S^2}$ an unbiased estimator of σ?

c. Is $\sqrt{\widehat{\sigma^2}}$ the maximum likelihood estimator of σ?

6.8. Let $Y \sim \mathcal{U}(-\pi/2, \pi/2)$ and define $Z = \tan(Y)$. Show, using transformation formula (3.22), that Z has a Cauchy distribution.

☞ 79
☞ 50

6.9. The following iid data, 0.685, 2.586, -1.969, -2.673, 1.464, 2.977, -1.120, 1.594, -0.543, 1.505, -1.266, 1.981, have been drawn from a **double exponential distribution**, with pdf:

$$f(x) = \frac{\lambda}{2}\, e^{-\lambda|x|}, \quad x \in \mathbb{R} .$$

Find the maximum likelihood estimate for λ.

6.10. The **Weibull distribution** with *rate* parameter $\lambda > 0$ and *shape* parameter $\alpha > 0$ has cdf

$$F(x) = 1 - e^{-(\lambda x)^\alpha}, \quad x \ge 0 .$$

Suppose $x_1, \ldots, x_n$ are the outcomes of an iid sample from a Weibull distribution with shape parameter $\alpha = 2$ and unknown rate parameter λ. Find the maximum likelihood estimate of λ.

6.11. Suppose $X_1, \ldots, X_n \sim_{\text{iid}}$ Geom(p). Show that the generalized likelihood ratio method for the hypothesis $H_0 : p = p_0$ versus $H_1 : p \ne p_0$ yields the test statistic:

$$\Lambda = \frac{\left(\dfrac{p_0}{1-p_0}\right)^n (1-p_0)^{(n\overline{X})}}{\left(\dfrac{1/\overline{X}}{1-1/\overline{X}}\right)^n (1-1/\overline{X})^{(n\overline{X})}} .$$

What is the approximate distribution of $-2\ln\Lambda$ for large n?

6.12. Let $X_1,\dots,X_n$ be an iid sample from the $\mathsf{Bin}(k,p)$ distribution, where k is given but $p \in [0,1]$ is unknown.

a. Find the maximum likelihood estimator $\widehat{p}$ of p.
b. Show that $\widehat{p}$ attains the Cramér–Rao lower bound.
c. Sketch the log-likelihood function for the case where $n = 1$, $k = 10$, and $x_1 = 5$.

6.13. Suppose that 100 observations are taken from the $\mathcal{N}(\mu,1)$ distribution with an unknown μ. Instead of recording all the observations, one records only whether the observation is less than 0. Suppose that 40 observations are less than 0. What is the maximum likelihood estimate for μ based on these observations?

6.14. Let $X_1,\dots,X_n$ be an iid sample from the $\mathsf{Exp}(1/v)$ distribution, where $v > 0$ is unknown. Let $\boldsymbol{X} = [X_1,\dots,X_n]^\top$.

a. Find the score $S(v;\boldsymbol{X})$.
b. Give the corresponding Fisher information.
c. Find the maximum likelihood estimator of v.
d. Give the maximum likelihood estimator of $\sin(v)$.

6.15. Let $X_1,\dots,X_n$ be an iid sample from the distribution with pdf $f(x;\theta)$, where

$$f(x;\theta) = \frac{1}{2\,\theta^3}\, x^2\, e^{-x/\theta}, \quad x > 0, \quad \theta > 0 .$$

a. Show that $\mathbb{E}X_i = 3\,\theta$ and $\mathrm{Var}(X_i) = 3\,\theta^2$.
b. Find a sufficient statistic for the parameter θ using the factorization Theorem 5.5.
c. Find the MLE of θ.
d. Find the Fisher information $I(\theta)$.
e. Give the asymptotic distribution of the MLE of θ.
f. What are the bias and the variance of the MLE of θ?
g. Determine whether or not the MLE of θ attains the Cramér–Rao lower bound.

6.16. An iid sample $X_1,\dots,X_n$ is taken from the $\mathcal{N}(0,\theta)$ distribution, where $\theta > 0$ is unknown. We wish to test the hypothesis $H_0 : \theta = 3$ against $H_1 : \theta \neq 3$ using an appropriate test statistic.

a. Show that the likelihood ratio test statistic is here a function of

$$T = \sum_{i=1}^{n} \frac{X_i^2}{3} .$$

b. What is the distribution of T under H_0?

6.17. Verify that the score function corresponding to the observed iid sample $x_1, \ldots, x_n$ from the Gamma(α, λ) distribution is

$$\boldsymbol{S}(\alpha, \lambda) = \begin{bmatrix} n(\ln \lambda - \psi(\alpha)) + \sum_{i=1}^{n} \ln x_i \\ \frac{n\alpha}{\lambda} - \sum_{i=1}^{n} x_i \end{bmatrix} ,$$

and that the corresponding Fisher information matrix is

$$\boldsymbol{I}(\alpha, \lambda) = n \begin{bmatrix} \psi'(\alpha) & -\frac{1}{\lambda} \\ -\frac{1}{\lambda} & \frac{\alpha}{\lambda^2} \end{bmatrix} ,$$

where $\psi'(\alpha)$ is the derivative of the **digamma** function $\psi(x) = \Gamma'(x)/\Gamma(x)$.

6.18. Suppose $x_1, \ldots, x_{10}$ are the outcomes of an iid sample from Exp(θ). Construct a score confidence interval for θ with confidence coefficient 0.90 if the sum of the $\{x_i\}$ is 10.

6.19. Let $X_1, \ldots, X_n$ and $Y_1, \ldots, Y_n$ be independent random samples from the Exp(λ) and Exp(μ) distributions, for unknown λ and μ. Suppose we wish to test the hypothesis $H_0 : \lambda = \mu$ against $H_1 : \lambda \neq \mu$.

a. Find the maximum likelihood estimators for λ and μ.
b. Find the maximum likelihood estimators for $\theta = \lambda = \mu$ under H_0.
c. Show that the following test statistic

$$T = \frac{\sum_{i=1}^{n} Y_i}{\sum_{i=1}^{n} X_i}$$

    can be derived from the generalized likelihood ratio procedure.
d. For large n, T has approximately a normal distribution. Find the param-
☞ 92   eters of this distribution via the delta method.

☞ 119 **6.20.** In (4.27) we introduced the Kullback–Leibler (KL) divergence to measure how far away a pdf g is from a pdf h, via

$$\mathcal{D}(g, h) = \mathbb{E}_g \ln \frac{g(\boldsymbol{X})}{h(\boldsymbol{X})} . \tag{6.42}$$

☞ 190 In the EM algorithm, it is used to derive the inequality (6.32) using the
following decomposition:

$$\ln f(\boldsymbol{x};\boldsymbol{\theta}) = \int g(\boldsymbol{z}) \ln f(\boldsymbol{x};\boldsymbol{\theta})\, \mathrm{d}\boldsymbol{z}$$

$$= \int g(\boldsymbol{z}) \ln \left(\frac{\widetilde{f}(\boldsymbol{x},\boldsymbol{z};\boldsymbol{\theta})/g(\boldsymbol{z})}{\widetilde{f}_{\boldsymbol{Z}|\boldsymbol{X}}(\boldsymbol{z}\,|\,\boldsymbol{x};\boldsymbol{\theta})/g(\boldsymbol{z})} \right) \mathrm{d}\boldsymbol{z}$$

$$= \underbrace{\int g(\boldsymbol{z}) \ln \left(\frac{\widetilde{f}(\boldsymbol{x},\boldsymbol{z};\boldsymbol{\theta})}{g(\boldsymbol{z})} \right) \mathrm{d}\boldsymbol{z}}_{\mathcal{L}(g,\boldsymbol{\theta})} + \mathcal{D}(g, \widetilde{f}_{\boldsymbol{Z}|\boldsymbol{X}}(\cdot\,|\,\boldsymbol{x};\boldsymbol{\theta})) . \qquad (6.43)$$

a. Using Jensen's inequality, show that $\mathcal{D}(g, h) \geq 0$ in (6.42). ☞ 33

b. Verify (6.43) and explain how g should be chosen such that the Kullback–Leibler term in (6.43) is minimized.

6.21. Let $X_1, \ldots, X_n$ be an iid sample from the discrete pdf:

$$f(x;\theta) = \frac{\theta^x \mathrm{e}^{-\theta}}{x!\,(1 - \mathrm{e}^{-\theta})}, \quad x \in \{1, 2, \ldots\}, \quad \theta > 0 .$$

Suppose that an iid sample of size $n = 16$ gives two 5s, four 4s, four 3s, four 2s, and two 1s. Plot the likelihood function and the log-likelihood function of the data and perform a **grid search** to obtain the maximum likelihood estimate; that is, of the plotted values, find the θ for which the likelihood (or log-likelihood) is maximal.

6.22. The data 1.1668, 0.0738, 0.7740, 1.0160, 0.4822, 1.4559, 0.1752, 0.5209, 0.1537, 0.2947 are the outcomes of an iid sample $X_1, \ldots, X_{10}$ from the pdf:

$$f(x) = c\,(b - x), \quad 0 \leq x \leq b ,$$

where $b > 0$ is unknown and c is a normalization constant.

a. Show that $c = 2/b^2$.

b. Estimate b via the method of moments.

c. Show that the maximum likelihood estimate $\widehat{b}$ satisfies:

$$\sum_{i=1}^{10} \frac{\widehat{b}}{\widehat{b} - x_i} - 20 = 0, \quad \widehat{b} \geq 1.4559 ,$$

if this equation has a solution. Determine $\widehat{b}$ numerically using Julia's `Roots` package.

6.23. Consider the score interval for the binomial distribution in Example 6.16. As in Problem 5.22, the exact coverage probability can be calculated as a function of p by means of total enumeration. Plot the coverage ☞ 18

probability for the score interval and compare it with the "standard" one in
Problem 5.22.

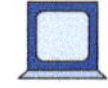

6.24. Using Problem 6.17, implement Fisher's scoring method:

$$\boldsymbol{\theta}_{t+1} = \boldsymbol{\theta}_t + \mathbf{I}^{-1}(\boldsymbol{\theta})\,\boldsymbol{S}(\boldsymbol{\theta})$$

to find the maximum likelihood estimate $\widehat{\boldsymbol{\theta}} = [\widehat{\alpha}, \widehat{\lambda}]$ for the following iid data
from $\mathsf{Gamma}(\alpha, \lambda)$.

29.7679	12.8406	105.3225	46.6101	75.7135	72.0340
33.9008	35.2510	50.9201	29.8086	32.6963	131.5229
29.1369	61.8774	31.0650	54.4877	103.6889	68.0230
30.1994	48.3140	54.4447	29.2253	27.0242	102.5929
43.0354	96.5552	64.1004	65.3381	89.6879	63.7344

Use the method of moment estimates as starting values for the Newton–
Raphson scheme. The function digamma function ψ is implemented in the
`SpecialFunctions` package of Julia as the `digamma` function and its derivative ψ' as as `trigamma`.

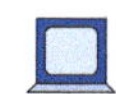

6.25. Consider the genetic linkage model in Example 6.21.

a. Show that the score and Hessian functions for θ are given by

$$S(\theta) = \frac{34}{\theta} + \frac{125}{\theta+2} - \frac{38}{1-\theta} \quad \text{and} \quad H(\theta) = -\frac{34}{\theta^2} - \frac{125}{(\theta+2)^2} - \frac{38}{(1-\theta)^2}.$$

b. Implement a Newton–Raphson procedure to find the MLE of θ.
c. Implement a simple grid search to find the MLE.
d. Do the Newton–Raphson, grid search, and EM approaches give the same
   estimate?

Chapter 7
Monte Carlo Sampling

Monte Carlo sampling—that is, random sampling on a computer—has become an important methodology in modern statistics. By simulating random variables from specified statistical models and probability distributions, one can often estimate certain statistical quantities that may otherwise be difficult to obtain. In Sect. 2.7 we already saw how random variables can be generated from common probability distributions via the *inverse-transform* and *acceptance–rejection* methods.

In this chapter we discuss two other important Monte Carlo sampling techniques: the *bootstrap method* and *Markov chain Monte Carlo* (MCMC). The bootstrap method is a sampling procedure in which new samples are generated by resampling the observed data. MCMC is used extensively in Bayesian statistics to sample from complicated multidimensional distributions. Bayesian statistics is introduced in Chap. 8.

The following example illustrates how random sampling can be used to estimate a p-value without having to derive the specific distribution of the test statistic.

Example 7.1 (Estimating a p-value). Suppose an iid sample of size 4 from a $\mathcal{N}(\mu, \sigma^2)$ distribution has a sample mean $\overline{x} = -0.7$ and sample standard deviation $s = 0.4$. We wish to test the hypothesis $H_0 : \mu = 0$ against $H_1 : \mu < 0$, using the test statistic $T = 2\overline{X}/S$, whereby we reject H_0 if the outcome of T is too small. The observed outcome of T is $t = 2 \times -0.7/0.4 = -3.5$. The corresponding $p\text{-value}$ is

$$p = \mathbb{P}_{H_0}(T \le -3.5) = \mathbb{E}_{H_0}\mathbb{1}_{\{T \le -3.5\}} \ .$$

© The Author(s), under exclusive license to Springer Science+Business Media, LLC, part of Springer Nature 2025
J. C. C. Chan, D. P. Kroese, *Statistical Modeling and Computation*,
Springer Texts in Statistics, https://doi.org/10.1007/978-1-0716-4132-3_7

This can be estimated by simulating, under H_0, a large iid sample $T_1, \ldots, T_N$ of copies of T and evaluating the sample average:

$$\widehat{p} = \frac{1}{N} \sum_{i=1}^{N} \mathbb{1}_{\{T_i \leq -3.5\}} ,$$

☞ 134   similar to the Monte Carlo integration procedure in Example 5.7. In the Julia program below, each T_i is generated by drawing an iid sample of size 4 from the *standard normal* distribution and evaluating T for that sample. The variable `count` contains the total number of test statistics with a value less than or equal to the observed value -3.5; the estimate $\widehat{p}$ is simply the value of `count` divided by N. A typical estimate for $\widehat{p}$ is 0.02. This indicates that there is fairly strong evidence that H_0 is not true. A huge advantage of this approach is that we do not have to analyze or evaluate the cdf of the test statistic under H_0; we only have to repeat the experiment under H_0 many ☞ 226   times. See Problem 7.1 for a further discussion.

```julia
pvalsim.jl

using Random, Statistics
xbar_obs = -0.7; s_obs = 0.4; t_obs = 2*xbar_obs/s_obs
N = 10^5;
count = 0;
for i in 1:N
    x = randn(4);
    xbar = mean(x); s = std(x); t = 2*xbar/s;
    global count = count + (t <= t_obs);
end
phat = count/N    # estimated p-value
```

Statistical sampling often involves generating an *iid* sample from some specified discrete or continuous pdf. Two important ways to analyze such data is to use the *empirical cdf* and *density estimation*.

7.1 Empirical Cdf

Definition 7.1. (Empirical Cdf). Let $x_1, \ldots, x_N$ be an iid real-valued sample from a cdf F. The function

$$F_N(x) = \frac{1}{N} \sum_{i=1}^{N} \mathbb{1}_{\{x_i \leq x\}}, \quad x \in \mathbb{R} , \tag{7.1}$$

is called the **empirical cdf** of the data.

Here, $\mathbb{1}_{\{x_i \leq x\}} = 1$ if $x_i \leq x$, and 0 otherwise. F_N is a nondecreasing step function which jumps up by an amount of $1/N$ at each of the points $\{x_i\}$. Moreover, F_N is right-continuous and bounded between 0 and 1. In other words, F_N is a cdf—see Sect. 2.1 It is the cdf of a random variable that takes 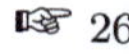 26 one of the values $x_1, \ldots, x_N$ with equal probability $1/N$, assuming that all the observations are different. In Fig. 7.1 the empirical cdf is shown of an iid sample of size 10 from the $\mathsf{Exp}(0.2)$ distribution. The true cdf is plotted as well.

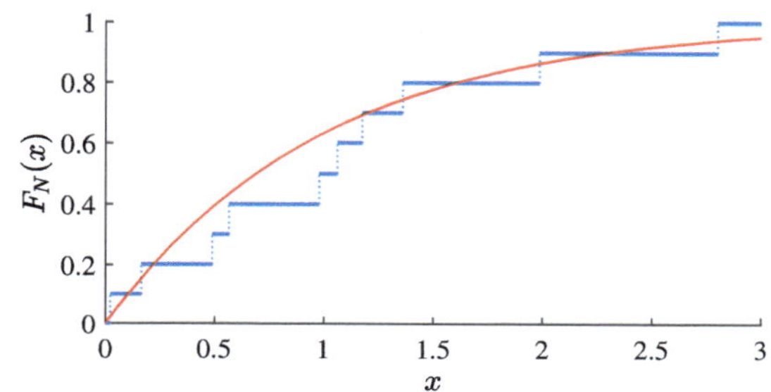

Fig. 7.1 The empirical cdf for a sample of size 10 from the $\mathsf{Exp}(0.2)$ distribution and the true cdf

We see that the empirical cdf follows the true cdf quite well. The fit becomes better and better as the sample size increases. In Fig. 7.2 the empirical and true cdfs are shown for the same distribution, but now for a sample size of 200.

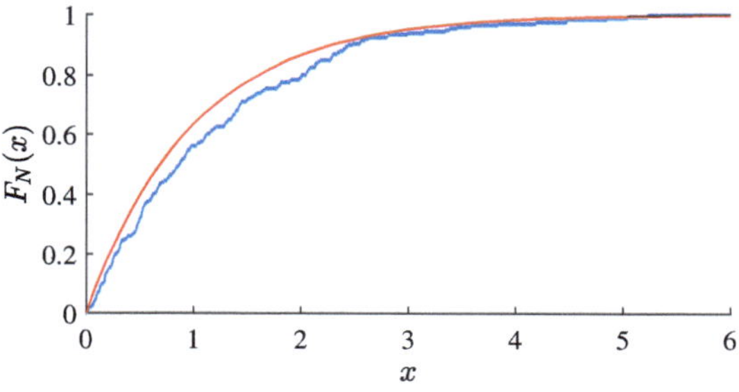

Fig. 7.2 The empirical cdf for a sample of size 200 from the $\mathsf{Exp}(0.2)$ distribution and the true cdf

If we order the sample as $x_{(1)} < x_{(2)} < \cdots < x_{(N)}$, then for each $i = 1, \ldots, N$,

$$F_N(x_{(i)}) = \frac{i}{N} , \tag{7.2}$$

assuming for simplicity that all $\{x_i\}$ take different values.

If instead of deterministic $\{x_i\}$ we take *random* X_i, in (7.1), then $F_N(x)$ becomes random as well. To distinguish between the deterministic and the random case, let us denote the random empirical cdf by $\widehat{F}_N(x)$. We now have:

$$\mathbb{P}\left(\widehat{F}_N(x) = \frac{i}{N}\right) = \mathbb{P}(X_{(i)} \leq x, X_{(i+1)} > x) = \binom{N}{i}(F(x))^i\,(1 - F(x))^{N-i}\,.$$

$$(7.3)$$

To see this, note that the event $\{X_{(i)} \leq x\} \cap \{X_{(i+1)} > x\}$ means that exactly i of the N random variables that we draw from F are less than or equal to x. Thus, the event is equivalent to having i successes in N independent Bernoulli experiments with success probability $F(x)$, which leads to (7.3).

Equation (7.3) can be summarized as: $N\,\widehat{F}_N(x) \sim \mathsf{Bin}(N, F(x))$. As a consequence

$$\mathbb{E}\widehat{F}_N(x) = F(x)$$

and

$$\mathrm{Var}(\widehat{F}_N(x)) = F(x)(1 - F(x))/N\,.$$

Moreover, by the law of large numbers and the central limit theorem, we have:

$$\mathbb{P}(\lim_{N\to\infty} \widehat{F}_N(x) = F(x)) = 1\,, \tag{7.4}$$

and

$$\lim_{N\to\infty} \mathbb{P}\left(\frac{\widehat{F}_N(x) - F(x)}{\sqrt{F(x)(1 - F(x))/N}} \leq z\right) = \Phi(z)\,, \tag{7.5}$$

where Φ is the cdf of the standard normal distribution.

Exactly as in (5.24), we see that an approximate $1 - \alpha$ confidence interval for $F(x)$ is

$$F_N(x) \pm z_{1-\alpha/2}\sqrt{\frac{F_N(x)(1 - F_N(x))}{N}}\,,$$

where $z_{1-\alpha/2}$ is the $1 - \alpha/2$ quantile of the standard normal distribution. Moreover, if we order the observations $x_{(1)} < \cdots < x_{(N)}$, then, by (7.2), an approximate $1 - \alpha$ confidence interval for $F(x_{(i)})$ is

$$\frac{i}{N} \pm z_{1-\alpha/2}\sqrt{\frac{i(1 - i/N)}{N^2}}\,, \quad i = 1, \ldots, N\,.$$

Example 7.2 (Confidence Interval for a Cdf). In Fig. 7.3 a 90% confidence interval (hence $z_{1-\alpha/2} = z_{0.95} = 1.645$) is given for the cdf of the $\mathsf{Exp}(1)$ distribution, based on an iid sample of size $N = 60$. The true cdf is given by the smooth line. We see that the true cdf lies convincingly within the confidence curves. However, the actual width of the confidence intervals (as a function of x) is quite sizable, due to the fact that N is not large.

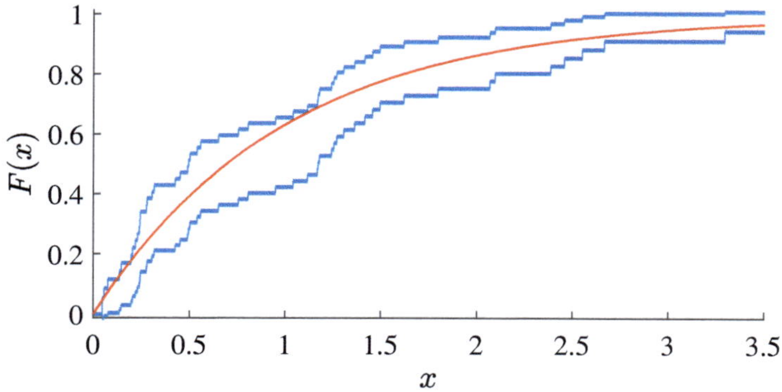

Fig. 7.3 A 90% confidence interval for the cdf $F(x) = 1 - e^{-x}$, $x \geq 0$

Let $X_1, \ldots, X_N \sim_{\text{iid}} F$, where F is continuous and strictly increasing. Define $U_1 = F(X_1), \ldots, U_N = F(X_N)$. From the inverse-transform method (see Sect. 2.7.2), we see that $U_1, \ldots, U_N$ is an iid sample from $\mathcal{U}(0, 1)$. Denote the empirical cdf of the $\{U_i\}$ by $\widehat{G}_N(u)$, and let x and u be related via $x = F^{-1}(u)$ and $u = F(x)$. Then,

$$\widehat{G}_N(u) = \frac{1}{N} \sum_{i=1}^{N} \mathbb{1}_{\{U_i \leq u\}} = \frac{1}{N} \sum_{i=1}^{N} \mathbb{1}_{\{F(X_i) \leq F(x)\}} = \frac{1}{N} \sum_{i=1}^{N} \mathbb{1}_{\{X_i \leq x\}} = \widehat{F}_N(x) .$$

$\widehat{G}_N$ is called the **reduced empirical cdf**. Note that $N\,\widehat{G}_N(u) \sim \mathsf{Bin}(N, u)$, irrespective of F. Define the maximum distance between the empirical and the true cdfs as

$$D_N = \sup_{x \in \mathbb{R}} |\widehat{F}_N(x) - F(x)| = \sup_{0 \leq u \leq 1} |\widehat{G}_N(u) - u| . \tag{7.6}$$

This is called the **Kolmogorov–Smirnov statistic** of the data. Note that this statistic does not depend on F. It can be used to test whether iid samples $X_1, \ldots, X_N$ come from a specified cdf F.

Example 7.3 (Kolmogorov–Smirnov Test). The Weibull distribution $\mathsf{Weib}(\alpha, \lambda)$ has cdf

$$F(x) = 1 - e^{-(\lambda x)^{\alpha}}, \quad x \geq 0 .$$

To generate from this distribution, we can use the inverse-transform method: generate $U \sim \mathcal{U}(0, 1)$ and output $X = \frac{1}{\lambda}(-\ln U)^{\frac{1}{\alpha}}$. Note that the $\mathsf{Weib}(1, \lambda)$ distribution is simply the $\mathsf{Exp}(\lambda)$ distribution.

Suppose we have an iid sample from the $\mathsf{Weib}(1.5, 1)$ distribution. Would the Kolmogorov–Smirnov statistic correctly reject the hypothesis H_0 that the sample is from the $\mathsf{Exp}(1)$ distribution? The following Julia program carries out this experiment. It generates an iid sample of size $N = 100$ from the

Weib(1.5, 1) distribution. It then evaluates the Kolmogorov–Smirnov statistic. Figure 7.4 shows the reduced empirical cdf $\widehat{G}_N(u)$. The maximum distance between $\widehat{G}_N(u)$ and u is $d_N \approx 0.1462$ in this case. The p-value $\mathbb{P}_{H_0}(D_N > d_N)$ is determined by Monte Carlo simulation, by repeating the experiment $K = 10000$ times under H_0, that is, using Exp(1) data. The estimated p-value is approximately 0.024. There is thus reasonable to strong evidence to suggest that the true distribution is not Exp(1).

```
kolsmirweib.jl

using Random, Plots, StatsBase , StatsPlots
Random.seed!(1234);
alpha = 1.5;
N = 100;
U = rand(N);
x = (-log.(U)).^(1/alpha); # generate data
y = sort(1 .- exp.(-x));
i = 1:N;

ecdfplot(y,legend=false)  # empirical cdf
plot!([0,1],[0,1])
dn_up = maximum(abs.(y -i/N));
dn_down = maximum(abs.(y -(i .- 1)/N));
dn = max(dn_up, dn_down);

# Use MC simulation to obtain the p-value
K = 10000;
DN = zeros(K);
for k in 1:K
    local i = 1:N;  # a global i already exists
    local y = sort(rand(N)); # same for y
    DN[k] = max( maximum(abs.(y-i/N)), maximum(abs.(y-(i .- 1)
        /N)));
end
p  = sum(DN .>= dn)/K
```

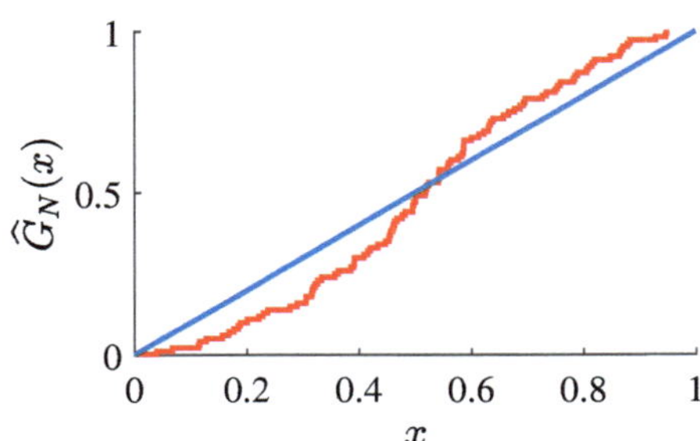

Fig. 7.4 The reduced empirical cdf $\widehat{G}_N(x)$

7.2 Density Estimation

Suppose that $x_1, \ldots, x_N$ is an iid sample from some unknown continuous pdf f—obtained from Monte Carlo sampling, for example. A useful approach to estimate f from the data is to use a Gaussian kernel density estimator.

> **Definition 7.2. (Gaussian Kernel Density Estimator).** Let $x_1, \ldots, x_N$ be the outcomes of an iid sample from a continuous pdf f. The **Gaussian kernel density estimator** of f with **bandwidth** $h > 0$ is given by
>
> $$\widehat{f}(x; h) = \frac{1}{N} \sum_{i=1}^{N} \frac{1}{\sqrt{2\pi h^2}} \, \mathrm{e}^{-\frac{(x - X_i)^2}{2h^2}}, \quad x \in \mathbb{R} . \tag{7.7}$$

The idea is illustrated in Fig. 7.5 for the case of $N = 5$ data points. The Gaussian kernel density estimate (KDE) is the equally weighed *mixture* (see (6.36)) of N Gaussian/normal pdfs, where each pdf is centered around a data point and has variance h^2.

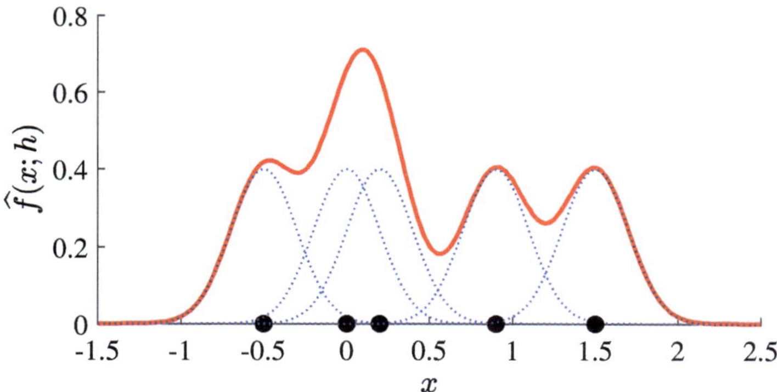

Fig. 7.5 The Gaussian KDE (solid line) is the equally weighted mixture of normal pdfs centered around the data and with standard deviation h (dashed)

How well the Gaussian KDE $\widehat{f}(\cdot; h)$ fits the true pdf f depends crucially on the choice of the bandwidth parameter h. If h is too small, the density estimate will be too spiky; if h is too large, the estimate will be too smooth. An often used *rule of thumb* is to take

$$h_{\mathrm{Rot}} = \left(\frac{4 \, S^5}{3 \, N} \right)^{4/5} ,$$

where S is the standard deviation of the data. This choice is based on a mathematical analysis of the discrepancy between $\widehat{f}(\cdot\,;h)$ and f as $N \to \infty$. There exist many sophisticated modifications of the basic Gaussian KDE in (7.7). In this book we use the fast and reliable **theta KDE** of Botev et al. (2010), with the new optimal bandwidth selection from Botev et al. (2025). The Julia module `ThetaKDE` can be downloaded from the book's homepage.

Example 7.4 (Kernel Density Estimate). The following Julia program draws an iid sample from the `Exp(1)` distribution and constructs a Gaussian kernel density estimate. We see in Fig. 7.6 that with an appropriate choice of the bandwidth, a good fit to the true pdf can be achieved, except at the boundary $x = 0$. The theta KDE, which can be viewed as a generalization of the Gaussian KDE, does not exhibit this boundary effect. Moreover, it chooses the bandwidth automatically and optimally, to achieve a superior fit.

```
gausthetakde.jl
```

```julia
include("ThetaKDE.jl") # make sure path is correct
using Random, Plots, .ThetaKDE  # dot is important
h = 0.1; h2 = h^2; c = 1/sqrt(2*pi)/h; # constants
phi(x,x0) = exp(-(x -x0)^2/(2*h2)) # unscaled kernel
f(x) = x >= 0 ? exp(-x) : 0 # true pdf
N = 10^4 # sample size
x = -log.(rand(N)) # generate the data

xmesh, density, bw = kde(x); # Determine theta KDE
phis = zeros(length(xmesh)) # Determine Gaussian KDE
for i=1:N
   global phis = phis + phi.(xmesh,x[i])
end
phis = c*phis/N
plot(xmesh,phis)        # Gaussian KDE
plot!(xmesh,density)    # theta KDE
plot!(xmesh,f.(xmesh)) # true pdf
```

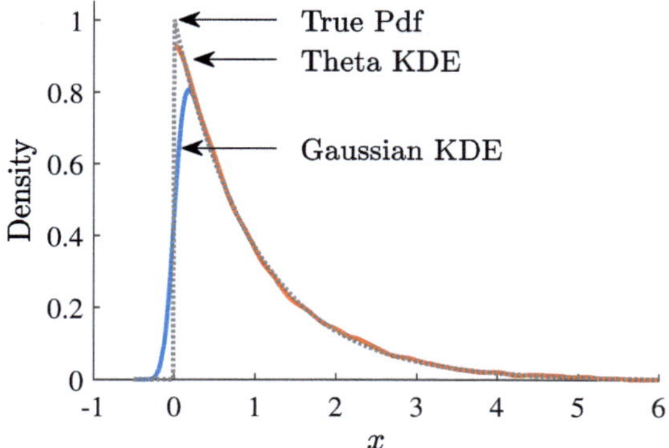

Fig. 7.6 Kernel density estimates for Exp(1)-distributed data

7.3 Resampling and the Bootstrap Method

The idea behind **resampling** is very simple: an iid sample $\boldsymbol{x} = (x_1, \ldots, x_N)$ from some unknown pdf f represents our best knowledge about f if we make no further a priori assumptions about f. So, the best way to "repeat" the experiment is to *resample* the $\{x_i\}$ by drawing from the empirical distribution. The following algorithm is a direct consequence of the inverse-transform method.

Algorithm 7.1. (Sampling from an Empirical Cdf). Let $x_1, \ldots,$ x_N be an iid sample from a continuous cdf F. To generate an iid sample of size M from the empirical cdf F_N, carry out the following steps:

1. Draw $U_1, \ldots, U_M \overset{\text{iid}}{\sim} \mathcal{U}(0, 1)$.
2. Set $I_i = \lceil N U_i \rceil, i = 1, \ldots, M$.
3. Return $x_{I_1}, \ldots, x_{I_M}$.

Here $\lceil x \rceil$ (the *ceiling* of x) is the smallest integer larger than or equal to x. The requirement that F be continuous is to rule out duplicate data points.

By sampling from the empirical cdf, we can thus repeat (approximately) the experiment that gave us the original data as many times as we like. This is useful if we want to assess the properties of certain statistics obtained from the data. For example, suppose that the original data $\boldsymbol{x}$ gave the statistic $t(\boldsymbol{x})$. By resampling we can gain information about the *distribution* of the corresponding random variable $t(\boldsymbol{X})$.

Example 7.5 (Resampling Cauchy Data). Suppose we have an iid sample of size $N = 100$ from the Cauchy distribution—that is, with pdf

$$f_X(x) = \frac{1}{\pi(1 + x^2)}, \quad x \in \mathbb{R} \; ;$$

☞ 188   see also Examples 6.3 and 6.20. We learned from the first example that the sample mean is a poor estimate of the mode (0) of the distribution. By resampling the data, we can get a good idea how the *distribution* of the sample mean compares with that of other estimators—for example, the **sample median** of the data. Ordering the data from smallest to largest, $x_{(1)} \le \cdots \le x_{(N)}$, the sample median $\widetilde{x}$ is defined as the "middle" observation; that is $\widetilde{x} = x_{((N+1)/2)}$ for odd N, and $\widetilde{x} = (x_{(N/2)} + x_{(N/2+1)})/2$ for even N.

Figure 7.7 depicts three graphs. The dashed line is the KDE of $K = 5000$ iid sample means, where each sample mean is obtained from a resampled data set of size $M = 100$ from the original iid Cauchy data of size $N = 100$. Similarly, the solid line represents the KDE of the sample medians.

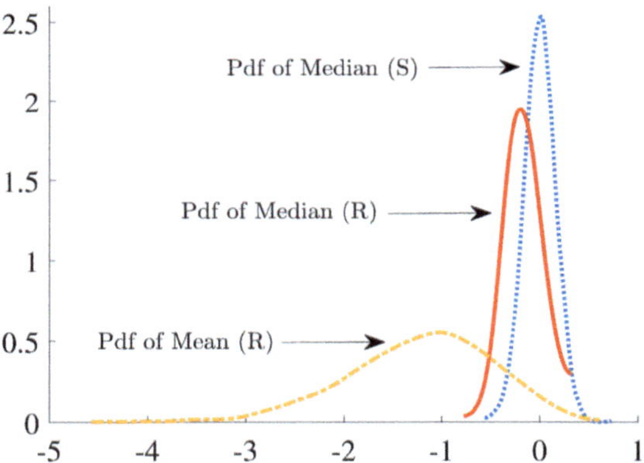

Fig. 7.7 Kernel density estimates for the mean (dashed line) and median (solid line) of resampled data, as well as for the median of newly sampled data (dotted line)

The figure shows that the sample median has much better statistical properties than the sample mean. In particular, the pdf of the sample median (estimated via the KDE) is much less spread out than that of the sample mean, and is (here) mostly concentrated in the interval $(-0.5, 0.5)$. For comparison, the figure also shows the KDE of the sample median obtained from $K = 5000$ iid samples from the original distribution (dotted line). Thus, instead of resampling the data, we draw each time the data from scratch. The following Julia program can be used to carry out the experiment. We again use the theta KDE. It is important that when using resampled data, the **res=true** flag is set. See Problem 7.6 for a further discussion of this example.

```julia
resampcauchy.jl

include("ThetaKDE.jl")
using Random, Plots, StatsBase, .ThetaKDE
N = 100; K = 5000
# Random.seed!(123)
xorg = tan.(pi*(0.5 .- rand(N))) # original data
medxorg = median(xorg); meanxorg = mean(xorg)
x = zeros(N); mx = zeros(K)
for i in 1:K
    ind = ceil.(Int64,N*rand(N)) # draw random indices
    x = xorg[ind]; # resampling the data (R)
    # x = tan(pi*(0.5 - rand(1,N))) # sampling new data (S)
    mx[i] = median(x)
    # mx[i] = mean(x);
end
xmesh,density,bw = kde(mx,res=true)
plot(xmesh,density)
```

The **bootstrap method** is a formalization of the resampling idea. Suppose we wish to estimate a number ℓ via some estimator $H = H(\boldsymbol{X})$, where $\boldsymbol{X} = [X_1, \ldots, X_N]^\top$ and the $\{X_i\}$ form an iid sample from some unknown cdf F. It is assumed that H does not depend on the order of the $\{X_i\}$. To assess the quality (e.g., accuracy) of the estimator H, one could draw independent replications $\boldsymbol{X}_1, \ldots, \boldsymbol{X}_K$ of $\boldsymbol{X}$ and find sample estimates for quantities such as the *variance* of the estimator:

$$\text{Var}(H) = \mathbb{E}H^2 - (\mathbb{E}H)^2 \,,$$

the *bias*

$$\text{Bias} = \mathbb{E}H - \ell \,,$$

and the *mean square error* (MSE)

☞ 159

$$\text{MSE} = \mathbb{E}(H - \ell)^2 \,.$$

However, it may be too time-consuming, or simply not feasible, to obtain such replications. An alternative is to resample the original data, as described above. To reiterate, given an outcome $(x_1, \ldots, x_N)$ of $\boldsymbol{X}$, we draw an iid sample $\boldsymbol{X}^* = [X_1^*, \ldots, X_N^*]^\top$ not from F but from the empirical cdf F_N, via Algorithm 7.1 (hence $M = N$ here).

The rationale is that the empirical cdf F_N is close to the actual distribution F and gets closer as N gets larger. Hence, any quantities depending on F, such as $\mathbb{E}_F h(H)$, where h is a function, can be approximated by $\mathbb{E}_{F_N} h(H)$. The latter is usually still difficult to evaluate, but it can be simply estimated via Monte Carlo simulation as

$$\frac{1}{K} \sum_{i=1}^{K} h(H_i^*) \, ,$$

where $H_1^*, \ldots, H_K^*$ are independent copies of $H^* = H(\boldsymbol{X}^*)$. This seemingly self-referent procedure is called **bootstrapping**—alluding to Baron von Münchhausen, who pulled himself out of a swamp by his own bootstraps. As an example, the bootstrap estimate of the expectation of H is

$$\widehat{\mathbb{E}H} = \overline{H}^* = \frac{1}{K} \sum_{i=1}^{K} H_i^* \, ,$$

which is simply the sample mean of $\{H_i^*\}$. Similarly, the bootstrap estimate for $\mathrm{Var}(H)$ is the sample variance

$$\widehat{\mathrm{Var}(H)} = \frac{1}{K-1} \sum_{i=1}^{K} (H_i^* - \overline{H}^*)^2 \, . \tag{7.8}$$

Bootstrap estimators for the bias and MSE are $\overline{H}^* - H$ and $\frac{1}{K} \sum_{i=1}^{K} (H_i^* - H)^2$, respectively. Note that for these estimators, the unknown quantity ℓ is replaced with the original estimator H. Confidence intervals can be constructed in the same fashion. We mention two variants: the **normal** method and the **percentile** method. In the normal method, a $1 - \alpha$ confidence interval for ℓ is given by

$$(H \pm z_{1-\alpha/2} S^*) \, ,$$

where S^* is the bootstrap estimate of the standard deviation of H, that is, the square root of (7.8). In the percentile method, the upper and lower bounds of the $1 - \alpha$ confidence interval for ℓ are given by the $1 - \alpha/2$ and $\alpha/2$ quantiles of H, which in turn are estimated via the corresponding sample quantiles of the bootstrap sample $\{H_i^*\}$.

Example 7.6 (Bootstrapping Regression Data). Bootstrapping can be applied to a variety of statistical models, including regression data. Suppose that we have linear regression data $\{(x_i, y_i), i = 1, \ldots, 10\}$ given in Table 7.1.

Table 7.1 Regression Data

x	y	x	y
13	5.0768	27	31.4085
16	21.1897	30	26.8648
19	17.1548	33	29.3894
21	22.8325	36	37.4476
24	26.5348	39	44.292

We wish to fit the data with a straight line. The least-squares method   ☞ 12
gives the following fitted regression line:

$$y = 3.3024\, x + 8.0561 \ .$$

We can assess the quality of this estimate by resampling the pairs $\{(x_i, y_i)\}$
independently, and then estimating the regression lines for the resampled
data. This is illustrated in Fig. 7.8 for 20 resampled regression lines. We see
that there is quite a lot of variability in the estimate.

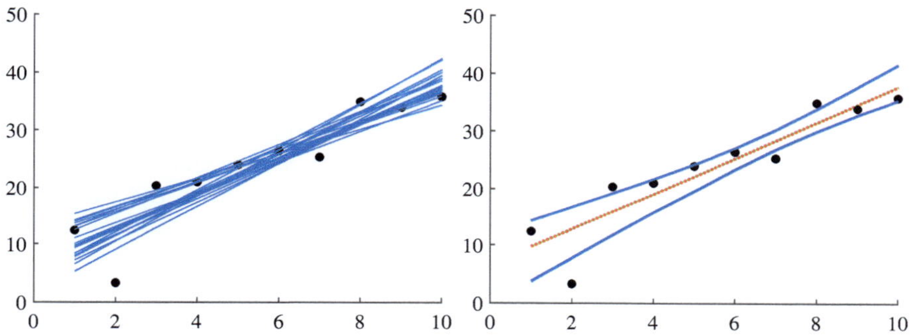

Fig. 7.8 Left: The linear regression data (10 points) and 20 resampled regression lines.
Right: A 90% bootstrapped confidence interval obtained from 1000 resampled regression
lines

Let us determine percentile confidence intervals for the regression line
$\beta_1 x + \beta_0$. We carry out the resampling many times, say 1000 times, and
calculate for each x the values $\widehat{\beta}_1 x + \widehat{\beta}_0$. A 90% bootstrap confidence interval
is then obtained by recording the 5% and the 95% quantile of these 1000 val-
ues for each x. The result is given in the right pane of Fig. 7.8. The straight
line through the middle is the estimated regression line. The curved lines
form the confidence interval—as a function of x.

Example 7.7 (Bootstrapping the Ratio Estimator). Suppose the data
consists of n iid copies $[X_1, Y_1]^\top, \ldots, [X_N, Y_N]^\top$ of a random vector $[X, Y]^\top$
with mean vector $[\mu_X, \mu_Y]^\top$ and covariance matrix Σ. We wish to estimate
the ratio μ_X / μ_Y. A straightforward estimator is the so-called **ratio estimator** $R = \overline{X}/\overline{Y}$.

As a particular example, consider the data in Fig. 7.9, where a sample of
size $N = 100$ of pairs (x, y) is plotted. The model that was used to generate
the data is

$$X \sim \mathcal{N}(11, 25) \quad \text{and} \quad (Y \mid X = x) \sim \mathcal{U}(0, x) \ .$$

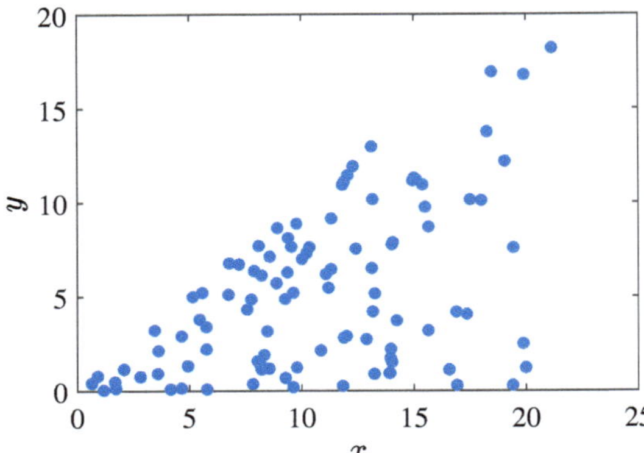

Fig. 7.9 An iid sample from a two-dimensional distribution

The estimate for μ_X/μ_Y is in this case $\overline{x}/\overline{y} = 2.0359$. But how accurate is this estimate? From Example 3.15 (delta method), we see that the estimator R has approximately a $\mathcal{N}(\mu_X/\mu_Y, \sigma^2/N)$ distribution, where the variance is given in (3.38). By replacing expectations, variances, and covariance with their sample means—that is, by using the method of moments—it is easy to estimate σ^2. The sample means and the covariance matrix of the $\{[X_i, Y_i]^\top\}$ are in this case:

$$\overline{x} = 10.3026, \quad \overline{y} = 5.0604, \quad \text{and} \quad \widehat{\boldsymbol{\Sigma}} = \begin{bmatrix} 19.7626 & 9.7052 \\ 9.7052 & 12.9859 \end{bmatrix},$$

which gives $\widehat{\sigma^2} = 1.3305$. Thus, R has approximately a $\mathcal{N}(2.0359, 1.3305)$ distribution. Its pdf is plotted in Fig. 7.10 (dotted graph). The 0.025 and 0.975 quantiles of this distribution give an approximate 95% confidence interval for μ_X/μ_Y:

$$2.0359 \pm 1.96\sqrt{1.33051/100} = (1.81, 2.26)\,.$$

The above analysis requires a good deal of mathematical sophistication. In contrast, the application of the bootstrap method for this data is relatively easy: independently resample the data K times and plot a kernel density estimate of the ratios, as in the following Julia code.

```julia
resampratio.jl

include("ThetaKDE.jl")
using Random, Plots, StatsBase, Distributions, .ThetaKDE
# Random.seed!(123)
N = 100 # size of data
K = 5000 # resample size
est = zeros(K)
```

```
xorg = 11 .+ 5*randn(N); yorg = rand(N).*xorg; # orig. data
estorg = mean(xorg)/mean(yorg)
x = zeros(N); y = zeros(N);
est = zeros(K);
for i in 1:K
    ind = ceil.(Int64,N*rand(N)) # draw random indices
    local x = xorg[ind]; local y = yorg[ind]; # resampled data
    est[i] = mean(x)/mean(y);
end
xmesh,density,bandwidth = kde(est,res=true)
plot(xmesh,density)
cv = cov(hcat(xorg,yorg))
sigma2 = estorg^2*(var(xorg)/mean(xorg)^2 + var(yorg)/mean(
    yorg)^2 - 2*cv[1,2]/mean(xorg)/mean(yorg));
t = estorg-4*sqrt(sigma2/N):0.01: estorg+4*sqrt(sigma2/N);
z = pdf.(Normal(estorg,sqrt(sigma2/N)),t);
plot!(t,z)
```

Figure 7.10 shows the kernel density estimate for the bootstrapped sample of size $K = 5000$. We see that the density estimate is in excellent agreement with that of the delta method.

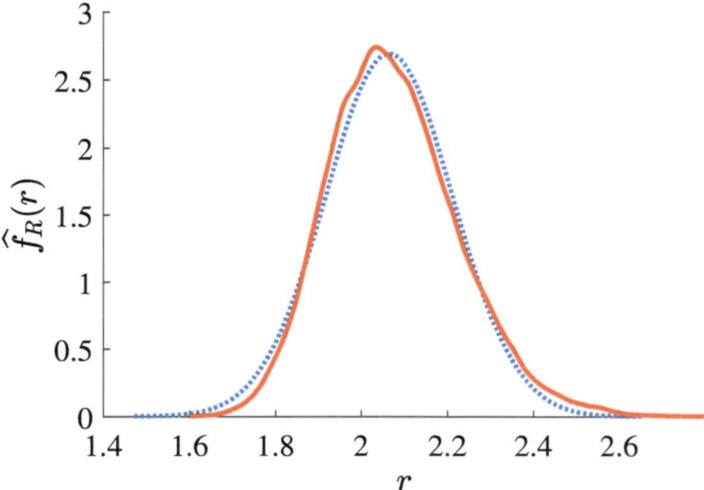

Fig. 7.10 Estimates of the pdf of the ratio estimator $R = \overline{X}/\overline{Y}$ using the delta method (dotted line) and the bootstrap method (solid line)

7.4 Markov Chain Monte Carlo

Markov chain Monte Carlo (MCMC) is a Monte Carlo sampling technique for (approximately) generating samples from an arbitrary distribution—often referred to as the **target** distribution. The basic idea is to run a Markov chain long enough such that its limiting distribution is close to the target distribution.

Before we discuss the method in more detail, let us go over some facts about Markov chains.

> **Definition 7.3. (Markov Chain).** A **Markov chain** is a collection $\{X_t, t = 0, 1, 2, \ldots\}$ of random variables (or random vectors) whose futures are conditionally independent of their pasts given their present values. That is,
>
> $$(X_{t+1} \mid X_s, s \leq t) \quad \sim \quad (X_{t+1} \mid X_t) \quad \text{for all } t . \tag{7.9}$$

In other words, the conditional distribution of the future variable X_{t+1}, given the entire past $\{X_s, s \leq t\}$, is the same as the conditional distribution of X_{t+1} given only the present X_t. Property (7.9) is called the **Markov property**.

The index t in X_t is usually seen as a "time" or "step" parameter. The index set $\{0, 1, 2, \ldots\}$ in the definition above was chosen out of convenience. It can be replaced by any countable index set. We restrict ourselves to Markov chains for which the conditional pdfs $f_{X_{t+1} \mid X_t}(y \mid x)$ do not depend on t; we abbreviate these as $q(y \mid x)$. The $\{q(y \mid x)\}$ are called the **(one-step) transition densities** of the Markov chain. Note that the random variables or vectors $\{X_t\}$ may be *discrete* (e.g., taking values in some set $\{1, \ldots, r\}$) or *continuous* (e.g., taking values in an interval $[0, 1]$ or $\mathbb{R}^d$). In particular, in the *discrete* case, each $q(y \mid x)$ is a probability: $q(y \mid x) = \mathbb{P}(X_{t+1} = y \mid X_t = x)$.

The distribution of X_0 is called the **initial distribution** of the Markov chain. The one-step transition densities and the initial distribution completely specify the distribution of the random vector $[X_0, X_1, \ldots, X_t]^\top$. Namely, we have by the product rule (3.10) and the Markov property (7.9) that the joint pdf is given by

☞ 72

$$
\begin{aligned}
f_{X_0, \ldots, X_t}&(x_0, \ldots, x_t) \\
&= f_{X_0}(x_0)\, f_{X_1 \mid X_0}(x_1 \mid x_0) \cdots f_{X_t \mid X_{t-1}, \ldots, X_0}(x_t \mid x_{t-1}, \ldots, x_0) \\
&= f_{X_0}(x_0)\, f_{X_1 \mid X_0}(x_1 \mid x_0) \cdots f_{X_t \mid X_{t-1}}(x_t \mid x_{t-1}) \\
&= f_{X_0}(x_0)\, q(x_1 \mid x_0)\, q(x_2 \mid x_1) \cdots q(x_t \mid x_{t-1}) .
\end{aligned}
$$

This leads to the following generic generation algorithm for Markov chains.

Algorithm 7.2. (Generating a Markov Chain). To generate a Markov chain $X_0, \ldots, X_N$ with transition densities $\{q(y\,|\,x)\}$ and initial pdf f_{X_0} execute the following steps

1 Draw $X_0 \sim f_0$.
2 **for** $t = 1$ **to** N **do**
3 $\quad$ Draw $X_t \sim q(\cdot\,|\,X_{t-1})$.
4 **return** $X_0, \ldots, X_N$

Example 7.8 (Stepping Stones). Imagine a pond with six stepping stones. From each stone one can step to a neighboring stone with a certain probability, indicated by the graph in Fig. 7.11. Let X_t be the position (stepping stone) after t steps, starting from position 1. Then, $\{X_t, t = 0, 1, 2, \ldots\}$ is a Markov chain. The graph in Fig. 7.11 is called the **transition graph** of the Markov chain. The arc weights indicate the transition probabilities. For example, $q(4\,|\,3) = 0.7, q(3\,|\,6) = 0.1$, and $q(3\,|\,4) = 0$.

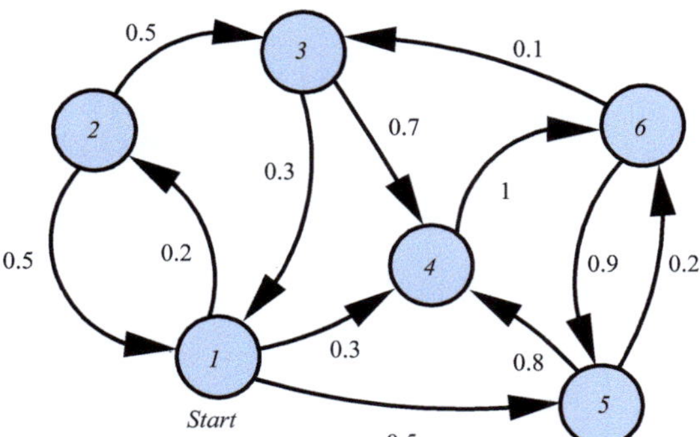

Fig. 7.11 The transition graph for the Markov chain $\{X_t, t = 0, 1, 2, \ldots\}$

The following Julia program generates the Markov chain for $N = 100$ steps. Note that the transition probabilities have been gathered into a matrix $\mathbf{P}$, with $\mathbf{P}(x, y) = q(y\,|\,x)$. $\mathbf{P}$ is called **one-step transition matrix** of the Markov chain. Given that $X_t = x$, state X_{t+1} is generated from the discrete distribution defined by the x-th row of $\mathbf{P}$. A typical outcome is depicted in Fig. 7.12. The program also keeps track of the fraction of visits to each state. We see that the Markov process spends most of its time in states 4, 5, and 6.

```
stepstone.jl
```

```julia
using Plots
N = 101; # times
P = [0     0.2 0    0.3 0.5 0;
     0.5 0   0.5 0   0   0;
     0.3 0   0   0.7 0   0;
     0   0   0   0   0   1;
     0   0   0   0.8 0   0.2;
     0   0   0.1 0   0.9 0];
x = zeros(Int64,N); x[1]= 1;
tot = zeros(6); tot[1] = 1;
for t in 1:N-1 # generate the Markov chain
    x[t+1] = minimum(findall(cumsum(P[x[t],:]) .> rand()));
    tot[x[t+1]] = tot[x[t+1]] + 1;
end
p = plot(0:N-1,x) # plot the path
scatter!(0:N-1,x)
println(tot/N) # fractions of visits to the states
```

```
[0.0297, 0.0, 0.0792, 0.2970, 0.2673, 0.3267
```

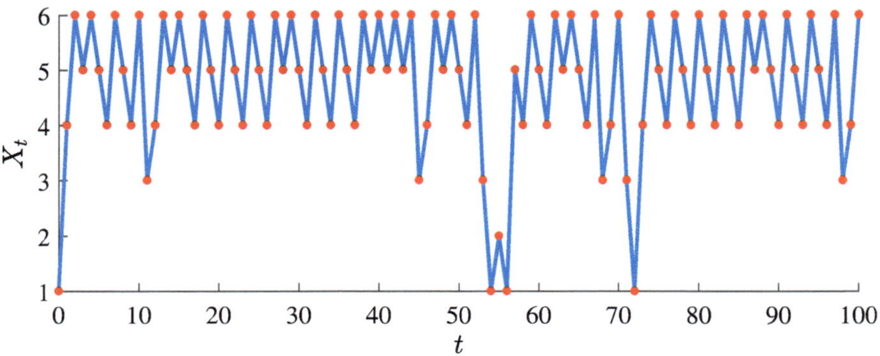

Fig. 7.12 A realization of the stepping stone Markov process $\{X_t, t = 0, 1, 2, \ldots, 100\}$

A Markov chain is said to be **ergodic** if the probability distribution of X_t converges to a fixed distribution as $t \to \infty$. Ergodicity is a natural property of Markov chains. For example, the Markov chain in Example 7.8 is ergodic. Intuitively, since this Markov chain cannot run off to infinity (which can only happen if the state space is infinite) and since each state can be reached from each other state, the probability $f_{X_t}(x) = \mathbb{P}(X_t = x)$ of encountering the chain in state x at time t far away in the future depends on x but not on t. In general, the pdf $f_{X_t}(x)$ of an ergodic Markov chain converges to a fixed **limiting pdf** $f(x)$ as $t \to \infty$, irrespective of the starting state. For the discrete case, $f(x)$ corresponds to the long-run fraction of times that the Markov process visits x.

The limiting pdf $f(x)$ can be found by solving the **global balance equations**:

$$f(x) = \begin{cases} \sum_y f(y)\, q(x \mid y) & \text{(discrete case)}, \\ \int f(y)\, q(x \mid y)\, \mathrm{d}y & \text{(continuous case)}. \end{cases} \tag{7.10}$$

For the discrete case, the rationale behind this is as follows. Since $f(x)$ is the long-run proportion of time that the Markov chain spends in x, the proportion of transitions *out of* x is $f(x)$. This should be balanced with the proportion of transitions *into* state x, which is $\sum_y f(y)\, q(x \mid y)$.

Example 7.9 (Limiting Probabilities for Stepping Stones Example). For the discrete case, the global balance equations can be written in matrix form as $\boldsymbol{f} = \boldsymbol{f}\mathbf{P}$, where $\mathbf{P}$ is the one-step transition matrix, and $\boldsymbol{f}$ the *row* vector of limiting probabilities. This leads to solving the linear equation $\boldsymbol{f}(\mathbb{I} - \mathbf{P}) = \mathbf{0}$, or equivalently $(\mathbb{I} - \mathbf{P}^{\top})\boldsymbol{f}^{\top} = \mathbf{0}$, where $\mathbb{I}$ denotes the identity matrix. In other words, $\boldsymbol{f}^{\top}$ lies in the *null space* of $(\mathbb{I} - \mathbf{P})^{\top}$. Also, the components of $\boldsymbol{f}$ must add to 1. By executing the following lines:

```julia
using LinearAlgebra
f = nullspace(I - P');
f = f/sum(f)
```

appended to the Julia code in Example 7.8, we find the limiting probabilities $\boldsymbol{f} = [0.0120, 0.0024, 0.0359, 0.2837, 0.3186, 0.3474]$.

In Markov chain Monte Carlo, one is often interested in a stronger type of balance equations. Imagine that we have taken a video of the evolution of the Markov chain, which we may run in forward and reverse time. If we cannot determine whether the video is running forward or backward (we cannot determine any systematic "looping"), the chain is said to be time-reversible or simply **reversible**.

Although not every Markov chain is reversible, each ergodic Markov chain, when run backward, gives another Markov chain—the **reverse Markov chain**—with transition densities $\widetilde{q}(y \mid x) = f(y)\, q(x \mid y)/f(x)$. To see this, first observe that $f(x)$ is the long-run proportion of time spent in x for both the original and reverse Markov chains. Second, the "probability flux" from x to y in the reversed chain must be equal to the probability flux from y to x in the original chain, meaning $f(x)\,\widetilde{q}(y \mid x) = f(y)\, q(x \mid y)$, which yields the stated transition probabilities for the reversed chain. In particular, for a *reversible* Markov chain, we have:

$$f(x)\, q(y \mid x) = f(y)\, q(x \mid y) \quad \text{for all } x, y \,. \tag{7.11}$$

These are the **detailed (or local) balance equations**. Note that the detailed balance equations imply the global balance equations. Hence, if a Markov chain is **irreducible** (i.e., every state can be reached from every other state) and there exists a pdf such that (7.11) holds, then $f(x)$ must be the limiting pdf. In the discrete state space case, an additional condition is that the chain must be **aperiodic**, meaning that the return times to the same state cannot always be a multiple of some integer ≥ 2; see Problem 7.13.

Example 7.10 (Random Walk on a Graph). Consider a Markov chain that performs a "random walk" on the graph in Fig. 7.13, at each step jumping from the current vertex (node) to one of the adjacent vertices, with equal probability. Clearly this Markov chain is reversible. It is also irreducible and aperiodic. Let $f(x)$ denote the limiting probability that the chain is in vertex x. By symmetry, $f(1) = f(2) = f(7) = f(8)$, $f(4) = f(5)$ and $f(3) = f(6)$. Moreover, by the detailed balance equations, $f(4)/5 = f(1)/3$, and $f(3)/4 = f(1)/3$. It follows that $f(1) + \cdots + f(8) = 4f(1) + 2 \times 5/3\, f(1) + 2 \times 4/3\, f(1) = 10\, f(1) = 1$, so that $f(1) = 1/10$, $f(3) = 2/15$, and $f(4) = 1/6$.

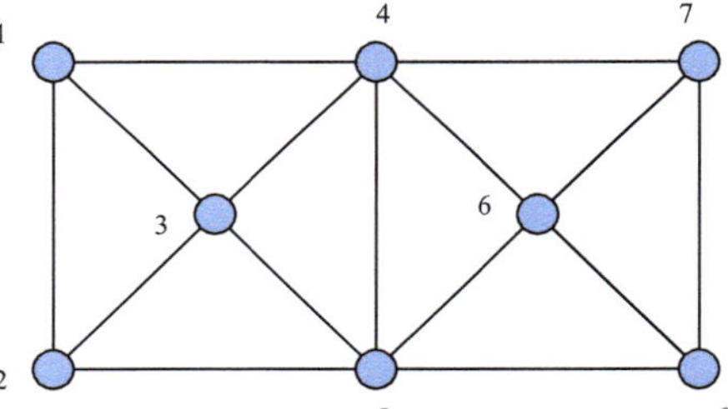

Fig. 7.13 The random walk on this graph is reversible

The idea behind Markov chain Monte Carlo can be summarized as follows. To draw approximately from an arbitrary pdf $f(x)$, run a Markov chain $\{X_t\}$ whose limiting distribution is $f(x)$. Often such a Markov chain is constructed to be reversible, so that the detailed balance equations (7.11) can be used. After a sufficiently long **burn-in period** from 0 to T, say, the random variables $X_{T+1}, X_{T+2}, \ldots$ form an *approximate* and *dependent* sample from $f(x)$.

In the next two sections, we discuss two specific MCMC samplers: the Metropolis–Hastings sampler and the Gibbs sampler.

7.5 Metropolis–Hastings Algorithm

Suppose we wish to sample from a discrete pdf $f(x)$, where x takes values in the set $\{1, \ldots, r\}$. Following Metropolis et al. (1953), we construct a Markov chain $\{X_t, t = 0, 1, \ldots\}$ in such a way that its limiting pdf is f. Suppose the Markov chain is in state x at time t. A transition of the Markov chain from state x is carried out in two phases. Similar to the acceptance–rejection

method, first a *trial* or *proposal* state Y is drawn from a transition density
$q(\cdot \mid x)$. This state is *accepted* as the new state, with probability $\alpha(x, Y)$, or
rejected otherwise. In the latter case, the chain remains in state x. For any
outcome $Y = y$, the one-step transition probabilities of the Markov chain are
thus

$$\widetilde{q}(y \mid x) = \begin{cases} q(y \mid x)\, \alpha(x, y), & \text{if } y \neq x \\ 1 - \sum_{z \neq x} q(z \mid x)\, \alpha(x, z), & \text{if } y = x\,. \end{cases} \tag{7.12}$$

By choosing the **acceptance probability** as

$$\alpha(x, y) = \min\left\{ \frac{f(y)\, q(x \mid y)}{f(x)\, q(y \mid x)}, 1 \right\}, \tag{7.13}$$

such a Markov chain can be made (see Problem 7.12) to satisfy the detailed
balance equations (7.11):

$$f(x)\, \widetilde{q}(y \mid x) = f(y)\, \widetilde{q}(x \mid y) \quad \text{for all } x, y\,. \tag{7.14}$$

Consequently, if this Markov chain is irreducible and aperiodic, its limiting
pdf is $f(x)$.

Note that in order to evaluate the acceptance probability $\alpha(x, y)$ in (7.13),
we only need to know the target pdf $f(x)$ *up to a constant*; that is $f(x) = c\overline{f}(x)$ for some known function $\overline{f}(x)$ but unknown constant c.

The extension of the above MCMC approach for generating samples from
an arbitrary joint pdf $f(\boldsymbol{x})$ is straightforward, giving the following algorithm.

Algorithm 7.3. (Metropolis–Hastings Sampler). Given a
transition density $q(\boldsymbol{y} \mid \boldsymbol{x})$:

1 Initialize $\boldsymbol{X}_0$.
2 **for** $t = 0$ **to** $N - 1$ **do**
3   Draw $\boldsymbol{Y} \sim q(\boldsymbol{y} \mid \boldsymbol{X}_t)$.   // draw a proposal
4     $\alpha = \alpha(\boldsymbol{X}_t, \boldsymbol{Y})$ // acceptance probability as in (7.13)
5   Draw $U \sim \mathcal{U}(0, 1)$.
6   **if** $U \leq \alpha$ **then** $\boldsymbol{X}_{t+1} = \boldsymbol{Y}$
7   **else** $\boldsymbol{X}_{t+1} = \boldsymbol{X}_t$
8 **return** $\boldsymbol{X}_1, \ldots, \boldsymbol{X}_N$

The above algorithm produces a sequence $\boldsymbol{X}_1, \boldsymbol{X}_2, \ldots$ of *dependent* random vectors, with $\boldsymbol{X}_t$ approximately distributed according to $f(\boldsymbol{x})$ for large t.

Since Algorithm 7.3 is of the acceptance–rejection type, its efficiency depends on the acceptance probability $\alpha(\boldsymbol{x}, \boldsymbol{y})$. Ideally, one would like the proposal transition density $q(\boldsymbol{y} \mid \boldsymbol{x})$ to reproduce the desired pdf $f(\boldsymbol{y})$ as faithfully as possible. Below we consider two particular choices of $q(\boldsymbol{y} \mid \boldsymbol{x})$.

☞ 55

Example 7.11 (Independence Sampler). The simplest Metropolis-type MCMC algorithm is obtained by choosing the proposal transition density $q(\boldsymbol{y}\,|\,\boldsymbol{x})$ to be independent of $\boldsymbol{x}$; that is, $q(\boldsymbol{y}\,|\,\boldsymbol{x}) = g(\boldsymbol{y})$ for some pdf $g(\boldsymbol{y})$. Thus, starting from a previous state $\boldsymbol{X}$, a candidate state $\boldsymbol{Y}$ is generated from $g(\boldsymbol{y})$ and accepted with probability:

$$\alpha(\boldsymbol{X}, \boldsymbol{Y}) = \min\left\{\frac{f(\boldsymbol{Y})\,g(\boldsymbol{X})}{f(\boldsymbol{X})\,g(\boldsymbol{Y})}, 1\right\}.$$

☞ 55　This procedure is very similar to the acceptance–rejection method of Sect. 2.7.3, and, as in that method, it is important that the proposal distribution g is close to the target f. Note, however, that in contrast to the acceptance–rejection method, this **independence sampler** produces *dependent* samples.

As a particular example, consider the pdf:

$$f(x) \propto x^2 \exp(-x^2 + \sin(x)), \quad x \in \mathbb{R},$$

where the normalization constant remains unspecified ($\propto$ means "is proportional to"). To sample from this pdf using the independence sampler, we choose the symmetric proposal pdf $g(x) = \mathrm{e}^{-|x|}/2, x \in \mathbb{R}$. Drawing from this
☞ 231　pdf is easy; see Problem 7.16. The program below provides a Julia implementation, and Fig. 7.14 shows a kernel density estimate of the data (as well as a graph of the true pdf f).

```julia
indepsamp.jl

include("ThetaKDE.jl")
using Random, Plots, QuadGK, .ThetaKDE
N = 10^5;   # sample size
f(x) = x^2*exp(-x^2 + sin(x)); # unnormalized target pdf
g(x) = exp(-abs(x))/2;         # proposal pdf
alpha(x,y) = min(f(y)*g(x)/(f(x)*g(y)), 1); # accept. prob.
x = 0; xx = zeros(N);
for t in 2:N
    global x
    y = -log(rand())*(2*(rand() < 1/2) - 1);  # proposal
    rand() < alpha(x,y) ? x = y : nothing
    xx[t] = x;
end
jx = xx[1:N] + randn(N)*0.05;
xmesh,density,bw = kde(jx);
plot(xmesh,density)  # plot the kde of the data
c = quadgk(f,-5,5)[1]; # determine the normalization constant
tt = -4:0.1:4;
plot!(tt,f.(tt)/c) # plot the target pdf
```

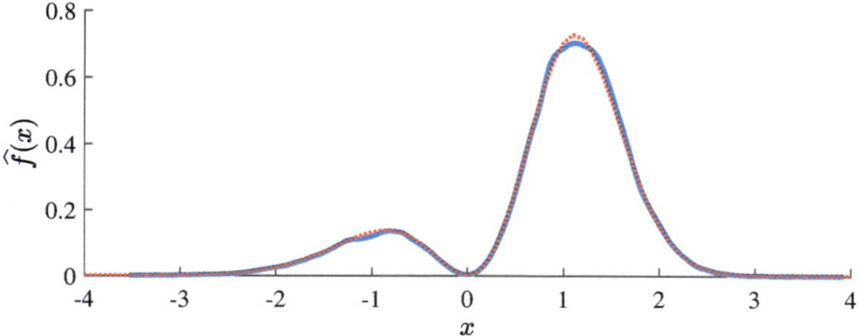

Fig. 7.14 The kernel density estimate $\widehat{f}(x)$ (smooth curve), obtained by the independence sampler, is practically indistinguishable from the target pdf $f(x)$ (dotted curve)

Example 7.12 (Random Walk Sampler). A popular Metropolis–Hastings-type sampler is the **random walk sampler**. Here, the proposal state $\boldsymbol{Y}$, for a given current state $\boldsymbol{x}$, is given by $\boldsymbol{Y} = \boldsymbol{x} + \boldsymbol{Z}$, where $\boldsymbol{Z}$ is typically generated from some spherically symmetric distribution, such as $\mathcal{N}(\boldsymbol{0}, \mathbb{I}_n)$. In that case the proposal transition density pdf is symmetric; that is, $q(\boldsymbol{y} \,|\, \boldsymbol{x}) = q(\boldsymbol{x} \,|\, \boldsymbol{y})$. It follows that the acceptance probability is

$$\alpha(\boldsymbol{x}, \boldsymbol{y}) = \min\left\{\frac{f(\boldsymbol{y})}{f(\boldsymbol{x})}, 1\right\}. \tag{7.15}$$

Example 7.13 (Sampling from a Pdf via Random Walk Sampler). Consider the two-dimensional pdf $f(x_1, x_2) = c\,\exp(-4(x_2 - x_1^2)^2 + (x_2 - 1)^2)$, $x_1 \in \mathbb{R}$, $x_2 \leq 2$, where c is an unknown normalization constant; see Fig. 7.15.

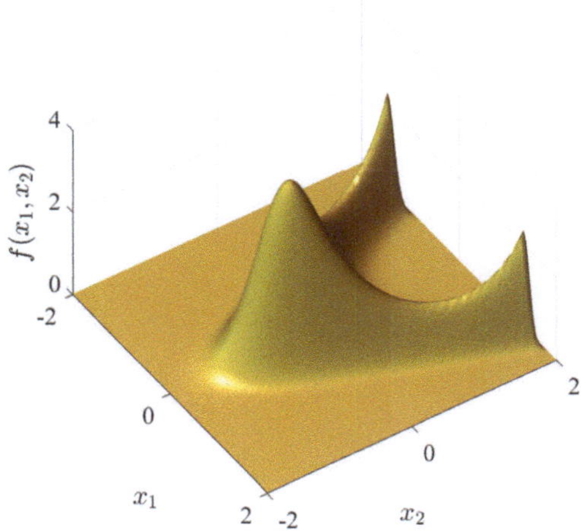

Fig. 7.15 The pdf $f(x_1, x_2) = c\,\exp(-4(x_2 - x_1^2)^2 + (x_2 - 1)^2)$, $\quad x_1 \in \mathbb{R}, x_2 \leq 2$

The following Julia program implements a random walk sampler to (approximately) draw $N = 10^4$ dependent samples from the pdf f. At each step, given a current state $\boldsymbol{x}$, a proposal $\boldsymbol{Y}$ is drawn from the $\mathcal{N}(\boldsymbol{x}, \mathbb{I}_2)$ distribution. That is, $\boldsymbol{Y} = \boldsymbol{x} + \boldsymbol{Z}$, with $\boldsymbol{Z}$ bivariate standard normal.

We see in Fig. 7.16 that the samples closely follow the contour plot of the pdf, indicating that the sampler works correctly. The starting point for the Markov chain is chosen as $(0, -1)$. Note that the normalization constant c is not used in the program.

```julia
rwsamp.jl
using Plots
f(x,y) = exp(-4*(y-x^2)^2 + (y-1)^2)*(y < 2)
N = 10000
xx = zeros(N,2); x = [0 -1]; xx[1,:] = x;
for i in 2:N
    y = x + randn(1,2); # proposal
    alpha = min(f(y[1],y[2])/f(x[1],x[2]),1); # acceptance
        prob
    r = (rand() < alpha);
    global x = r*y + (1-r)*x; # next value of the Markov chain
    xx[i,:] = x;
end
scatter(xx[:,1],xx[:,2],markersize = 1)
x = range(-2, stop=2, length=50)
y = range(-2, stop=2, length=50)
contour!(x,y,f)
```

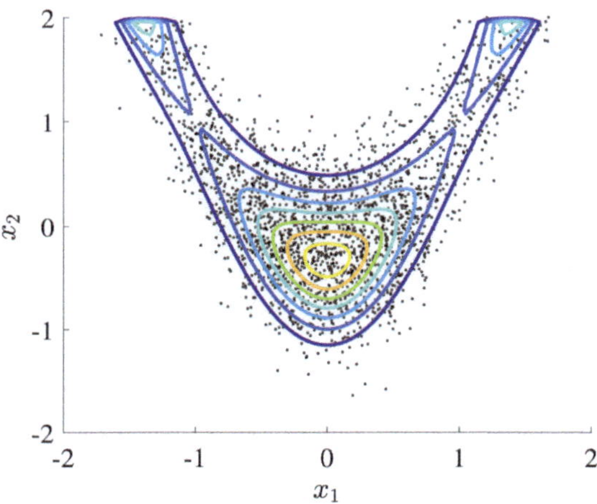

Fig. 7.16 Approximate samples from pdf f produced via the random walk sampler

7.6 Gibbs Sampler

Suppose that $\boldsymbol{X} = [X_1, \ldots, X_n]^\top$ is a random vector with joint pdf $f(\boldsymbol{x})$. Direct sampling from f may be difficult, especially if n is large. However, often sampling from the conditional pdf of X_i given $X_j = x_j, j \neq i$ is feasible. Let us denote these one-dimensional pdfs by $f_i(x_i \,|\, x_1, \ldots, x_{i-1}, x_{i+1}, \ldots, x_n)$, $i = 1, \ldots, n$. If drawing from each f_i is easy, then one can use the **Gibbs sampler** to construct a Markov chain $\boldsymbol{X}_1, \boldsymbol{X}_2, \ldots$ with limiting pdf f. This Markov chain is generated as follows. As in the Metropolis–Hastings sampler, at each step t, given a current state $\boldsymbol{X}_t = \boldsymbol{x}$, a proposal $\boldsymbol{Y}$ is drawn from a transition density $q_{1 \to n}(\boldsymbol{y} \,|\, \boldsymbol{x})$ given by

$$q_{1 \to n}(\boldsymbol{y} \,|\, \boldsymbol{x}) = f_1(y_1 \,|\, x_2, \ldots, x_n) f_2(y_2 \,|\, y_1, x_3, \ldots, x_n) \cdots f_n(y_n \,|\, y_1, \ldots, y_{n-1}) \,.$$

Thus, draw Y_1 from the conditional pdf $f_1(y_1 \,|\, x_2, \ldots, x_n)$, draw Y_2 from $f_2(y_2 \,|\, y_1, x_3, \ldots, x_n)$, and so on. However, unlike the Metropolis–Hastings sampler, this proposal is *always accepted*; so $\boldsymbol{X}_{t+1} = \boldsymbol{Y}$. The algorithm is summarized as follows.

Algorithm 7.4. (Gibbs Sampler)

1 Initialize $\boldsymbol{X}_0 = (X_{0,1}, \ldots, X_{0,n})$.
2 **for** $t = 0$ **to** $N - 1$ **do**
3 $\quad$ Draw Y_1 from $f(y_1 \,|\, X_{t,2}, \ldots, X_{t,n})$.
4 $\quad$ **for** $i = 2$ **to** n **do**
5 $\quad\quad$ Draw Y_i from $f(y_i \,|\, Y_1, \ldots, Y_{i-1}, X_{t,i+1}, \ldots, X_{t,n})$.
6 $\quad$ $\boldsymbol{X}_{t+1} \leftarrow \boldsymbol{Y}$
7 **return** $\boldsymbol{X}_0, \ldots, \boldsymbol{X}_N$

$\quad$ To verify that the Markov chain $\boldsymbol{X}_0, \boldsymbol{X}_1, \ldots$ indeed has limiting pdf $f(\boldsymbol{x})$, we need to check that the global balance equations (7.10) hold. In general the detailed balance equations (7.11) do *not* hold—$f(\boldsymbol{x}) \, q_{1 \to n}(\boldsymbol{y} \,|\, \boldsymbol{x}) \neq f(\boldsymbol{y}) \, q_{1 \to n}(\boldsymbol{x} \,|\, \boldsymbol{y})$. However, a similar result, due to Hammersley and Clifford, does hold: if $q_{n \to 1}(\boldsymbol{x} \,|\, \boldsymbol{y})$ denotes the transition density of the reverse move, in the order $n \to n - 1 \to \cdots \to 1$, that is,

$$q_{n \to 1}(\boldsymbol{x} \,|\, \boldsymbol{y})$$
$$= f_n(x_n \,|\, y_1, \ldots, y_{n-1}) f_{n-1}(x_{n-1} \,|\, y_1, \ldots, y_{n-2}, x_n) \cdots f_1(x_1 \,|\, x_2, \ldots, x_n) \,,$$

then

$$f(\boldsymbol{x}) \, q_{1 \to n}(\boldsymbol{y} \,|\, \boldsymbol{x}) = f(\boldsymbol{y}) \, q_{n \to 1}(\boldsymbol{x} \,|\, \boldsymbol{y}) \,. \tag{7.16}$$

Intuitively, the long-run proportion of transitions $\boldsymbol{x} \to \boldsymbol{y}$ for the "forward move" chain is equal to the long-run proportion of transitions $\boldsymbol{y} \to \boldsymbol{x}$ for the "reverse move" chain. By integrating (in the continuous case) both sides in (7.16) with respect to $\boldsymbol{x}$, we see that the global balance equations hold:

$$\int f(\boldsymbol{x})\, q_{1\to n}(\boldsymbol{y}\,|\,\boldsymbol{x})\, \mathrm{d}\boldsymbol{x} = f(\boldsymbol{y})\ .$$

Example 7.14 (Sampling from Pdf via Gibbs Sampler). Consider the two-dimensional pdf:

$$f(x_1, x_2) = c\, \mathrm{e}^{-x_1 x_2 - x_1 - x_2}, \quad x_1 \geq 0, x_2 \geq 0\ ,$$

where the normalization constant c remains unspecified. Let (X_1, X_2) be distributed according to f. The conditional pdf of X_1 given $X_2 = x_2$ is

$$f_1(x_1\,|\,x_2) \overset{\mathrm{def}}{=} f_{X_1\,|\,X_2}(x_1\,|\,x_2) = \frac{f(x_1, x_2)}{f_{X_2}(x_2)} \propto f(x_1, x_2) \propto \mathrm{e}^{-x_1(x_2 + 1)}\ .$$

It follows that X_1 given $X_2 = x_2$ has an $\mathsf{Exp}(x_2 + 1)$ distribution; and, by symmetry, X_2 given $X_1 = x_1$ has an $\mathsf{Exp}(x_1 + 1)$ distribution. Sampling from the joint pdf can thus be established via the Gibbs sampler by alternately generating from $\mathsf{Exp}(x_2 + 1)$ and $\mathsf{Exp}(x_1 + 1)$, as implemented in the following Julia program.

```
gibbssamp.jl
```

```julia
using Plots
f(x,y) = exp(-(x*y + x + y))*(x > 0 && y > 0)
N = 10^4; x = zeros(N,2); x2 = 1;
for i  in  2:N
    x1 = -log(rand())/(x2+1);
    global x2 = -log(rand())/(x1+1);
    global x[i,:] = [x1 x2];
end
scatter(x[:,1],x[:,2],markersize=0.2)
```

7.7 Problems

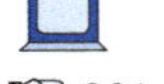

7.1. Consider the estimation of the p-value in Example 7.1

a. Under H_0 we have $\mu = 0$, but σ^2 remains unspecified. Why is it allowed to take $\sigma = 1$ to generate the sample $T_1, \ldots, T_N$?

b. Show, using Theorem 5.1, that T under H_0 has a t_3 distribution, and calculate the true p-value.

c. Speed up the given Julia code by "vectorizing" the **for** loop.

7.2. Monte Carlo sampling methods are useful for calculating p-values for a **goodness-of-fit test**, where the data $X_1, \ldots, X_k$ is assumed to come from a multinomial distribution $\mathsf{Mnom}(n, p_1, \ldots, p_k)$.

As an example, consider a racetrack with eight starting boxes. Out of 200 races, the numbers of winning horses that started from boxes $1, 2, \ldots, 8$ are 39, 29, 24, 20, 21, 24, 21, and 22, respectively. Is this an indication that the winning probabilities $p_1, \ldots, p_8$ are not all equal to $1/8$? The test statistic that is typically used for a goodness-of- fit test is

$$T = \sum_{i=1}^{k} \frac{(O_i - E_i)^2}{E_i} \, ,$$

where O_i $(=X_i)$ is the *observed* number of observations in class i and E_i $(= \mathbb{E}X_i)$ is the *expected* number of observations in class i. In this case $E_i = 25$ for all i and the observed counts are given above. The hypothesis $H_0 : p_1 = \ldots = p_8 = 1/8$ is rejected in favor of the negation of H_0 for large values of the test statistic.

a. Write a Monte Carlo sampling program to estimate the p-value for this test. Do you reject the null hypothesis or not? Hint: to draw a vector $\boldsymbol{X} = [X_1, \ldots, X_8]^\top \sim \mathsf{Mnom}(200, 1/8, \ldots, 1/8)$, you can use:

```
using NaNStatistics
winner = ceil.(8*rand(200))
X, bins = histcountindices(winner,0:8);
```

b. It can be shown that under H_0 the test statistic, T has approximately a χ_7^2 distribution. Verify this by drawing an iid sample from T and comparing the empirical cdf with that of the χ_7^2 distribution:

7.3. Let F_N be the empirical cdf of $x_1, \ldots, x_N$, and let X be a random variable with cdf F_N. Show that $\mathbb{E}X = \bar{x}$ and $\mathrm{Var}(X) = \sum_{i=1}^{N} (x_i - \bar{x})^2/N$, where $\bar{x} = (x_1 + \cdots + x_N)/N$.

7.4. Consider a mixture pdf:

$$f(x) = w_1 f_1(x) + \cdots + w_k f_k(x), \quad w_j \geq 0, j = 1, \ldots, k, \quad \sum_{j=1}^{k} w_j = 1 \, , \quad (7.17)$$

where each f_j is itself a pdf. Let J be a discrete random variable taking values $1, \ldots, k$ with probabilities $w_1, \ldots, w_k$, respectively. Let X be a random variable such that the conditional pdf of X given $J = j$ is f_j.

a. Show that X has mixture pdf (7.17).
b. Using (a.) describe how one could generate a random variable from the mixture pdf (7.17).

c. Suppose pdf f_j has mean μ_j and variance σ_j^2, $j = 1, \ldots, n$. Express $\mathbb{E}X$ and $\mathrm{Var}(X)$ in terms of these parameters.

7.5. It can be shown that the Kolmogorov–Smirnov statistic D_N in (7.6) satisfies

$$\lim_{N \to \infty} \mathbb{P}(\sqrt{N}\,D_N \le x) = \sum_{k=-\infty}^{\infty} (-1)^k e^{-2(kx)^2}, \quad x > 0 . \tag{7.18}$$

Compare the estimated p-value in Example 7.3 with an approximated one calculated via (7.18).

7.6. In Example 7.5 we considered the quality of various estimators for the mode of the Cauchy distribution using (re)sampling techniques.

a. Instead of estimating the pdf of the sample mean using resampled data (dashed line in Fig. 7.7), estimate the pdf of the sample mean by sampling new data from the Cauchy distribution. How do the kernel density estimates compare?
b. Another possible estimator for the mode of the Cauchy distribution is the **trimmed mean** estimator, which is given by the sample mean of all outcomes x_i with $|x_i| \le \beta$, where β is some positive number. Carry out a bootstrap procedure for the trimmed mean with $\beta = 100$ and $\beta = 10$. How do the pdfs compare with those of the sample median and sample mean?

7.7. In Example 7.7 we saw that for a sample size of $N = 100$ the bootstrap and delta method gave identical results for the ratio estimator $\overline{X}/\overline{Y}$. Repeat the analysis and compare the two methods for a sample size $N = 10$, with x-values

$$
\begin{array}{ccccc}
16.4321 & 2.4334 & 14.3433 & 7.9650 & 14.1052 \\
6.7660 & 0.1430 & 10.0420 & 7.1071 & 13.5305
\end{array}
$$

and y-values

$$
\begin{array}{ccccc}
14.9151 & 0.4312 & 11.5407 & 4.4538 & 8.7741 \\
0.8462 & 0.0302 & 1.7955 & 1.4568 & 7.8052
\end{array}
$$

7.8. The **median** of a distribution with pdf f is the number m such that $\int_{-\infty}^{m} f(x)\,dx = 1/2$. The data

$$
\begin{array}{cccccc}
1.4066 & 1.2917 & 1.4080 & 4.2801 & 1.2136 & 2.7461 \\
11.1076 & 0.9247 & 5.8833 & 10.2513 & 3.8285 & 3.2116 \\
0.5451 & 0.9896 & 1.1602 & 7.7723 & 0.1702 & 0.8907 \\
0.2276 & 3.1197 & 11.4909 & 0.6475 & 11.2279 & 0.7639
\end{array}
$$

form an iid sample from an $\mathsf{Exp}(\lambda)$ distribution.

a. Show that the median of $\mathsf{Exp}(\lambda)$ is $\ln(2)/\lambda$.

b. This suggests that we could estimate λ via the estimator $T = \ln(2)/\widetilde{X}$, where $\widetilde{X}$ is the sample median. Find the corresponding estimate. What is the maximum likelihood estimate of λ?

c. Carry out a bootstrap analysis of both estimators and compare their accuracies.

7.9. The concentration of a certain chemical is measured at times $1, 2, 3, \ldots,$ 20. The measurements are

```
18.9506    41.4228    52.0253    63.5451    71.9634
79.0504    80.9685    84.6222    89.6391    93.5085
95.8680    91.3177    97.7423    97.1969    96.7448
96.8155    96.4435    98.2087    98.3126    97.8173
```

(e.g., at time $t = 12$ the concentration is 91.3177). Suppose the data are modeled by the following nonlinear regression model:

$$Y_i = a\,(1 - e^{-b\,t_i}) + \varepsilon_i\,, \quad i = 1, \ldots, n\,, \tag{7.19}$$

where $\{\varepsilon_i\} \overset{\text{iid}}{\sim} \mathcal{N}(0, \sigma^2)$, and a, b, and σ^2 are unknown. To fit the model (7.19) to the points $\{(t_i, y_i)\}$, we can apply a *least-squares* approach, where a and b are chosen such that the sum of the squared deviations   ☞ 12

$$r(a, b) = \sum_{i=1}^{n} (y_i - a\,(1 - e^{-b\,t_i}))^2\,, \tag{7.20}$$

is minimized. This requires numerical minimization.

a. Plot the points (t_i, y_i), $i = 1, \ldots, n = 20$.

b. Show that the values $\widehat{a}$ and $\widehat{b}$ that minimize the function r in (7.20) are the maximum likelihood estimates of a and b. Express the maximum likelihood estimate of σ^2 in terms of $\widehat{a}$ and $\widehat{b}$.

c. Implement a Julia program to find the optimal values $\widehat{a} = 99.14$ and $\widehat{b} = 0.255$, using the following code snippet (`yorg` and `torg` store the original data):

```julia
using Optim
r(x) =  sum((yorg .- x[1]*(1 .- exp.(-x[2]*torg))).^2);
res = optimize(r,[100.0,1.0])
mle = res.minimizer
ahat = mle[1]; bhat=mle[2];
```

d. To assess how accurate the estimates for a and b are, resample the data 1000 times. For each resampled dataset, estimate a and b via `optimize`, as above. Plot kernel density estimates for the pdfs of $\widehat{a}$ and $\widehat{b}$, and determine 95% bootstrap intervals for a and b.

7.10. Let $X_1, \ldots, X_n$ and $Y_1, \ldots, Y_n$ be independent random samples from the $\mathsf{Exp}(\lambda)$ and $\mathsf{Exp}(\mu)$ distribution, respectively, for unknown λ and μ. Suppose outcomes of $X_1, \ldots, X_n$ are given by the data in Problem 7.8 (so $n = 24$), and outcomes of $Y_1, \ldots, Y_n$ are

23.9618	4.9055	6.0424	0.5870	4.0856	1.6503
10.1976	4.0208	25.9484	15.3954	19.5160	0.5937
11.5481	18.3895	30.4093	7.6527	9.7329	8.6130
6.2353	5.5157	9.9489	21.3850	5.1142	28.2284

The maximum likelihood estimator for $\ell = \lambda/\mu$ is $\sum_{i=1}^{n} Y_i / \sum_{i=1}^{n} X_i$. Find a 95% bootstrap confidence interval (percentile method) for ℓ.

7.11. Let $X_1, \ldots, X_n$ be an iid sample from a $\mathcal{U}(0, \theta)$ distribution, where $\theta > 0$ is unknown. The maximum likelihood estimator of θ is $M = \max\{X_1, \ldots, X_n\}$. Suppose $M_1^*, \ldots, M_K^*$ is a bootstrap sample of M, based on an outcome $x_1, \ldots, x_n$. Explain why it is a bad idea to construct a confidence interval for θ on the basis of the $\{M_i^*\}$.

☞ 221

7.12. For the Metropolis–Hastings sampler, verify that the local balance equations (7.14) hold if the acceptance probability is chosen as in (7.13). Hint: consider two cases: $f(y)q(x\,|\,y) \le f(x)q(y\,|\,x)$ and $f(y)q(x\,|\,y) \ge f(x)q(y\,|\,x)$.

7.13. Let $X_t, t = 0, 1, 2, \ldots$ be a random walk on the graph in Fig. 7.17. From each state the random walk chooses one of the adjacent states with equal probability. The starting state is 1.

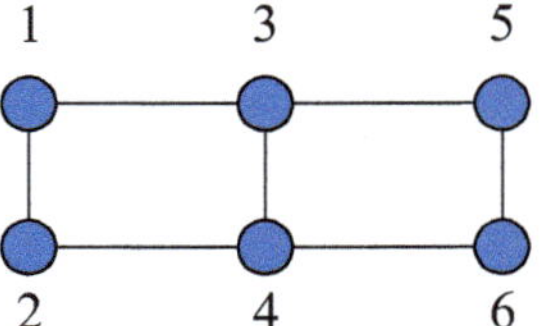

Fig. 7.17 The graph on which the random walk is performed

a. Is the chain irreducible and aperiodic?
b. Do the local balance equations hold? If so, find the solution $f(1), \ldots, f(6)$.
c. Explain why the probabilities $\mathbb{P}(X_t = x)$, $x = 1, \ldots, 6$, do not converge as $t \to \infty$.

7.14. Run the random walk sampler with a $\mathcal{N}(10, 2)$ target distribution and $\mathcal{N}(x, 0.01)$ proposal, drawing the initial point from the $\mathcal{N}(0, 0.01)$ distribution. Take a sample size of $N = 5000$ and plot $\{X_t\}$ against $t = 1, \ldots, N$. Based on the graph, give a rough estimate of the burn-in period.

We can estimate $\ell = \mathbb{E}\ln(X^2)$, where $X \sim \mathcal{N}(10,2)$, by taking the sample average of $\ln(X_{B+1}^2), \ldots, \ln(X_N^2)$, where B is the burn-in size. By independently generating $K = 100$ such estimates, find an approximate 95% confidence interval for ℓ. Generate 20 such intervals and show that the true value for ℓ (which is $4.58453\ldots$) is contained in these intervals with a probability much smaller than 95%. Hence, the combination of a burn-in size of $B = 1000$ and a sample size of $N = 5000$ is inadequate to provide an accurate estimate for ℓ.

7.15. Let $\mathscr{X}$ be a finite set on which a *neighborhood* structure is defined; that is, each $\boldsymbol{x} \in \mathscr{X}$ has a set of neighbors $\mathcal{N}(\boldsymbol{x})$. Let $n_{\boldsymbol{x}}$ be the number of neighbors of $\boldsymbol{x} \in \mathscr{X}$. Consider a Metropolis–Hastings algorithm with proposal density $q(\boldsymbol{y} \,|\, \boldsymbol{x}) = 1/n_{\boldsymbol{x}}$ for all $\boldsymbol{y} \in \mathcal{N}(\boldsymbol{x})$. That is, from a current state $\boldsymbol{x}$, the proposal state is drawn from the set of neighbors with equal probability. Let the acceptance probability be $\alpha(\boldsymbol{x}, \boldsymbol{y}) = \min\{n_{\boldsymbol{x}}/n_{\boldsymbol{y}}, 1\}$.

Assuming the chain is irreducible and aperiodic, what is its limiting distribution?

7.16. Let $U_1, U_2 \sim_{\text{iid}} \mathcal{U}(0,1)$. Explain why $X = -\ln U_1 \times (2\mathbb{1}_{\{U_2 \leq 1/2\}} - 1)$ has pdf $g(x) = \mathrm{e}^{-|x|}/2, x \in \mathbb{R}$.

7.17. A **Langevin Metropolis–Hastings** sampler is a random walk sampler where the proposal state, for a current state $\boldsymbol{x}$, is given by

$$\boldsymbol{Y} = \boldsymbol{x} + \frac{h}{2}\nabla \ln f(\boldsymbol{x}) + \sqrt{h}\,\boldsymbol{Z}, \quad \boldsymbol{Z} \sim \mathcal{N}(\boldsymbol{0}, \mathbb{I}),$$

where $h > 0$ is a step size, f is the target pdf, and $\nabla \ln f$ is the gradient of $\ln f$. Note that the proposal distribution is not symmetric around $\boldsymbol{x}$. Use this sampler to draw $N = 10^5$ dependent samples from the $\mathsf{Gamma}(2,1)$ distribution. Use the `kde` function (with `res = true` flag) to assess how well the estimated pdf fits the true pdf. Investigate how the step size h and the length of the burn-in period affect the fit.

7.18. Let $\boldsymbol{X} = [X, Y]^\top$ be a random column vector with a bivariate normal distribution with expectation vector $\boldsymbol{0} = [0,0]^\top$ and covariance matrix:

$$\Sigma = \begin{bmatrix} 1 & \varrho \\ \varrho & 1 \end{bmatrix}.$$

a. Show that $(Y \,|\, X = x) \sim \mathcal{N}(\varrho x, 1 - \varrho^2)$ and $(X \,|\, Y = y) \sim \mathcal{N}(\varrho y, 1 - \varrho^2)$.
b. Write a Gibbs sampler to draw 10^4 samples from the bivariate distribution $\mathcal{N}(\boldsymbol{0}, \Sigma)$ and plot the data for $\varrho = 0, 0.7$, and 0.9.

7.19. Consider the two-dimensional pdf:

$$f(\boldsymbol{x}) = c\, \exp(-(x_1^2 x_2^2 + x_1^2 + x_2^2 - 8x_1 - 8x_2)/2)\,, \quad \boldsymbol{x} \in \mathbb{R}^2\,. \qquad (7.21)$$

a. Give a 3D plot and a contour plot for this function (ignoring c).
b. Implement a random walk sampler with proposals of the form $\boldsymbol{Y} = \boldsymbol{x} + \sigma \boldsymbol{Z}$, where $\boldsymbol{Z} \sim \mathsf{N}(\boldsymbol{0}, \mathbb{I}_2)$. Start the sampler at the point $[0, 4]$.
c. Plot the progression of the first component of the Markov chain against time, for $\sigma = 0.2$ and $\sigma = 2$. Comment on the difference.
d. Give a kernel density estimate of the pdf X_1 if $\boldsymbol{X} = [X_1, X_2]^\top \sim f$.

7.20. Consider the two-dimensional pdf (7.21) in Problem 7.19.

a. Show that conditional on $X_2 = x_2$, X_1 has a normal distribution with expectation $4/(1 + x_2^2)$ and variance $1/(1 + x_2^2)$.
b. Implement a Gibbs sampler to sample from f.

7.21. In Algorithm 7.4 the vector $\boldsymbol{X}$ is updated in a *systematic* order: $1, 2, \ldots, n, 1, 2, \ldots$. A variant of the algorithm is to update the coordinates in *random* order. Specifically, Steps 3–5 of the algorithm are replaced by

Given the current state $\boldsymbol{X}_t$, generate $\boldsymbol{Y}$ as follows:

1. Draw J uniformly from $\{1, \ldots, n\}$.
2. Given $J = j$, draw $Y_j \sim f_j(y_j \mid X_{t,1}, \ldots, X_{t,j-1}, X_{t,j+1}, \ldots, X_{t,n})$.
3. For $i \neq j$ set $Y_i = X_{t,i}$.

a. Show that, given $\boldsymbol{X}_t = \boldsymbol{x}$, $\boldsymbol{Y}$ has pdf (in the continuous case)

$$q(\boldsymbol{y} \mid \boldsymbol{x}) = \frac{1}{n} \frac{f(\boldsymbol{y})}{\int_{-\infty}^{\infty} f(\boldsymbol{y})\, \mathrm{d}y_j}\,, \qquad (7.22)$$

where $\boldsymbol{y} = (x_1, \ldots, x_{j-1}, y_j, x_{j+1}, \ldots, x_n)$.
b. Show that the random-order Gibbs sampler can be viewed as an instance of the Metropolis–Hastings sampler, with transition density $q(\boldsymbol{y} \mid \boldsymbol{x})$ given in (7.22) and with acceptance probability $\alpha(\boldsymbol{x}, \boldsymbol{y}) = 1$.

Chapter 8
Bayesian Inference

Bayesian statistics is a branch of statistics that is centered around Bayes' formula (1.8), which is repeated in (8.1). To fully appreciate Bayesian inference, it is important to understand that the type of statistical reasoning here is somewhat different from that in frequentist statistics. In particular, model parameters are usually treated as *random* rather than fixed quantities. Moreover, Bayesian statistics uses a notation system that deviates from the frequentist one in two aspects:

☞ 16

1. Pdfs and conditional pdfs always use the *same letter f* (sometimes p is used instead of f). For example, instead of writing $f_X(x)$ and $f_Y(y)$ for the pdfs of X and Y, one simply writes $f(x)$ and $f(y)$. Similarly, the conditional pdf $f_{X \mid Y}(x \mid y)$ of X given Y is denoted in Bayesian notation as $f(x \mid y)$. This style of notation can be of great descriptive value, despite its apparent ambiguity, and we will use it in this book whenever we work in a Bayesian setting. As an example, the Bayesian formula (1.8) in terms of (conditional) pdfs can be written in Bayesian notation as

$$f(\boldsymbol{y} \mid \boldsymbol{x}) = \frac{f(\boldsymbol{x} \mid \boldsymbol{y}) \, f(\boldsymbol{y})}{\int f(\boldsymbol{x} \mid \boldsymbol{y}) \, f(\boldsymbol{y}) \, \mathrm{d}\boldsymbol{y}} \propto f(\boldsymbol{x} \mid \boldsymbol{y}) \, f(\boldsymbol{y}) \,. \tag{8.1}$$

   (Replace the integral with a sum in the discrete case.)
2. In Bayesian statistics the notation does not make a distinction between random variables and their outcomes. Both are usually indicated by *lowercase* letters. It is assumed that it is clear from the context whether a variable x or θ should be interpreted as an outcome (a number) or a random variable.

J. C. C. Chan, D. P. Kroese, *Statistical Modeling and Computation*,
Springer Texts in Statistics, https://doi.org/10.1007/978-1-0716-4132-3_8

The general framework for Bayesian statistics is as follows (compare with
the frequentist framework in Chap. 5): it is assumed that the data vector, $\boldsymbol{x}$
say, has been drawn from a conditional pdf $f(\boldsymbol{x}\,|\,\boldsymbol{\theta})$, where $\boldsymbol{\theta}$ is a random[1]
vector of parameters. The pdf of $\boldsymbol{\theta}$ conveys the a priori (existing beforehand,
before any experience) information about $\boldsymbol{\theta}$. Observing the data $\boldsymbol{x}$ will affect
our knowledge of $\boldsymbol{\theta}$, and the way to update this information is to use Bayes'
formula (8.1). The main concepts are summarized in the following definition.

Definition 8.1. (Prior, Likelihood, and Posterior). Let $\boldsymbol{x}$ and $\boldsymbol{\theta}$
denote the data and parameters in a Bayesian statistical model:

- The pdf of $\boldsymbol{\theta}$ is called the **prior** pdf.
- The conditional pdf $f(\boldsymbol{x}\,|\,\boldsymbol{\theta})$ is called the Bayesian **likelihood** func-
  tion.
- The central object of interest is the **posterior** pdf $f(\boldsymbol{\theta}\,|\,\boldsymbol{x})$ which,
  by Bayes' theorem, is proportional to the product of the prior and
  likelihood:

$$f(\boldsymbol{\theta}\,|\,\boldsymbol{x}) \propto f(\boldsymbol{x}\,|\,\boldsymbol{\theta})\, f(\boldsymbol{\theta})\,.$$

The posterior pdf thus conveys the knowledge of $\boldsymbol{\theta}$ after taking into account the information $\boldsymbol{x}$. Note that the likelihood function in Bayesian statistics differs slightly from that in frequentist statistics. In Bayesian statistics
the likelihood $f(\boldsymbol{x}\,|\,\boldsymbol{\theta})$ is a conditional pdf of the data $\boldsymbol{x}$, whereas in the fre-
quentist case the likelihood $L(\boldsymbol{\theta};\boldsymbol{x}) = f(\boldsymbol{x};\boldsymbol{\theta})$ is viewed as a function of $\boldsymbol{\theta}$
for fixed $\boldsymbol{x}$. The posterior pdf can be viewed as a scaled version of the fre-
quentist likelihood. Indeed, if the prior pdf is constant, then the posterior pdf
coincides with the frequentist likelihood, up to a multiplicative constant.

Example 8.1 (Bayesian Inference for Coin Toss Experiment). Consider the basic random experiment where we toss a biased coin n times. Suppose that the outcomes are $x_1, \ldots, x_n$, with $x_i = 1$ if the i-th toss is Heads
and $x_i = 0$ otherwise, $i = 1, \ldots, n$. Let θ denote the probability of Heads.
We wish to obtain information about θ from the data $\boldsymbol{x} = [x_1, \ldots, x_n]^\top$. For
example, we wish to construct a confidence interval.

The a priori information about θ is described by the prior pdf $f(\theta)$. For
example, the choice of a *uniform* prior $f(\theta) = 1, 0 \le \theta \le 1$ indicates no prior
knowledge about θ. We assume that conditional on θ the $\{x_i\}$ are independent
and $\mathsf{Ber}(\theta)$ distributed. Thus, the Bayesian likelihood is

$$f(\boldsymbol{x}\,|\,\theta) = \prod_{i=1}^{n} \theta^{x_i}(1-\theta)^{1-x_i} = \theta^s\,(1-\theta)^{n-s}\,,$$

---

[1] Strict Bayesians would insist that $\boldsymbol{\theta}$ is not random, but that the information on $\boldsymbol{\theta}$
is summarized by a probability distribution. However, for computational and analysis
purposes, we can treat $\boldsymbol{\theta}$ as if it were a random vector.

where $s = x_1 + \cdots + x_n$ represents the total number of successes. Using a uniform prior gives the posterior pdf:

$$f(\theta \mid \boldsymbol{x}) = c\,\theta^s\,(1-\theta)^{n-s}\,, \quad 0 \le \theta \le 1\,.$$

This is the pdf of the $\mathsf{Beta}(s+1, n-s+1)$ distribution. The normalization constant is $c = (n+1)\binom{n}{s}$. The graph of the posterior pdf for $n = 100$ and $s = 1$ is given in Fig. 8.1.

☞ 74

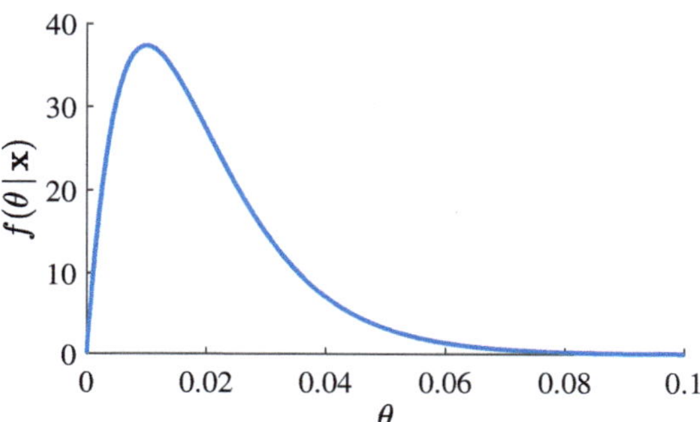

Fig. 8.1 Posterior pdf for θ, with $n = 100$ and $s = 1$

A Bayesian confidence interval, called a **credible interval**, for θ is formed by taking the appropriate quantiles of the posterior pdf. As an example, suppose that $n = 100$ and $s = 1$. Then, a left one-sided 95% credible interval for θ is $[0, 0.0461]$, where 0.0461 is the 0.95 quantile of the $\mathsf{Beta}(2, 100)$ distribution. As an estimate for θ, one often takes the **posterior mean**, that is, the expectation corresponding to the posterior pdf. In this case, for general n and s, the posterior mean is $(s+1)/(s+1+n-s+1) = (s+1)/(n+2)$; see also Problem 8.1. An alternative estimate for θ is the value for which the posterior pdf is maximal—the so-called **posterior mode**. The posterior mode is here $\widehat{\theta} = s/n$, which coincides with the (frequentist) sample mean.

☞ 26?

8.1 Hierarchical Bayesian Models

In the coin flipping example, both the parameter θ and the data $\boldsymbol{x}$ are random variables, and the joint distribution of θ and $\boldsymbol{x}$ is specified in a "hierarchical" way:

$$\theta \sim f(\theta)$$
$$(\boldsymbol{x} \mid \theta) \sim f(\boldsymbol{x} \mid \theta)\,.$$

By the product rule of probability, the joint pdf is simply the product $f(\theta)\,f(\boldsymbol{x} \mid \theta)$, and the posterior pdf is proportional to this last product (viewed a function of θ). For models involving more than one parameter, a similar hierarchical structure is often used to specify the model. For example, a three-parameter model could be specified as follows:

$$\alpha \sim f(\alpha)$$
$$(\beta \,|\, \alpha) \sim f(\beta \,|\, \alpha)$$
$$(\gamma \,|\, \alpha, \beta) \sim f(\gamma \,|\, \alpha, \beta)$$
$$(\boldsymbol{x} \,|\, \alpha, \beta, \gamma) \sim f(\boldsymbol{x} \,|\, \alpha, \beta, \gamma) \,.$$

That is, first specify the prior pdf of α, then given α specify the pdf of β, etc., until finally the likelihood as a function of all the parameters is given. Often in practice the reverse order is used: the likelihood is specified first and the priors are defined last. The hierarchical model approach allows for an easy
☞ 72   evaluation of the joint pdf: it is simply the product of the (conditional) pdfs:

$$f(\boldsymbol{x}, \alpha, \beta, \gamma) = f(\boldsymbol{x} \,|\, \alpha, \beta, \gamma)\, f(\gamma \,|\, \alpha, \beta)\, f(\beta \,|\, \alpha) f(\alpha) \,.$$

To find the posterior

$$f(\alpha, \beta, \gamma \,|\, \boldsymbol{x}) \,,$$

view $f(\boldsymbol{x}, \alpha, \beta, \gamma)$ as a function of α, β, and γ for fixed $\boldsymbol{x}$. To find the marginal
☞ 70   posterior pdfs, $f(\alpha \,|\, \boldsymbol{x}), f(\beta \,|\, \boldsymbol{x}), f(\gamma \,|\, \boldsymbol{x})$, *integrate out* the other parameters. For example,

$$f(\gamma \,|\, \boldsymbol{x}) = \iint f(\alpha, \beta, \gamma \,|\, \boldsymbol{x}) \, \mathrm{d}\alpha \, \mathrm{d}\beta \,.$$

This may not always be easy or feasible. An alternative is to use the *Gibbs*
☞ 225   *sampler* to sample from the posterior pdf. After initializing α, β, γ, iterate the following steps:

1. Draw α from $f(\alpha \,|\, \beta, \gamma, \boldsymbol{x})$.
2. Draw β from $f(\beta \,|\, \alpha, \gamma, \boldsymbol{x})$.
3. Draw γ from $f(\gamma \,|\, \alpha, \beta, \boldsymbol{x})$.

After a (dependent) sample $\{(\alpha_t, \beta_t, \gamma_t)\}$ from $f(\alpha, \beta, \gamma \,|\, \boldsymbol{x})$ is generated, output only the variables of interest, e.g., only the $\{\alpha_t\}$.

Example 8.2 (Ticket Inspector).   A ticket inspector has the option of taking three different routes for inspection of parking violations. Each route is characterized by the time it takes to complete the route and the intensity of ticket violations. Suppose the time t spent on route k is exponentially distributed with mean $k/2$ (hours), $k = 1, 2, 3$. For example, route 2 takes on average 1 hour to complete. Suppose further that the number of traffic violations encountered, x say, has a Poisson distribution with mean $10\,k\,t$. So if route 3 takes 2 hours, an average of 60 tickets will be issued. Suppose that on a particular day the ticket inspector has issued 60 tickets. Which route has she/he taken?

Assuming that our prior information about k is that each of the routes is taken with equal probability, we obtain the following hierarchical model:

$$k \sim \mathsf{DU}\{1, 2, 3\} \quad \text{(discrete uniform)}$$
$$(t \mid k) \sim \mathsf{Exp}(2/k)$$
$$(x \mid k, t) \sim \mathsf{Poi}(10\, k\, t) \, .$$

It follows that the joint pdf is

$$f(k, t, x) = f(k) f(t \mid k) f(x \mid t, k) = \frac{1}{3} \frac{2}{k} \, \mathrm{e}^{-\frac{2}{k} t} \mathrm{e}^{-10kt} \frac{(10kt)^x}{x!} \tag{8.2}$$

for $k = 1, 2, 3$, $t \geq 0$, and $x = 0, 1, 2, \ldots$. Note that k and x are discrete random variables and t is continuous. The posterior pdf $f(k, t \mid x = 60)$ is thus of the form:

$$f(k, t \mid x = 60) \propto \frac{1}{k} \, \mathrm{e}^{-\frac{2}{k} t} \mathrm{e}^{-10kt} (kt)^{60} \, . \tag{8.3}$$

The marginal posterior pdf of k can be found by integrating out t in (8.3). That is, for each $k = 1, 2, 3$, calculate:

$$\frac{1}{k} \int_0^\infty \mathrm{e}^{-\frac{2}{k} t} \mathrm{e}^{-10kt} (kt)^{60} \, \mathrm{d}t \, ,$$

and normalize. Numerical evaluation yields the following posterior probabilities (rounded):

$$0.000353516, \quad 0.30469, \quad \text{and} \quad 0.694957 \, .$$

Hence, we have deduced from Bayes formula that the most likely route that was followed is route 3. But route 2 is also quite possible. It is very unlikely that route 1 was used.

In a similar manner, to find $f(t \mid x = 60)$, we sum (8.3) with respect to k, giving

$$f(t \mid x = 60) = c^{-1} t^{60} \left(3^{59} \mathrm{e}^{-92t/3} + 2^{59} \mathrm{e}^{-21t} + \mathrm{e}^{-12t} \right) \, .$$

The normalization constant (which can be expressed in terms of the gamma function) evaluates to $c \approx 3.481048347 \times 10^{19}$. The graph of this marginal posterior pdf is shown in Fig. 8.2 (solid line).

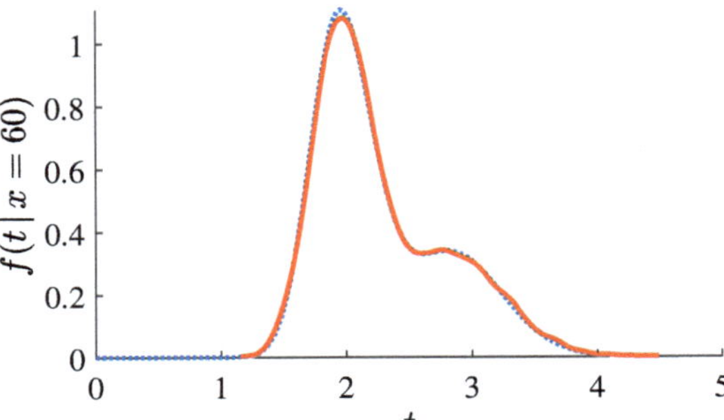

Fig. 8.2 Posterior pdf of t given $x = 60$ (solid line) and its estimate obtained via Gibbs sampling (dotted line)

To (approximately) sample from $f(k, t \mid x = 60)$, we can use the Gibbs sampler (Algorithm 7.4). For this we need to specify:

☞ 225

1. the conditional distribution of k given t and x;
2. the conditional distribution of t given k and x.

By viewing t and x as constants in (8.2), we see that, given t and x, k has a discrete distribution on $\{1, 2, 3\}$ with probabilities proportional to

$$\mathrm{e}^{-12\,t}, \qquad 2^{x-1}\mathrm{e}^{-21t}, \qquad \text{and} \quad 3^{x-1}\mathrm{e}^{-92t/3} \, .$$

Similarly, by viewing k and x as constants in (8.2), we have:

$$f(t \mid x, k) \propto t^x \exp\left\{ -t\left(\frac{2}{k} + 10k\right) \right\} ,$$

which is the pdf of the $\mathsf{Gamma}(x + 1, \frac{2}{k} + 10k)$ distribution. By alternatively sampling from $f(k \mid t, x)$ and $f(t \mid k, x)$, we obtain a dependent sample from $f(k, t \mid x)$. The following Julia program implements the Gibbs sampler. The burn-in period was ignored. Throughout this chapter we use the theta KDE

☞ 208

function **kde** to display a kernel density estimate of the simulated data.

```julia
ticketinspector.jl

include("ThetaKDE.jl")
using Plots, Distributions, .ThetaKDE
n = 10000;
x = 60; # number of tickets
p = [1/3, 1/3, 1/3] # initial value
kk = zeros(Int64,n);
tt = zeros(n);
k = minimum(findall(cumsum(p) .> rand()));
for i in 1:n
    a = x + 1;
```

```
      b = 2/k + 10*k;
      t = rand(Gamma(a,1/b));
      tt[i] = t;
      global p = [exp(-12*t), 2.0^(x-1)*exp(-21*t),  3.0^(x-1)*
          exp(-92*t/3)];
      p = p/sum(p);
      global k = minimum(findall(cumsum(p) .> rand()));
      kk[i] = k;
  end
p1est = sum(kk .== 1)/n # estimate of post. prob. 1
p2est = sum(kk .== 2)/n # estimate of post. prob. 2
p3est = sum(kk .== 3)/n # estimate of post. prob 3
xmesh, density, bw = kde(tt)
plot(xmesh,density)
f1(t) = t^60
f2(t) = 3.0^59*exp(-92*t/3)
f3(t) = 2.0^59*exp(-21*t)
f4(t) = exp(-12*t)
tickf(t) = f1(t)*(f2(t) + f3(t)+f4(t))/3.481048347e19
plot!(xmesh,tickf.(xmesh))
```

Typical outcomes of the posterior probabilities for route k are 10^{-4}, 0.32, and 0.68. These probabilities are in close correspondence with the actual probabilities. The KDE of the posterior pdf of t is given in Fig. 8.2 (dotted line). This is in excellent agreement with the true posterior pdf.

8.2 Common Bayesian Models

The common statistical models in Chap. 4 can also be formulated and ana- ☞ 10:
lyzed in a Bayesian framework. In this section we give various examples of how this is done. Note that inference in a Bayesian setting depends on the prior information, in contrast to the frequentist case.

8.2.1 Normal Model with Unknown μ and σ^2

Let $x_1,\ldots,x_n$ be a random sample from the $\mathcal{N}(\mu,\sigma^2)$ distribution. Let $x = [x_1,\ldots,x_n]^\top$. In frequentist statistics the model can be written as $x \sim \mathcal{N}(\mu\mathbf{1}, \sigma^2\,\mathbb{I}_n)$, where $\mathbf{1}$ is the n-dimensional vector of 1s and $\mathbb{I}_n$ the n-dimensional identity matrix. To formulate the corresponding Bayesian model, we start with a similar likelihood as in the frequentist case; that is,

$$(\boldsymbol{x} \mid \mu, \sigma^2) \sim \mathcal{N}(\mu \mathbf{1}, \sigma^2 \, \mathbb{I}_n) \, .$$

In the Bayesian setting, both μ and σ^2 are random, and we need to specify their prior distributions to complete the model. In practice the choice of the prior distribution is governed by two considerations. Firstly, the prior should be simple enough to facilitate the computation or simulation of the posterior pdf. Secondly, the prior distribution should be general enough to model complete ignorance of the parameter of interest. Priors that do not convey any preknowledge of the parameter are said to be **uninformative**. The uniform or **flat** prior in Example 8.1 is an example.

For the present model, a standard prior for μ is

$$\mu \sim \mathcal{N}(0, \sigma_0^2) \, , \tag{8.4}$$

where $\sigma_0^2 > 0$ is a constant. The larger σ_0^2 is, the more uninformative is the the prior. A standard prior for σ^2 is

$$\sigma^2 \sim \mathsf{InvGamma}(\alpha_0, \lambda_0) \, , \tag{8.5}$$

where $\alpha_0 > 0$ and $\lambda_0 > 0$ are constants and $\mathsf{InvGamma}(\alpha, \lambda)$ denotes the **inverse-gamma** distribution.

Definition 8.2. (Inverse-Gamma Distribution). A random variable Z is said to have an **inverse-gamma** distribution with **shape** parameter $\alpha > 0$ and **rate** parameter $\lambda > 0$ if its pdf is given by

$$f(z; \alpha, \lambda) = \frac{\lambda^\alpha z^{-\alpha-1} e^{-\lambda z^{-1}}}{\Gamma(\alpha)}, \quad z > 0 \, . \tag{8.6}$$

This is the pdf of the random variable $Z = 1/X$ with $X \sim \mathsf{Gamma}(\alpha, \lambda)$.

Thus, (8.5) is equivalent to

$$\frac{1}{\sigma^2} \sim \mathsf{Gamma}(\alpha_0, \lambda_0) \, . \tag{8.7}$$

The smaller the α_0 and λ_0 are, the less informative is the prior. It is further assumed that μ and σ^2 are independent. The joint pdf of $\boldsymbol{x}, \mu$ and σ^2 is therefore

$$f(\boldsymbol{x}, \mu, \sigma^2) = f(\mu) \times f(\sigma^2) \times f(\boldsymbol{x} \mid \mu, \sigma^2)$$

$$= \left(2\pi\sigma_0^2\right)^{-1/2} \exp\left\{-\frac{1}{2}\frac{\mu^2}{\sigma_0^2}\right\}$$

$$\times \frac{\lambda_0^{\alpha_0}(\sigma^2)^{-\alpha_0-1}\exp\left\{-\lambda_0\,(\sigma^2)^{-1}\right\}}{\Gamma(\alpha_0)}$$

$$\times \left(2\pi\sigma^2\right)^{-n/2}\exp\left\{-\frac{1}{2}\frac{\sum_i(x_i-\mu)^2}{\sigma^2}\right\}.$$

It follows that the posterior pdf is given by

$$f(\mu, \sigma^2 \mid \boldsymbol{x}) \propto \left(\sigma^2\right)^{-n/2-\alpha_0-1}\exp\left\{-\frac{1}{2}\frac{\sum_i(x_i-\mu)^2}{\sigma^2} - \frac{1}{2}\frac{\mu^2}{\sigma_0^2} - \frac{\lambda_0}{\sigma^2}\right\}. \quad (8.8)$$

To simulate from it using the Gibbs sampler, we need the distributions of both $(\mu \mid \sigma^2, \boldsymbol{x})$ and $(\sigma^2 \mid \mu, \boldsymbol{x})$. To find $f(\mu \mid \sigma^2, \boldsymbol{x})$, view the right-hand side of (8.8) as a function of μ. This gives:

$$f(\mu \mid \sigma^2, \boldsymbol{x}) \propto \exp\left\{-\frac{n\mu^2 - 2\mu\sum_i x_i}{2\sigma^2} - \frac{1}{2}\frac{\mu^2}{\sigma_0^2}\right\}$$

$$= \exp\left\{-\frac{1}{2}\left(\frac{(n\mu^2 - 2\mu\sum_i x_i)\sigma_0^2 + \mu^2\sigma^2}{\sigma^2\,\sigma_0^2}\right)\right\}$$

$$= \exp\left\{-\frac{1}{2}\left(\frac{\mu^2 - 2\mu\,\sigma_0^2\sum_i x_i/(n\sigma_0^2+\sigma^2)}{\sigma^2\sigma_0^2/(n\sigma_0^2+\sigma^2)}\right)\right\}. \quad (8.9)$$

This shows that $(\mu \mid \sigma^2, \boldsymbol{x})$ has a normal distribution with mean $\sigma_0^2\sum x_i/(n\sigma_0^2 +\sigma^2)$ and variance $\sigma^2\sigma_0^2/(n\sigma_0^2+\sigma^2)$. By defining $\kappa_n = \sigma^2/(\sigma_0^2\,n)$, we can write this succinctly as

$$(\mu \mid \sigma^2, \boldsymbol{x}) \sim \mathcal{N}\left(\frac{\overline{x}}{1+\kappa_n}, \frac{\sigma^2/n}{1+\kappa_n}\right),$$

where $\overline{x}$ is the sample mean. Similarly, to find $f(\sigma^2 \mid \mu, \boldsymbol{x})$, view (8.8) as a function of σ^2. This gives:

$$f(\sigma^2 \mid \mu, \boldsymbol{x}) \propto (\sigma^2)^{-n/2-\alpha_0-1}\exp\left\{-\frac{1}{2}\sum_{i=1}^{n}(x_i-\mu)^2/\sigma^2 - \lambda_0/\sigma^2\right\}. \quad (8.10)$$

In other words,

$$(\sigma^2 \mid \mu, \boldsymbol{x}) \sim \mathsf{InvGamma}\left(\alpha_0 + n/2, \sum_{i=1}^{n}(x_i-\mu)^2/2 + \lambda_0\right).$$

It is interesting to note that in the limit $\sigma_0^2 \to \infty$, $\alpha_0 \to 0$, and $\lambda_0 \to 0$, the right-hand sides of (8.10) and (8.9) define valid probability distributions; namely,

$$(\mu \mid \sigma^2, \boldsymbol{x}) \sim \mathcal{N}\left(\overline{x},\, \sigma^2/n\right)$$

$$(\sigma^2 \mid \mu, \boldsymbol{x}) \sim \mathsf{InvGamma}\left(n/2,\, \sum_{i=1}^{n}(x_i - \mu)^2/2\right).$$

The two distributions above correspond to the following simplified Bayesian model:

$$f(\mu, \sigma^2) = 1/\sigma^2$$

$$(\boldsymbol{x} \mid \mu, \sigma^2) \sim \mathcal{N}(\mu \mathbf{1}, \sigma^2 \, \mathbb{I}_n).$$

Here the prior for (μ, σ^2) is **improper**. That is, it is not a pdf in itself, but by obstinately applying Bayes' formula it does yield a proper posterior pdf. In some sense this prior conveys the least amount of information about μ and σ^2.

In the following Julia script, an iid sample of size $n = 10$ is drawn from $\mathcal{N}(0, 1)$, and a dependent sample from the posterior distribution for the simplified model is obtained, using the Gibbs sampler with $N = 10^5$ samples.

```julia
bayesnorm.jl

using Distributions, .ThetaKDE, Plots
n = 10;
X = randn(n); # generate the data
sample_mean = mean(X);
sample_var = var(X);
sig2 = var(X); mu = sample_mean; # initial state
N = 10^5; # sample size for Gibbs sampler
gibbs_sample = zeros(N,2);
for k in 1:N
    global mu = sample_mean + sqrt(sig2/n)*randn();  # draw mu
    V = sum((X .- mu).^2)/2;
    global sig2 = 1/rand(Gamma(n/2,1/V)); # draw sigma^2
    gibbs_sample[k,:] = [mu sig2];
end
p1 = xmesh,density,bw = kde(gibbs_sample[:,1]);
p2 = xmesh,density,bw = kde(gibbs_sample[:,2]);
plot([p1,p2],layout=(1,2))
```

The estimated posterior pdfs of μ and σ^2 are given in Fig. 8.3. In this case the sample mean and sample variance are 0.1298 and 0.5221, respectively. The

0.05 and 0.95 sample quantiles of the simulated posterior values for μ give the 90% credible interval $(-0.2919, 0.5464)$. This is in close agreement with the frequentist confidence interval (5.19), which in this case is $(-0.2891, 0.5487)$. Similarly, an estimated 90% credible interval for σ^2 is $(0.2773, 1.4128)$, which is in close agreement with the frequentist confidence interval (5.20), which here is $(0.2777, 1.4132)$. See Problem 8.10 for a further discussion of this model.

☞ 13
☞ 264

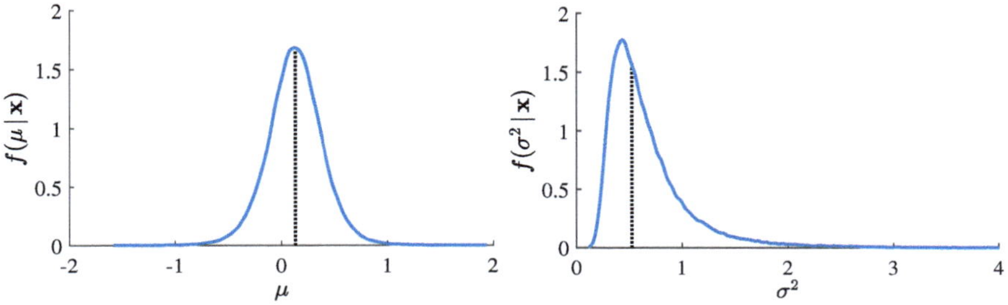

Fig. 8.3 The estimated posterior pdfs of μ and σ^2. The dashed lines correspond to the sample mean (left) and the sample variance (right)

8.2.2 Bayesian Normal Linear Model

Suppose $\boldsymbol{y} = [y_1, \ldots, y_n]^\top$ is described via a *normal linear model*. That is (see (6.23)) the likelihood is specified by

☞ 179

$$(\boldsymbol{y} \mid \boldsymbol{\beta}, \sigma^2) \sim \mathcal{N}(\mathbf{X}\boldsymbol{\beta}, \sigma^2 \mathbb{I}_n) \,,$$

where $\mathbf{X} = [x_{ij}]$ is the (known) $n \times m$ design matrix and $\boldsymbol{\beta} = [\beta_1, \ldots, \beta_m]^\top$ and σ^2 are unknown parameters. Again, both $\boldsymbol{\beta}$ and σ^2 are random in the Bayesian setting, and we need to specify their prior distributions. The prior for σ^2 is the same as in the normal model:

$$\sigma^2 \sim \mathsf{InvGamma}(\alpha_0, \lambda_0) \,,$$

with $\alpha_0 > 0$ and $\lambda_0 > 0$ known. A standard prior for $\boldsymbol{\beta}$ is

$$\boldsymbol{\beta} \sim \mathcal{N}(\boldsymbol{\beta}_0, \boldsymbol{\Sigma}_0),$$

where $\boldsymbol{\Sigma}_0$ is a known covariance matrix and $\boldsymbol{\beta}_0$ a known mean vector. The joint pdf of $\boldsymbol{y}, \boldsymbol{\beta}$ and σ^2 is thus

$$f(\boldsymbol{y}, \boldsymbol{\beta}, \sigma^2) = f(\boldsymbol{\beta}) \times f(\sigma^2) \times f(\boldsymbol{y} \mid \boldsymbol{\beta}, \sigma^2)$$

$$= ((2\pi)^m |\boldsymbol{\Sigma}_0|)^{-1/2} \exp\left\{ -\frac{1}{2}(\boldsymbol{\beta} - \boldsymbol{\beta}_0)^\top \boldsymbol{\Sigma}_0^{-1}(\boldsymbol{\beta} - \boldsymbol{\beta}_0) \right\}$$

$$\times \frac{\lambda_0^{\alpha_0} (\sigma^2)^{-\alpha_0 - 1} \exp\left\{ -\lambda_0 (\sigma^2)^{-1} \right\}}{\Gamma(\alpha_0)}$$

$$\times \left(2\pi\sigma^2\right)^{-n/2} \exp\left\{ -\frac{1}{2\sigma^2}(\boldsymbol{y} - \mathbf{X}\boldsymbol{\beta})^\top (\boldsymbol{y} - \mathbf{X}\boldsymbol{\beta}) \right\} .$$

It follows that the posterior pdf is given by

$$f(\boldsymbol{\beta}, \sigma^2 \mid \boldsymbol{y}) \propto \left(\sigma^2\right)^{-n/2 - \alpha_0 - 1} \exp\left\{ -\frac{1}{2\sigma^2}(\boldsymbol{y} - \mathbf{X}\boldsymbol{\beta})^\top (\boldsymbol{y} - \mathbf{X}\boldsymbol{\beta}) \right.$$
$$\left. -\frac{1}{2}(\boldsymbol{\beta} - \boldsymbol{\beta}_0)^\top \boldsymbol{\Sigma}_0^{-1}(\boldsymbol{\beta} - \boldsymbol{\beta}_0) - \frac{\lambda_0}{\sigma^2} \right\} . \tag{8.11}$$

As before, we use the Gibbs sampler to simulate from this posterior pdf. To that end, we need to derive the distributions of both $(\boldsymbol{\beta} \mid \sigma^2, \boldsymbol{y})$ and $(\sigma^2 \mid \boldsymbol{\beta}, \boldsymbol{y})$.

Following the same argument in Sect. 8.2.1, we can show that

$$(\sigma^2 \mid \boldsymbol{\beta}, \boldsymbol{y}) \sim \mathsf{InvGamma}\left(\alpha_0 + n/2, \ (\boldsymbol{y} - \mathbf{X}\boldsymbol{\beta})^\top (\boldsymbol{y} - \mathbf{X}\boldsymbol{\beta})/2 + \lambda_0 \right) .$$

Next, to find $f(\boldsymbol{\beta} \mid \sigma^2, \boldsymbol{y})$, view the right-hand side of (8.11) as a function of $\boldsymbol{\beta}$. This gives:

$$f(\boldsymbol{\beta} \mid \sigma^2, \boldsymbol{y}) \propto \exp\left\{ -\frac{1}{2\sigma^2}(\boldsymbol{y} - \mathbf{X}\boldsymbol{\beta})^\top (\boldsymbol{y} - \mathbf{X}\boldsymbol{\beta}) - \frac{1}{2}(\boldsymbol{\beta} - \boldsymbol{\beta}_0)^\top \boldsymbol{\Sigma}_0^{-1}(\boldsymbol{\beta} - \boldsymbol{\beta}_0) \right\}$$

$$\propto \exp\left\{ -\frac{1}{2\sigma^2}(\boldsymbol{\beta}^\top \mathbf{X}^\top \mathbf{X}\boldsymbol{\beta} - 2\boldsymbol{\beta}^\top \mathbf{X}^\top \boldsymbol{y}) + \boldsymbol{\beta}^\top \boldsymbol{\Sigma}_0^{-1} \boldsymbol{\beta}_0 - \frac{1}{2}\boldsymbol{\beta}^\top \boldsymbol{\Sigma}_0^{-1} \boldsymbol{\beta} \right\}$$

$$= \exp\left\{ -\frac{1}{2}\left[\boldsymbol{\beta}^\top (\mathbf{X}^\top \mathbf{X}/\sigma^2 + \boldsymbol{\Sigma}_0^{-1})\boldsymbol{\beta} - 2\boldsymbol{\beta}^\top (\mathbf{X}^\top \boldsymbol{y}/\sigma^2 + \boldsymbol{\Sigma}_0^{-1}\boldsymbol{\beta}_0) \right] \right\} . \tag{8.12}$$

Note that the exponent is quadratic in $\boldsymbol{\beta}$, and thus $(\boldsymbol{\beta} \mid \sigma^2, \boldsymbol{y}) \sim \mathcal{N}(\boldsymbol{\mu}, \mathbf{D})$ for some mean vector $\boldsymbol{\mu}$ and covariance matrix $\mathbf{D}$. Therefore,

$$f(\boldsymbol{\beta} \mid \sigma^2, \boldsymbol{y}) \propto \exp\left\{ -\frac{1}{2}(\boldsymbol{\beta} - \boldsymbol{\mu})^\top \mathbf{D}^{-1}(\boldsymbol{\beta} - \boldsymbol{\mu}) \right\}$$

$$\propto \exp\left\{ -\frac{1}{2}\left(\boldsymbol{\beta}^\top \mathbf{D}^{-1}\boldsymbol{\beta} - 2\boldsymbol{\beta}^\top \mathbf{D}^{-1}\boldsymbol{\mu} \right) \right\} .$$

To determine $\boldsymbol{\mu}$ and $\mathbf{D}$, we only need to compare the linear and quadratic terms in (8.12) to those of the $\mathcal{N}(\boldsymbol{\mu}, \mathbf{D})$ density above. This process is sometimes called **completing the squares**. Comparing the quadratic terms gives $\mathbf{D} = (\mathbf{X}^\top \mathbf{X}/\sigma^2 + \boldsymbol{\Sigma}_0^{-1})^{-1}$. Similarly, equating the linear terms in the two expressions gives $\mathbf{D}^{-1}\boldsymbol{\mu} = \mathbf{X}^\top \boldsymbol{y}/\sigma^2 + \boldsymbol{\Sigma}_0^{-1}\boldsymbol{\beta}_0$. In summary, we have the following result.

> **Theorem 8.1. (Conditional Posteriors for the Linear Model).**
> Consider the Bayesian model
>
> $$\boldsymbol{\beta} \sim \mathcal{N}(\boldsymbol{\beta}_0, \boldsymbol{\Sigma}_0)\,, \tag{8.13}$$
>
> $$\sigma^2 \sim \mathsf{InvGamma}(\alpha_0, \lambda_0)\,, \tag{8.14}$$
>
> $$(\boldsymbol{y}\,|\,\boldsymbol{\beta}, \sigma^2) \sim \mathcal{N}(\mathbf{X}\boldsymbol{\beta}, \sigma^2\,\mathbb{I}_n)\,, \tag{8.15}$$
>
> where $\mathbf{X}$ is a fixed $n \times m$ design matrix, $\boldsymbol{\Sigma}_0$ is a fixed $n \times n$ covariance matrix, $\boldsymbol{\beta}_0$ is a fixed vector, and α_0 and λ_0 are fixed constants. Then,
>
> $$(\boldsymbol{\beta}\,|\,\sigma^2, \boldsymbol{y}) \sim \mathcal{N}(\boldsymbol{\mu}, \mathbf{D})\,,$$
>
> where $\boldsymbol{\mu} = \mathbf{D}(\mathbf{X}^\top \boldsymbol{y}/\sigma^2 + \boldsymbol{\Sigma}_0^{-1}\boldsymbol{\beta}_0)$, with $\mathbf{D} = (\mathbf{X}^\top \mathbf{X}/\sigma^2 + \boldsymbol{\Sigma}_0^{-1})^{-1}$, and
>
> $$(\sigma^2\,|\,\boldsymbol{\beta}, \boldsymbol{y}) \sim \mathsf{InvGamma}\left(\alpha_0 + n/2,\ (\boldsymbol{y} - \mathbf{X}\boldsymbol{\beta})^\top(\boldsymbol{y} - \mathbf{X}\boldsymbol{\beta})/2 + \lambda_0\right)\,.$$

Note that as the prior precision matrix $\boldsymbol{\Sigma}_0^{-1}$ approaches the zero matrix, the prior for $\boldsymbol{\beta}$ becomes more non-informative. For $\boldsymbol{\Sigma}_0^{-1} = \mathbf{O}$ (zero matrix), the prior for $\boldsymbol{\beta}$ is improper. However, the conditional density $f(\boldsymbol{\beta}\,|\,\sigma^2, \boldsymbol{y})$ is still a proper pdf. In fact, for $\boldsymbol{\Sigma}_0^{-1} = \mathbf{O}$, we have $\boldsymbol{\mu} = \mathbf{D}\mathbf{X}^\top \boldsymbol{y}/\sigma^2$, with $\mathbf{D} = \sigma^2(\mathbf{X}^\top \mathbf{X})^{-1}$, so that

$$(\boldsymbol{\beta}\,|\,\sigma^2, \boldsymbol{y}) \sim \mathcal{N}(\mathbf{X}^+ \boldsymbol{y}, \sigma^2(\mathbf{X}^\top \mathbf{X})^{-1})\,,$$

where $\mathbf{X}^+ = (\mathbf{X}^\top \mathbf{X})^{-1}\mathbf{X}^\top$ is the (right) pseudo-inverse of $\mathbf{X}$. Using this improper prior for $\boldsymbol{\beta}$, the conditional expectation $\mathbb{E}[\boldsymbol{\beta}\,|\,\sigma^2, \boldsymbol{y}]$ therefore coincides with the least-squares estimate in (5.12).   ☞ 13

The following corollary presents an important generalization of Theorem 8.1 for the situation where $\boldsymbol{y} - \mathbf{X}\boldsymbol{\beta}$ is an affine transformation of $\boldsymbol{y}$; that is, $\boldsymbol{y} - \mathbf{X}\boldsymbol{\beta} = \boldsymbol{a} + \mathbf{A}\boldsymbol{y}$ for some vector $\boldsymbol{a}$ and matrix $\mathbf{A}$. The result will   ☞ 83 be heavily relied on in later parts of the book.

Corollary 8.1. (Conditional Posteriors for the Linear Model with General Error Covariance Matrix). Consider the Bayesian model

$$\boldsymbol{\beta} \sim \mathcal{N}(\boldsymbol{\beta}_0, \boldsymbol{\Sigma}_0) \,, \tag{8.16}$$

$$\sigma^2 \sim \mathsf{InvGamma}(\alpha_0, \lambda_0) \,, \tag{8.17}$$

$$(\boldsymbol{y} - \mathbf{X}\boldsymbol{\beta} \,|\, \boldsymbol{\beta}, \sigma^2) \sim \mathcal{N}(\mathbf{0}, \sigma^2 \mathbf{R}) \,, \tag{8.18}$$

where $\boldsymbol{y} - \mathbf{X}\boldsymbol{\beta}$ is an affine transformation of $\boldsymbol{y}$, $\mathbf{R}$ and $\boldsymbol{\Sigma}_0$ are fixed $n \times n$ (covariance) matrices, $\boldsymbol{\beta}_0$ is a fixed vector, and α_0 and λ_0 are fixed constants. Then,

$$(\boldsymbol{\beta} \,|\, \sigma^2, \boldsymbol{y}) \sim \mathcal{N}(\boldsymbol{\mu}, \mathbf{D}) \,,$$

where $\boldsymbol{\mu} = \mathbf{D}(\mathbf{X}^\top \mathbf{R}^{-1} \boldsymbol{y}/\sigma^2 + \boldsymbol{\Sigma}_0^{-1} \boldsymbol{\beta}_0)$, with $\mathbf{D} = (\mathbf{X}^\top \mathbf{R}^{-1} \mathbf{X}/\sigma^2 + \boldsymbol{\Sigma}_0^{-1})^{-1}$, and

$$(\sigma^2 \,|\, \boldsymbol{\beta}, \boldsymbol{y}) \sim \mathsf{InvGamma}\left(\alpha_0 + n/2, \, (\boldsymbol{y} - \mathbf{X}\boldsymbol{\beta})^\top \mathbf{R}^{-1}(\boldsymbol{y} - \mathbf{X}\boldsymbol{\beta})/2 + \lambda_0\right) \,.$$

Proof. By assumption we have $\boldsymbol{y} - \mathbf{X}\boldsymbol{\beta} = \boldsymbol{a} + \mathbf{A}\boldsymbol{y} \overset{\text{def}}{=} \boldsymbol{z}$ for some vector $\boldsymbol{a}$ and matrix $\mathbf{A}$, where $(\boldsymbol{z} \,|\, \sigma^2, \boldsymbol{\beta}) \sim \mathcal{N}(\mathbf{0}, \sigma^2 \mathbf{R})$. It follows that

$$f(\boldsymbol{y} \,|\, \sigma^2, \boldsymbol{\beta}) \propto f(\boldsymbol{z} \,|\, \sigma^2, \boldsymbol{\beta}) \propto (2\pi\sigma^2)^{-n/2} \exp\left\{ -\frac{1}{2\sigma^2}(\boldsymbol{y} - \mathbf{X}\boldsymbol{\beta})^\top \mathbf{R}^{-1}(\boldsymbol{y} - \mathbf{X}\boldsymbol{\beta}) \right\} \,.$$

The rest of the proof follows exactly the same reasoning as for Theorem 8.1.
$\square$

8.2.3 Bayesian Multinomial Model

In this section we extend the Bayesian analysis of the binomial model in Example 8.1 to the multinomial case. Recall (see Definition 3.4) that a random vector $\boldsymbol{X} = [X_1, X_2, \ldots, X_k]^\top$ has a **multinomial** distribution, with parameters n and $p_1, p_2, \ldots, p_k$ (probabilities summing up to 1), if

$$\mathbb{P}(X_1 = x_1, \ldots, X_k = x_k) = \frac{n!}{x_1! \, x_2! \cdots x_k!} \, p_1^{x_1} p_2^{x_2} \cdots p_k^{x_k} \,, \tag{8.19}$$

for all $x_1, \ldots, x_k \in \{0, 1, \ldots, n\}$ such that $x_1 + x_2 + \cdots + x_k = n$. We can think of $\boldsymbol{X} \sim \mathsf{Mnom}(n, \boldsymbol{p})$ representing the configuration of n balls in k urns when the balls are thrown independently into the urns according to a vector of probabilities $\boldsymbol{p} = [p_1, \ldots, p_k]^\top$. For the binomial case, there are only two urns and $\boldsymbol{p} = [p, 1-p]^\top$.

Suppose we are given data $\boldsymbol{x}$ from an $\mathsf{Mnom}(n, \boldsymbol{p})$ distribution and wish to gain information about $\boldsymbol{p}$ on the basis of $\boldsymbol{x}$. Assuming uniform priors, the Bayesian model is

$$f(\boldsymbol{p}) \propto 1 \,, \qquad f(\boldsymbol{x}\,|\,\boldsymbol{p}) = \frac{n!}{x_1!\,x_2!\cdots x_k!}\, p_1^{x_1} p_2^{x_2} \cdots p_k^{x_k}\,.$$

It follows that the posterior pdf is of the form:

$$f(\boldsymbol{p}\,|\,\boldsymbol{x}) \propto p_1^{x_1} p_2^{x_2} \ldots p_k^{x_k}\,, \quad \boldsymbol{p} \in [0,1]^k\,, \quad \sum_{i=1}^{k} p_i = 1\,.$$

Since $\sum_{i=1}^{k} x_i = n$ and $\sum_{i=1}^{k} p_i = 1$, we can drop p_k from the analysis and look instead at the posterior pdf of $p_1, \ldots, p_{k-1}$ given $\boldsymbol{x}$, which is given by

$$f(p_1, \ldots, p_{k-1}\,|\,\boldsymbol{x}) \propto p_1^{x_1} \ldots p_{k-1}^{x_{k-1}} \Big(1 - \sum_{i=1}^{k-1} p_i\Big)^{x_k}\,,$$

where $p_i \geq 0, i = 1, \ldots, k-1$ and $\sum_{i=1}^{k-1} p_i \leq 1$. This is the pdf of a Dirichlet distribution:

$$(p_1, \ldots, p_{k-1}\,|\,\boldsymbol{x}) \sim \mathsf{Dirichlet}(x_1 + 1,\ x_2 + 1,\ \ldots, x_k + 1).$$

Definition 8.3. (Dirichlet Distribution). A random vector $\boldsymbol{Z} = [Z_1, \ldots, Z_m]^\top$ is said to have a **Dirichlet** distribution with **shape** parameter $\boldsymbol{\alpha} = [\alpha_1, \ldots, \alpha_{m+1}]^\top$ if its pdf is given by

$$f(\boldsymbol{z}; \boldsymbol{\alpha}) = \frac{\Gamma\big(\sum_{i=1}^{m+1} \alpha_i\big)}{\prod_{i=1}^{m+1} \Gamma(\alpha_i)} \prod_{i=1}^{m} z_i^{\alpha_i - 1} \Big(1 - \sum_{i=1}^{m} z_i\Big)^{\alpha_{m+1} - 1}\,, \quad \boldsymbol{z} \in [0,1]^m\,, \sum_{i=1}^{m} z_i \leq 1\,.$$

We write this distribution as $\mathsf{Dirichlet}(\alpha_1, \ldots, \alpha_{m+1})$ or $\mathsf{Dirichlet}(\boldsymbol{\alpha})$.

The m-dimensional $\mathsf{Dirichlet}(1, \ldots, 1)$ distribution has a constant density on the set $\{\boldsymbol{z} \in \mathbb{R}^m : z_i \geq 0, i = 1, \ldots, m, \sum_{i=1}^{m} z_i \leq 1\}$ and thus corresponds to the uniform distribution on that set. The $\mathsf{Dirichlet}(\alpha_1, \alpha_2)$ distribution is the $\mathsf{Beta}(\alpha_1, \alpha_2)$ distribution. Moreover, if $\boldsymbol{Z} = [Z_1, \ldots, Z_m]^\top \sim \mathsf{Dirichlet}(\alpha_1, \ldots, \alpha_{m+1})$, the marginal distribution of Z_i is $\mathsf{Beta}(\alpha_i, \sum_{j \neq i} \alpha_j)$; see Problem 8.6. The following theorem shows how one can simulate from the Dirichlet distribution using **Gamma** random variables.

Theorem 8.2. (Sampling from the Dirichlet Distribution). Let $Y_1, \ldots, Y_{m+1}$ be independent random variables with $Y_i \sim \mathsf{Gamma}(\alpha_i, 1)$, $i = 1, \ldots, m + 1$, and define

$$Z_j = \frac{Y_j}{\sum_{i=1}^{m+1} Y_i}, \quad j = 1, \ldots, m . \tag{8.20}$$

Then, $\boldsymbol{Z} = [Z_1, \ldots, Z_m]^\top \sim \mathsf{Dirichlet}(\alpha_1, \ldots, \alpha_{m+1})$.

☞ 81   *Proof.* This is a direct consequence of the transformation rule (3.26). In particular, consider the transformation $\boldsymbol{g} : [y_1, \ldots, y_{m+1}]^\top \mapsto [z_1, \ldots, z_{m+1}]^\top$ defined by (8.20) and $z_{m+1} = y_1 + \cdots + y_{m+1}$. By rewriting the $\{y_i\}$ in terms of the $\{z_i\}$, we see that the inverse transformation is given by

$$y_i = z_i\, z_{m+1}, \; i = 1, \ldots, m \quad \text{and} \quad y_{m+1} = (1 - (z_1 + \cdots + z_m))\, z_{m+1} .$$

The determinant of the corresponding Jacobian matrix is z_{m+1}^m; see Problem 8.5. Using frequentist notation for clarity and defining $\boldsymbol{Y} = [Y_1, \ldots,$
☞ 48 $Y_{m+1}]^\top$, we have by the transformation rule and the definition (2.20) of the Gamma pdf:

$$
\begin{aligned}
f_{\boldsymbol{Z}, Z_{m+1}}(\boldsymbol{z}, z_{m+1}) = f_{\boldsymbol{Y}}(\boldsymbol{y}) z_{m+1}^m &= \frac{\left(\prod_{i=1}^{m+1} y_i^{\alpha_i - 1}\right) \mathrm{e}^{-\sum_{i=1}^{m+1} y_i} z_{m+1}^m}{\prod_{i=1}^{m+1} \Gamma(\alpha_i)} \\
&= \frac{\left(\prod_{i=1}^{m} y_i^{\alpha_i - 1}\right) y_{m+1}^{\alpha_{m+1} - 1} \mathrm{e}^{-z_{m+1}} z_{m+1}^m}{\prod_{i=1}^{m+1} \Gamma(\alpha_i)} \\
&= \frac{\left(\prod_{i=1}^{m} z_i^{\alpha_i - 1}\right) \left(1 - \sum_{i=1}^{m} z_i\right)^{\alpha_{m+1} - 1}}{\prod_{i=1}^{m+1} \Gamma(\alpha_i)} \underbrace{z_{m+1}^{\left(\sum_{i=1}^{m+1} \alpha_i\right) - 1} \mathrm{e}^{-z_{m+1}}}_{(\star)} .
\end{aligned}
\tag{8.21}
$$

To obtain the pdf of $\boldsymbol{Z}$, we need to integrate out z_{m+1} in (8.21). Since $(\star)$ is proportional to the pdf of a $\mathsf{Gamma}(\sum_{i=1}^{m+1} \alpha_i, 1)$ distribution, this integral is $\Gamma(\sum_{i=1}^{m+1} \alpha_i)$, which completes the proof. $\qquad\square$

Example 8.3 (Bayesian Inference for the Multinomial Model). Five hundred and one people are randomly selected from a large population. They are asked if they like, dislike, or are indifferent to the current anti-smoking campaign. Table 8.1 lists the data.

    Let x_{ij} be the count in row i and column j in Table 8.1; for example, $x_{13} = 147$ and $x_{22} = 38$. Denote by $\boldsymbol{x} = [x_{11}, \ldots, x_{23}]^\top$ the vector of counts, and let $\boldsymbol{p} = [p_{11}, p_{12}, p_{13}, p_{21}, p_{22}, p_{23}]^\top$ be the corresponding vector of probabilities.

Table 8.1 Opinions on smoking campaign, by gender.

		Opinion	
Gender	Dislike	Neutral	Like
Male	53	57	147
Female	93	38	113

Thus, p_{13} is the probability that a randomly selected person is male and likes the campaign. A natural Bayesian model for the data is that $(\boldsymbol{x} \mid \boldsymbol{p}) \sim$ $\mathsf{Mnom}(501, \boldsymbol{p})$, with a uniform prior for $\boldsymbol{p}$. It follows that $([p_{11}, \ldots, p_{22}]^\top \mid \boldsymbol{x})$ (i.e., the vector $\boldsymbol{p}$ with component p_{23} removed) has a Dirichlet distribution with parameter $\boldsymbol{\alpha} = [x_{11} + 1, \ldots, x_{23} + 1]^\top$.

Can we conclude from the data that opinion is independent of gender? For this to be true, it must hold that

$$p_{ij} = p_i^{(r)} p_j^{(c)}, \quad i = 1, 2, \quad j = 1, 2, 3 \, ,$$

where the row totals $p_i^{(r)} = p_{i1} + p_{i2} + p_{i3}$, $i = 1, 2$ give the probability that a selected person is male $(i = 1)$ or female $(i = 2)$; similarly, the column totals $p_j^{(c)} = p_{1j} + p_{2j}$, $j = 1, 2, 3$ give the probabilities of the opinions. It thus makes sense to investigate the posterior distribution of

$$a_{ij} = p_{ij} - p_i^{(r)} p_j^{(c)}, \quad i = 1, 2, \quad j = 1, 2, 3 \tag{8.22}$$

and check if 0 lies within a reasonable (say 95%) credible interval of each a_{ij}. The following Julia program generates $N = 10000$ vectors $\boldsymbol{p}$ drawn from the posterior distribution. For each $\boldsymbol{p}$ the row and column totals are calculated, and subsequently realizations from the posterior distribution of $a_{1j}, j = 1, 2, 3$ are obtained via (8.22). Since $a_{1j} = -a_{2j}$, it suffices to consider only $a_{1j}, j = 1, 2, 3$. Kernel density plots of the posterior pdfs are shown in Fig. 8.4. We see that opinion and gender are likely to be *dependent*, as 0 is not contained in, for example, a 0.99 credible interval of the posterior pdf of a_{11}.

```julia
multinomex.jl

include("ThetaKDE.jl")
using Distributions, .ThetaKDE, Plots
x = [53,57,147,93,38,113];
N = 10000;
p = zeros(N,2,3); a = zeros(N,2,3);
p_row = zeros(2,N); p_col=zeros(3,N);
alpha = x .+ 1;
for i in 1:N
```

```
    h = rand(Dirichlet(alpha));
    p[i,:,:] = reshape(h',3,2)';
end
for i in 1:2
    p_row[i,:] = sum(p[:,i,:],dims=2);
end
for j in 1:3
    p_col[j,:] = sum(p[:,:,j],dims=2);
end
for k in 1:N
    for i in 1:2
        for j in 1:3
            a[k,i,j] = p[k,i,j] - p_row[i,k]*p_col[j,k];
        end
    end
end
p = plot()
for j in 1:3
    xmesh, density, h = kde(a[:,1,j])
    p = plot!(xmesh,density)
    display(p)
end
```

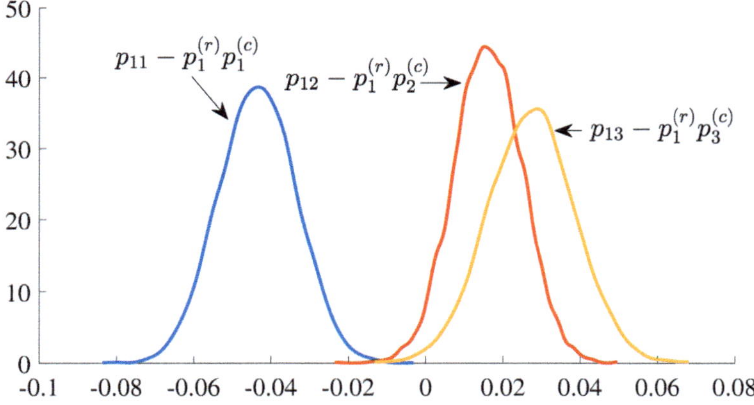

Fig. 8.4 Posterior pdfs of $a_{1j} = p_{1j} - p_1^{(r)} p_j^{(c)}, j = 1, 2, 3$, indicating that opinion and gender are not independent

8.3 Bayesian Networks

The formulation and analysis of a Bayesian model can often be facilitated
through the use of **Bayesian networks**. Mathematically, a Bayesian network
is a **directed acyclic graph**, that is, a collection of **vertices** (nodes) and
arcs (arrows between nodes) such that arcs, when put head-to-tail, do not
create loops. Figure 8.5 shows two directed acyclic graphs ((a) and (b)) and
a counterexample (c).

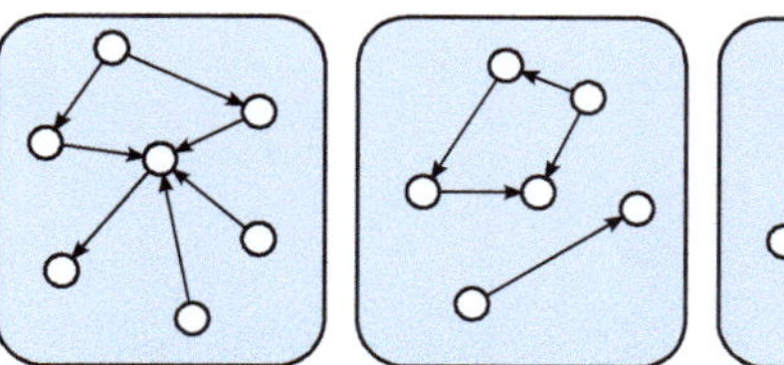

Fig. 8.5 The directed
graphs in (**a**) and (**b**) are
acyclic. Graph (**c**) has a
(directed) cycle and can
therefore not represent a
Bayesian network

Bayesian networks can be used to graphically represent the joint probability distribution of a collection of random variables. In particular, consider
a Bayesian network with vertices labeled $x_1, \ldots, x_n$. Let $\mathcal{P}_j$ denote the set of
parents of x_j, that is, the vertices x_i for which there exist an arc from x_i to
x_j in the graph. We can associate with this network a joint pdf:

$$f(x_1, \ldots, x_n) = \prod_{j=1}^{n} f(x_j \mid \mathcal{P}_j) \,.$$

Note that any pdf can be represented by a Bayesian network in this way
because, by the product rule (3.10),   ☞ 72

$$f(x_1, \ldots, x_n) = f(x_1)f(x_2 \mid x_1) \cdots f(x_n \mid x_1, \ldots, x_{n-1}) \,.$$

As an example, the left pane of Fig. 8.6 shows a Bayesian network with five
variables, representing the following structure for the pdf:

$$f(x_1, \ldots, x_n) = f(x_1)f(x_2 \mid x_1)f(x_3 \mid x_2)f(x_4 \mid x_2)f(x_5 \mid x_3, x_4) \,.$$

In the same figure, two small black nodes have been added with labels θ_1 and
θ_2. This is a way of representing fixed parameters of the distribution. Thus,
in this case the (frequentist) pdf is of the form

$$f(x_1, \ldots, x_n) = f(x_1; \theta_1)f(x_2 \mid x_1; \theta_2)f(x_3 \mid x_2)f(x_4 \mid x_2)f(x_5 \mid x_3, x_4) \,.$$

In the right pane of Fig. 8.6, the corresponding Bayesian model is depicted.
It is useful to distinguish between random variables and their observations,
by using a dark color or gray scale for the latter one. For example, the right

pane of Fig. 8.6 represents the situation where the "data" $x_1, \ldots, x_n$ have been observed. The aim is to find the posterior pdf of θ_1 and θ_2 given the data.

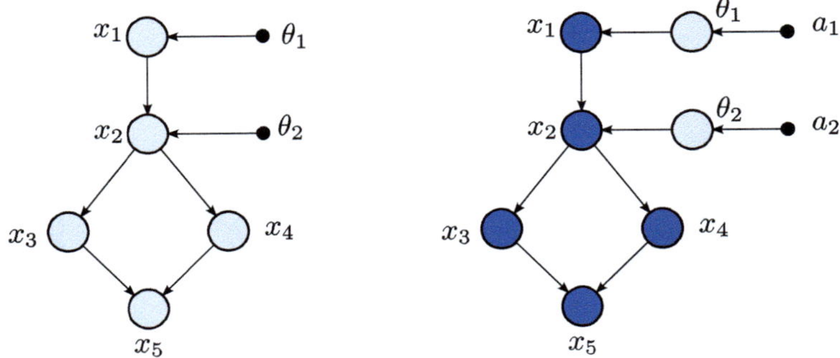

Fig. 8.6 Left: a graphical representation of a *frequentist* statistical model with random variables $x_1, \ldots, x_5$ and fixed parameters θ_1, θ_2. The representation is in the form of a directed acyclic graph (Bayesian network). Right: the graphical representation of the corresponding *Bayesian* model with *observed* (i.e., fixed) data $x_1, \ldots, x_n$, indicated by shaded nodes. In this case the parameters θ_1 and θ_2 are random and depend on fixed parameters a_1 and a_2 (sometimes called **hyperparameters**)

Figure 8.7 gives two more examples of Bayesian networks. The first corresponds to the ticket inspector model in Example 8.2; the second refers to the normal Bayesian model in Sect. 8.2.1.

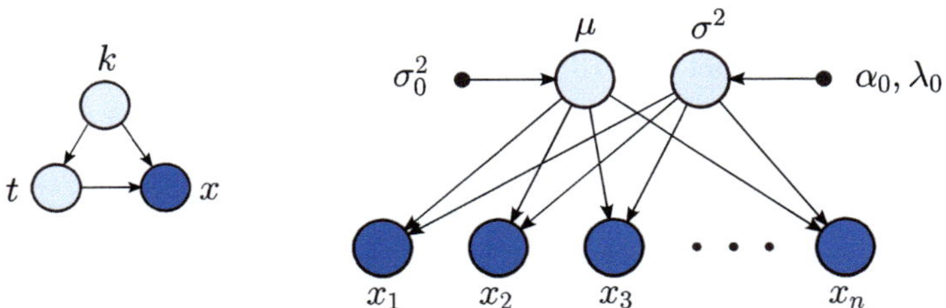

Fig. 8.7 Left: the Bayesian network for the ticket inspector model in Example 8.2. Right: a representation of the Bayesian model for iid normal data

Example 8.4 (Belief Nets). Bayesian networks are frequently used for medical diagnosis and statistical classification. In this context they are sometimes called *belief nets*. An example belief net is shown in Fig. 8.8. The purpose of this belief net is to determine if a patient is to be diagnosed with heart disease, based on several factors and symptoms. Two important factors in heart disease are smoking and age, and two main symptoms are chest pains and shortness of breath. The belief net in Fig. 8.8 shows the prior probabilities of smoking and age, the conditional probabilities of heart disease given age and smoking, and the conditional probabilities of chest pains and shortness of breath given heart disease.

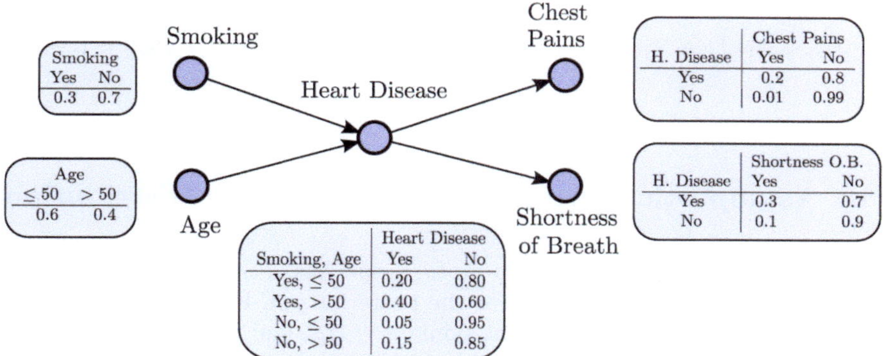

Smoking, Age	Heart Disease Yes	No
Yes, ≤ 50	0.20	0.80
Yes, > 50	0.40	0.60
No, ≤ 50	0.05	0.95
No, > 50	0.15	0.85

H. Disease	Chest Pains Yes	No
Yes	0.2	0.8
No	0.01	0.99

H. Disease	Shortness O.B. Yes	No
Yes	0.3	0.7
No	0.1	0.9

Fig. 8.8 A Bayesian belief net for the diagnosis of heart disease

Suppose a person experiences chest pains and shortness of breath, but we do not know her/his age and if she/he is smoking. How likely is it that she/he has a heart disease?

Define the variables s (smoking), a (age), h (heart disease), c (chest pains), and b (shortness of breath). We assume that s and a are independent. We wish to calculate

$$\mathbb{P}(h = \text{Yes} \mid b = \text{Yes},\, c = \text{Yes}) \, .$$

From the Bayesian network structure, we see that the joint pdf of $s, a, h, c,$ and b can be written as

$$f(s, a, h, c, b) = f(s)f(a)f(h \mid s, a)f(c \mid h)f(b \mid h) \, .$$

It follows that

$$f(h \mid b, c) \propto f(c \mid h)f(b \mid h) \underbrace{\sum_{a,s} f(h \mid s, a)f(s)f(a)}_{f(h)} \, .$$

We have:

$$f(h = \text{Yes}) = 0.2 \times 0.3 \times 0.6 + 0.4 \times 0.3 \times 0.4$$
$$+ \, 0.05 \times 0.7 \times 0.6 + 0.15 \times 0.7 \times 0.4 = 0.147 \, .$$

Consequently,

$$f(h = \text{Yes} \mid b = \text{Yes}, c = \text{Yes}) = \beta \times 0.2 \times 0.3 \times 0.147 = \beta \, 0.00882$$

and

$$f(h = \text{No} \,|\, b = \text{Yes}, c = \text{Yes}) = \beta \times 0.01 \times 0.1 \times (1 - 0.147) = \beta\, 0.000853$$

for some normalization constant β. Thus,

$$f(h = \text{Yes} \,|\, b = \text{Yes}, c = \text{Yes}) = \frac{0.00882}{0.00882 + 0.000853} = 0.911816 \approx 0.91 \;.$$

8.4 Asymptotic Normality of the Posterior Distribution

☞ 182　We saw in Sect. 6.3.2 various asymptotic properties of the likelihood function. Similar results can be obtained for the posterior pdf. For clarity we identify the (conditional) pdfs by different symbols: f, f_Θ, and $\mathring{f}$.

> **Theorem 8.3. (Asymptotic Distribution of the Posterior Pdf).**
> Let $\boldsymbol{x} = [x_1, \ldots, x_n]^\top$ be an iid sample from $\mathring{f}(x \,|\, \theta_0)$, where θ_0 is fixed. The posterior pdf with prior pdf $f_\Theta(\theta)$:
>
> $$f(\theta \,|\, \boldsymbol{x}) \propto f_\Theta(\theta) \prod_{i=1}^{n} \mathring{f}(x_i \,|\, \theta) \tag{8.23}$$
>
> is approximately normal with mean θ_0 and variance $\mathring{I}^{-1}(\theta_0)/n$, where $\mathring{I}(\theta_0)$ is the information number of $\mathring{f}(x \,|\, \theta_0)$.

Proof. (Sketch). Let $\widehat{\theta}$ be the mode of the posterior pdf in (8.23). The proof
☞ 182　of Theorem 6.7 can be mimicked to show that $\widehat{\theta}$ is consistent; that is, $\widehat{\theta} \to \theta_0$
☞ 477　as $n \to \infty$. A second-order Taylor expansion of $\ln f(\theta \,|\, \boldsymbol{x})$ around $\widehat{\theta}$ gives:

$$\ln f(\theta \,|\, \boldsymbol{x}) = \ln f(\widehat{\theta} \,|\, \boldsymbol{x}) + (\theta - \widehat{\theta})\frac{\mathrm{d}}{\mathrm{d}\theta} \ln f(\widehat{\theta} \,|\, \boldsymbol{x}) + \frac{1}{2}(\theta - \widehat{\theta})^2 \frac{\mathrm{d}^2}{\mathrm{d}\theta^2} \ln f(\widehat{\theta} \,|\, \boldsymbol{x}) + R$$

$$= \ln f(\widehat{\theta} \,|\, \boldsymbol{x}) + \frac{n}{2}(\theta - \widehat{\theta})^2 \underbrace{\left(\frac{1}{n}\frac{\mathrm{d}^2}{\mathrm{d}\theta^2} \ln\big(c(\boldsymbol{x}) f_\Theta(\widehat{\theta})\big) + \frac{1}{n}\sum_{i=1}^{n} \frac{\mathrm{d}^2}{\mathrm{d}\theta^2} \ln \mathring{f}(x_i \,|\, \widehat{\theta}) \right)}_{(\star)} + R \;,$$

where $c(\boldsymbol{x})$ is the normalization constant of the posterior and R is the remainder term, which includes higher-order polynomials $(\theta - \widehat{\theta})^k, k = 3, 4, \ldots$. Note that the linear term in the Taylor expansion can be omitted since the derivative of $\ln(f(\theta \,|\, \boldsymbol{x})$ at $\theta = \widehat{\theta}$ is 0. For large n the first term in $(\star)$ be-
☞ 183　comes negligible compared to the second one. Moreover, similar to (6.27) the

second term converges to $-\mathring{I}(\theta_0)$. Since R/n remains bounded as $n \to \infty$ and $\ln f(\widehat{\theta} \,|\, \boldsymbol{x})$ is a constant with respect to θ, the posterior pdf $f(\theta \,|\, \boldsymbol{x})$ becomes more and more concentrated around θ_0, and tends to the form:

$$f(\theta \,|\, \boldsymbol{x}) \propto e^{-\frac{1}{2}(\theta-\theta_0)^2 \, n\mathring{I}(\theta_0)} \,,$$

which is the pdf of the $\mathcal{N}(\theta_0, \mathring{I}^{-1}(\theta_0)/n)$ distribution, in accordance with Theorem 6.8. $\qquad\square$ ☞ 18

8.5 Priors and Conjugacy

In Bayesian analysis it is often useful to choose the prior pdf in the same family of distributions as the posterior pdf. Consider, for example, the binomial model in Example 8.1. Using a uniform prior, the posterior pdf belongs to Beta family of distributions. Suppose we choose the prior in the same family, giving the Bayesian model:

$$\theta \sim \mathsf{Beta}(a, b)$$
$$(x \,|\, \theta) \sim \mathsf{Bin}(n, \theta)$$

for some fixed a and b. By Bayes' formula the posterior pdf satisfies:

$$f(\theta \,|\, x) \propto \theta^{a-1}(1-\theta)^{b-1}\theta^x(1-\theta)^{n-x} = \theta^{a+x-1}(1-\theta)^{b+n-x-1} \,,$$

which corresponds to the $\mathsf{Beta}(a+x,\, b+n-x)$ distribution. We see that the posterior and prior are in the same family of distributions. This property is called **conjugacy**. The advantage of conjugacy is that only the parameters of the distribution need to be considered. We say that the **Beta** family is a **conjugate family** for the binomial distribution.

Exponential families provide natural conjugate priors. Recall (see Definition 5.3) that a random variable x is said to belong to an m-dimensional exponential family if its pdf is of the form: ☞ 15

$$\mathring{f}(x \,|\, \boldsymbol{\theta}) = c(\boldsymbol{\theta})\exp\left(\sum_{i=1}^{m}\eta_i(\boldsymbol{\theta})\,t_i(x)\right)h(x)\,, \tag{8.24}$$

where we have used the Bayesian notation $\mathring{f}(x \,|\, \boldsymbol{\theta})$ instead of the frequentist notation $\mathring{f}(x; \boldsymbol{\theta})$.

Theorem 8.4. (Conjugate Prior for an Exponential Family).
Let $\boldsymbol{x} = [x_1, \ldots, x_n]^\top$ be an iid sample from $\mathring{f}(x \,|\, \boldsymbol{\theta})$ of the form (8.24).
The prior

$$f(\boldsymbol{\theta}) \propto c(\boldsymbol{\theta})^b \exp\left(\sum_{i=1}^{m} \eta_i(\boldsymbol{\theta}) a_i \right), \tag{8.25}$$

where the proportionality constant only depends on $(a_1, \ldots, a_m, b)$, is
conjugate to the conditional pdf

$$f(\boldsymbol{x} \,|\, \boldsymbol{\theta}) = c(\boldsymbol{\theta})^n \exp\left(\sum_{i=1}^{m} \eta_i(\boldsymbol{\theta}) \sum_{k=1}^{n} t_i(x_k) \right) \prod_{k=1}^{n} h(x_k). \tag{8.26}$$

Proof. By Bayes' theorem the posterior pdf satisfies:

$$f(\boldsymbol{\theta} \,|\, \boldsymbol{x}) \propto f(\boldsymbol{\theta}) f(\boldsymbol{x} \,|\, \boldsymbol{\theta}) \propto c(\boldsymbol{\theta})^{n+b} \exp\left(\sum_{i=1}^{m} \eta_i(\boldsymbol{\theta}) \Big(a_i + \sum_{k=1}^{n} t_i(x_k) \Big) \right),$$

where the proportionality constant does not depend on $\boldsymbol{\theta}$. This shows
that the posterior pdf lies in the same m-dimensional exponential family as the prior (8.25). In particular, if the prior is specified by parameters $(a_1, \ldots, a_m, b)$, then the corresponding parameters for the posterior are
$(\widetilde{a}_1, \ldots, \widetilde{a}_m, \widetilde{b})$, with $\widetilde{a}_i = a_i + \sum_{k=1}^{n} t_i(x_k)$, $i = 1, \ldots, m$, and $\widetilde{b} = b + n$. $\qquad\square$

Example 8.5 (Conjugate Prior for Bernoulli Likelihood). In Example 8.1 we are dealing with independent Bernoulli random variables whose
joint pdf conditional on θ is

$$f(\boldsymbol{x} \,|\, \theta) = \theta^{\sum_{k=1}^{n} x_k} (1 - \theta)^{n - \sum_{k=1}^{n} x_k},$$

which is of the form (8.26), with $m = 1$, $\eta(\theta) = \ln(\theta/(1 - \theta))$, $t(x_k) = x_k$,
and $c(\theta) = 1 - \theta$. The corresponding conjugate class is therefore of the form

$$c(\theta)^b \mathrm{e}^{\eta(\theta)a} = (1 - \theta)^b \left(\frac{\theta}{1 - \theta} \right)^a \propto \theta^a (1 - \theta)^b,$$

which corresponds to the **Beta** family of distributions.

Example 8.6 (Conjugate Prior for Poisson Likelihood). Let $x_1, \ldots, x_n$
be an iid sample from the Poisson distribution $\mathsf{Poi}(\lambda)$. This is an exponential
family, and the joint pdf can be written as

$$f(\boldsymbol{x} \,|\, \lambda) = \mathrm{e}^{-n\lambda} \mathrm{e}^{n\overline{x} \ln \lambda} \prod_{k=1}^{n} \frac{1}{x_k!}.$$

This is of the form (8.26), which suggests a conjugate prior of the form

$$f(\lambda) \propto e^{-b\lambda} e^{a \ln \lambda} = e^{-b\lambda} \lambda^a \,.$$

This corresponds to the gamma density. In particular, if we take a $\mathsf{Gamma}(a, b)$ prior for λ, that is,

$$f(\lambda) \propto e^{-b\lambda} \lambda^{a-1} \,,$$

(notice λ is the variable here, not the parameter), then the posterior pdf is

$$f(\lambda \mid \boldsymbol{x}) \propto e^{-(n+b)\lambda} \lambda^{a-1+n\overline{x}} \,,$$

which corresponds to the $\mathsf{Gamma}(a + n\overline{x}, b + n)$ distribution.

8.6 Bayesian Model Comparison

Under the Bayesian framework, hypothesis testing, or more generally comparing models, is straightforward. Suppose we wish to compare two possibly non-nested models M_1 and M_2. Each model $M_i, i = 1, 2$, is formally defined by a likelihood function $f(\boldsymbol{x} \mid \boldsymbol{\theta}_i, M_i)$ and a prior distribution on the model-specific parameter vector $\boldsymbol{\theta}_i$ denoted as $f(\boldsymbol{\theta}_i \mid M_i)$. Note that in both the likelihood function and the prior distribution, we make the dependence on the model M_i explicit.

A popular criterion for comparing models M_1 and M_2 is the **Bayes factor** in favor of model M_1 against model M_2:

$$\mathrm{BF}_{12} \stackrel{\text{def}}{=} \frac{f(\boldsymbol{x} \mid M_1)}{f(\boldsymbol{x} \mid M_2)} \,,$$

where

$$f(\boldsymbol{x} \mid M_i) = \int f(\boldsymbol{x} \mid \boldsymbol{\theta}_i, M_i) \, f(\boldsymbol{\theta}_i \mid M_i) \, \mathrm{d}\boldsymbol{\theta}_i \tag{8.27}$$

is the **marginal likelihood** under model $M_i, i = 1, 2$.

The marginal likelihood $f(\boldsymbol{x} \mid M_i)$ is simply the marginal density of the data $\boldsymbol{x}$ under model M_i. If the actual data are likely under model M_i, then the associated marginal likelihood will be large, and vice versa. Hence, a Bayes factor BF_{12} greater than 1 indicates that model M_1 better predicts the observed data than M_2. It is therefore taken as evidence in favor of model M_1.

The Bayes factor between the two models is related to their **posterior odds ratio**:

$$\mathrm{PO}_{12} \stackrel{\text{def}}{=} \frac{\mathbb{P}(M_1 \mid \boldsymbol{x})}{\mathbb{P}(M_2 \mid \boldsymbol{x})} = \frac{\mathbb{P}(M_1)}{\mathbb{P}(M_2)} \times \frac{f(\boldsymbol{x} \mid M_1)}{f(\boldsymbol{x} \mid M_2)} \,,$$

where $\mathbb{P}(M_i)$ and $\mathbb{P}(M_i \mid \boldsymbol{x})$ are respectively the prior and posterior model probabilities of model $M_i, i = 1, 2$. If both models are equally probable a priori, i.e., $\mathbb{P}(M_1) = \mathbb{P}(M_2)$, the posterior odds ratio between the two models is then the same as the Bayes factor. In that case, if, for example, $\mathrm{BF}_{12} = 50$, we can say that model M_1 is 50 times more likely than model M_2 given the data.

☞ 248 **Example 8.7 (Comparing Multinomial Models).** In Example 8.3 we investigated if opinions on an anti-smoking campaign are independent of gender. Using the data in Table 8.1, we found evidence that suggests opinions differ by gender. In this example we perform a formal model comparison exercise to quantity the weight of evidence.

Let M_1 denote the multinomial model $(\boldsymbol{x} \mid \boldsymbol{p}, M_1) \sim \mathsf{Mnom}(501, \boldsymbol{p})$, where $\boldsymbol{p} = [p_{11}, p_{12}, p_{13}, p_{21}, p_{22}, p_{23}]^\top$, with a uniform prior for $\boldsymbol{p}$, or equivalently, $(p_{11}, \ldots, p_{22} \mid M_1) \sim \mathsf{Dirichlet}(1, \ldots, 1)$. Hence, the prior density is given by

$$f(p_{11}, \ldots, p_{22} \mid M_1) = \Gamma(6) = 5! \, .$$

It follows that the marginal likelihood $f(\boldsymbol{x} \mid M_1)$ can be directly computed using the definition (8.27):

$$
\begin{aligned}
f(\boldsymbol{x} \mid M_1) &= \int \frac{501!}{x_{11}! \cdots x_{23}!} \, p_{11}^{x_{11}} \cdots p_{23}^{x_{23}} \times 5! \, \mathrm{d}(p_{11}, \ldots, p_{22}) \\
&= \frac{501! \, 5!}{x_{11}! \cdots x_{23}!} \int p_{11}^{x_{11}} \cdots p_{23}^{x_{23}} \, \mathrm{d}(p_{11}, \ldots, p_{22}) \\
&= \frac{501! \, 5!}{x_{11}! \cdots x_{23}!} \times \frac{\Gamma(x_{11} + 1) \cdots \Gamma(x_{23} + 1)}{\Gamma(507)} \\
&= \frac{501! \, 5!}{506!} \approx 3.6901 \times 10^{-12} \, .
\end{aligned}
$$

Next, if opinion is independent of gender, we must have:

$$p_{ij} = p_i^{(r)} p_j^{(c)}, \quad i = 1, 2, \quad j = 1, 2, 3 \, ,$$

where $p_1^{(r)} + p_2^{(r)} = 1$ and $p_1^{(c)} + p_2^{(c)} + p_3^{(c)} = 1$. Let $r_i = x_{i1} + x_{i2} + x_{i3}, i = 1, 2$, and $c_i = x_{1j} + x_{2j}, j = 1, 2, 3$, denote the row and column counts, respectively. Then, the likelihood function under the model M_2 (in which opinion is independent of gender) is given by

$$
\begin{aligned}
f(\boldsymbol{x} \mid \widetilde{\boldsymbol{p}}, M_2) &= \frac{501!}{x_{11}! \cdots x_{23}!} \, (p_1^{(r)} p_1^{(c)})^{x_{11}} \cdots (p_2^{(r)} p_3^{(c)})^{x_{23}} \\
&= \frac{501!}{x_{11}! \cdots x_{23}!} \, (p_1^{(r)})^{r_1} (p_2^{(r)})^{r_2} (p_1^{(c)})^{c_1} (p_2^{(c)})^{c_2} (p_3^{(c)})^{c_3} \, ,
\end{aligned}
$$

where $\widetilde{\boldsymbol{p}} = (p_1^{(r)}, p_2^{(r)}, p_1^{(c)}, p_2^{(c)}, p_3^{(c)})$. Further, we assume independent and uniform priors for $(p_1^{(r)}, p_2^{(r)})$ and $(p_1^{(c)}, p_2^{(c)}, p_3^{(c)})$. Hence, the prior density is

$$f(p_1^{(r)}, p_1^{(c)}, p_2^{(c)} \mid M_2) = \Gamma(2)\Gamma(3) = 2 .$$

Following a similar computation as before, the marginal likelihood for model M_2 is given by

$$\begin{aligned}
f(\boldsymbol{x} \mid M_2) &= \frac{2 \times 501!}{x_{11}! \cdots x_{23}!} \frac{\Gamma(r_1+1)\Gamma(r_2+1)\Gamma(c_1+1)\Gamma(c_2+1)\Gamma(c_3+1)}{\Gamma(r_1+r_2+2)\Gamma(c_1+c_2+c_3+3)} \\
&= \frac{2 \times r_1! \, r_2! \, c_1! \, c_2! \, c_3!}{502 \times x_{11}! \cdots x_{23}! \, 503!} \approx 9.2122 \times 10^{-15} .
\end{aligned}$$

Finally, the Bayes factor is $\mathrm{BF}_{12} = f(\boldsymbol{x} \mid M_1)/f(\boldsymbol{x} \mid M_2) \approx 400$, showing overwhelming evidence for M_1 against M_2. In other words, given the data it is highly likely (400 times more so) that opinion varies with gender.

The computation of the marginal likelihood in (8.27) involves "integrating out" all the model parameters, and an analytic expression is often unavailable. In those cases, Monte Carlo methods are required to estimate the marginal likelihood. One popular method to do so using posterior output is Chib's method (Chib, 1995; Chib and Jeliazkov, 2001).

However, when comparing *nested* models, i.e., when one model is a restricted version of the other model, the Bayes factor has an alternative expression that can often be easily estimated using posterior output. To set the stage, let M_u denote the *unrestricted* model, where the model parameters are partitioned into two subsets $\boldsymbol{\theta} = (\boldsymbol{\psi}, \boldsymbol{\omega})$. Suppose M_r is the *restricted* version of M_u, where $\boldsymbol{\theta} = (\boldsymbol{\psi}, \boldsymbol{\omega}_0)$ for some constant vector $\boldsymbol{\omega}_0$. Clearly, comparing M_u and M_r is equivalent to testing the hypothesis $\boldsymbol{\omega} = \boldsymbol{\omega}_0$.

Now, suppose $f(\boldsymbol{\psi}, \boldsymbol{\omega} \mid M_u)$ is the prior distribution under the unrestricted model. Then, the induced prior for $\boldsymbol{\psi}$ under the restricted model M_r is simply the marginal distribution $f(\boldsymbol{\psi} \mid M_r) = \int f(\boldsymbol{\psi}, \boldsymbol{\omega} \mid M_u) \, d\boldsymbol{\omega}$. It turns out that if this induced prior is the same as the conditional prior for $\boldsymbol{\psi}$ given $\boldsymbol{\omega} = \boldsymbol{\omega}_0$, then the Bayes factor is equivalent to the ratio of posterior and prior densities under M_u evaluated at $\boldsymbol{\omega} = \boldsymbol{\omega}_0$. This is referred to as the **Savage–Dickey density ratio**. The result is summarized in the following theorem. Its proof can be found in, for example, Verdinelli and Wasserman (1995).

Theorem 8.5. (Savage–Dickey Density Ratio). Let M_u denote the unrestricted model with model parameters $\boldsymbol{\theta} = (\boldsymbol{\psi}, \boldsymbol{\omega})$, and let M_r be a restricted version of M_u, with $\boldsymbol{\omega} = \boldsymbol{\omega}_0$ and free parameter vector $\boldsymbol{\psi}$. Suppose the priors in the two models satisfy

$$f(\boldsymbol{\psi} \mid M_r) = f(\boldsymbol{\psi} \mid \boldsymbol{\omega} = \boldsymbol{\omega}_0, M_u) \,. \tag{8.28}$$

Then, the Bayes factor in favor of model M_r can be written as

$$\mathrm{BF}_{ru} = \frac{f(\boldsymbol{\omega} = \boldsymbol{\omega}_0 \mid \boldsymbol{x}, M_u)}{f(\boldsymbol{\omega} = \boldsymbol{\omega}_0 \mid M_u)} \,.$$

In particular, (8.28) holds if $\boldsymbol{\psi}$ and $\boldsymbol{\omega}$ are a priori independent under M_u; that is, $f(\boldsymbol{\psi}, \boldsymbol{\omega} \mid M_u) = f(\boldsymbol{\psi} \mid M_u) f(\boldsymbol{\omega} \mid M_u)$.

Writing the Bayes factor as such a ratio of densities avoids the often difficult task of computing marginal likelihoods. The denominator $f(\boldsymbol{\omega} = \boldsymbol{\omega}_0 \mid M_u)$ can frequently be calculated analytically, when the conditional prior $f(\boldsymbol{\omega} \mid M_u)$ is of a standard form. In addition, the numerator can often be estimated from posterior output of model M_u. In particular, the numerator can be estimated via $\frac{1}{N} \sum_{i=1}^{N} f(\boldsymbol{\omega} = \boldsymbol{\omega}_0 \mid \boldsymbol{x}, \boldsymbol{\psi}_i, M_u)$, where $\boldsymbol{\psi}_1, \ldots, \boldsymbol{\psi}_N$ are posterior draws from model M_u.

Example 8.8 (Comparing Polynomial Regression Models). In Example 5.18 we considered five different polynomial regression models for fitting the data in Table 5.4, and compared the models using cross-validation. In this example, we perform a Bayesian model comparison on the same data. Let model M_i denote the i-th order polynomial regression model, $i = 1, \ldots, 5$:

$$y_k = \beta_0 + \beta_1 x_k + \cdots + \beta_i x_k^i + \varepsilon_k \,,$$

where $\{\varepsilon_k\} \sim_{\mathrm{iid}} \mathcal{N}(0, \sigma^2)$. Clearly, models $M_1, \ldots, M_4$ are all nested within model M_5. To complete the model specification (of model M_5), we take the following independent priors: $\boldsymbol{\beta} = [\beta_0, \ldots, \beta_5]^\top \sim \mathcal{N}(\boldsymbol{0}, 100 \, \mathbb{I}_6)$ and $\sigma^2 \sim \mathsf{InvGamma}(2, 1)$.

To compare models via the Bayes factor, we can obtain posterior draws from model M_5 and estimate the relevant Savage–Dickey density ratio (since $\beta_0, \ldots, \beta_5$ are independent under the prior, the condition (8.28) is satisfied). For example, model M_3 is obtained by imposing $[\beta_4, \beta_5]^\top = \boldsymbol{0}$. Hence, the Bayes factor BF_{35} can be written as

$$\mathrm{BF}_{35} = \frac{f([\beta_4, \beta_5] = \boldsymbol{0} \mid \boldsymbol{y}, M_5)}{f([\beta_4, \beta_5] = \boldsymbol{0} \mid M_5)} \,.$$

Using the properties of the multivariate normal distribution (see Theorem 3.7), the marginal prior $f(\beta_4, \beta_5 \mid M_5)$ is a bivariate normal density and can be evaluated easily. The conditional posterior $f(\boldsymbol{\beta} \,|\, \boldsymbol{y}, \sigma^2, M_5)$ is also a normal density, by Theorem 8.1. Hence, the numerator in the ratio can be estimated using posterior draws for σ^2.

☞ 24

The following Julia script estimates the log-Bayes factors $\ln \mathrm{BF}_{i5}, i = 1, \ldots, 4$, via the Savage–Dickey density ratio approach. Note that the statement `logpdf(MvNormal(mu,Sig),x)` evaluates the log density of the $\mathcal{N}(\boldsymbol{\mu}, \boldsymbol{\Sigma})$ distribution at $\boldsymbol{x}$.

```julia
polyreg_bayes.jl

using LinearAlgebra, Distributions
x = [4.7,2,2.7,0.1,4.7,3.7,2,3.4,1.3,
3.8,4.8,1.7,-0.4,4.5,1.3,0.4,2.6,4,2.9,1.6];
y = [6.57,5.15,7.15,0.18,6.48,8.95,5.24,10.54,1.24,8.05,
3.56,3.4,2.18,7.16,2.32,-0.23,7.68,9.09,9.13,4.04];
n = length(x);
X = hcat(ones(n), x, x.^2, x.^3, x.^4, x.^5);
XX = X'*X;
Xy = X'*y;
m = 6;
N = 10^5;    # Gibbs sample size
IM = diagm(ones(m))
V0 = 100*IM     # prior for beta
invV0 = V0\IM;
alp0 = 2; lam0 = 1;   # prior for sig2
beta = XX\Xy;
sig2 = sum((y -X*beta).^2)/n
gibbs_sample = zeros(N,m+1);
lpostden_sample = zeros(N,4);

for k in 1:N
   global beta, sig2
   D = (invV0 + XX/sig2)\IM;
   betahat = D*(Xy/sig2)
   beta = betahat + cholesky(Hermitian(D)).L*randn(m);
   sig2 = 1/rand(Gamma(alp0+n/2,1/(lam0+sum((y-X*beta).^2)/2)
      ));
   gibbs_sample[k,:]=[beta' sig2];
   lp1 = logpdf(MvNormal(betahat[3:end],
             Hermitian(D[3:end,3:end])),zeros(4))
   lp2 = logpdf(MvNormal(betahat[4:end],
             Hermitian(D[4:end,4:end])),zeros(3))
   lp3 = logpdf(MvNormal(betahat[5:end],
             Hermitian(D[5:end,5:end])),zeros(2))
   lp4 = logpdf(Normal(betahat[6],sqrt(D[6,6])),0)
```

```
        lpostden_sample[k,:] = [lp1 lp2 lp3 lp4];
end
lpostden = zeros(4,1);
for i in 1:4
    maxpden = maximum(lpostden_sample[:,i]);
    lpostden[i]=log.(mean(exp.(lpostden_sample[:,i].-maxpden))
        ) + maxpden;
end
lpriden = zeros(4,1);
lpriden[1] = logpdf(MvNormal(zeros(4),
                     V0[3:end,3:end]),zeros(4));
lpriden[2] = logpdf(MvNormal(zeros(3),
                     V0[4:end,4:end]),zeros(3));
lpriden[3] = logpdf(MvNormal(zeros(2),
                     V0[5:end,5:end]),zeros(2));
lpriden[4] = logpdf(Normal(0,sqrt(V0[6,6])),0);
lBF = lpostden - lpriden;
```

The log-Bayes factors $\ln \mathrm{BF}_{15}, \ldots, \ln \mathrm{BF}_{45}$ are estimated to be, respectively, -2.08, -2.63, 10.69, and 5.72. In other words, compared to model M_5, the data favor models M_3 and M_4, but not models M_1 and M_2. Furthermore, note that the Bayes factor BF_{34} can be written as

$$\mathrm{BF}_{34} = \frac{f(\boldsymbol{y} \mid M_3)}{f(\boldsymbol{y} \mid M_4)} = \frac{f(\boldsymbol{y} \mid M_3)}{f(\boldsymbol{y} \mid M_5)} \times \frac{f(\boldsymbol{y} \mid M_5)}{f(\boldsymbol{y} \mid M_4)} = \frac{\mathrm{BF}_{35}}{\mathrm{BF}_{45}} .$$

Hence, an estimate of BF_{34} is $e^{10.69-5.72} \approx 144$. To conclude, the data decisively prefer the cubic polynomial regression model. If we assume equal prior probabilities for all the models, the cubic polynomial is about 144 times more likely than the next best model (4*th*-order polynomial) given the data.

8.7 Problems

☞ 74 **8.1.** Let $f(x), x \in (0,1)$ be the pdf of $X \sim \mathsf{Beta}(\alpha, \beta)$:

a. Prove that the derivative of f (or, equivalently, of $\ln f$) has a unique zero at $x^* = (\alpha - 1)/(\alpha + \beta - 2)$ in the interval $(0,1)$, provided that either $\alpha > 1, \beta > 1$ or $\alpha < 1, \beta < 1$. For which of these two regimes is x^* a maximum point?

☞ 74 b. Show that $\mathbb{E}X = B(\alpha+1, \beta)/B(\alpha, \beta)$, where B is the *beta* function (3.11).

☞ 48   Using the properties of the *gamma* function (2.21), show that $\mathbb{E}X = \alpha/(\alpha + \beta)$.

8.2. Suppose $x_1 = 1.1065, x_2 = 0.5343, x_3 = 11.1438, x_4 = 0.4893, x_5 = 2.4748$ is an observed iid sample from the $\mathsf{Exp}(\lambda)$ distribution. Consider Bayesian inference for the parameter λ, using an improper prior $f(\lambda) = 1/\lambda$.

a. Show that the posterior pdf of λ has a $\mathsf{Gamma}(5, 15.7487)$ distribution.
b. Give the expectation of the posterior pdf.

8.3. Let $(x \mid \lambda) \sim \mathsf{Poi}(\lambda)$, and suppose that the prior distribution for λ is $\mathsf{Gamma}(a, b)$, where a and b are known. Find the posterior pdf of λ.

8.4. Let $x \sim \mathsf{Gamma}(\alpha, \lambda)$. Show that the pdf of $z = 1/x$ is given by (8.6). ☞ 24

8.5. Consider the transformation $[z_1, \ldots, z_{m+1}]^\top \mapsto [y_1, \ldots, y_{m+1}]^\top$ defined by $y_i = z_i\, z_{m+1}$, $i = 1, \ldots, m$ and $y_{m+1} = (1 - (z_1 + \cdots + z_m))\, z_{m+1}$. Show that the determinant of the corresponding matrix of Jacobi is z_{m+1}^m. This is used in the proof of Theorem 8.2. ☞ 24

8.6. Let $\mathbf{Z} = (Z_1, \ldots, Z_m) \sim \mathsf{Dirichlet}(\alpha_1, \ldots, \alpha_{m+1})$. Show that the marginal distribution of Z_i is $\mathsf{Beta}(\alpha_i, \sum_{j \neq i} \alpha_j)$. Hint: use Theorem 8.2. ☞ 24

8.7. Let $(x \mid p) \sim \mathsf{Geom}(p)$. Suppose that the prior distribution of p is $\mathcal{U}(0, 1)$.

a. Find the posterior pdf of p.
b. Find the posterior mode.
c. Find the posterior expectation.

8.8. The data 0.4453, 9.2865, 0.4077, 2.0623, 10.4737, 5.7525, 2.7159, 0.1954, 0.1608, 8.3143 were drawn from an $\mathsf{Exp}(1/\theta)$ distribution. Consider a Bayesian model with a constant prior for θ:

a. Show that the posterior distribution of θ is inverse-gamma, and determine the parameters.
b. Determine estimates of the 0.025 and 0.975 quantiles of the posterior distribution, using $N = 10^5$ simulated samples from the posterior distribution.

8.9. Suppose $\mathbf{x} = [x_1, \ldots, x_n]^\top$ is an iid sample from $\mathcal{N}(\mu, \sigma^2)$ with *known* variance σ^2. As a prior for μ take the $\mathcal{N}(\mu_0, \sigma_0^2)$ distribution for some fixed parameters μ_0 and σ_0^2. The Bayesian model is therefore

$$\mu \sim \mathcal{N}(\mu_0, \sigma_0^2)\,,$$

$$(x_1, \ldots, x_n \mid \mu) \overset{\text{iid}}{\sim} \mathcal{N}(\mu, \sigma^2)\,.$$

Show that the posterior pdf $f(\mu \mid \mathbf{x})$ corresponds to the pdf of the $\mathcal{N}(\mu_1, \sigma_1^2)$ distribution with

$$\mu_1 = \frac{\frac{1}{\sigma_0^2}\mu_0 + \frac{n}{\sigma^2}\overline{x}}{\frac{1}{\sigma_0^2} + \frac{n}{\sigma^2}} \qquad \text{and} \qquad \frac{1}{\sigma_1^2} = \frac{1}{\sigma_0^2} + \frac{n}{\sigma^2}\,.$$

8.10. Consider the simplified Bayesian model for normal data in Sect. 8.2.1; that is,

$$f(\mu, \sigma^2) = 1/\sigma^2 \,,$$
$$(\boldsymbol{x} \mid \mu, \sigma^2) \sim \mathcal{N}(\mu \mathbf{1}, \sigma^2 \, \mathbb{I}_n) \,.$$

The joint posterior pdf is

$$f(\mu, \sigma^2 \mid \boldsymbol{x}) \propto \left(\sigma^2\right)^{-n/2-1} \exp\left\{ -\frac{1}{2} \frac{\sum_{i=1}^n (x_i - \mu)^2}{\sigma^2} \right\} \,. \tag{8.29}$$

The marginal posterior pdfs of μ and σ^2 can be obtained by integrating out the other variable.

a. Prove that

$$\sum_{i=1}^n (x_i - \mu)^2 = \sum_{i=1}^n (x_i - \overline{x})^2 + n(\mu - \overline{x})^2 \,. \tag{8.30}$$

b. By using (8.30), show that

$$f(\sigma^2 \mid \boldsymbol{x}) \propto \left(\sigma^2\right)^{-n/2-1/2} \exp\left\{ -\frac{1}{2} \frac{\sum_{i=1}^n (x_i - \overline{x})^2}{\sigma^2} \right\} \,. \tag{8.31}$$

c. Show that (8.31) corresponds to the $\mathsf{InvGamma}\left((n-1)/2,\ s_x^2(n-1)/2\right)$ distribution, where s_x^2 is the frequentist sample variance of the $\{x_i\}$.

d. Let q_1 and q_2 be the $\gamma/2$ and $1-\gamma/2$ quantiles of (8.31). Show that the $1-\gamma$ credible interval (q_1, q_2) is *identical* to the classic confidence interval (5.20) (with α replaced by γ).

☞ 136

☞ 240

e. By using (8.30) and (8.6) show that

$$f(\mu \mid \boldsymbol{x}) \propto \left(\sum_{i=1}^n (x_i - \mu)^2 \right)^{-n/2} \propto \left(\frac{(\mu - \overline{x})^2 n}{s_x^2 \nu} + 1 \right)^{-(\nu+1)/2} \,,$$

☞ 50

where $\nu = n - 1$. Verify that, in view of (2.24), this means that

$$\left(\frac{\mu - \overline{x}}{s_x/\sqrt{n}} \,\Big|\, \boldsymbol{x} \right) \sim \mathsf{t}_{n-1} \,.$$

f. Let q_1 and q_2 be the $\gamma/2$ and $1 - \gamma/2$ quantiles of $f(\mu \mid \boldsymbol{x})$. Show that the $1 - \gamma$ credible interval (q_1, q_2) is *identical* to the classic confidence interval (5.19) (with α replaced by γ).

☞ 135

8.11. In Problem 8.10 compare the simulated densities in Fig. 8.3 with the exact ones. In particular, plot the pdf of $(\sigma^2 \mid \boldsymbol{x})$, that is, the pdf of the random variable $(n-1)s_x^2 \, Y$, where $Y \sim \mathsf{InvGamma}((n-1)/2, 1/2)$. Similarly, plot the pdf of $(\mu \mid \boldsymbol{x})$; that is, of the random variable $\overline{x} + T s_x/\sqrt{n}$, where $T \sim \mathsf{t}_{n-1}$.

8.12. In the *zero-inflated Poisson* model, random data $x_1, \ldots, x_n$ are assumed to be of the form $x_i = r_i\, y_i$, where the $\{y_i\}$ have a $\mathsf{Poi}(\lambda)$ distribution and the $\{r_i\}$ have a $\mathsf{Ber}(p)$ distribution, all independent of each other. Given an outcome $\boldsymbol{x} = [x_1, \ldots, x_n]^\top$, the objective is to estimate both λ and p. Consider the following hierarchical Bayesian model:

$$p \sim \mathcal{U}(0, 1)\,,$$
$$(\lambda \,|\, p) \sim \mathsf{Gamma}(a, b)\,,$$
$$(r_i \,|\, p, \lambda) \sim \mathsf{Ber}(p) \quad \text{independently}\,,$$
$$(x_i \,|\, \boldsymbol{r}, \lambda, p) \sim \mathsf{Poi}(\lambda\, r_i) \quad \text{independently}\,,$$

where $\boldsymbol{r} = (r_1, \ldots, r_n)$ and a and b are known parameters. We wish to sample from the posterior pdf $f(\lambda, p, \boldsymbol{r} \,|\, \boldsymbol{x})$ using the Gibbs sampler.

a. Show that

$$f(\boldsymbol{r}, \lambda, p \,|\, \boldsymbol{x}) \propto \lambda^{a-1} \mathrm{e}^{-b\lambda} \prod_{i=1}^{n} \mathrm{e}^{-\lambda\, r_i} (\lambda\, r_i)^{x_i}\, p^{r_i} (1 - p)^{1 - r_i}\,.$$

b. Show that

$$(\lambda \,|\, p, \boldsymbol{r}, \boldsymbol{x}) \sim \mathsf{Gamma}\left(a + \sum_{i=1}^{n} x_i, b + \sum_{i=1}^{n} r_i \right),$$

$$(p \,|\, \lambda, \boldsymbol{r}, \boldsymbol{x}) \sim \mathsf{Beta}\left(1 + \sum_{i=1}^{n} r_i, 1 + n - \sum_{i=1}^{n} r_i \right)$$

and, for $k = 1, \ldots, n$,

$$(r_k \,|\, \lambda, p, \boldsymbol{x}) \sim \mathsf{Ber}\left(\frac{p\, \mathrm{e}^{-\lambda}}{p\, \mathrm{e}^{-\lambda} + (1 - p)\, \mathbb{1}_{\{x_k = 0\}}} \right).$$

c. Generate an iid sample of size $n = 100$ for the zero-inflated Poisson model using parameters $p = 0.3$ and $\lambda = 2$.

d. Implement the Gibbs sampler, generate a large (dependent) sample from the posterior distribution, and use this to construct 95% credible intervals for p and λ using the data in (c). Compare these with the true values.

8.13. For a Markov chain $x_1, \ldots, x_n$, the joint pdf is of the form:

$$f(x_1, \ldots, x_n) = f(x_1) f(x_2 \,|\, x_1) f(x_3 \,|\, x_2) \cdots f(x_n \,|\, x_{n-1})\,.$$

The corresponding Bayesian network is given in the left pane of Figure 8.9. An alternative Bayesian network for the same Markov chain is given in the right pane of the figure, where the arcs have been turned around. Show that both networks represent the same joint pdf. Hint: write $f(x_{t+1} \mid x_t)$ in terms of $f(x_t \mid x_{t+1})$.

Fig. 8.9 Bayesian networks for a Markov chain

8.14. Figure 8.10 shows the Bayesian network for a **hidden Markov model**. Here $x_1, \ldots, x_n$ is a Markov chain on $\{1, \ldots, K\}$, defined by an initial (discrete) pdf $f(x_1)$ and transition probabilities $f(x_t \mid x_{t-1})$, which are here assumed to be known. For each time $t = 1, 2, \ldots, n$, the state of the chain, x_t, remains *hidden*. Instead, a variable y_t is observed, whose (known) distribution depends only on x_t; for example, $(y_t \mid x_t) \sim \mathcal{N}(x_t, 1)$.

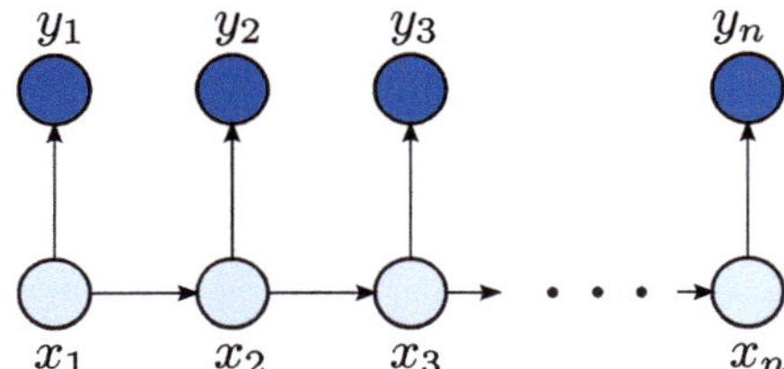

Fig. 8.10 Bayesian network for a hidden Markov model

A typical object of interest for such models is the posterior pdf $f(x_t \mid \boldsymbol{y}_{1:t})$, where $\boldsymbol{y}_{1:t} = (y_1, \ldots, y_t)$. That is, we wish to assess the state at time t given all the observations at and before time t.

a. Prove that

$$f(x_t, \boldsymbol{y}_{1:t}) = \sum_{x_{t-1}} f(x_t, y_t \mid x_{t-1}, \boldsymbol{y}_{1:t-1}) f(x_{t-1}, \boldsymbol{y}_{1:t-1}) \,. \tag{8.32}$$

b. Further, show that

$$f(x_t, y_t \mid x_{t-1}, \boldsymbol{y}_{1:t-1}) = f(x_t \mid x_{t-1}) f(y_t \mid x_t) \,. \tag{8.33}$$

c. Express $f(x_1, y_1)$ in terms of $f(x_1)$ and $f(y_1 \mid x_1)$. Explain how, with $f(x_1, y_1)$, (8.32), and (8.33), the posterior distribution of x_t given $\boldsymbol{y}_{1:t}$ can be determined recursively for $t = 2, 3, \ldots, n$.

8.15. Find an appropriate conjugate family for the $\mathsf{Exp}(\lambda)$ distribution, using

☞ 255 Theorem 8.4.

8.16. Let $\boldsymbol{x} = [x_1, \ldots, x_n]^\top$ be an iid sample from $\mathsf{Exp}(1/\theta)$ for some θ. Show that $\theta \sim \mathsf{InvGamma}(\alpha_0, \lambda_0)$ is a conjugate prior for this distribution. Determine the resulting posterior distribution.

8.17. Suppose $f(\boldsymbol{\theta} \mid \boldsymbol{x})$ is the posterior pdf for some Bayesian estimation problem. For example, $\boldsymbol{\theta}$ could represent the parameters of a regression model based on the data $\boldsymbol{x}$. An important use for the posterior pdf is to make predictions about the distribution of other random variables. For example, suppose that, conditional on $\boldsymbol{x}$, some random vector $\boldsymbol{y}$ depends on $\boldsymbol{\theta}$ via the conditional pdf $f(\boldsymbol{y} \mid \boldsymbol{\theta}, \boldsymbol{x}) = f(\boldsymbol{y} \mid \boldsymbol{\theta})$. Thus, conditional on $\boldsymbol{\theta}$, the random vector $\boldsymbol{y}$ is independent of $\boldsymbol{x}$. The **predictive pdf** of $\boldsymbol{y}$ given $\boldsymbol{x}$ is defined as $f(\boldsymbol{y} \mid \boldsymbol{x})$, which can be written as

$$f(\boldsymbol{y} \mid \boldsymbol{x}) = \int f(\boldsymbol{y} \mid \boldsymbol{\theta}) f(\boldsymbol{\theta} \mid \boldsymbol{x}) \, \mathrm{d}\boldsymbol{\theta} \, . \tag{8.34}$$

This can be viewed as the expectation of $f(\boldsymbol{y} \mid \boldsymbol{\theta})$ under the posterior pdf. Therefore, we can use Monte Carlo simulation to approximate $f(\boldsymbol{y} \mid \boldsymbol{x})$ via

$$f(\boldsymbol{y} \mid \boldsymbol{x}) \approx \frac{1}{N} \sum_{i=1}^{N} f(\boldsymbol{y} \mid \boldsymbol{\theta}_i) \, ,$$

where the sample $\{\boldsymbol{\theta}_i, i = 1, \ldots, N\}$ is obtained from $f(\boldsymbol{\theta} \mid \boldsymbol{x})$; for example, via MCMC.

a. Prove (8.34).
b. As a concrete example, suppose that the iid data $-0.4326, -1.6656,$ $0.1253, 0.2877, -1.1465$ come from some $\mathcal{N}(\mu, \sigma^2)$ distribution. Define $\boldsymbol{\theta} = [\mu, \sigma^2]$. Let $Y \sim \mathcal{N}(\mu, \sigma^2)$ be a new measurement. Estimate and plot the predictive pdf $f(y \mid \boldsymbol{x})$, using a sample $\boldsymbol{\theta}_1, \ldots, \boldsymbol{\theta}_N$ obtained via the Gibbs sampler of Example 8.2.1. Take $N = 1000$. Compare this with the "common-sense" Gaussian pdf with expectation $\overline{x}$ (sample mean) and variance s^2 (sample variance). ☞ 23

8.18. The **bag of words** method is a popular procedure for classification. Given are k *objects* that are each characterized by n *features*. For example, the objects could be k different people, and the features could be various facial measurements, such as the width of the eyes divided by the distance between the eyes, or the ratio of the nose height and mouth width. The features, $x_1, \ldots, x_n$ say, have a known distribution and are assumed to be conditionally independent of each other given the object p; that is, $f(x_1, \ldots, x_n \mid p) = f(x_1 \mid p) \cdots f(x_n \mid p)$. Assuming a uniform prior for p, the posterior pdf is thus given by

$$f(p \mid x_1, \ldots, x_n) \propto \prod_{i=1}^{n} f(x_i \mid p) \, .$$

To classify the object on the basis of the features, simply take the p that maximizes the unnormalized posterior pdf:

a. Give the Bayesian network for the joint pdf of $p, x_1, \ldots, x_n$.
b. Suppose the i-th feature distribution of object p is $\mathcal{N}(\mu_{pi}, \sigma^2)$, $p = 1, \ldots, k$, $i = 1, \ldots, n$. Define $\boldsymbol{\mu}_p = [\mu_{p1}, \ldots, \mu_{pn}]^\top$, $p = 1, \ldots, k$. Let $\boldsymbol{x} = [x_1, \ldots, x_n]^\top$ be the vector of observed features. Let $p^* = \operatorname{argmin}_p \|\boldsymbol{\mu}_p - \boldsymbol{x}\|$; that is, among all feature vectors $\{\boldsymbol{\mu}_p\}$ the vector $\boldsymbol{\mu}_{p^*}$ is closest to $\boldsymbol{x}$. Show that p^* also maximizes the posterior pdf.
c. Next, consider the case where the i-th feature of object p is $\mathcal{N}(\mu_{pi}, \sigma_{pi}^2)$ distributed. Table 8.2 lists the means μ and standard deviations σ of the normal feature distributions of four objects. The observed features of an object are $[x_1, x_2, x_3]^\top = [1.67, 2.00, 4.23]^\top$. How should this object be classified?

Table 8.2 Feature parameters

Object	Feature 1		Feature 2		Feature 3	
	μ	σ	μ	σ	μ	σ
1	1.6	0.1	2.4	0.5	4.3	0.2
2	1.5	0.2	2.9	0.6	6.1	0.9
3	1.8	0.3	2.5	0.3	4.2	0.3
4	1.1	0.2	3.1	0.7	5.6	0.3

Part III

Advanced Models and Inference

In Part III of the book, we consider estimation and inference for a wide variety of advanced models. Topics include shrinkage and regularization, generalized linear models with discrete responses, nonparametric models, autoregressive moving average models for time series, Gaussian models for data arising from repeated measurements, and state space models for data exhibiting time-varying persistence and volatility. Both classical and Bayesian estimation of these models are covered. It is assumed that the reader is familiar with the statistical concepts and computational techniques discussed in Part II.

Chapter 9
Shrinkage and Regularization

For some modern statistical analyses, it may be useful to *combine* frequentist and Bayesian techniques. Noticeable examples are found in the theory of shrinkage estimation and regularization.

Classical (i.e., frequentist) estimation methods focus on obtaining *unbiased* estimators. However, when many parameters need to be estimated, unbiasedness may not always lead to the best estimators, in terms of their distance to the true parameters.

9.1 James–Stein Estimator

Consider n estimation problems, where in the i-th estimation problem, there is a single datum $X_i \sim \mathcal{N}(\mu_i, 1)$, and it is assumed that the $\{X_i\}$ are independent. The maximum likelihood estimator for μ_i is simply X_i, $i = 1, \ldots, n$. Similarly, the maximum likelihood estimator for the vector $\boldsymbol{\mu} = [\mu_1, \ldots, \mu_n]^\top$ is $\boldsymbol{X} = [X_1, \ldots, X_n]^\top$. This estimator has a total mean square error (MSE) of

$$\sum_{i=1}^{n} \mathbb{E}(X_i - \mu_i)^2 = \sum_{i=1}^{n} \mathrm{Var}(X_i) = n \ .$$

Can we do better, in terms of MSE, by using some *biased* estimator of $\boldsymbol{\mu}$? To that end, let us examine the corresponding Bayesian model, with prior

$$\mu_i \sim \mathcal{N}(\alpha, \tau^2), \quad i = 1, \ldots, n, \text{independently} \ ,$$

© The Author(s), under exclusive license to Springer Science+Business Media, LLC, part of Springer Nature 2025
J. C. C. Chan, D. P. Kroese, *Statistical Modeling and Computation*,
Springer Texts in Statistics, https://doi.org/10.1007/978-1-0716-4132-3_9

where α and τ^2 are given hyperparameters, and with likelihood

$$(X_i \mid \mu_i) \sim \mathcal{N}(\mu_i, 1), \quad i = 1, \ldots, n, \text{independently} .$$

It follows, by integrating out the μ_i, that

$$X_i \sim \mathcal{N}(\alpha, 1 + \tau^2), \quad i = 1, \ldots, n, \text{ independently} . \tag{9.1}$$

Moreover, the posterior pdf of $\boldsymbol{\mu}$ is

$$f(\boldsymbol{\mu} \mid \boldsymbol{x}) \propto p(\boldsymbol{x} \mid \boldsymbol{\mu})p(\boldsymbol{\mu}) \propto \prod_{i=1}^{n} \mathrm{e}^{-\frac{1}{2}(x_i - \mu_i)^2} \mathrm{e}^{-\frac{1}{2}\frac{(\mu_i - \alpha)^2}{\tau^2}} ,$$

which shows that conditional on $\boldsymbol{x}$, the $\{\mu_i\}$ are independent, and

$$(\mu_i \mid x_i) \sim \mathcal{N}\left(\frac{\tau^2 x_i + \alpha}{\tau^2 + 1}, \frac{\tau^2}{\tau^2 + 1}\right) = \mathcal{N}(\alpha + \sigma^2(x_i - \alpha), \sigma^2) ,$$

where $\sigma^2 = \tau^2/(\tau^2 + 1)$. In particular, the posterior mean for μ_i is

$$\alpha + \sigma^2(x_i - \alpha) . \tag{9.2}$$

The idea is now to estimate α and σ^2 from the data, using the (9.1). We can estimate these parameters in a purely frequentist way. Namely, α can be estimated unbiasedly via the sample mean:

$$\widehat{\alpha} \stackrel{\text{def}}{=} \overline{X}$$

and σ^2 can be estimated unbiasedly via the estimator:

$$\widehat{\sigma^2} \stackrel{\text{def}}{=} 1 - \frac{n - 3}{\sum_{i=1}^{n}(X_i - \overline{X})^2} , \tag{9.3}$$

for $n \geq 4$; see Problem 9.1. If we plug $\widehat{\alpha}$ and $\widehat{\sigma^2}$ into (9.2), we obtain the famous James–Stein estimator (James and Stein, 1961):

$$\widetilde{\mu}_i = \overline{X} + \left(1 - \frac{n - 3}{\sum_{i=1}^{n}(X_i - \overline{X})^2}\right)(X_i - \overline{X}), \quad i = 1, \ldots, n . \tag{9.4}$$

Depending on the spread of the $\{\mu_i\}$, the James–Stein estimator can yield a significant reduction of the MSE. The most striking fact is that for $n \geq 4$, it always improves on the total MSE for the unbiased case, no matter what $\boldsymbol{\mu}$ is! You can try it out yourself in the following Julia code.

```
jamesstein.jl
```
```julia
using StatsBase, LinearAlgebra,Plots
n = 100
# mu = rand(n)*100 .- 50 # not much difference
mu = rand(n)*0.1 .- 0.05 # a lot of difference
K = 10000
mse_js = zeros(K)
mse = zeros(K)
for k=1:K
  global mu,n
  X = mu + randn(n)
  mu_js = mean(X) .+ (1 - (n-3)/(var(X)*(n-2)))*(X .- mean(X))
  mse_js[k] = norm(mu_js - mu)^2 mse[k] = norm(X - mu)^2
end
m1 = mean(mse_js)
m2 = mean(mse)
print("MSE JS =", m1," MSE MLE = ",m2)
```

That the James–Stein is a shrinkage estimator, which shrinks the unbiased estimator toward values which are closer to the true mean, is illustrated in Fig. 9.1. The $\{\mu_i\}_{i=1}^{10}$ were here drawn uniformly on $[-2, 2]$.

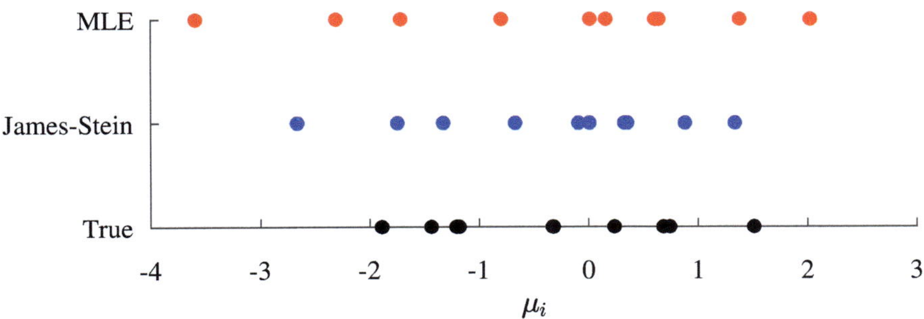

Fig. 9.1 The James–Stein estimator shrinks the estimates toward the true means

The moral of this story is that for high-dimensional parameter estimation problems, shrinkage estimators may provide better overall estimates than unbiased ones. In the next section, we derive shrinkage estimators for linear regression.

9.2 Ridge Regression

Ridge regression is a simple modification of ordinary regression that yields shrinkage estimators.

We motivate the method via the Bayesian normal linear model of Sect. 8.2.2. In particular, suppose the likelihood of the data $\boldsymbol{y} = [y_1, \ldots, y_n]^\top$ is specified by

$$(\boldsymbol{y} \mid \boldsymbol{\beta}, \sigma^2) \sim \mathcal{N}(\mathbf{X}\boldsymbol{\beta}, \sigma^2 \mathbb{I}_n) \, ,$$

where $\mathbf{X} = [x_{ij}]$ is the (known) $n \times m$ design matrix and $\boldsymbol{\beta} = [\beta_1, \ldots, \beta_m]^\top$ and σ^2 are unknown parameters.

We put an improper prior $1/\sigma^2$ on σ^2, and, given σ^2, the prior distribution for $\boldsymbol{\beta}$ is $\mathcal{N}(\mathbf{0}, \sigma^2/\lambda \, \mathbb{I}_m)$, where $\lambda > 0$ is a **regularization parameter**. Thus, the (joint) prior density of $\boldsymbol{\beta}$ and σ^2 is given by

$$f(\boldsymbol{\beta}, \sigma^2) \propto \frac{1}{\sigma^2} \times (2\pi\sigma^2)^{-m/2} \exp\left\{ -\frac{\lambda \|\boldsymbol{\beta}\|^2}{2\sigma^2} \right\} \, .$$

Consequently, similar to the derivation of (8.11), the posterior density is of the form:

$$f(\boldsymbol{\beta}, \sigma^2 \mid \boldsymbol{y}) \propto \left(\sigma^2\right)^{-(n+m)/2-1} \exp\left\{ -\frac{\|\boldsymbol{y} - \mathbf{X}\boldsymbol{\beta}\|^2}{2\sigma^2} - \frac{\lambda\|\boldsymbol{\beta}\|^2}{2\sigma^2} \right\} \, . \tag{9.5}$$

By integrating out σ^2, we find:

$$f(\boldsymbol{\beta} \mid \boldsymbol{y}) \propto \left(\|\boldsymbol{y} - \mathbf{X}\boldsymbol{\beta}\|^2 + \lambda\|\boldsymbol{\beta}\|^2\right)^{-(n+m)/2} \, . \tag{9.6}$$

The **ridge regression estimator** $\widehat{\boldsymbol{\beta}}$ is taken to be the *maximum posterior estimate* of $\boldsymbol{\beta}$, that is, the value of $\boldsymbol{\beta}$ for which the posterior pdf is maximal. Thus,

$$\widehat{\boldsymbol{\beta}} = \underset{\boldsymbol{\beta}}{\operatorname{argmin}} \underbrace{\|\boldsymbol{y} - \mathbf{X}\boldsymbol{\beta}\|^2 + \lambda\|\boldsymbol{\beta}\|^2}_{L(\boldsymbol{\beta})} \, . \tag{9.7}$$

The objective function L in (9.7) is strictly convex and differentiable (see Problem 9.4), so the solution of this optimization problem can be found by identifying the stationary points of L; that is, by solving $\nabla L(\boldsymbol{\beta}) = \mathbf{0}$. This leads to the system of linear equations:

$$\mathbf{X}^\top(\mathbf{X}\boldsymbol{\beta} - \boldsymbol{y}) + \lambda\boldsymbol{\beta} = \mathbf{0} \, . \tag{9.8}$$

☞ 130 If $\lambda = 0$, these are simply the *normal equations* (5.9), so that then $\widehat{\boldsymbol{\beta}}$ is the ordinary least-squares estimate. For any $\lambda > 0$, the matrix $\mathbf{X}^\top\mathbf{X} + \lambda\mathbb{I}_m$ is invertible (see Problem 9.2), even if $\mathbf{X}^\top\mathbf{X}$ is not. This is of particular relevance when there are more explanatory variables than observations, i.e., $m > n$. In that case the normal equations have multiple solutions. However, the ridge regression estimator is still unique for any $\lambda > 0$, and is given by

$$\widehat{\boldsymbol{\beta}} = (\mathbf{X}^\top\mathbf{X} + \lambda\mathbb{I}_m)^{-1}\mathbf{X}^\top\boldsymbol{y} \, . \tag{9.9}$$

In fact, by taking the limit of $(\mathbf{X}^\top\mathbf{X} + \lambda\mathbb{I}_m)^{-1}\mathbf{X}^\top$ as $\lambda \to 0$, we obtain the *pseudo-inverse* $\mathbf{X}^+$ of $\mathbf{X}$. Thus, even in the case where $m > n$, the corresponding estimator is of the form $\mathbf{X}^+\boldsymbol{y}$, as in (5.12), although $\mathbf{X}^+$ is no longer defined by (5.11). Moreover, it can be shown that this estimator is the solution to the normal equations with the smallest squared norm $\|\boldsymbol{\beta}\|^2 = \sum_{i=1}^{m} \beta_i^2$.

For $\lambda > 0$, and a given $\mathbf{X}$, an optimal choice for the parameter λ is typically determined from test data or via cross-validation.

Example 9.1 (Ridge Regression). Let us examine a ridge regression scenario in which the design matrix $\mathbf{X}$ is of dimension 100×20 and where its entries are drawn independently from the $\mathcal{U}(0,1)$ distribution. Let the i-th component of the 20-dimensional true parameter vector $\boldsymbol{\beta}$ be $\beta_i = i/10$ if $i \in \{1,\ldots,10\}$ and $\beta_i = 0$ if $i \in \{11,\ldots,20\}$. The 100-dimensional data vector $\boldsymbol{y}$ is generated from the model:

$$Y = \mathbf{X}\boldsymbol{\beta} + \sigma\boldsymbol{\varepsilon} \, ,$$

where $\sigma = 3$ and $\boldsymbol{\varepsilon} \sim \mathcal{N}(\mathbf{0}, \mathbb{I}_{100})$. Figure 9.2 shows the components of $\boldsymbol{\beta}$ as a function of the regularization parameter λ, as determined from (9.9). We see the shrinkage of the vector $\widehat{\boldsymbol{\beta}}$ with increasing λ.

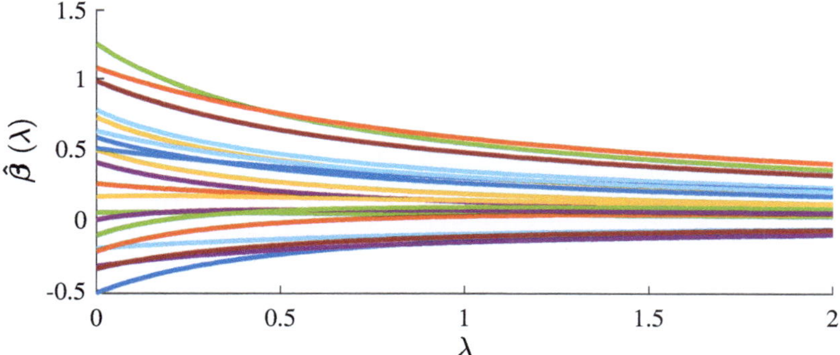

Fig. 9.2 Ridge regression estimates as a function of the regularization parameter λ

Figure 9.3 shows the true values of each β_i as well as the ordinary least-squares (OLS) estimates and the ridge regression estimates, for $\lambda = 0.74$. We see that the ridge regression estimates are on average significantly closer to the true parameter values.

Finally, Fig. 9.4 shows how the squared error $\|\widehat{\boldsymbol{\beta}} - \boldsymbol{\beta}\|^2$ varies with λ. In this case the optimal value for λ was 0.74, which was used in Fig. 9.4. Compared with the ordinary least-squares case, the ridge estimate has a decidedly reduced squared error (around 2.5 times smaller). Of course, in practical situations the true $\boldsymbol{\beta}$ is not known.

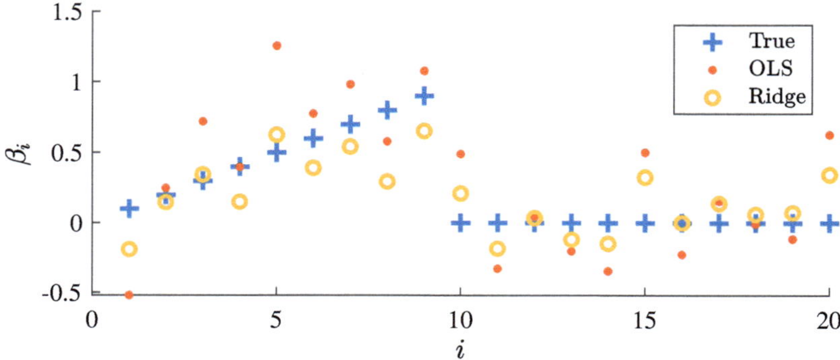

Fig. 9.3 True and estimated parameters for the linear model

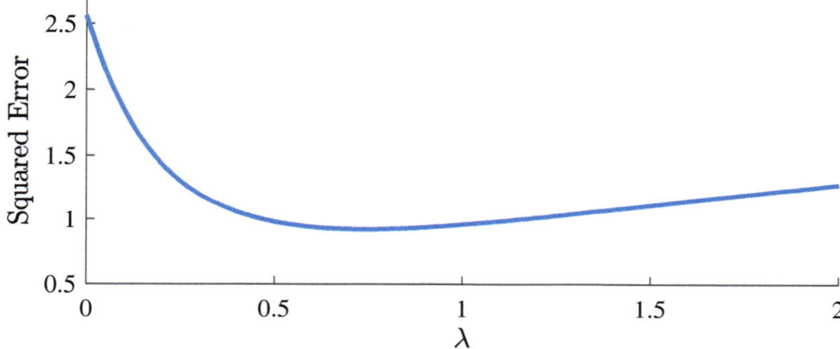

Fig. 9.4 Ridge regression solutions for a simple linear regression problem

As the $m > n$ case illustrates, the ridge estimator (9.9) can be useful when the matrix $\mathbf{X}\mathbf{X}^\top$ is singular or ill-conditioned, e.g., comprised of highly correlated explanatory variables. Moreover, for cases that are at risk of overfitting, i.e., when $\|\boldsymbol{y} - \mathbf{X}\widetilde{\boldsymbol{\beta}}\|$ is 0 or very small for some $\widetilde{\boldsymbol{\beta}} \in \mathbb{R}^m$, imposing a penalty on the squared norm of $\boldsymbol{\beta}$, as in (9.7), may benefit the predictive performance of the prediction function $\boldsymbol{x} \mapsto \boldsymbol{x}^\top\widehat{\boldsymbol{\beta}}$. Note that for large λ, the squared-norm penalty will be the dominant term in the optimization problem (9.7), and therefore $\widehat{\boldsymbol{\beta}} \to \mathbf{0}$ as $\lambda \to \infty$.

Finally, using optimization theory (see, e.g., Boyd and Vandenberghe 2004), it is possible to recast the regularized minimization program:

$$\min_{\boldsymbol{\beta}} \|\boldsymbol{y} - \mathbf{X}\boldsymbol{\beta}\|^2 + \lambda\|\boldsymbol{\beta}\|^2$$

in (9.7) as the *constrained* minimization program

$$\min_{\boldsymbol{\beta}} \|\boldsymbol{y} - \mathbf{X}\boldsymbol{\beta}\|^2$$
$$\text{subject to } \|\boldsymbol{\beta}\|^2 \leq b \tag{9.10}$$

for some $b \geq 0$. In fact, the relation between the regularization constant λ and the bound b is that $b = \|\widehat{\boldsymbol{\beta}}\|^2$, where $\widehat{\boldsymbol{\beta}}$ is the minimizer of the objective function L in (9.7). Thus, regularization forces $\boldsymbol{\beta}$ to lie in a restricted class of parameters, and as a result the class of candidate prediction functions $\boldsymbol{x} \mapsto \boldsymbol{x}^\top \boldsymbol{\beta}$ is reduced.

9.2.1 Gram Matrix

Suppose that $n \geq m$ and that $\mathbf{X}$ has full rank m. Then, any vector $\boldsymbol{\beta} \in \mathbb{R}^m$ can be written as a linear combination of the features $\{\boldsymbol{x}_i\}$; that is

$$\boldsymbol{\beta} = \sum_{i=1}^{n} \alpha_i \, \boldsymbol{x}_i$$

for some vector $\boldsymbol{\alpha} = [\alpha_1, \ldots, \alpha_n]^\top \in \mathbb{R}^n$. For $n > m$ there is a whole subspace of solutions $\boldsymbol{\alpha}$. As the feature vectors form the rows of $\mathbf{X}$, and thus the columns of $\mathbf{X}^\top$, we can write $\boldsymbol{\beta} = \mathbf{X}^\top \boldsymbol{\alpha}$. Equation (9.8) then leads to

$$(\mathbf{X}\mathbf{X}^\top + \lambda \mathbb{I}_n)\boldsymbol{\alpha} = \boldsymbol{y} \,. \tag{9.11}$$

This is now a system of n equations and n unknowns, as opposed to (9.8), which has m equations and m unknowns. The $n \times n$ matrix $\mathbf{K} = \mathbf{X}\mathbf{X}^\top$ is called the **Gram matrix** of the feature vectors, that is, the matrix of inner product terms $\langle \boldsymbol{x}_i, \boldsymbol{x}_j \rangle = \boldsymbol{x}_i^\top \boldsymbol{x}_j$. The Gram matrix is symmetric and not invertible for $n > m$. Do not confuse it with the matrix $\mathbf{X}^\top \mathbf{X}$, which has dimension $m \times m$. Assuming invertibility of $\mathbf{K} + \lambda \mathbb{I}_n$ (again, which is always the case when $\lambda > 0$), the solution to (9.11) is

$$\widehat{\boldsymbol{\alpha}} = (\mathbf{K} + \lambda \mathbb{I}_n)^{-1} \boldsymbol{y} \,,$$

which only depends on the training features through the Gram matrix. See also Problem 9.13. For $\lambda = 0$ the matrix $\mathbf{K}$ is not invertible. Note that (with $\lambda > 0$) the optimal prediction function based on the training data $\tau = \{(\boldsymbol{x}_i, y_i)\}$ is a linear combination of inner products:

$$g_\tau(\boldsymbol{x}) = \boldsymbol{x}^\top \widehat{\boldsymbol{\beta}} = \boldsymbol{x}^\top \mathbf{X}^\top \widehat{\boldsymbol{\alpha}} = \sum_{i=1}^{n} \widehat{\alpha}_i \langle \boldsymbol{x}_i, \boldsymbol{x} \rangle \,. \tag{9.12}$$

9.2.2 Not Penalizing the Constant Feature

When $\lambda \to \infty$, the optimal prediction function shrinks to 0, and has no merit for prediction. It would be better if it were to shrink to the constant $\overline{y}$ (the average of the response data), as this would correspond to the default model $Y \sim \mathcal{N}(\mu, \sigma^2)$, rather than $Y = 0$. To achieve this, we modify the optimization problem (9.7) in such a way that the constant feature is not penalized. This requires a slight alteration of the notation. In particular, we are interested in prediction functions of the form $\boldsymbol{x} \mapsto \beta_0 \mathbf{1} + \boldsymbol{x}^\top \boldsymbol{\beta}$, where $\mathbf{1}$ is the $n \times 1$ vector of 1s and $\boldsymbol{x} = [x_1, \ldots, x_m]^\top$. We thus have $m + 1$ features, rather than m. The optimal β_0 and $\boldsymbol{\beta}$ are found from the modified optimization problem:

$$\min_{\beta_0, \boldsymbol{\beta}} \| \boldsymbol{y} - \beta_0 \mathbf{1} - \mathbf{X}\boldsymbol{\beta} \|^2 + \lambda \|\boldsymbol{\beta}\|^2 \,. \tag{9.13}$$

Note that the optimal prediction function converges to $\overline{y}$ as $\lambda \to \infty$. The objective function in (9.13) is strictly convex and differentiable, so the solution follows again by identification of the stationary points, which leads to the linear equations:

$$\mathbf{X}^\top (\beta_0 \mathbf{1} + \mathbf{X}\boldsymbol{\beta} - \boldsymbol{y}) + \lambda \boldsymbol{\beta} = \mathbf{0} \,, \tag{9.14}$$

and

$$n\beta_0 = \mathbf{1}^\top (\boldsymbol{y} - \mathbf{X}\boldsymbol{\beta}) \,. \tag{9.15}$$

This means that we can solve $\boldsymbol{\beta}$ from

$$(\mathbf{X}^\top \mathbf{X} - n^{-1}\mathbf{X}^\top \mathbf{1}\mathbf{1}^\top \mathbf{X} + \lambda \mathbb{I}_m)\boldsymbol{\beta} = (\mathbf{X}^\top - n^{-1}\mathbf{X}^\top \mathbf{1}\mathbf{1}^\top)\boldsymbol{y} \,, \tag{9.16}$$

and determining β_0 from (9.15). By making the substitution (9.15) in the quadratic form $\|\boldsymbol{y} - \beta_0 \mathbf{1} - \mathbf{X}\boldsymbol{\beta}\|^2$ in (9.13), we can effectively eliminate β_0 from our optimization problem by *centering* the data, that is, by premultiplying $\boldsymbol{y}$ and $\mathbf{X}$ with the **centering** matrix $\mathbf{C} = \mathbb{I}_n - n^{-1}\mathbf{1}\mathbf{1}^\top$, which subtracts the mean from $\boldsymbol{y}$ and each column of $\mathbf{X}$. Written out, we have:

$$\boldsymbol{y} - \beta_0 \mathbf{1} - \mathbf{X}\boldsymbol{\beta} = \boldsymbol{y} - n^{-1}\mathbf{1}^\top \mathbf{1}(\boldsymbol{y} - \mathbf{X}\boldsymbol{\beta}) - \mathbf{X}\boldsymbol{\beta} = \mathbf{C}\boldsymbol{y} - \mathbf{C}\mathbf{X} \,.$$

To find a Gram matrix representation as in Sect. 9.2.1, let us assume again that $n \geq m$ and that $\mathbf{X}$ has full (column) rank m. Then, with $\boldsymbol{\beta} = \mathbf{X}^\top \boldsymbol{\alpha}$, (9.16) reduces to

$$(\mathbf{C}\mathbf{K} + \lambda \mathbb{I}_n)\boldsymbol{\alpha} = \mathbf{C}\boldsymbol{y} \,,$$

where $\mathbf{K} = \mathbf{X}\mathbf{X}^\top$ is the Gram matrix. Assuming invertibility of $\mathbf{C}\mathbf{K} + \lambda \mathbb{I}_n$, we have the solution:

$$\widehat{\boldsymbol{\alpha}} = (\mathbf{C}\mathbf{K} + \lambda \mathbb{I}_n)^{-1}\mathbf{C}\boldsymbol{y} \,,$$

which depends on the training feature vectors $\{x_i\}$ only through the Gram matrix. From (9.15), the solution for the constant term is $\widehat{\beta}_0 = \mathbf{1}^\top(y - \mathbf{K}\widehat{\alpha})/n$.

Thus, similar to (9.12), the optimal prediction function is an affine combination of inner products:

$$g_\tau(x) = \widehat{\beta}_0 + x^\top \mathbf{X}^\top \widehat{\alpha} = \widehat{\beta}_0 + \sum_{i=1}^{n} \widehat{\alpha}_i \langle x_i, x \rangle \,,$$

where the coefficients $\widehat{\beta}_0$ and $\widehat{\alpha}_i$ only depend on the inner products $\{\langle x_i, x_j \rangle\}$.

Example 9.2 (Not Penalizing the Constant Feature). We illustrate in Fig. 9.5 how the solutions of the two differently penalized ridge regression problems behave as a function of the regularization parameter λ. The data used is that of the elementary normal linear regression model

$$Y_i = \beta_0 + \beta_1 x_i + \varepsilon_i, \quad i = 1, \ldots, n \,,$$

with $\{\varepsilon_i\} \sim_{\text{iid}} \mathcal{N}(0, 1)$, $n = 30$, $\beta_0 = 1$ and $\beta_1 = -2$. The explanatory variables were independently drawn from the uniform distribution on the interval $[0, 10]$.

The left panel of Fig. 9.5 shows the positions (indicated by the "+" symbols) of the ridge regression estimates for various values of λ; specifically, $\lambda/n \in \{0.0, 0.1, 1, 10, 30, 100\}$. The contours are those of the squared-error loss (actually the logarithm thereof), which is minimized with respect to the model parameters β_0 and β_1. We see that for large values of λ, the estimates tend to the origin $(0, 0)$. The circles in the figure are centered at $(0, 0)$ and have a radius equal to the norm of $\widehat{\beta}$. They illustrate the important point that the regularization in ridge regression is equivalent to imposing a bound on the (squared) norm of the parameter vector β. For large λ there is a heavy restriction on the norm of β, while for $\lambda = 0$, there is no restriction, so that in this case the solution corresponds to the ordinary least-squares solution (indicated by the symbol "o").

The right panel of Fig. 9.5 also displays the positions of the ridge regression estimates for various values of λ, but now regularization is only applied to the parameter β_1, not to β_0, which corresponds to the constant feature. The regularization parameters are here $\lambda/n \in \{0.0, 0.8, 3, 8, 20, 100\}$. The red line segments depict the allowed intervals in which β_1 can lie, for each λ. For large λ, β_1 goes to 0, while β_0 goes to $\overline{y}$, which in this case is -8.88. For $\lambda = 0$, we obtain again the ordinary least-squares solution.

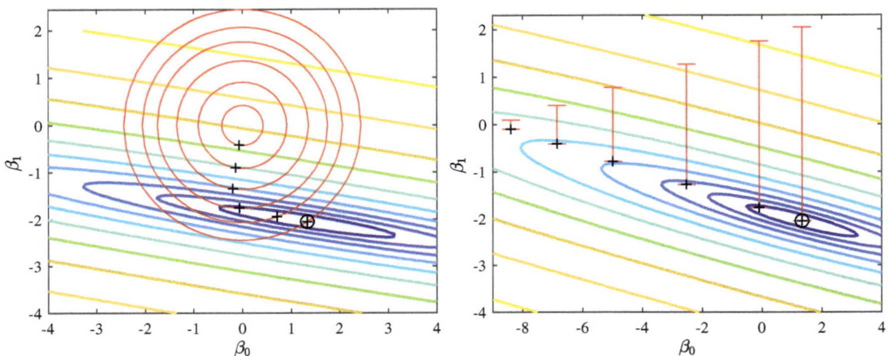

Fig. 9.5 Ridge regression solutions for a simple linear regression problem. Left: both β_0 and β_1 are regularized. Right: only β_1 is regularized

9.3 Lasso Regression

We motivated the ridge regression estimator in (9.7) via a Bayesian normal linear model. Let us repeat the arguments, but now with a joint prior density

$$f(\boldsymbol{\beta}, \sigma^2) \propto \frac{1}{\sigma^2} \left(\frac{\lambda}{4\sigma^2} \right)^m \exp\left\{ -\frac{\lambda \|\boldsymbol{\beta}\|_1}{2\sigma^2} \right\},$$

where $\|\boldsymbol{\beta}\|_1 = \sum_{i=1}^{m} |\beta_i|$. The distribution with pdf $\boldsymbol{x} \mapsto 2^{-m} \exp(-\|\boldsymbol{x}\|_1)$ is called the **Laplace distribution** and is the multivariate equivalent of the double exponential distribution. A dotplot from the two-dimensional Laplace distribution is given in Fig. 9.6. In contrast to the spherical contours of the multivariate normal distribution, the Laplace distribution has square contours. Using a Laplace rather than a normal prior assigns more credibility to the corner points, that is, to the case where one or more coordinates are 0.

The posterior density is now given by

$$f(\boldsymbol{\beta}, \sigma^2 \mid \boldsymbol{y}) \propto \left(\sigma^2 \right)^{-(n+m)-1} \exp\left\{ -\frac{\|\boldsymbol{y} - \mathbf{X}\boldsymbol{\beta}\|^2}{2\sigma^2} - \frac{\lambda \|\boldsymbol{\beta}\|_1}{2\sigma^2} \right\} \qquad (9.17)$$

and is of the same form as in (9.5), except that the squared Euclidean norm $\|\boldsymbol{\beta}\|^2$ is replaced with the **1-norm** of $\boldsymbol{\beta}$. By taking again the maximum posterior estimate of $\boldsymbol{\beta}$, we arrive at

$$\widehat{\boldsymbol{\beta}} = \operatorname*{argmin}_{\boldsymbol{\beta}} \|\boldsymbol{y} - \mathbf{X}\boldsymbol{\beta}\|^2 + \lambda \|\boldsymbol{\beta}\|_1 . \qquad (9.18)$$

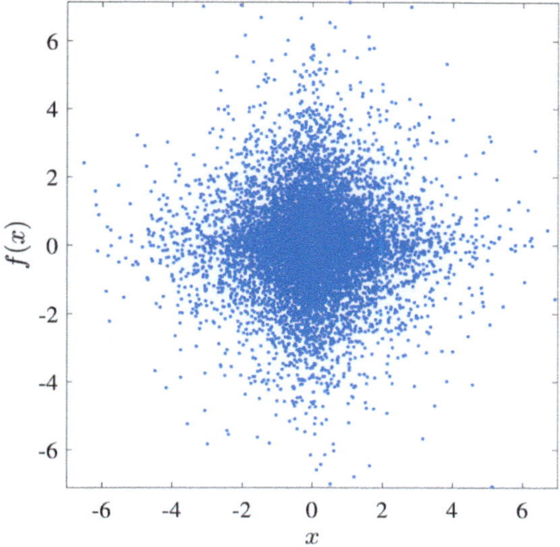

Fig. 9.6 10000 realizations from the bivariate Laplace distribution. Compare with Fig. 3.6

This gives the so-called **lasso** (least absolute shrinkage and selection operator) estimator. Similar to (9.10), the minimization program

$$\min_{\boldsymbol{\beta}} \|\boldsymbol{y} - \mathbf{X}\boldsymbol{\beta}\|^2 + \lambda \|\boldsymbol{\beta}\|_1 \tag{9.19}$$

is equivalent to the constrained minimization program

$$\min_{\boldsymbol{\beta}} \|\boldsymbol{y} - \mathbf{X}\boldsymbol{\beta}\|^2$$
$$\text{subject to } \|\boldsymbol{\beta}\|_1 \leq b \,, \tag{9.20}$$

where the connection between b and λ is that $b = \|\widehat{\boldsymbol{\beta}}\|_1$, with $\widehat{\boldsymbol{\beta}}$ being the solution to (9.18). Note that the constraint region matches the (square) contours of the Laplace distribution.

One could of course create many different regularization problems by changing the regularization term with some other function of $\boldsymbol{\beta}$. However, using the lasso estimator has particular advantages. The first is that the optimization problem in (9.18) is, as in ridge regression, a *convex* optimization problem. Although no explicit solution exists, such as in (9.9), the lasso estimator can be found very efficiently, as described next.

By introducing an auxiliary variable $\boldsymbol{z}$, we can write (9.19) as

$$\min_{\boldsymbol{x},\boldsymbol{z}} \|\boldsymbol{y} - \mathbf{X}\boldsymbol{\beta}\|^2 + \lambda \|\boldsymbol{z}\|_1$$
$$\text{subject to } \boldsymbol{\beta} - \boldsymbol{z} = \boldsymbol{0} \,. \tag{9.21}$$

One way to solve such problems efficiently is to minimize the **augmented Lagrangian**:

$$L(\boldsymbol{\beta}, \boldsymbol{z}, \boldsymbol{\mu}) = \|\boldsymbol{y} - \mathbf{X}\boldsymbol{\beta}\|^2 + \lambda\|\boldsymbol{z}\|_1 + \boldsymbol{\mu}^{\top}(\boldsymbol{\beta} - \boldsymbol{z}) + \varrho\|\boldsymbol{\beta} - \boldsymbol{z}\|^2$$

for some $\varrho > 0$, where $\boldsymbol{\mu}$ is a Lagrange multiplier. The **alternating direction method of multipliers** (ADMM) algorithm (Boyd et al., 2010) updates the components iteratively as follows:

$$\boldsymbol{\beta}^{(t+1)} = \underset{\boldsymbol{\beta}}{\operatorname{argmin}}\, L(\boldsymbol{\beta}, \boldsymbol{z}^{(t)}, \boldsymbol{\mu}^{(t)}) \tag{9.22}$$

$$\boldsymbol{z}^{(t+1)} = \underset{\boldsymbol{z}}{\operatorname{argmin}}\, L(\boldsymbol{\beta}^{(t+1)}, \boldsymbol{z}, \boldsymbol{\mu}^{(t)}) \tag{9.23}$$

$$\boldsymbol{\mu}^{(t+1)} = \boldsymbol{\mu}^{(t)} + 2\varrho\left(\boldsymbol{\beta}^{(t+1)} - \boldsymbol{z}^{(t+1)}\right). \tag{9.24}$$

Explicitly, the ADMM updates are (see Problem 9.6)

$$\boldsymbol{\beta}^{(t+1)} = (\mathbf{X}^{\top}\mathbf{X} + \varrho\,\mathbb{I}_m)^{-1}(\mathbf{X}^{\top}\boldsymbol{y} + \varrho(\boldsymbol{z}^{(t)} - \boldsymbol{u}^{(t)})) \tag{9.25}$$

$$\boldsymbol{z}^{(t+1)} = \left(\boldsymbol{\beta}^{(t+1)} + \boldsymbol{u}^{(t)} - \lambda/(2\varrho)\right)^{+} - \left(-\boldsymbol{\beta}^{(t+1)} - \boldsymbol{u}^{(t)} - \lambda/(2\varrho)\right)^{+} \tag{9.26}$$

$$\boldsymbol{u}^{(t+1)} = \boldsymbol{u}^{(t)} + \boldsymbol{\beta}^{(t+1)} - \boldsymbol{z}^{(t+1)}, \tag{9.27}$$

where $\boldsymbol{u}^{(t)} = \boldsymbol{\mu}^{(t)}/(2\varrho)$, and the notation a^{+} means $\max\{a, 0\}$.

Example 9.3 (Lasso Regression). We repeat the estimation of β_0 and β_1 in Example 9.2, but now using lasso regression and including both β_0 and β_1 in the regularization. The ADMM method was used to find the estimates. The results are displayed in Fig. 9.7; compare with the left panel in Fig. 9.5.

The squares in the figure are centered at $(0, 0)$ corresponding to points (β_0, β_1) with $\|\boldsymbol{\beta}\|_1 = |\beta_0| + |\beta_1| = b$ for various values of b, exhibiting the square constraint region in (9.20). The given solutions correspond to $\lambda/n \in \{0.0, 0.1, 0.5, 20, 75, 50, 100\}$. We see that the optimal solutions for large λ lie exactly in a corner point of the constraint region. In particular, the estimate for β_0 is 0 for large value of λ.

When it is undesirable to regularize the constant term, one can center the data to eliminate β_0 from the analysis, in the same way as described in Sect. 9.2.2 for ridge regression. That is, to solve the modified program

$$\min_{\beta_0, \boldsymbol{\beta}} \| \boldsymbol{y} - \beta_0 \mathbf{1} - \mathbf{X}\boldsymbol{\beta} \|^2 + \lambda \|\boldsymbol{\beta}\|_1 , \tag{9.28}$$

first center the data via $\mathbf{X} = \mathbf{C}\mathbf{X}$ and $\boldsymbol{y} = \mathbf{C}\boldsymbol{y}$ and then solve the original lasso program (9.19). In addition, if components of $\boldsymbol{\beta}$ are vastly different in magnitude, it is often recommended to further *scale* the input matrix $\mathbf{X}$ to have columns with standard deviation 1.

Example 9.3 hints at a second reason why the lasso estimator has merit: it can be used for *model selection*. Namely, the solutions of (9.18) tend to lie

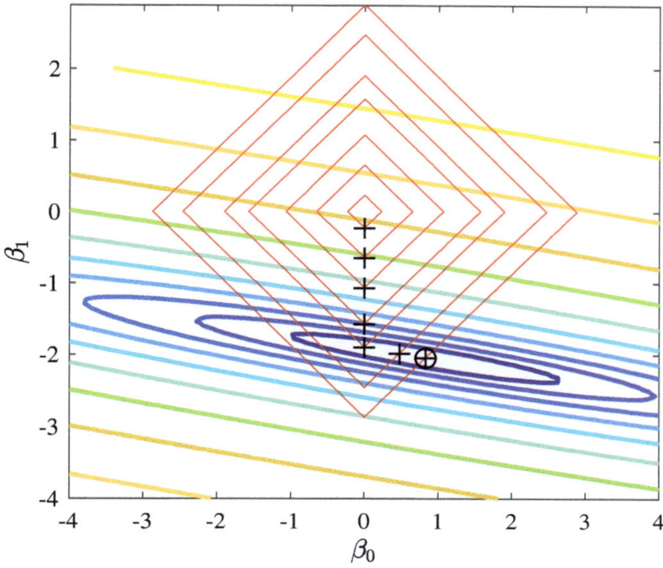

Fig. 9.7 Lasso regression solutions. Compare with Fig. 9.5

on the corners of the constraint region $\|\boldsymbol{\beta}\|_1 \leq b$. Consequently, a significant number of components may be exactly zero, especially for larger values of λ. Such *sparsity* is desirable in models that contain many parameters. A graphical methodology for model selection is to plot $\widehat{\boldsymbol{\beta}}$ against λ or, more transparently, $\widehat{\boldsymbol{\beta}}$ against $\|\widehat{\boldsymbol{\beta}}\|_1$ for λ ranging from 0 to some large enough value where $\widehat{\boldsymbol{\beta}} = \mathbf{0}$. Inspection of such **regularization paths** or **coefficient profiles** may help assess which parameters should be included in a more *parsimonious* (i.e., simpler) model to explain the variability in the observed responses.

Example 9.4 (Regularization Paths). Figure 9.8 shows the regularization paths for $p = 20$ coefficients from the same linear model and data as in Example 9.1. In particular, we have $\beta_i = i/10$ for $i = 1, \ldots, 10$ and $\beta_i = 0$ for $i = 11, \ldots, 20$. Before applying the ADMM algorithm, the data was centered, but not standardized.

As the 1-norm of the parameter vector $\boldsymbol{\beta}$ increases, more and more coefficients become non-zero. The order in which this happens is roughly the same as the magnitude of the components; so first $\beta_{10} = 1$ is selected as a non-zero component, then $\beta_9 = 0.9$, and so on. When the 1-norm reaches around 3, all the non-zero components except $\beta_1 = 0.1$ have been correctly identified as being significant, and the remaining 10 parameters are estimated as exactly 0. The regularization parameter λ varied here from 0 to 2000. For $\lambda = 0$, the 1-norm of the ordinary least-squares solution was here 6.1. The parameter ϱ was taken to be equal to 100.

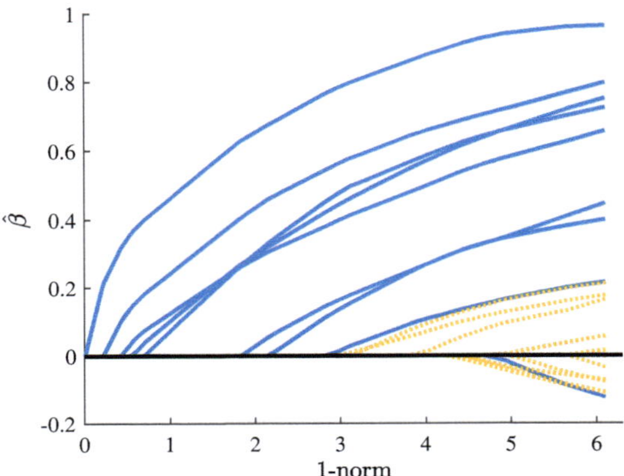

Fig. 9.8 Regularization paths for lasso regression solutions as a function of the 1-norm of the solutions. The solid blue lines correspond to the non-zero components and the dotted orange lines to the components that are 0

9.4 False-Discovery Rate

Suppose we perform a large number of statistical tests, such as the two-sample t-test in Example 5.16, providing an outcome of the test statistic for each test. For example, the data could be measurements on n different genes for a group of cancer patients and a control (reference) group. For each of the n genes, a different two-sample t-test is performed, and the objective is to determine which are the principal genes associated with having cancer. Simply rejecting/accepting each of the n on the basis of a fixed significance level α will introduce many *false -positive* results. In particular, if none of the n genes have any effect on the cancer, the expected number of false positives is $n\alpha$.

To reduce the number of false positives, we can use a mix of Bayesian and frequentist reasoning (Efron and Hastie, 2016). Let $Z_1, \ldots, Z_n$ denote the test statistics of the n statistical tests. Under H_0 each Z_i is assumed to have a known continuous distribution, such as $\mathcal{N}(0, 1)$, χ_n^2 or t_n, with cdf F_0 and pdf f_0. For simplicity, we can assume that we are dealing with right one-sided tests, so that the p-value corresponding to an outcome z of Z is given by $1 - F_0(z)$.

Consider the following Bayesian model:

$$\begin{aligned}
(M_1, \ldots, M_n) &\overset{\text{iid}}{\sim} \mathsf{Ber}(1 - \pi_0) \\
(Z_i \mid M_1, \ldots, M_n) &\sim f_{M_i}, \quad i = 1, \ldots, n \,,
\end{aligned}$$

(9.29)

where n is large, π_0 is close to 1, and f_1 is unknown. Here, $\{M_i = 0\}$ denotes the event that the i-th null hypothesis is accepted, and π_0 is the prior probability of this happening. The second line of the model specifies that if the null hypothesis holds true, each test statistic Z has pdf f_0, and under the alternative hypothesis, it has pdf f_1, which is typically unknown.

Using Bayes' formula, the probability of a "false discovery" for test statistic z is

$$\mathrm{pfd}(z) = \mathbb{P}(M_i = 0 \mid Z_i \geq z) = \frac{\pi_0(1 - F_0(z))}{1 - F(z)} \, ,$$

which may be estimated via

$$\widehat{\mathrm{pfd}}(z) = \frac{\pi_0(1 - F_0(z))}{1 - F_n(z)} \, ,$$

where F_n is the empirical cdf of the $z_1, \ldots, z_n$, as in (7.1). Ordering the p-values as $p_{(1)} \leq p_{(2)} \leq \cdots \leq p_{(n)}$ and z-values as $z^{(1)} \geq z^{(2)} \geq \cdots \geq z^{(n)}$, we have:

$$\widehat{\mathrm{pfd}}(z^{(i)}) = \frac{\pi_0 p_{(i)}}{i/n} \, .$$

Remembering that π_0 is close to 1, the above suggests the following rule: reject the null hypothesis if the estimated false discovery rate is less than or equal to a threshold q. In other words, reject the null hypothesis for the i-th smallest p-value if

$$p_{(i)} \leq \frac{i}{n} q \, .$$

Algorithm 9.1. (Benjamini–Hochberg (BH) Method).

1. Order the p-values from smallest to largest: $p_{(1)} \leq p_{(2)} \leq \cdots \leq p_{(n)}$.
2. Reject the null hypothesis corresponding to the i-th smallest p-value if $p_{(i)} \leq iq/n$.

An alternative, but equivalent, procedure is to first "adjust" the p-values, and then accept or reject the null hypotheses based on q as significance level, just as in ordinary hypothesis testing. The adjusted p-values $p^*_{(i)}, i = 1, \ldots, n$ of the original sorted p-values $p_{(i)}, i = 1, \ldots, n$ are found as follows:

1. Initialize $c = 1$ and $i = n$.
2. Set $p^*_{(i)} = \min\{c, p_{(i)} n/i\}$
3. Set $c = p^*_{(i)}$ and $i = i - 1$.
4. If $i = 0$ stop; otherwise, return to Step 2.

Example 9.5 (FDR). We simulated $n = 5000$ test statistics and p-values from the Bayesian model (9.29), with $\pi_0 = 0.95$, where f_0 is the pdf of the $\mathcal{N}(0, 1)$ distribution and f_1 is the pdf of the $\mathcal{N}(4, 4)$ distribution. Figure 9.9

shows a kernel density estimate (blue line) of the test statistics. The null density f_0 is shown as the dotted red line. The figure indicates that there are a large number of null cases, but also implies the existence of non-null cases that are deserving to be identified.

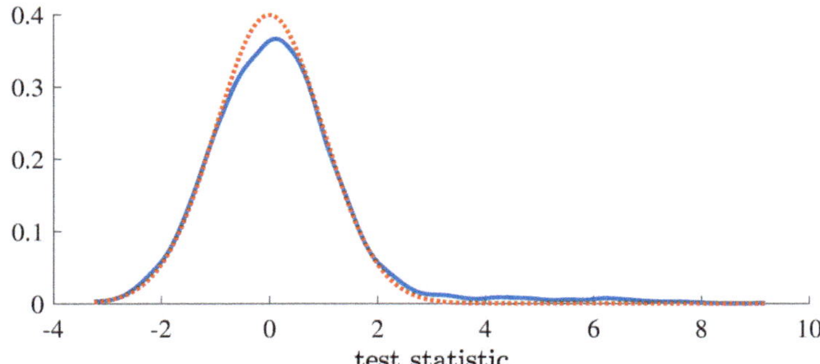

Fig. 9.9 Kernel density estimate of 5000 test statistics and the pdf of the $\mathcal{N}(0,1)$ distribution under the null hypothesis

The top panel of Fig. 9.10 illustrates the BH method with $q = 0.05$. The number of identified non-null cases is here 143. Thus, $p_{(143)} \leq 143q/n = 0.00143$, but $p_{(144)} > 0.00143$. The bottom panel shows the adjusted sorted p-values. We see exactly the same cutoff 143.

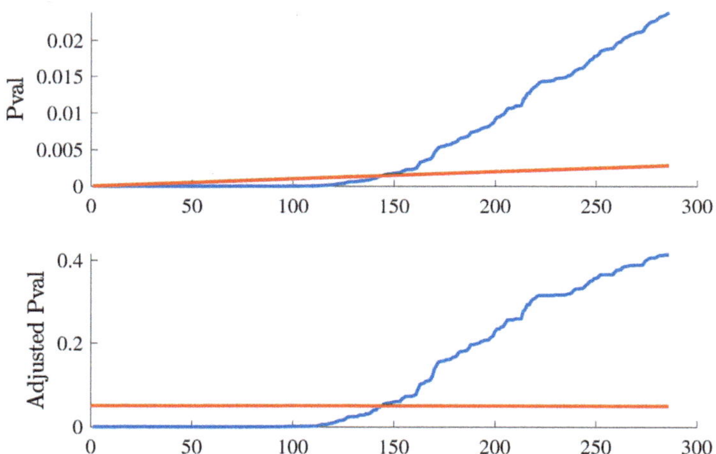

Fig. 9.10 Illustration of the BH method. Top: sorted p-values (blue). Bottom: sorted adjusted p-values

The p-values corresponded to a two-sided test; so for a test statistic z, the p-value is $2(1 - \Phi(z))$, where Φ is the cdf of the $\mathcal{N}(0,1)$ distribution. For the particular outcome in Fig. 9.10, the actual number of non-null cases was 213.

The BH method can also be analyzed in a purely probabilistic way. Denoting the p-values of the null cases by $P_1, \ldots, P_{n_0}$ and of the non-null cases by $P_{n_0+1}, \ldots, P_n$, the model assumption is that the null p-values are independent and $\mathcal{U}(0,1)$ distributed, which is an appropriate assumption; see Problem 9.10. The key stochastic processes to investigate are

$$V_t = \sum_{i=1}^{n_0} \mathbb{1}\{P_i \le t\} \quad \text{and} \quad R_t = \sum_{i=1}^{n} \mathbb{1}\{P_i \le t\}, \quad t \in [0,1] .$$

Thus, V_t is the number of null p-values less than or equal to threshold t, and R_t is the number of all p-values less than or equal to t. Under the above assumptions, the random process $(V_t/t, t \in [0,1])$ is a *martingale* with "time" t running backward and with *filtration* $\mathcal{F}_t = \sigma(V_u, R_u, u \ge t), t \in [0,1]$. The precise meaning (see Problem 9.11) is that

$$\mathbb{E}\left[\frac{V_s}{s} \,\middle|\, V_u, R_u, u \ge t\right] = \frac{V_t}{t}, \quad s \le t . \tag{9.30}$$

Since (V_t/t) is a martingale, it has the same expectation for all t; in particular it holds that $\mathbb{E}V_t/t = \mathbb{E}V_1 = n_0$. By *Doob's stopping theorem* (see, e.g., Kroese and Botev 2023, Chapter 5), the same holds if t is replaced with any (bounded) random *stopping time* T relative to the filtration $(\mathcal{F}_t)$, meaning that every event $\{T \ge t\}$ can be discerned from the information on $V_u, R_u, u \ge t$. The random time

$$T = \sup\{t \in [0,1] : R_t \ge \frac{tn}{q}\}$$

is such a bounded stopping time, with $R_T = Tn/q$. Using these definitions, we can express the proportion of false discoveries found by the BH method as

$$\frac{V_T}{R_T} = \frac{q}{n} \frac{V_T}{T} .$$

The expectation of this random variable is called the **false-discovery rate**. Consequently, by Doob's stopping theorem, we have:

$$\mathbb{E}\frac{V_T}{R_T} = \frac{q}{n}\mathbb{E}\frac{V_T}{T} = \frac{q}{n}\mathbb{E}V_1 = \frac{n_0}{n}q \le q.$$

That is, the false-discovery rate is bounded by q .

9.5 Problems

9.1. Show that $\widehat{\sigma^2}$ in (9.3) is an unbiased estimator for σ^2.

9.2. Show that $\mathbf{X}\mathbf{X}^\top + \lambda \mathbb{I}_m$ is invertible for any $\lambda > 0$.

9.3. In the Bayesian setting of ridge regression in Sect. 9.2, the posterior expectation of $\boldsymbol{\beta}$ is identical to $\widehat{\boldsymbol{\beta}}$ in (9.7). Prove this, using Theorem 8.1.

9.4. We can extend the definition of convexity in (2.9) to the n-dimensional case as follows. Let $\mathcal{X} \subseteq \mathbb{R}^n$. A function $h : \mathcal{X} \to \mathbb{R}$ is said to be **convex** on $\mathcal{X}$ if for each $\boldsymbol{x}$ in the interior of $\mathcal{X}$, there exists a vector $\boldsymbol{v}$ (depending on $\boldsymbol{x}$) such that

$$h(\boldsymbol{y}) \geq h(\boldsymbol{x}) + (\boldsymbol{y} - \boldsymbol{x})^\top \boldsymbol{v}, \quad \boldsymbol{y} \in \mathcal{X} . \tag{9.31}$$

The vector $\boldsymbol{v}$ is typically the gradient of h at $\boldsymbol{x}$, but can be more general, and is thus called a **subgradient**:

a. Show that the function h defined by $h(\boldsymbol{x}) = \|\mathbf{A}\boldsymbol{x} + \boldsymbol{b}\|^2$, where $\mathbf{A}$ is a matrix and $\boldsymbol{b}$ a vector, is convex.
b. Show that the sum of two convex functions is again convex.

9.5.

a. Show that the function

$$g(z) = (\beta - z)^2 + \mu(\beta - z) + \lambda |z|, \quad z \in \mathbb{R} \tag{9.32}$$

is convex for any choice of β, μ, and λ.
b. Show that

$$\underset{z}{\text{argmin}} \; g(z) = (\beta + \mu/2 - \lambda/2)^+ - (-\beta - \mu/2 - \lambda/2)^+ , \tag{9.33}$$

where $x^+ = \max\{x, 0\}$.
c. The **lasso shrinkage function** for parameter $\lambda \geq 0$ is given by

$$S_\gamma(x) = x \left(1 - \frac{\gamma}{|x|} \right)^+ , \quad x \in \mathbb{R} . \tag{9.34}$$

Draw a plot of S_1 and show that (9.33) implies that

$$\underset{z}{\text{argmin}} \left\{ (z - x)^2 + \lambda |z| \right\} = S_{\lambda/2}(x) . \tag{9.35}$$

9.6. Using Problem 9.5 verify that the ADMM updates in (9.25)–(9.27) follow from (9.22)–(9.24).

9.7.

a. Write a Julia function that implements the ADMM algorithm, taking as input $\mathbf{X}, \boldsymbol{y}$ and λ, and returning the solution, $\boldsymbol{b}$ say, of (9.19).

b. Apply the ADMM function to the data

$$\boldsymbol{y} = \mathbf{X}\boldsymbol{\beta} + \boldsymbol{e}\,,$$

with

$$\mathbf{X} = \begin{bmatrix} 8.46 & 4.73 & 6.26 \\ 5.29 & 0.98 & 5.54 \\ 6.99 & 2.96 & 0.38 \\ 9.87 & 4.67 & 8.89 \\ 9.58 & 9.22 & 5.98 \end{bmatrix}\,,$$

$\boldsymbol{\beta} = [0.1, 0.2, 0.3]^\top$ and $\boldsymbol{e} = [-0.83, 0.93, -0.24, -0.40, -0.02]^\top$. Before applying the ADMM algorithm, center the matrix $\mathbf{X}$ and the vector $\boldsymbol{y}$. Verify that for $\lambda = 10$, the solution to (9.19) is given by $\boldsymbol{b} = [0, 0.05088, 0.22403]^\top$, with 1-norm 0.27492.

c. For λ ranging from 0 to 30, produce the regularization paths in Fig. 9.11.

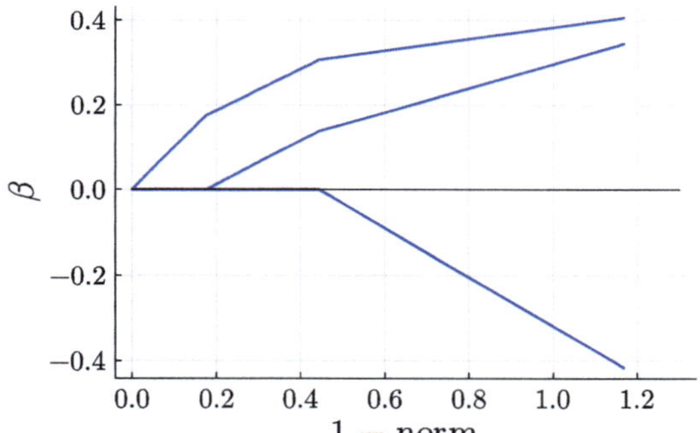

Fig. 9.11 Regularization paths for the lasso estimates as a function of their 1-norm

9.8. Let

$$L(\boldsymbol{\beta}) \stackrel{\text{def}}{=} \|\boldsymbol{y} - \mathbf{X}\boldsymbol{\beta}\|^2 + \lambda\,\|\boldsymbol{\beta}\|_1\,.$$

An alternative approach to solve the lasso minimization problem (9.19) is the **coordinate descent** method, which iteratively solves the one-dimensional optimization problems $\min_{\beta_j} L(\boldsymbol{\beta})$ for $j = 1, \ldots, m$. These optimization problems can be solved exactly, as will be shown next:

a. Let $\boldsymbol{v}_j$ be the j-th column of $\mathbf{X}$ and let $\boldsymbol{u}_{\neg j} = \boldsymbol{y} - \mathbf{X}\boldsymbol{\beta} + \beta_j \boldsymbol{v}_j$ be the vector of residuals with the j-th residual set to 0. For a fixed $\boldsymbol{\beta}$, we wish to minimize $L(\boldsymbol{\beta} + (x - \beta_j)\boldsymbol{e}_j)$ with respect to x, where $\boldsymbol{e}_j$ is the j-th unit vector. With $z_j = \|\boldsymbol{v}_j\|^2$, show that

$$L(\boldsymbol{\beta} + (x - \beta_j)\boldsymbol{e}_j) = z_j\left[(x - \boldsymbol{u}_{\neg j}^\top \boldsymbol{v}/z_j)^2 + \lambda|x|/z_j\right] + \text{const}\,. \qquad (9.36)$$

b. Show that (9.36) is minimized for

$$\beta_j^* = S_{\lambda/(2z_j)}(\boldsymbol{u}_{-j}^\top \boldsymbol{v}_j/z_j) = S_{\lambda/(2z_j)}(\beta_j + \boldsymbol{u}^\top \boldsymbol{v}_j/z_j)\,, \qquad (9.37)$$

where $\boldsymbol{u} = \boldsymbol{y} = \mathbf{X}\boldsymbol{\beta}$ is the full vector of residuals and S_γ is the lasso shrinkage function in (9.34).

c. The coordinate descent method proceeds by iteratively updating β_j with (9.37) as in:

Algorithm 9.2. (Coordinate Descent)

1 Initialize $\boldsymbol{\beta}$ and $\boldsymbol{u} = \boldsymbol{y} - \mathbf{X}\boldsymbol{\beta}$
2 Set $z_j = \|\boldsymbol{v}_j\|^2$, $j = 1,\ldots,m$
3 **repeat**
4 $\quad$ $\boldsymbol{\beta}_{\mathrm{old}} = \boldsymbol{\beta}$
5 $\quad$ **for** $j = 1,\ldots,m$ **do**
6 $\quad\quad$ $b = S_{\lambda/(2z_j)}(\beta_j + \boldsymbol{u}^\top \boldsymbol{v}_j/z_j)$
7 $\quad\quad$ $\boldsymbol{u} = \boldsymbol{u} + (\beta_j - b)\boldsymbol{v}_j$
8 $\quad\quad$ $\beta_j = b$
9 **until** $\|\boldsymbol{\beta} - \boldsymbol{\beta}_{\mathrm{old}}\| < \varepsilon$
10 **return** $\boldsymbol{\beta}$

Implement this algorithm as a Julia function and apply it to the same data as in Problem 9.7.

9.9. Using the generic CE algorithm **CEmin** in Sect. A.7, verify the solution to (9.19) for the data in Problem 9.7b.

9.10. Let T be the test statistic for a right one-sided statistical test. Recall from Sect. 5.3 that the null hypothesis is then rejected for large values of the test statistic. Suppose that T is a continuous random variable with cdf F under the null hypothesis. The p-value for an outcome t or T is in this case given by $\mathbb{P}_{H_0}(T \geq t) = 1 - F(t)$. Explain why under the null hypothesis the random p-value (i.e., the random variable $1 - F(X)$, where $X \sim F$) has a $\mathcal{U}(0,1)$ distribution:

9.11. Show that (9.30) holds.

9.12. Reproduce Fig. 9.10 using Julia.

9.13. Suppose $\mathbf{X}$ is an $n \times m$ matrix and $\boldsymbol{y}$ is an n-vector. Show that for $\lambda > 0$,

$$\mathbf{X}^\top(\mathbf{X}\mathbf{X}^\top + \lambda\mathbb{I}_n)^{-1} = (\mathbf{X}^\top\mathbf{X} + \lambda\mathbb{I}_m)^{-1}\mathbf{X}^\top\,.$$

Hence, the ridge regression estimator in (9.9) can be represented as $\widehat{\boldsymbol{\beta}} = \mathbf{X}^\top\widehat{\boldsymbol{\alpha}}$, where $\widehat{\boldsymbol{\alpha}} = (\mathbf{X}\mathbf{X}^\top + \lambda\mathbb{I}_n)^{-1}\boldsymbol{y}$.

Chapter 10
Generalized Linear Models

☞ 101

☞ 115

The linear models introduced in Chap. 4 deal with *continuous* response variables—such as height and crop yield—and continuous or discrete explanatory variables. For example, under a normal linear model , the responses $\{Y_i\}$ are independent of each other, and each has a normal distribution with mean $\mu_i = \boldsymbol{x}_i^\top \boldsymbol{\beta}$, where $\boldsymbol{x}_i^\top$ is the i-th row of the design matrix $\mathbf{X}$. However, these continuous models are obviously not suitable for data that take on *discrete* values. For example, we might want to analyze women's labor market participation decision (whether to work or not), voters' opinion of the government (rating on the government performance on a scale of five), or the choice among a few cereal brands, as a function of one or more explanatory variables. In this chapter we discuss models that are suitable for analyzing these discrete response variables. We will first introduce the flexible framework of *generalized linear models*.

10.1 Generalized Linear Models

Definition 10.1. (Generalized Linear Model). A vector of (response) data $\boldsymbol{Y} = [Y_1, \ldots, Y_n]^\top$ is said to satisfy a **generalized linear model** if the expectation vector $\boldsymbol{\mu} = \mathbb{E}\boldsymbol{Y}$ can be written in the form:

$$\boldsymbol{\mu} = \boldsymbol{g}^{-1}(\mathbf{X}\boldsymbol{\beta}) \, ,$$

where $\mathbf{X}$ is an $n \times m$ **design matrix** (i.e., a matrix of explanatory variables), $\boldsymbol{\beta}$ is an m-dimensional vector of **parameters**, and $\boldsymbol{g}^{-1}$ is

J. C. C. Chan, D. P. Kroese, *Statistical Modeling and Computation*,
Springer Texts in Statistics, https://doi.org/10.1007/978-1-0716-4132-3_10

the inverse of a **link function** g. The distribution of $\boldsymbol{Y}$ may depend on additional **dispersion** parameters that model the randomness in the data that is not explained by the explanatory variables.

A common assumption for $\boldsymbol{Y}$ is that its components $Y_1, \ldots, Y_n$ are independent and come from some exponential family. The central focus is the parameter vector $\boldsymbol{\beta}$, which summarizes how the matrix of explanatory variables $\mathbf{X}$ affects the response vector $\boldsymbol{Y}$. By choosing different members of the exponential family and different link functions, the class of generalized linear models can encompass a wide variety of popular models as special cases, some of which are discussed below.

Example 10.1 (Normal Linear Model). The normal linear model $\boldsymbol{Y} = \mathbf{X}\boldsymbol{\beta} + \boldsymbol{\varepsilon}$ in Sect. 4.5 is a special case of a generalized linear model. Here, $\boldsymbol{\mu} = \mathbf{X}\boldsymbol{\beta}$, so that the link function is simply the identity function: $g(\boldsymbol{z}) = \boldsymbol{z}$. The vector $\boldsymbol{Y}$ has a multivariate normal distribution:

$$\boldsymbol{Y} \sim \mathcal{N}(\boldsymbol{\mu}, \sigma^2 \, \mathbb{I}_n) \, ,$$

where σ^2 is a dispersion parameter that models the residual randomness in the data.

Example 10.2 (Binary Variable Regression Model). Suppose we are interested in the effectiveness of a certain insecticide. For this purpose an experiment is carried out as follows: the i-th insect is exposed to the insecticide with dose level x_i, and we observe Y_i, whether the insect is killed or not. Thus, $Y_i \sim \mathsf{Ber}(\mu_i)$, where $\mu_i = \mathbb{E}Y_i$ is the "success" probability, which has to lie in the interval $(0, 1)$. Let $\boldsymbol{Y}$ and $\boldsymbol{x}$ be the response and explanatory vectors. One way to link the expectation vector $\boldsymbol{\mu} = [\mu_1, \ldots, \mu_n]^\top$ to $\boldsymbol{x}$ is to specify μ_i as

$$\mu_i = F(\beta_0 + \beta_1 x_i)$$

for some cdf F and "regression" parameters β_0 and β_1. Defining the $n \times 2$ design matrix $\mathbf{X} = [\mathbf{1} \, \boldsymbol{x}]$ and $\boldsymbol{\beta} = [\beta_0, \beta_1]^\top$, the distribution of $\boldsymbol{Y} = [Y_1, \ldots, Y_n]^\top$ is completely specified by $\boldsymbol{\mu}$, which in turn is determined by $\mathbf{X}\boldsymbol{\beta}$. For different choices of F, we have different binary variable models. Common choices for F are (1) the cdf of the standard normal distribution and (2) the cdf of the logistic distribution. These are discussed in detail in the next section. The choice

$$F_{\mathrm{ex}}(x) = 1 - \mathrm{e}^{-\mathrm{e}^x}$$

gives the cdf of the **extreme value distribution**. The corresponding link function for each component is $F^{-1}(z) = \ln(-\ln(1 - z))$. Finally, by taking F as the cdf of the Student's t distribution with parameter ν, we obtain the so-called **t-link model**. One attractive feature of the t-link model is its flexibility; in particular, it includes the popular probit model (see next section) as a limiting case.

10.2 Logit and Probit Models

In this section we discuss two popular specifications for binary data: the **probit** model and the **logit** or **logistic** model. Both models are binary variable regression models of the form discussed in Example 10.2. More precisely, the responses $Y_1, \ldots, Y_n$ are assumed to be independent Bernoulli random variables with success probabilities:

$$\mu_i = F(\boldsymbol{x}_i^\top \boldsymbol{\beta}), \quad i = 1, \ldots, n ,$$

where $\boldsymbol{x}_i$ is the vector of explanatory variables corresponding to the i-th response, $\boldsymbol{\beta}$ is the parameter vector of interest, and F is a cdf.

10.2.1 Logit Model

Definition 10.2. (Logit Model). Let Y_i denote the i-th binary response, and let $\boldsymbol{x}_i$ represent the vector of explanatory variables and $\boldsymbol{\beta}$ the associated parameter vector. In a **logistic regression** or **logit model**, the $\{Y_i\}$ are independent and $Y_i \sim \mathsf{Ber}(\mu_i)$, with $\mu_i = F(\boldsymbol{x}_i^\top \boldsymbol{\beta})$, where F is the cdf of **logistic distribution**:

$$F(x) = \frac{1}{1 + \mathrm{e}^{-x}} .$$

In other words, the component link function is $g(x) = \ln(x/(1 - x))$.

Example 10.3 (Logit Model). Figure 10.1 shows the outcomes of 500 independent binary response variables for a logistic regression model. The explanatory variables $\boldsymbol{x}_i = [x_{i1}, x_{i2}]^\top$, $i = 1, \ldots, 500$ were chosen uniformly on the unit square, and $\boldsymbol{\beta} = [-8, 8]^\top$. The S-shaped surface depicts the graph of the function:

$$p(x_1, x_2) = F(\boldsymbol{x}^\top \boldsymbol{\beta}) = (1 + \exp(8(x_2 - x_1)))^{-1} .$$

For each given vector of explanatory variables $[x_{i1}, x_{i2}]^\top$, the response Y_i is generated from a Bernoulli distribution with success probability $p(x_{i1}, x_{i2})$.

Using the same notation as in Definition 10.2, we now derive the log-likelihood function, score function, and the information matrix for this model. Since the responses are independent Bernoulli random variables, the log-likelihood function is given by

$$l(\boldsymbol{\beta}; \boldsymbol{y}) = \sum_{i=1}^{n} \left[y_i \ln \mu_i + (1 - y_i) \ln(1 - \mu_i) \right] ,$$

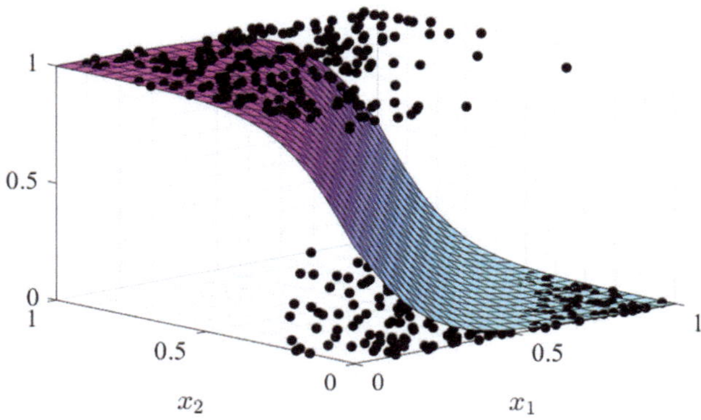

Fig. 10.1 Responses (0 or 1) for a logistic regression model, with two explanatory variables for each response

where $\mu_i = (1 + e^{-\boldsymbol{x}_i^\top \boldsymbol{\beta}})^{-1}$ and $1 - \mu_i = e^{-\boldsymbol{x}_i^\top \boldsymbol{\beta}}/(1 + e^{-\boldsymbol{x}_i^\top \boldsymbol{\beta}})$. It follows that $\ln \mu_i = -\ln(1 + e^{-\boldsymbol{x}_i^\top \boldsymbol{\beta}})$ and $\ln(1 - \mu_i) = -\boldsymbol{x}_i^\top \boldsymbol{\beta} - \ln(1 + e^{-\boldsymbol{x}_i^\top \boldsymbol{\beta}})$. After some algebra, the log-likelihood function can be rewritten as

$$l(\boldsymbol{\beta}; \boldsymbol{y}) = \sum_{i=1}^{n} \left[(y_i - 1)\boldsymbol{x}_i^\top \boldsymbol{\beta} - \ln(1 + e^{-\boldsymbol{x}_i^\top \boldsymbol{\beta}}) \right] . \tag{10.1}$$

☞ 476   Taking the gradient of the log-likelihood function, we obtain the score function

$$\boldsymbol{S}(\boldsymbol{\beta}; \boldsymbol{y}) = \nabla_{\boldsymbol{\beta}}\, l(\boldsymbol{\beta}; \boldsymbol{y}) = \sum_{i=1}^{n} \left[(y_i - 1)\boldsymbol{x}_i + \frac{\boldsymbol{x}_i\, e^{-\boldsymbol{x}_i^\top \boldsymbol{\beta}}}{1 + e^{-\boldsymbol{x}_i^\top \boldsymbol{\beta}}} \right]$$

$$= \sum_{i=1}^{n} \left[y_i - (1 + e^{-\boldsymbol{x}_i^\top \boldsymbol{\beta}})^{-1} \right] \boldsymbol{x}_i$$

$$= \sum_{i=1}^{n} (y_i - \mu_i)\, \boldsymbol{x}_i .$$

Differentiating the score function with respect to $\boldsymbol{\beta}$ and multiplying by -1, we obtain the **observed information matrix**:

$$
\begin{aligned}
\mathbf{I}(\boldsymbol{\beta};\boldsymbol{y}) = -\nabla_{\boldsymbol{\beta}}^2\, l(\boldsymbol{\beta};\boldsymbol{y}) &= \sum_{i=1}^{n} \frac{e^{-\boldsymbol{x}_i^{\top}\boldsymbol{\beta}}}{(1+e^{-\boldsymbol{x}_i^{\top}\boldsymbol{\beta}})^2}\, \boldsymbol{x}_i\,\boldsymbol{x}_i^{\top} \\
&= \sum_{i=1}^{n} \mu_i(1-\mu_i)\,\boldsymbol{x}_i\,\boldsymbol{x}_i^{\top}\ .
\end{aligned}
\tag{10.2}
$$

It is worth noting that the observed information matrix does not depend on the data $\boldsymbol{y}$, and therefore it coincides with the Fisher information matrix $\mathbf{I}(\boldsymbol{\beta})$. Now, the maximum likelihood estimate can be computed numerically using, say, Fisher's scoring method. Specifically, given an initial value $\boldsymbol{\beta}_0$, for $t = 1, 2, \ldots$, iteratively compute

$$
\boldsymbol{\beta}_t = \boldsymbol{\beta}_{t-1} + [\mathbf{I}(\boldsymbol{\beta}_{t-1})]^{-1} \boldsymbol{S}(\boldsymbol{\beta}_{t-1};\boldsymbol{y})\ ,
$$

until the sequence $\boldsymbol{\beta}_0, \boldsymbol{\beta}_1, \boldsymbol{\beta}_2, \ldots$ is found to have converged, using some pre-fixed convergence criterion. Once the maximum likelihood estimate $\widehat{\boldsymbol{\beta}}$ is obtained, one can readily compute the corresponding asymptotic covariance matrix as $\mathbf{I}^{-1}(\widehat{\boldsymbol{\beta}})$; see also Theorem 6.8.

Example 10.4 (MLE for the Logit Model). In the development of drugs, bioassay experiments are often carried out on animals to test the potential toxicity of the drugs. Various dose levels are given to batches of animals, and the animals' responses—typically characterized by a binary outcome, say alive or dead—are recorded. The aim is to describe the probability of "success," μ, as a function of the dose, x, via a link function $g(\mu) = \beta_0 + x\beta_1$. In this example we analyze the data with a logit model with

$$
\mu = g^{-1}(\beta_0 + x\beta_1) = (1 + e^{-(\beta_0+\beta_1 x)})^{-1}.
$$

The outcomes of such an experiment are given in Table 10.1: a total of 20 animals were tested, 5 at each of the 4 dose levels.

Table 10.1 Animal mortality data

Dose (log g/ml)	Number of animals	Number of deaths
-0.863	5	0
-0.296	5	1
-0.053	5	3
0.727	5	5

One obvious quantity of interest is the estimate for β_1. In particular, we are interested to know whether or not it is positive (i.e., if the drug is toxic). In addition, we might also want to learn about the effect of a specific dose level. Since we only have two parameters, we first obtain a contour plot for the likelihood function to get a rough estimate for $\boldsymbol{\beta} = [\beta_0, \beta_1]^\top$. From Fig. 10.2 it can be seen that the maximum likelihood estimate for $\boldsymbol{\beta}$ is around $[1, 8]^\top$.

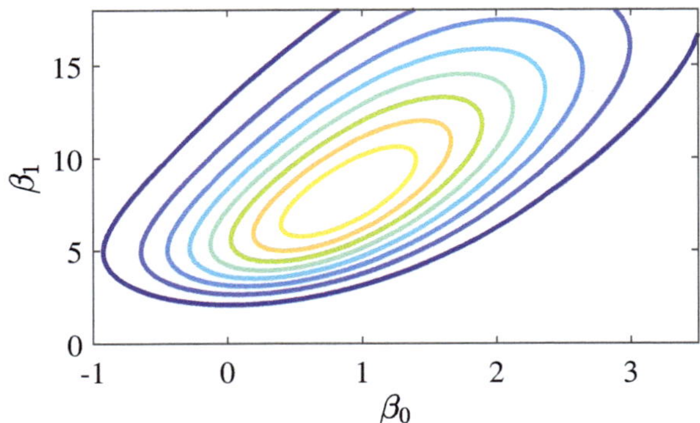

Fig. 10.2 Contour plot for the likelihood function of the parameters in the bioassay example

We use the following Julia code to implement Fisher's scoring method to obtain the maximum likelihood estimate $\widehat{\boldsymbol{\beta}}$ and the information matrix evaluated at $\widehat{\boldsymbol{\beta}}$.

bioassay.jl

```julia
using LinearAlgebra
y = [0 0 0 0 0 1 0 0 0 0 1 1 1 0 0 1 1 1 1 1]';
x = repeat([-0.863 -0.296 -0.053 0.727], inner = (1,5));
X = [ones(20, 1) x'];        # design matrix
betat = (X' * X) \ (X' * y); # initial guess
S = ones(2, 1);              # score
IM = zeros(2,2)              # info matrix
e = 10^(-5); # tolerance level
while sum(abs.(S)) > e       # stopping criterion
    global betat, S, IM
    mu = 1 ./ (1 .+ exp.(-X * betat))
    S = sum(repeat((y - mu), outer=(1,2)) .* X, dims=1)'
    IM = X' * diagm(vec(mu .* (1 .- mu))) * X
    betat = betat + IM \ S
end
V = IM \ I
println(betat)
println(V)
```

Note that we have vectorized the computation of the score and information matrix in the code to avoid for-loops. For example, the information matrix $\mathbf{I}$ in (10.2) can be written as $\mathbf{I} = \mathbf{X}^{\top}\mathbf{B}\mathbf{X}$, with

$$
\mathbf{X} = \begin{bmatrix} 1 & x_1 \\ \vdots & \vdots \\ 1 & x_{20} \end{bmatrix} \quad \text{and} \quad \mathbf{B} = \begin{bmatrix} \mu_1(1-\mu_1) & \cdots & 0 \\ & \ddots & \\ 0 & \cdots & \mu_{20}(1-\mu_{20}) \end{bmatrix}.
$$

The maximum likelihood estimate for $\boldsymbol{\beta}$ and the associated covariance matrix $\mathbf{V} = \mathbf{I}^{-1}(\boldsymbol{\beta})$ are

$$
\widehat{\boldsymbol{\beta}} = \begin{bmatrix} 0.873 \\ 7.912 \end{bmatrix} \quad \text{and} \quad \mathbf{V} = \begin{bmatrix} 1.081 & 3.833 \\ 3.833 & 25.624 \end{bmatrix}. \tag{10.3}
$$

In particular, a 95% (approximate) confidence interval for β_1 is given as $7.912 \pm 1.96\sqrt{25.624}$ or $(-2, 17.83)$. It is interesting to note that we cannot reject the null hypothesis $\beta_1 = 0$ at significance level 0.05, even though the contour plot suggests that most of the mass of the likelihood lies in the region $2 - 20$. One reason might be because the normal distribution is not a good approximation due to the small sample size.

Further, suppose that we are interested in the "success" rate at dose level -0.1 log g/ml. An estimate can be computed as $\widehat{\mu} = [1, -0.1]\widehat{\boldsymbol{\beta}} = 0.082$, or 8.2%.

For *Bayesian* estimation of the logit model, we need to have an efficient way to obtain draws from the posterior distribution $f(\boldsymbol{\beta} \mid \boldsymbol{y})$ for a given prior $f(\boldsymbol{\beta})$. Since the likelihood function for the logit model is highly nonlinear, the posterior distribution is typically nonstandard, and estimation requires more work. One feasible approach to obtaining posterior draws is to use Markov chain Monte Carlo. In particular, we will use an independence sampler (see Example 7.11) with a multivariate Student's t proposal distribution. The reason for sampling from a Student's t proposal is that the samples tend to be less concentrated around the mode of the distribution than is the case for the normal distribution, for example. As a result the samples from the independence sampler tend to be less correlated.

☞ 22

Definition 10.3. (Multivariate Student's t Distribution). An n-dimensional random vector $\boldsymbol{X}$ is said to have a **multivariate Student's t** distribution with **mean vector** $\boldsymbol{\mu}$ and **scale matrix** $\boldsymbol{\Sigma}$ if its pdf is given by

$$f(\boldsymbol{x}; \nu, \boldsymbol{\mu}, \boldsymbol{\Sigma}) = \frac{c}{\sqrt{\det(\boldsymbol{\Sigma})}} \left(1 + \frac{1}{\nu}(\boldsymbol{x} - \boldsymbol{\mu})^\top \boldsymbol{\Sigma}^{-1}(\boldsymbol{x} - \boldsymbol{\mu})\right)^{-\frac{\nu + n}{2}}, \quad (10.4)$$

where $c = \frac{\Gamma\left(\frac{\nu + n}{2}\right)}{(\pi\nu)^{n/2}\,\Gamma\left(\frac{\nu}{2}\right)}$ and $\nu > 0$ is the **degrees of freedom** parameter. We write the distribution as $\boldsymbol{t}_\nu(\boldsymbol{\mu}, \boldsymbol{\Sigma})$.

☞ 83   Similar to the multivariate $\mathcal{N}(\boldsymbol{\mu}, \boldsymbol{\Sigma})$ distribution, a vector $\boldsymbol{X} \sim \boldsymbol{t}_\nu(\boldsymbol{\mu}, \boldsymbol{\Sigma})$ can be viewed as an affine transformation $\boldsymbol{X} = \boldsymbol{\mu} + \mathbf{B}\,\boldsymbol{Z}$ of a random vector $\boldsymbol{Z} \sim \boldsymbol{t}_\nu(\mathbf{0}, \mathbb{I}_n)$ from the *standard* multivariate Student's t distribution, where $\mathbf{BB}^\top = \boldsymbol{\Sigma}$. To simulate draws from the latter distribution, one can use the following theorem. The proof is left as an exercise; see Problem 10.1.

Theorem 10.1. (Generating from the Multivariate Student's t Distribution). Let $\boldsymbol{R} \sim \mathcal{N}(\mathbf{0}, \mathbb{I}_n)$ and $W \sim \chi_\nu^2$ be independent. Then,

$$\boldsymbol{Z} = \sqrt{\frac{\nu}{W}}\,\boldsymbol{R} \sim \mathsf{t}_\nu(\mathbf{0}, \mathbb{I}_n)\ .$$

To sample from the posterior pdf $f(\boldsymbol{\beta}\,|\,\boldsymbol{y})$ of the logit model, we draw the proposal from a $\mathsf{t}_\nu(\widehat{\boldsymbol{\beta}}, \mathbf{V})$ distribution, where $\widehat{\boldsymbol{\beta}}$ is the maximum likelihood estimate and $\mathbf{V}$ the inverse information matrix evaluated at $\widehat{\boldsymbol{\beta}}$.

Denote the pdf of the $\mathsf{t}_\nu(\widehat{\boldsymbol{\beta}}, \mathbf{V})$ distribution by $f_{\mathsf{t}}(\boldsymbol{\beta})$. In the independence sampler, given a current draw $\boldsymbol{\beta}$, the candidate $\boldsymbol{\beta}^*$ is accepted with probability:

$$\alpha(\boldsymbol{\beta}, \boldsymbol{\beta}^*) = \min\left\{\frac{f(\boldsymbol{y}\,|\,\boldsymbol{\beta}^*)f(\boldsymbol{\beta}^*)f_{\mathsf{t}}(\boldsymbol{\beta})}{f(\boldsymbol{y}\,|\,\boldsymbol{\beta})f(\boldsymbol{\beta})f_{\mathsf{t}}(\boldsymbol{\beta}^*)}, 1\right\},$$

where $f(\boldsymbol{y}\,|\,\boldsymbol{\beta})$ is the likelihood function and $f(\boldsymbol{\beta})$ is the prior density.

Example 10.5 (Bayesian Inference for Logit Model). We continue Example 10.4. Taking a uniform prior for $\boldsymbol{\beta}$ (i.e., $f(\boldsymbol{\beta}) \propto 1$), the posterior pdf is proportional to the likelihood function. In other words, Fig. 10.2 is also a contour plot for the posterior distribution. For this example, the posterior pdf is proper even though the prior pdf is not. To compute other useful summary statistics, we use the independence sampler with $\mathsf{t}_\nu(\widehat{\boldsymbol{\beta}}, \mathbf{V})$ proposal, as described above. Note that both the proposal pdf f_{t} and the likelihood only have to be specified up to a multiplicative normalization constant. In fact, it is easier to specify the natural logarithms of both pdfs (up to an additive constant) and evaluate

$$\varrho(\boldsymbol{\beta}, \boldsymbol{\beta}^*) = \ln f(\boldsymbol{y} \mid \boldsymbol{\beta}^*) + \ln f_{\mathsf{t}}(\boldsymbol{\beta}) - \ln f(\boldsymbol{y} \mid \boldsymbol{\beta}) - \ln f_{\mathsf{t}}(\boldsymbol{\beta}^*) \,,$$

and accept $\boldsymbol{\beta}^*$ with probability $\min\{\exp(\varrho(\boldsymbol{\beta}, \boldsymbol{\beta}^*)), 1\}$. To obtain a draw from the proposal distribution, we first sample $\boldsymbol{Z} = [Z_1, Z_2]^\top \sim \mathcal{N}(\boldsymbol{0}, \mathbb{I}_n)$ and $W \sim \chi^2_\nu = \mathsf{Gamma}(\nu/2, 1/2)$, and return

$$\boldsymbol{\beta}^* = \widehat{\boldsymbol{\beta}} + \mathbf{B}\,\boldsymbol{Z}\,\sqrt{\nu/W}\,, \tag{10.5}$$

where $\mathbf{B}\mathbf{B}^\top = \mathbf{V}$. Then, $\boldsymbol{\beta}^*$ follows the desired t distribution, by Theorem 10.1.

The following Julia code—to be appended to the code of Example 10.4—implements the independence sampler, and is used to obtain 10,000 draws from the posterior distribution after a burn-in period of 500. We use $\nu = 5$, giving samples that are spread out relatively far around the mode $\widehat{\boldsymbol{\beta}}$.

```
bioassay_bayes.jl
```

```julia
using Distributions
B = cholesky(V).L
burnin = 500
nloop = 10000 + burnin
store_beta = zeros(nloop, 2)
nu = 5;    # df for the proposal
# log posterior density
logf(b)=(sum((y .- 1) .* (X*b) - log.((1 .+ exp.(-X*b)))))[1]
# log density of the t proposal
logprop(b) = (-0.5*(nu+2)*log(1 .+
              (b - betat)' * (V \ (b - betat)) / nu))[1]
beta = betat      # initialize the chain
for i = 1:nloop
    global beta
    # candidate draw from the t proposal
    betac = betat + B * randn(2, 1) *
              sqrt(nu / rand(Gamma(nu / 2, 2)))
    rho = logf(betac) - logf(beta) + logprop(beta) -
              logprop(betac)
    exp(rho) > rand()   ? beta = betac : nothing
    store_beta[i, :] = beta'
end
store_beta = store_beta[burnin+1:end, :]   # discard the burnin
cov(store_beta)
mean(store_beta, dims=1)
```

The posterior mean and posterior covariance matrix are estimated to be

$$\mathbb{E}(\boldsymbol{\beta}\,|\,\boldsymbol{y}) = \begin{bmatrix} 1.36 \\ 11.98 \end{bmatrix}, \quad \mathrm{Var}(\boldsymbol{\beta}\,|\,\boldsymbol{y}) = \begin{bmatrix} 1.25 & 4.47 \\ 4.47 & 35.62 \end{bmatrix}.$$

It is interesting to note that even though the posterior mode coincides with the maximum likelihood estimate under the flat prior, the posterior mean of β_1 is substantially larger than the corresponding maximum likelihood estimate, reflecting the fact that the marginal distribution of β_1 is positively skewed. Further, a 95% credible interval for β_1 is estimated to be $(3.52, 26.18)$, which excludes the value 0.

10.2.2 Probit Model

Definition 10.4.   (Probit Model). Let Y_i denote the i-th binary response, and let $\boldsymbol{x}_i$ represent the vector of explanatory variables and $\boldsymbol{\beta}$ the associated parameter vector. In a **probit model**, the $\{Y_i\}$ are independent, and $Y_i \sim \mathsf{Ber}(\mu_i)$, with $\mu_i = \Phi(\boldsymbol{x}_i^\top \boldsymbol{\beta})$, where Φ is the cdf of the standard normal distribution. That is, the component link function is $g(x) = \Phi^{-1}(x)$.

As in the logit model, we first derive the log-likelihood function, score function, and information matrix. Let $\varphi(x)$ denote the pdf of the standard normal distribution. Note that since the standard normal distribution is symmetric around 0, it follows that $\varphi(x) = \varphi(-x)$ and $1 - \Phi(x) = \Phi(-x)$. Now, given the independent Bernoulli responses and the component link function $g(x) = \Phi^{-1}(x)$, the log-likelihood function for the probit model is

$$l(\boldsymbol{\beta};\boldsymbol{y}) = \sum_{i=1}^{n} \left[y_i \ln \Phi(\boldsymbol{x}_i^\top \boldsymbol{\beta}) + (1 - y_i) \ln \Phi(-\boldsymbol{x}_i^\top \boldsymbol{\beta}) \right] . \tag{10.6}$$

The score function is the gradient of the log-likelihood function:

$$\begin{aligned}
\boldsymbol{S}(\boldsymbol{\beta}) = \nabla_{\boldsymbol{\beta}}\, l(\boldsymbol{\beta};\boldsymbol{y}) &= \sum_{i=1}^{n} \left[y_i \frac{\varphi(\boldsymbol{x}_i^\top \boldsymbol{\beta})}{\Phi(\boldsymbol{x}_i^\top \boldsymbol{\beta})} \boldsymbol{x}_i - (1 - y_i) \frac{\varphi(-\boldsymbol{x}_i^\top \boldsymbol{\beta})}{\Phi(-\boldsymbol{x}_i^\top \boldsymbol{\beta})} \boldsymbol{x}_i \right] \\
&= \sum_{i=1}^{n} \varphi(\boldsymbol{x}_i^\top \boldsymbol{\beta}) \left[\frac{y_i}{\Phi(\boldsymbol{x}_i^\top \boldsymbol{\beta})} - \frac{1 - y_i}{\Phi(-\boldsymbol{x}_i^\top \boldsymbol{\beta})} \right] \boldsymbol{x}_i .
\end{aligned}$$

Noting that $\frac{\mathrm{d}}{\mathrm{d}x}\varphi(x) = -x\,\varphi(x)$, we differentiate the score function again with respect to $\boldsymbol{\beta}$ to obtain:

$$\nabla_{\boldsymbol{\beta}}^2 \, l(\boldsymbol{\beta}; \boldsymbol{y}) = - \sum_{i=1}^{n} (\boldsymbol{x}_i^{\top} \boldsymbol{\beta}) \, \varphi(\boldsymbol{x}_i^{\top} \boldsymbol{\beta}) \left[\frac{y_i}{\varPhi(\boldsymbol{x}_i^{\top} \boldsymbol{\beta})} - \frac{1 - y_i}{\varPhi(-\boldsymbol{x}_i^{\top} \boldsymbol{\beta})} \right] \boldsymbol{x}_i \boldsymbol{x}_i^{\top}$$

$$- \sum_{i=1}^{n} \varphi(\boldsymbol{x}_i^{\top} \boldsymbol{\beta}) \left[\frac{y_i \, \varphi(\boldsymbol{x}_i^{\top} \boldsymbol{\beta})}{\varPhi(\boldsymbol{x}_i^{\top} \boldsymbol{\beta})^2} + \frac{(1 - y_i) \, \varphi(-\boldsymbol{x}_i^{\top} \boldsymbol{\beta})}{\varPhi(-\boldsymbol{x}_i^{\top} \boldsymbol{\beta})^2} \right] \boldsymbol{x}_i \boldsymbol{x}_i^{\top} .$$

Using the fact that $\mathbb{E}(Y_i) = \varPhi(\boldsymbol{x}_i^{\top} \boldsymbol{\beta})$, the information matrix is therefore

$$\mathbf{I}(\boldsymbol{\beta}) = \sum_{i=1}^{n} \frac{\varphi(\boldsymbol{x}_i^{\top} \boldsymbol{\beta})^2}{\varPhi(\boldsymbol{x}_i^{\top} \boldsymbol{\beta}) \, \varPhi(-\boldsymbol{x}_i^{\top} \boldsymbol{\beta})} \, \boldsymbol{x}_i \boldsymbol{x}_i^{\top} .$$

Given the score function and the information matrix, one can then obtain the maximum likelihood estimate via Fisher's scoring method as before.

For a Bayesian analysis, we can sample from the posterior pdf using MCMC; for example, using a similar independence sampler as in the logit model. If we use a normal prior $\boldsymbol{\beta} \sim \mathcal{N}(\boldsymbol{b}_0, \mathbf{V}_0)$, then the logarithm of the posterior pdf $f(\boldsymbol{\beta} \,|\, \boldsymbol{y}) \propto f(\boldsymbol{\beta}) f(\boldsymbol{y} \,|\, \boldsymbol{\beta})$ is

$$\ln f(\boldsymbol{\beta} \,|\, \boldsymbol{y}) = l(\boldsymbol{\beta}; \boldsymbol{y}) - \frac{1}{2} (\boldsymbol{\beta} - \boldsymbol{b}_0)^{\top} \mathbf{V}_0^{-1} (\boldsymbol{\beta} - \boldsymbol{b}_0) + \text{const} , \qquad (10.7)$$

with $l(\boldsymbol{\beta}; \boldsymbol{y})$ given in (10.6). From the (dependent) sample of the posterior pdf, it is straightforward to estimate the posterior mean, standard deviation, and quantiles. One can also estimate the marginal posterior pdfs $\{f(\beta_i \,|\, \boldsymbol{y})\}$, using a kernel density estimator.

☞ 20

Other quantities of interest include the **marginal effects** of the covariates, that is, how a change in the covariate affects the response. To make the discussion concrete, let x_j be the j-th element of a covariate vector $\boldsymbol{x}$. If x_j is a continuous explanatory variable, then

$$\frac{\partial}{\partial x_j} \mathbb{E}(Y \,|\, \boldsymbol{\beta}) = \frac{\partial}{\partial x_j} \varPhi(\boldsymbol{x}^{\top} \boldsymbol{\beta}) = \varphi(\boldsymbol{x}^{\top} \boldsymbol{\beta}) \beta_j , \qquad (10.8)$$

where β_j is the j-th element of $\boldsymbol{\beta}$. This depends on both $\boldsymbol{\beta}$ and $\boldsymbol{x}$. For the "average" marginal effect of x_j, one could consider $\varphi(\overline{\boldsymbol{x}}^{\top} \boldsymbol{\beta}) \beta_j$, where $\overline{\boldsymbol{x}}$ is the average of the explanatory vectors $\boldsymbol{x}_1, \ldots, \boldsymbol{x}_n$ corresponding to the responses $Y_1, \ldots, Y_n$. Similarly, if x_j is a binary explanatory variable, the average marginal effect of x_j is

$$\varPhi(\boldsymbol{z}_1^{\top} \boldsymbol{\beta}) - \varPhi(\boldsymbol{z}_0^{\top} \boldsymbol{\beta}) ,$$

where $\boldsymbol{z}_x = [\overline{x}_1, \ldots, \overline{x}_{j-1}, x, \overline{x}_{j+1}, \ldots, \overline{x}_n]^{\top}$ for $x \in \{0, 1\}$.

Note that the marginal effect is a (continuous) function of the regression parameter vector $\boldsymbol{\beta}$, and so it is a random variable. Given the posterior draws for $\boldsymbol{\beta}$, the posterior distribution of the marginal effect can be obtained readily.

Example 10.6 (Modeling Extramarital Affairs with Probit Model).
Fair (1978) analyzed the decision to have an extramarital affair with a probit model, using surveys conducted by *Psychology Today* and *Redbook*. The data used in this example are obtained from Koop et al. (2007) and contain 601 independent observations. All observations are taken from individuals currently married and married for the first time.

The response is a binary variable that indicates if the respondent has (had) an extramarital affair; the seven explanatory variables are an intercept (CONST), a male indicator (MALE), number of years married (YEAR), a binary variable to indicate if the respondent has children from the marriage (KIDS), a binary variable for classifying one's self as "religious" (RELIGIOUS), years of schooling completed (ED), and a final binary variable denoting whether the person views the marriage as happier than an average marriage (HAPPY).

We first obtain the maximum likelihood estimate $\widehat{\boldsymbol{\beta}}$ via Fisher's scoring method, as well as the information matrix $\mathbf{V}$ evaluated at $\widehat{\boldsymbol{\beta}}$. The following Julia code accomplishes this task.

```
probit_mle.jl
```

```julia
using DelimitedFiles, Distributions, LinearAlgebra
affair = readdlm("affair.csv", ',')
y = affair[:,1];
X = affair[:,2:end];
n, k = size(X);
# find the MLE and the information matrix
S = ones(k,1); # score
betat = (X'*X)(X'*y); # initial guess
e = 10^(-5);  # tolerance level
while sum(abs.(S)) > e  # stopping criterion
    Xbetat = X*betat;
    phi = pdf.(Normal(0,1),Xbetat);
    Phi = cdf.(Normal(0,1),Xbetat);
    global S = sum(repeat(y.*phi./Phi-(1 .- y).*phi./(1 .-Phi)
        ,outer = [1,k]).*X,dims=1)';
    d = phi.^2 ./ (Phi.*(1 .-Phi));
    IM = X'*diagm(vec(d))*X; # information matrix
    global betat = betat + IM\S;
end
println(round.(betat,digits=4))
```

```
[-0.7379; 0.1504; 0.0287; 0.2491; -0.5103; 0.0064; -0.5136;;]
```

To sample from the posterior distribution, we use the same MCMC approach as for the logit model. That is, we use an independence sampler with a $t_\nu(\widehat{\boldsymbol{\beta}}, \mathbf{V})$ proposal distribution. The hyperparameters for the normal prior are chosen as $\boldsymbol{b}_0 = \boldsymbol{0}$ and $\mathbf{V}_0 = 10\,\mathbb{I}_7$, where $\mathbb{I}_7$ is the identity matrix. This gives a relatively non-informative prior which is centered around zero. The logarithm of the posterior pdf is given in (10.7). The degrees of freedom is set to $\nu = 5$. We use the method described in (10.5) to generate a draw from the proposal distribution, and run the sampler for 5500 iterations, discarding the first 500 as burn-in. Add the following to the previous code.

```
probit_bayes.m

burnin = 500;
nloop = 5000+burnin;
V = IM\I;   # scale matrix for the proposal
B = cholesky(Hermitian(V)).L;
nu = 5; # df for the proposal
b0 = zeros(k,1); # prior mean
V0 = 10*I; # prior covariance
# log-posterior density
logf(b)= (y'*log.(cdf.(Normal(0,1),X*b)) + (1 .-y)'*log.(cdf.(
    Normal(0,1),-X*b))- 0.5*(b-b0)'*(V0(b-b0)))[1];
# log-proposal density
logprop(b)  = (-0.5*(k+nu)*log.(1 .+ (b-betat)'*(V(b-betat))/
    nu))[1];
store_beta = zeros(nloop,k);
beta = betat;
for i = 1:nloop
# candidate draw from the t proposal
    global beta
    betac = betat + B*randn(k,1)*sqrt(nu/rand(Gamma(nu/2,2)));
    rho = logf(betac)-logf(beta) + logprop(beta)-logprop(betac
        );
    if exp(rho) > rand()
        beta = betac;
    end
    store_beta[i,:] = beta';
end
store_beta = store_beta[burnin+1:end,:]; # discard the burn-in
println(mean(store_beta,dims=1))
println(std(store_beta,dims=1))
```

Table 10.2 lists various summary statistics of the posterior distribution, including the means, standard deviations, and 2.5- and 97.5-percentiles, based on the 5000 (dependent) samples from the posterior distribution. Of the six variables (excluding the intercept), only three seem to have a substantial impact on the response. In particular, the 95% credible intervals for the coefficients associated with YEAR, RELIGIOUS, and HAPPY exclude zero, while the other three do not. On average, people reporting themselves as religious or in happy marriages are less likely to have affairs, while the longer someone is in a marriage, the more likely he or she has an affair.

Table 10.2 Coefficient posterior means, standard deviations, 2.5- and 97.5-percentile for the probit model

Variable	Mean	Std. dev.	2.5-percentile	97.5-percentile
CONST	−0.728	0.408	−1.528	0.061
MALE	0.150	0.126	−0.098	0.392
YEAR	0.029	0.013	0.004	0.054
KIDS	0.249	0.161	−0.065	0.561
RELIGIOUS	−0.516	0.122	−0.757	−0.277
ED	0.005	0.025	−0.045	0.055
HAPPY	−0.517	0.124	−0.760	−0.269

To assess the quantitative impacts of the covariates, we estimate the average marginal effects of the covariates, using the following code, again added to the previous.

```
margeff.jl

N = size(store_beta,1);
store_ME = zeros(nloop-burnin,6);
xbar = mean(X,dims=1)';
for loop in 1:N
  global beta = store_beta[loop,:]; # ME for cont. vars.
  store_ME[loop,[2 5]] = pdf.(Normal(0,1),xbar'*beta) .*
      beta[[3,6]];
  for j in [1 3 4 6] # ME for discrete variables
    z0 = copy(xbar); z0[j+1] = 0;  # using copy is important!
    z1 = copy(xbar); z1[j+1] = 1;
    store_ME[loop,j] = (cdf(Normal(0,1),z1'*beta) -
        cdf(Normal(0,1),z0'*beta))[1];
  end
end
mean(store_ME,dims=1)
```

The summary statistics of the posterior distribution for the marginal effects are reported in Table 10.3. For example, people who report themselves as religious are 15 percent less likely to have affairs (fixing the other covariates at the sample means), and those who report to be happy in their marriages are 17 percent less likely.

Table 10.3 Posterior means, standard deviations, 2.5- and 97.5-percentile for the marginal effects

variable	mean	std. dev.	2.5-percentile	97.5-percentile
MALE	0.045	0.038	−0.030	0.121
YEAR	0.009	0.004	0.001	0.016
KIDS	0.071	0.046	−0.024	0.157
RELIGIOUS	−0.150	0.035	−0.217	−0.082
ED	0.002	0.008	−0.014	0.017
HAPPY	−0.167	0.043	−0.255	−0.084

10.2.3 Latent Variable Representation

Estimation and inference under the logit and probit models can be simplified by using *data augmentation*. The general idea behind data augmentation is to include "hidden" variables in the model for the data in order to simplify the analysis of the model. A prime example of data augmentation is found in the EM algorithm in Sect. 6.6.

For the logit and probit models, data augmentation can be introduced by thinking of an observed binary response in terms of whether or not an underlying continuous latent (i.e., hidden) variable crosses a particular threshold: if it does, then we observe, say, 1; otherwise, we observe 0. The advantage of the latent variable representation is that it is often easier to work with the continuous latent variables than the observed binary variable. To be mathematically precise, consider again the probit model: each binary response Y_i is distributed as $Y_i \sim \mathsf{Ber}(\mu_i)$, where $\mu_i = \varPhi(\boldsymbol{x}_i^\top \boldsymbol{\beta})$, and $\boldsymbol{x}_i$ is a vector of covariates.

Now, introduce the latent variables $\{Z_i\}$, each is distributed independently according to the normal distribution with mean $\boldsymbol{x}_i^\top \boldsymbol{\beta}$ and variance 1:

$$Z_i \sim \mathcal{N}(\boldsymbol{x}_i^\top \boldsymbol{\beta}, 1) . \tag{10.9}$$

These latent variables are then linked to the observed binary variables $\{Y_i\}$ as follows:

$$Y_i = \begin{cases} 1 \text{ if } Z_i > 0, \\ 0 \text{ if } Z_i \leq 0. \end{cases} \tag{10.10}$$

The values of the binary variables $\{Y_i\}$ are observed and the covariates $\{\boldsymbol{x}_i\}$ are fixed. However, the latent variables $\{Z_i\}$ are unobserved.

To check that this latent variable representation (10.9)–(10.10) does indeed give the same probit model, we need to show that it implies the same likelihood function. To this end, note that under the latent variable representation, each Y_i is an independent Bernoulli random variable with success probability:

$$\mathbb{P}(Y_i = 1) = \mathbb{P}(Z_i > 0) = 1 - \varPhi(-\boldsymbol{x}_i^\top \boldsymbol{\beta}) = \varPhi(\boldsymbol{x}_i^\top \boldsymbol{\beta}) ,$$

which is the same success probability under the probit model. Hence, the latent variable representation in (10.9)–(10.10) implies the same probit model.

Introducing more unobserved variables might seem to be odd as they give rise to exactly the same model. However, as it turns out, by augmenting the data with these latent variables, computation becomes more tractable. In fact, we can use the expectation–maximization algorithm discussed in Sect. 6.6 to obtain the maximum likelihood estimate easily.

We first determine the complete-data log-likelihood—using frequentist rather than Bayesian notation. Since conditional on $\boldsymbol{Z}$ the vector $\boldsymbol{Y}$ is deterministic, the joint pdf of $\boldsymbol{Y}$ and $\boldsymbol{Z}$ has the same form as the pdf of $\boldsymbol{Z}$. It follows that

$$l(\boldsymbol{\beta}; \boldsymbol{y}, \boldsymbol{z}) = \ln f_{\boldsymbol{Z}}(\boldsymbol{z}; \boldsymbol{\beta}) = -\frac{n}{2} \ln(2\pi) - \frac{1}{2} \sum_{i=1}^{n} (z_i - \boldsymbol{x}_i^\top \boldsymbol{\beta})^2$$

$$= -\frac{1}{2} \sum_{i=1}^{n} \left\{ (\boldsymbol{x}_i^\top \boldsymbol{\beta})^2 - 2 z_i \boldsymbol{x}_i^\top \boldsymbol{\beta} \right\} + \text{const} . \quad (10.11)$$

Now, suppose $\boldsymbol{\beta}_{t-1}$ is the current value for $\boldsymbol{\beta}$. To implement the E-step, we derive the conditional density:

$$g_t(\boldsymbol{z}) = f_{\boldsymbol{Z} \mid \boldsymbol{Y}}(\boldsymbol{z} \mid \boldsymbol{y}; \boldsymbol{\beta}_{t-1}) = \prod_{i=1}^{n} f_{Z_i \mid Y_i}(z_i \mid y_i; \boldsymbol{\beta}_{t-1}) ,$$

where we use the fact that the latent variables $Z_1, \ldots, Z_n$ are conditionally independent. If $y_i = 1$, the only extra information we have is that $Z_i > 0$. What this means is that given $y_i = 1$, Z_i follows the normal distribution with mean $\boldsymbol{x}_i^\top \boldsymbol{\beta}_{t-1}$ and variance 1, left-truncated at 0. So, $f_{Z_i \mid Y_i}(z_i \mid y_i = 1; \boldsymbol{\beta}_{t-1}) = 0$ for $z < 0$ and proportional to $\exp(-\frac{1}{2}(z_i - \boldsymbol{x}_i^\top \boldsymbol{\beta}_{t-1})^2)$ for $z_i \geq 0$. We write

$$(Z_i \mid y_i = 1; \boldsymbol{\beta}_{t-1}) \sim \mathsf{TN}_{(0,\infty)}(\boldsymbol{x}_i^\top \boldsymbol{\beta}_{t-1}, 1) . \quad (10.12)$$

Similarly, if $y_i = 0$, then

$$(Z_i \mid y_i = 0; \boldsymbol{\beta}_{t-1}) \sim \mathsf{TN}_{(-\infty,0)}(\boldsymbol{x}_i^\top \boldsymbol{\beta}_{t-1}, 1) . \quad (10.13)$$

In particular, (see Problem 10.7), we have:

$$\mathbb{E}[Z_i \mid y_i = 1; \boldsymbol{\beta}_{t-1}] = \boldsymbol{x}_i^\top \boldsymbol{\beta}_{t-1} + \frac{\varphi(\boldsymbol{x}_i^\top \boldsymbol{\beta}_{t-1})}{\Phi(\boldsymbol{x}_i^\top \boldsymbol{\beta}_{t-1})} , \quad (10.14)$$

$$\mathbb{E}[Z_i \mid y_i = 0; \boldsymbol{\beta}_{t-1}] = \boldsymbol{x}_i^\top \boldsymbol{\beta}_{t-1} - \frac{\varphi(\boldsymbol{x}_i^\top \boldsymbol{\beta}_{t-1})}{\Phi(-\boldsymbol{x}_i^\top \boldsymbol{\beta}_{t-1})} . \quad (10.15)$$

Writing $v_i = \mathbb{E}_{g_t}[Z_i \mid y_i; \boldsymbol{\beta}_{t-1}]$, it follows from (10.11) that

$$Q_t(\boldsymbol{\beta}) = \mathbb{E}_{g_t} l(\boldsymbol{\beta}; \boldsymbol{y}, \boldsymbol{Z}) = -\frac{1}{2} \sum_{i=1}^{n} \left\{ (\boldsymbol{x}_i^\top \boldsymbol{\beta})^2 - 2\,v_i\,\boldsymbol{x}_i^\top \boldsymbol{\beta} \right\} + \text{const}.$$

Next, to implement the M-step, we simply solve $\nabla Q_t(\boldsymbol{\beta}) = \mathbf{0}$. Since Q_t is quadratic in $\boldsymbol{\beta}$, we can use the differentiation rules in Sect. B.1 to find (see ☞ 47 also Problem 10.8) the solution:

$$\boldsymbol{\beta}_t = \left(\sum_{i=1}^{n} \boldsymbol{x}_i \boldsymbol{x}_i^\top \right)^{-1} \sum_{i=1}^{n} v_i\,\boldsymbol{x}_i . \tag{10.16}$$

Finally, the maximum likelihood estimate for $\boldsymbol{\beta}$ can be obtained by going through the E- and M-steps iteratively until convergence.

For *Bayesian* estimation, the probit model can be fitted using the Gibbs sampler with data augmentation. Specifically, if we have draws from the joint posterior pdf $f(\boldsymbol{z}, \boldsymbol{\beta} \mid \boldsymbol{y})$ and retain only the draws for $\boldsymbol{\beta}$, then those draws are from the desired marginal pdf $f(\boldsymbol{\beta} \mid \boldsymbol{y})$. Therefore, we can construct a Gibbs sampler by sequentially drawing from $f(\boldsymbol{\beta} \mid \boldsymbol{y}, \boldsymbol{z})$ followed by $f(\boldsymbol{z} \mid \boldsymbol{y}, \boldsymbol{\beta})$. As it turns out, both conditional densities are of standard form and samples from each can be obtained quickly.

For concreteness, assume the prior $\boldsymbol{\beta} \sim \mathcal{N}(\mathbf{0}, \boldsymbol{\Sigma}_0)$. First, to derive $f(\boldsymbol{\beta} \mid \boldsymbol{y}, \boldsymbol{z})$ note that, given the latent vector $\boldsymbol{z}$, we in fact have a linear regression model; see (10.9). Hence, using Theorem 8.1 we have: ☞ 24

$$(\boldsymbol{\beta} \mid \boldsymbol{y}, \boldsymbol{z}) \sim \mathcal{N}(\widehat{\boldsymbol{\beta}}, \mathbf{D}) ,$$

where

$$\mathbf{D} = (\mathbf{X}^\top \mathbf{X} + \boldsymbol{\Sigma}_0^{-1})^{-1} \qquad \text{and} \qquad \widehat{\boldsymbol{\beta}} = \mathbf{D}\mathbf{X}^\top \boldsymbol{z} ,$$

and $\mathbf{X}$ is the design matrix with i-th row $\boldsymbol{x}_i^\top$, $i = 1, \ldots, n$.

Second, the conditional density $f(\boldsymbol{z} \mid \boldsymbol{y}, \boldsymbol{\beta}) = \prod_{i=1}^{n} f(z_i \mid y_i, \boldsymbol{\beta})$ is given in (10.12)–(10.13). A draw from a truncated normal distribution can be obtained, say, via the inverse-transform method or (faster) the acceptance– ☞ 53 rejection method.

Example 10.7 (Gibbs Sampler for Probit Model). To demonstrate fitting the probit model using the Gibbs sampler with data augmentation, we revisit Example 10.6. We use the **Truncated** function to draw from truncated distributions; see also Problem 10.7.

In the main script, we implement a Gibbs sampler by alternatively drawing from $f(\boldsymbol{\beta} \mid \boldsymbol{y}, \boldsymbol{z})$ and $f(\boldsymbol{z} \mid \boldsymbol{y}, \boldsymbol{\beta})$. The estimation results are similar to those obtained in Example 10.6, and they are not repeated here.

```
probit_bayes_gibbs.jl
```

```julia
using DelimitedFiles, Distributions, LinearAlgebra
affair = readdlm("affair.csv", ',')
y = Int64.(affair[:,1]); # convert to integers
X = affair[:,2:end];
XX = X'*X;
n, k = size(X);
V0 = 10*diagm(ones(k)); # prior covariance
invV0 = V0\I;
burnin = 500;
nloop = 5000+burnin;
store_beta = zeros(nloop,k);
z = 1.0*y; # initial guess, new float copy
beta = XX(X'*z);
# compute a few things before the loop
id0 = findall(y .== 0); id1 = findall(y .==1);
n0 = length(id0); n1=n-n0;
V = (invV0 + XX)\I; # posterior covariance
for i in  1:nloop
    # sample z
    global beta
    global Xb = X*beta;
   for k in id0
        z[k] = rand(Truncated(Normal(Xb[k],1), -Inf,0))
    end
    for k in id1
        z[k] = rand(Truncated(Normal(Xb[k],1), 0, Inf))
    end
    # sample beta
    dbeta = X'*z;
    beta = V*dbeta + cholesky(Hermitian(V)).L * randn(k,1);
    store_beta[i,:] = beta';
end
store_beta = store_beta[burnin+1:end,:]; # discard the burn-in
mean(store_beta,dims=1)
```

10.3 Poisson Regression

Poisson regression deals with *count* data Y, for example, the number of cars in
a household. We are interested in how some observed characteristics $\boldsymbol{x}$—e.g.,
household income, number of children in the household, whether it is a single-
parent household, etc.—affect the response Y. Since Y takes values on the set

of nonnegative integers, one natural specification for Y is the Poisson model $Y \sim \mathsf{Poi}(\mu)$. In terms of a generalized linear model (see Definition 10.1), it remains to link $\boldsymbol{x}^\top\boldsymbol{\beta}$ to the mean μ, which has to be positive. One easy way to guarantee this is to specify μ as

☞ 29

$$\mu = e^{\boldsymbol{x}^\top \boldsymbol{\beta}} \;.$$

This leads to the following definition.

> **Definition 10.5. (Poisson Regression Model).** Let Y_i denote the i-th response (count) and let $\boldsymbol{x}_i$ represent the vector of explanatory variables and $\boldsymbol{\beta}$ the associated parameter vector. In a **Poisson regression model**, the $\{Y_i\}$ are independent, and $Y_i \sim \mathsf{Poi}(\mu_i)$, with $\mu_i = e^{\boldsymbol{x}_i^\top \boldsymbol{\beta}}$. In other words, the component link function is $g(x) = \ln x$.

Let $\boldsymbol{x}_i^\top$ be the i-th row of the design matrix $\mathbf{X}$, and let $\boldsymbol{g} = [g, \ldots, g]^\top$. We see that the distribution of $\boldsymbol{Y} = [Y_1, \ldots, Y_n]^\top$ is completely specified by $\boldsymbol{\mu} = \boldsymbol{g}^{-1}(\mathbf{X}\boldsymbol{\beta})$. In this case no additional dispersion parameters are used.

Example 10.8 (MLE for the Poisson Regression Model). Suppose we are interested in determining the impact of research and development (R&D) on the number of patents obtained by firms in a certain industry. For this purpose a total of $n = 14$ firms are interviewed. For each firm we record its number of patents obtained over the last 3 years, as well as its R&D budget (in tens of thousands of dollars) over the same period. The data are presented in Table 10.4.

To investigate the effectiveness of R&D, let Y_i denote the number of patents obtained by the i-th firm and let $\boldsymbol{x}_i = [1, x_i]^\top$ be a 2×1 vector of explanatory variables, where x_i is the i-th firm's R&D budget. We consider the Poisson regression $Y_i \sim \mathsf{Poi}(\mu_i)$, where $\mu_i = e^{\boldsymbol{x}_i^\top \boldsymbol{\beta}}$ and $\boldsymbol{\beta} = [\beta_1, \beta_2]^\top$ is a 2×1 vector of regression coefficients.

Table 10.4 Number of patents and R&D

Number of patents	R & D budget	Number of patents	R&D budget
6	26	8	29
3	21	2	13
2	19	0	5
1	11	2	3
3	21	6	29
1	16	1	3
1	19	3	21

The log-likelihood function for the Poisson regression model is given by

$$l(\boldsymbol{\beta}; \boldsymbol{y}) = \sum_{i=1}^{n} \left[y_i \boldsymbol{x}_i^\top \boldsymbol{\beta} - \mathrm{e}^{\boldsymbol{x}_i^\top \boldsymbol{\beta}} - \ln y_i! \right] .$$

Moreover, it can be shown that the score function and the information matrix are respectively (see Problem 10.2):

$$\boldsymbol{S}(\boldsymbol{\beta}) = \sum_{i=1}^{n} (y_i - \mathrm{e}^{\boldsymbol{x}_i^\top \boldsymbol{\beta}}) \boldsymbol{x}_i \quad \text{and} \quad \mathbf{I}(\boldsymbol{\beta}) = \sum_{i=1}^{n} \mathrm{e}^{\boldsymbol{x}_i^\top \boldsymbol{\beta}} \boldsymbol{x}_i \boldsymbol{x}_i^\top .$$

Hence, the maximum likelihood estimate of $\boldsymbol{\beta}$ can be computed using Fisher's scoring method, which is implemented in the following Julia script.

☞ 187

```
poissonreg.jl

using SparseArrays, LinearAlgebra
y = [6 3 2 1 3 1 1 8 2 0 2 6 1 3]'
RD = [26 21 19 11 21 16 19 29 13 5 3 29 3 21]'
n = length(y)
X = [ones(n,1) RD]
betat = (X'*X)(X'*log.(y .+ .001)) # initial guess
S = ones(2,1)                      # score
e = 10^(-5)   # tolerance level
IM = zeros(2,2)
while sum(abs.(S)) > 10^(-5) # stopping criterion
    global S, betat, IM
    mu = exp.(X*betat)
    S = sum(repeat((y - mu), 1,2).*X,dims=1)'
    IM =   X'*sparse(1:n,1:n,vec(mu))*X # info matrix
    betat = betat + IM\S
end
println(round.(betat,digits=4))
V = IM\I  # inverse of the info matrix
println(round.(V,digits=4))
```

```
[-0.7947; 0.0919;;]
[0.3109 -0.0128; -0.0128 0.0006]
```

10.4 Problems

10.1. Prove Theorem 10.1; that is, show that if $\boldsymbol{R} \sim \mathcal{N}(\boldsymbol{0}, \mathbb{I}_n)$ and $W \sim \mathrm{Gamma}(\nu/2, 1/2)$ are independent, then the random vector $\boldsymbol{Z} = \sqrt{\nu/W}\,\boldsymbol{R}$ has pdf

$$f(\boldsymbol{z}) = \frac{\Gamma(\frac{\nu+n}{2})}{\Gamma(\nu/2)(\pi\nu)^{n/2}}\left(1 + \frac{\|\boldsymbol{z}\|^2}{\nu}\right)^{-\frac{\nu+1}{2}}.$$

Hint: consider the coordinate transformation:

$$\begin{bmatrix} z_1 \\ \vdots \\ w \end{bmatrix} \mapsto \begin{bmatrix} z_1\sqrt{w/\nu} \\ \vdots \\ z_n\sqrt{w/\nu} \\ w \end{bmatrix} = \begin{bmatrix} r_1 \\ \vdots \\ r_n \\ w \end{bmatrix}$$

and determine the determinant of the corresponding Jacobian matrix. Next, apply the transformation rule (3.26) to find the joint pdf of $[\boldsymbol{Z}, W]$. Finally integrate out W to obtain the pdf of $\boldsymbol{Z}$.   ☞ 81

10.2. Consider the Poisson regression model in Definition 10.5. Given the data $[y_1, \boldsymbol{x}_n^\top], \dots [y_n, \boldsymbol{x}_n^\top]$, show that the log-likelihood function is given by

$$l(\boldsymbol{\beta}; \boldsymbol{y}) = \sum_{i=1}^{n}\left[y_i\boldsymbol{x}_i^\top\boldsymbol{\beta} - \mathrm{e}^{\boldsymbol{x}_i^\top\boldsymbol{\beta}} - \ln y_i!\right].$$

Further, show that the score function and the information matrix are, respectively,

$$\boldsymbol{S}(\boldsymbol{\beta}) = \sum_{i=1}^{n}(y_i - \mathrm{e}^{\boldsymbol{x}_i^\top\boldsymbol{\beta}})\boldsymbol{x}_i \quad \text{and} \quad \mathbf{I}(\boldsymbol{\beta}) = \sum_{i=1}^{n}\mathrm{e}^{\boldsymbol{x}_i^\top\boldsymbol{\beta}}\boldsymbol{x}_i\boldsymbol{x}_i^\top.$$

10.3. It is generally believed that births by Caesarean section are more frequent in private hospitals than in public ones. To investigate if there is any evidence for this claim, data are collected on the number of Caesarean sections carried out in three private hospitals (type 0) and seven public hospitals (type 1), as well as the total number of births in each of the hospitals. These are presented in Table 10.5.

Table 10.5 Poisson regression example

Number of Caesarean sections	Number of births	Hospital type	Number of Caesarean sections	Number of births	Hospital type
8	236	0	13	679	1
16	739	1	4	26	0
15	970	1	19	1272	1
23	2371	1	33	3246	1
5	309	1	2	28	0

Use the data to fit a Poisson regression: regress the response variable "number of Caesarean sections" on an intercept, "number of births," and "hospital type." Are births by Caesarean section more frequent in private hospitals? Hint: use the results in Problem 10.2.

10.4. Consider again Example 10.6 where we use the probit model to analyze the decision to have an extramarital affair. For a nonreligious, college-educated (16 years of education) male who has married for 10 years with one child from the marriage, and who reports that his marriage is happier than average, what is the probability that he has an extramarital affair? Use the `kde` function to plot a kernel density estimate of the posterior probability.

10.5. In the linear regression model $Y = \boldsymbol{x}^\top \boldsymbol{\beta} + \varepsilon$, the parameter vector $\boldsymbol{\beta}$ can be interpreted as the marginal effects of the (continuous) covariates, that is, the rate at which the response changes as the result of an infinitesimal change in the covariate:

$$\boldsymbol{\beta} = \nabla_{\boldsymbol{x}} \mathbb{E}Y \ .$$

However, for the probit model, the marginal effects depend on *both* the parameter vector $\boldsymbol{\beta}$ and the covariates $\boldsymbol{x}_i$ in a nonlinear functional form: $\varphi(\boldsymbol{x}^\top\boldsymbol{\beta})\boldsymbol{\beta}$; see (10.8). What are the marginal effects for the *logit* model?

☞ 298 **10.6.** In Definition 10.3 the matrix $\boldsymbol{\Sigma}$ was intentionally called the *scale* matrix rather than *covariance* matrix, because the covariance matrix of $\boldsymbol{X}$ (i.e., $\mathbb{E}[(\boldsymbol{X} - \boldsymbol{\mu})(\boldsymbol{X} - \boldsymbol{\mu})^\top])$ is not equal to $\boldsymbol{\Sigma}$:

a. Show that the covariance matrix of $\boldsymbol{X}$ is $\boldsymbol{\Sigma}\,\mathbb{E}[\boldsymbol{Z}\boldsymbol{Z}^\top]$, where $\boldsymbol{Z}$ has a standard multivariate Student's t distribution.

b. Use Theorem 10.1 to show that the covariance matrix of $\boldsymbol{Z}$, that is $\mathbb{E}[\boldsymbol{Z}\boldsymbol{Z}^\top]$, is equal to $c\,\nu\,\mathbb{I}_n$, where $\mathbb{I}_n$ is the identity matrix and

$$c = \int_0^\infty \frac{1}{w} \frac{\left(\frac{1}{2}\right)^{\frac{\nu}{2}} w^{\frac{\nu}{2}-1} e^{-\frac{1}{2}w}}{\Gamma\left(\frac{\nu}{2}\right)} \, \mathrm{d}w \ .$$

c. Evaluate c.

10.7. Let $Z \sim \mathsf{TN}(\mu, \sigma^2, a, b)$, where $a < b$. Thus, the distribution of Z is that of a random variable $X \sim \mathsf{N}(\mu, \sigma^2)$ conditioned on X lying in $[a, b]$:

a. Show that the pdf of Z is

$$f_Z(z) = \frac{\varphi((z - \mu)/\sigma)/\sigma}{\Phi((b - \mu)/\sigma) - \Phi((a - \mu)/\sigma)} \ ,$$

where φ and Φ are respectively the pdf and cdf of the standard normal distribution.

b. For $\sigma = 1$, $a = -\infty$, and $b = 0$, show that $\mathbb{E}Z = \mu - \varphi(\mu)/\Phi(-\mu)$.

c. For $\sigma = 1$, $a = 0$, and $b = \infty$, show that $\mathbb{E}Z = \mu + \varphi(\mu)/\Phi(\mu)$.

d. Show that the cdf of Z is

$$F_Z(z) = \frac{\Phi((z-\mu)/\sigma) - \Phi((a-\mu)/\sigma)}{\Phi((b-\mu)/\sigma) - \Phi((a-\mu)/\sigma)} .$$

e. Explain why the function **tnormrnd** in Example 10.7 can be used to simulate Z.

10.8. Prove (10.16).

Chapter 11
Nonparametric Methods

The standard frequentist and Bayesian models involve parameterized distributions for the data that contain a small number of parameters. For example, if the data are represented by $\boldsymbol{X}$, then a typical model is of the form

$$\boldsymbol{X} \sim \mathsf{Dist}(\boldsymbol{\theta}) , \tag{11.1}$$

depending on a known distribution (multivariate normal, binomial, gamma, and so on) up to an unknown parameter vector $\boldsymbol{\theta}$ of small dimension. In this section we relax the requirement that the form of the distribution needs to be specified in advance. The resulting models are often said to be **nonparametric**. The nonparametric counterpart of (11.1) is that $\boldsymbol{X} \sim \mathsf{Dist}$, where Dist is left unspecified. The quintessential case is where the data vector $\boldsymbol{X} = [X_1, \ldots, X_n]$ is comprised of an iid sample from a distribution with an unknown cdf F:

$$X_1, \ldots, X_n \overset{\text{iid}}{\sim} F . \tag{11.2}$$

Even though the model (11.2) might not seem to carry much information, it is still feasible to do inference on the data. In particular, we saw in Sect. 7.1 that it is possible to estimate the unknown cdf F via the empirical cdf of the data. In a similar way, density estimation (Sect. 7.2) is considered to be a nonparametric method, as the model for the data is of the form (11.2), where F is assumed to have a density f. Nonparametric methods may still involve parameterized distributions, but the dimension of the parameter vector is unbounded. Using the general framework for statistical learning in Sect. 4.6, the same principle applies to nonparametric regression.

    We consider various nonparametric methods in this section. Nonparametric statistical tests often involve the ordering and ranking of data, giving rise to *order statistics*, which are discussed in Sect. 11.1. We present nonparamet-

J. C. C. Chan, D. P. Kroese, *Statistical Modeling and Computation,* Springer Texts in Statistics, https://doi.org/10.1007/978-1-0716-4132-3_11

ric equivalents to the standard one- and two-sample t-tests in Sect. 11.2. Section 11.3 deals with nonparametric regression using the versatile framework of *kernel* functions. Another common approach to nonparametric regression is to employ *spline* functions, as treated in Sect. 11.4. Finally, Sect. 11.5 discusses a Bayesian analysis of nonparametric regression via *Gaussian process regression*.

11.1 Order Statistics

Let $X_1, \ldots, X_n$ be a sequence of iid random variables from some cdf F, which may be known or unknown. Arrange these in order and denote the ordered sample by $X_{(1)}, \ldots, X_{(n)}$. For example, $X_{(1)}$ is the smallest, and $X_{(n)}$ is the largest. Then, $X_{(r)}$ is called the **r-th order statistic**. The order statistics are neither independent nor identically distributed, but their marginal and joint distributions are easy to derive.

First consider the marginal distribution of the r-th order statistic. We have

$$
\begin{aligned}
F_{X_{(r)}}(x) &= \mathbb{P}(X_{(r)} \leq x) \\
&= \mathbb{P}(\text{At least } r \text{ of } X_1, \ldots, X_n \text{ are } \leq x) \\
&= \sum_{j=r}^{n} \mathbb{P}(\text{Exactly } j \text{ of } X_1, \ldots, X_n \text{ are } \leq x) \\
&= \sum_{j=r}^{n} \binom{n}{j} (F(x))^j (1 - F(x))^{n-j} .
\end{aligned}
$$

Consequently, if $X_1, \ldots, X_n$ are continuous random variables with common pdf f, then

$$
f_{X_{(r)}}(x) = F'_{X_{(r)}}(x) = n \binom{n-1}{r-1} (F(x))^{r-1} (1 - F(x))^{n-r} f(x) . \tag{11.3}
$$

While (11.3) can be derived in a purely combinatorial fashion, it is easier to show it probabilistically as follows. The most likely way in which the event $\{x \leq X_{(r)} \leq x + \varepsilon\}$ happens is that *exactly one* of the n variables falls in the interval $[x, x + \varepsilon]$, while $r - 1$ variables fall in $(-\infty, x)$ and the remaining $n - r$ fall in $(x + \varepsilon, \infty)$. The probability of having more than one variable in $[x, x + \varepsilon]$ is negligible as ε goes to 0. In particular, we have

$$
\begin{aligned}
f_{X_{(r)}}(x)\,\varepsilon + o(\varepsilon) &= \mathbb{P}(x \leq X_{(r)} \leq x + \varepsilon) \\
&= n \times \binom{n-1}{r-1} (F(x))^{r-1} (1 - F(x))^{n-r} \times f(x)\,\varepsilon + o(\varepsilon) ,
\end{aligned}
$$

where $o(\varepsilon)/\varepsilon \downarrow 0$ as $\varepsilon \downarrow 0$. Dividing both sides by ε and letting $\varepsilon \downarrow 0$ now gives the stated result.

In particular, the *minimum* of the sample has distribution function

$$F_{X_{(1)}}(x) = 1 - (1 - F(x))^n \,,$$

and, in the continuous case,

$$f_{X_{(1)}}(x) = n(1 - F(x))^{n-1} f(x) \,,$$

while for the *maximum* we have

$$F_{X_{(n)}}(x) = (F(x))^n \,,$$

and, in the continuous case,

$$f_{X_{(n)}}(x) = n(F(x))^{n-1} f(x) \,.$$

Using a symmetry argument, if $X_1, \ldots, X_n$ are continuous random variables with common pdf f, then the order statistics $X_{(1)}, \ldots, X_{(n)}$ have joint pdf

$$h(x_1, \ldots, x_n) = \begin{cases} n! \prod_{i=1}^{n} f(x_i) & \text{if } x_1 < x_2 < \cdots < x_n \\ 0 & \text{otherwise} \,. \end{cases} \tag{11.4}$$

This is intuitively obvious because h is just the joint pdf of $X_1, \ldots, X_n$ multiplied by $n!$ (being the number of arrangements of the sample).

11.2 Nonparametric Statistical Tests

Making assumptions about the distribution of the data is fraught with risks, in case the assumptions are not true. This may lead to incorrect conclusions. In *nonparametric* tests, we still may make assumptions about the data (e.g., independence), but we do not model the data via a specific parametric class of distributions. Nonparametric tests tend to be more "robust" to outliers in the data. The downside is that they are less "powerful" than parametric tests, in the sense that it is more difficult to reject the null hypothesis when it indeed should be rejected. We discuss a number of nonparametric versions of the standard tests (e.g., one- and two-sample t-tests).

11.2.1 One-Sample Nonparametric Tests

For the one-sample setting, suppose $Z_1, \ldots, Z_n$ are iid random variables from an unknown continuous distribution that is symmetric around some μ. Hence, μ is the median of the distribution and also its expectation, if the latter exists. We wish to assess via a statistical test whether the hypothesis $H_0 : \mu = 0$ should be accepted or not versus some two- or one-sided alternative; e.g., $H_1 : \mu \neq 0$ or $H_1 : \mu > 0$. The simplest nonparametric test statistic to use in this situation is

$$T = \sum_{i=1}^{n} \mathbb{1}_{\{Z_i > 0\}} . \tag{11.5}$$

This gives the **sign test** statistic, where we simply count the total number of positive observations. Under H_0 the test statistic T has a $\mathsf{Bin}(n, 1/2)$ distribution, and for the alternative $H_1 : \mu \neq 0$, we reject H_0 for large or small values of T. This is simply the one-sample binomial test in disguise, where we test $H_0 : p = 1/2$ against $H_1 : p \neq 1/2$, with $p = \mathbb{P}(Z > 0)$.

Example 11.1 (Sign Test for Paired Data). We return to the weight loss data in Example 5.15, which is replicated in Table 11.1.

☞ 146

Table 11.1 Weight loss data

Before	280	140	90	128	135	98	111	97	89	156
After	240	135	89	135	120	95	99	103	87	140
Loss	40	5	1	-7	15	3	12	-6	2	16
Sign	$+$	$+$	$+$	$-$	$+$	$+$	$+$	$-$	$+$	$+$

For the one-sample t-test, it was assumed that the weight loss data came from some normal distribution. If instead we carry out a sign test, with alternative $H_1 : \mu > 0$, then the corresponding p-value is $\mathbb{P}(X \geq 8) = 1 - \mathbb{P}(X \leq 7)$, where $X \sim \mathsf{Bin}(10, 1/2)$. Using Julia:

```
using Distributions
1 - cdf(Binomial(10,0.5),7)
```

```
0.0546875
```

Again, there is modest, but not compelling, evidence that the weight loss program works.

The sign test uses only minimal information about the values $\{Z_i\}$—it records only if the values are positive or negative. To better exploit the symmetry assumption in the model, more sophisticated nonparametric tests also include information on the *ranking* of the data, as well as the sign of the data. In particular, by ordering the absolute values $\{|Z_i|\}$ from smallest to largest, we can assign a rank R to each absolute value $|Z|$, where $R = r$ means that $|Z|$ is the r-th smallest of the $\{|Z_i|\}$. Note that from the symmetry and continuity assumption, it follows that under $H_0 : \mu = 0$ the vector $[R_1, \ldots, R_n]$ is a random permutation of $[1, \ldots, n]$, where all of the $n!$ possible permutations are equally likely.

We consider test statistics of the form

$$T = \sum_{r=1}^{n} \alpha_r B_r , \qquad (11.6)$$

where $\alpha_1, \ldots, \alpha_n$ are given numbers and, for $r = 1, \ldots, n,$

$$B_r = \begin{cases} 1 & \text{if the variable whose absolute value has rank } r \text{ is positive,} \\ 0 & \text{otherwise.} \end{cases}$$

Under $H_0 : \mu = 0$ the $\{B_i\}$ are independent and $\mathsf{Ber}(1/2)$ distributed. It follows that the expectation of T under H_0 is

$$\mathbb{E}T = \frac{1}{2} \sum_{r=1}^{n} \alpha_r = \frac{n}{2}\, \overline{\alpha} , \qquad (11.7)$$

where $\overline{\alpha} = \frac{1}{n} \sum_{r=1}^{n} \alpha_r$ is the average of the $\{\alpha_r\}$. Similarly, the variance of T under H_0 is

$$\mathrm{Var}(T) = \sum_{r=1}^{n} \alpha_r^2 \, \mathrm{Var}(B_r) = \frac{1}{4} \sum_{r=1}^{n} \alpha_r^2 . \qquad (11.8)$$

For small n, the probability distribution of T under H_0 can be obtained by full enumeration, as

$$\mathbb{P}(T \le t) = 2^{-n} \sum_{b} \mathbb{1}_{\{T(b) \le t\}} ,$$

where the enumeration is over all 2^n binary vectors $b = [b_1, \ldots, b_n]$ and $T(b) = \sum_{r=1}^{n} \alpha_r b_r$. When total enumeration is not feasible one can instead estimate $\mathbb{P}(T \le t)$ via the Monte Carlo estimator

$$\frac{1}{K} \sum_{i=1}^{K} \mathbb{1}_{\{T^{(i)} \le t\}} ,$$

where $T^{(1)}, \ldots, T^{(K)}$ are iid copies of T.

Note that if $a_r = 1$ for all r, then (11.6) simply yields the test statistic for the sign test in (11.5). If instead $a_r = r, r = 1, \ldots, n$, the resulting test statistic

$$T^+ = \sum_{r=1}^{n} r B_r \qquad (11.9)$$

is called the (Wilcoxon) **positive-rank sum test** statistic. The test statistic
is thus obtained as follows:

1. First rank the absolute values.
2. The test statistic T^+ is the sum of the ranks of the positive values.

From (11.7) and (11.8) the expectation and variance of T^+ under the null
hypothesis are

$$\mathbb{E}T^+ = \frac{n(n+1)}{4} \quad \text{and} \quad \text{Var}(T^+) = \frac{n(n+1)(2n+1)}{24}. \tag{11.10}$$

Moreover, it can be shown that under the null hypothesis and for large sample
size n, the test statistic has approximately a normal distribution.

Under the model assumption of a symmetric continuous distribution, there
are no ties. When ties do occur in practical situations, the method is modified
by giving equal fractional ranks to the tied values.

Example 11.2 (Wilcoxon Positive-Rank Sum Test). Consider again
the weight loss data in Table 11.1. The last row in Table 11.2 gives the ranks
of the absolute values.

Table 11.2 Weight loss data with ranks

Loss	40	5	1	−7	15	3	12	−6	2	16
Sign	+	+	+	−	+	+	+	−	+	+
Rank	10	4	1	6	8	3	7	5	2	9

The outcome of the test statistic is $t^+ = 10+4+1+8+3+7+2+9 = 44$.
Under H_0, T^+ has approximately a normal distribution with expectation 27.5
and standard deviation 9.810708, so that the p-value for this right one-sided
test can be approximated as follows:

```
using Distributions
n = 10; t = 44
et = n*(n+1)/4
sdt = sqrt(n*(n+1)*(2*n+1)/24)
pval = 1 - cdf(Normal(et,sdt), t)
print(pval)
```
```
0.0463
```

In fact, the exact p-value is a bit larger. The following Julia program
computes the ranks using the Julia function **sortperm** and **invperm** and
determines the true p-value via complete enumeration.

```
pvalposrank.jl
```

```julia
using Distributions
z =    [40 , 5,  1 , -7, 15 , 3 , 12 , -6 , 2 , 16]
ind = sortperm(abs.(z))
ranks = invperm(ind)
t = sum(ranks .* (z .> 0))

function pval(t)
    tot = 0
    a = 1:10
    for i = 0:2^10-1
        b = digits(i, base=2, pad=10)
        tot = tot + (sum(b .* a) >= t)
    end
    return tot / 2^10
end

pval(t)
```

```
0.052734375
```

11.2.2 Two-Sample Nonparametric Tests

The use of rankings for statistical tests is more natural in a two-sample setting. Consider a two-sample data model, where the measurements $X_1, \ldots, X_m$ from Group 1 are iid from a continuous distribution with cdf F and the measurements $Y_1, \ldots, Y_n$ from Group 2 are iid with cdf G, where F and G are unspecified. It is assumed that the $\{X_i\}$ and $\{Y_j\}$ are independent. We wish to test if the distributions of the two groups are the same or not.

Sort pooled data $X_1, \ldots, X_m, Y_1, \ldots, Y_n$ as $Z_{(1)} < \cdots < Z_{(N)}$, where $N = m + n$. This gives a rank to each measurement. For ranks $r = 1, \ldots, N$, let

$$B_r = \begin{cases} 1 & \text{if the variable with rank } r \text{ belongs to Group 1,} \\ 0 & \text{otherwise.} \end{cases}$$

Under H_0 the $\{B_r\}$ are $\mathsf{Ber}(p)$ distributed with success probability $p = m/N$, but note that in this case the $\{B_r\}$ are *dependent* random variables, in contrast to the one-sample scenario in the previous section. In particular, under H_0 we have $B_1, \ldots, B_N \sim_{\text{iid}} \mathsf{Ber}(p)$ *conditional on* $B_1 + \cdots + B_N = m$.

Similar to (11.6), we consider test statistics of the form

$$T = \sum_{r=1}^{N} \alpha_r B_r \tag{11.11}$$

for some fixed $\{\alpha_r\}$. As in the one-sample case, the expectation and variance of T under H_0 are readily evaluated. The expectation of T is

$$\mathbb{E}T = \sum_{r=1}^{N} \alpha_r \, \mathbb{E}B_r = \frac{m}{N} \sum_{r=1}^{N} \alpha_r = m\,\overline{\alpha}\,,$$

where $\overline{\alpha} = \frac{1}{N} \sum_{r=1}^{N} \alpha_r$.

For the variance, observe that under H_0, it holds that $\mathrm{Cov}(B_r, B_s) = \mathrm{Cov}(B_1, B_2)$ for all $r \neq s$. If we denote $v = \mathrm{Cov}(B_r, B_r) = \mathrm{Var}(B_r)$ and $c = \mathrm{Cov}(B_r, B_s)$ for $r \neq s$, then

$$v = \mathrm{Var}(B_1) = p(1 - p) = \frac{m\,n}{N^2}$$

and

$$\begin{aligned}
c = \mathrm{Cov}(B_1, B_2) &= \mathbb{E}[B_1 B_2] - p^2 \\
&= \mathbb{P}(B_2 = 1 \mid B_1 = 1)\mathbb{P}(B_1 = 1) - p^2 \\
&= \frac{m-1}{N-1}p - p^2 = -\frac{m\,n}{N^2(N-1)}\,.
\end{aligned}$$

Noting that $v - c = m\,n/(N(N - 1))$, it follows that

$$\begin{aligned}
\mathrm{Var}(T) &= \sum_{r=1}^{N}\sum_{s=1}^{N} \alpha_r \alpha_s \, \mathrm{Cov}(B_r, B_s) \\
&= v \sum_{r=1}^{N} \alpha_r^2 + c \sum_{r=1}^{N}\sum_{\substack{s=1 \\ s \neq r}}^{N} \alpha_r \alpha_s \\
&= (v - c) \sum_{r=1}^{N} \alpha_r^2 + cN^2 \overline{\alpha}^2 \\
&= \frac{m\,n}{N-1}\left(\frac{1}{N}\sum_{r=1}^{N} \alpha_r^2 - \overline{\alpha}^2\right) = \frac{m\,n\,V_\alpha}{N-1}\,,
\end{aligned}$$

where $V_\alpha = \frac{1}{N}\sum_{r=1}^{N}(\alpha_r - \overline{\alpha})^2$ is the average squared deviation of the $\{\alpha_r\}$.

The main instance is where $\alpha_r = r$, which yields the **Wilcoxon's rank sum test**, where the test statistic is the sum of the ranks of the first group. In this case, $\overline{\alpha} = (N + 1)/2$ and $V_\alpha = N(N^2 - 1)/12$, so

$$\mathbb{E}T = \frac{m(N+1)}{2} \quad \text{and} \quad \mathrm{Var}(T) = \frac{m\,n(N+1)}{12}\,.$$

An intuitive way to derive the expectation is that under the null hypothesis, all ranks are equally likely, so the rank R of one observation is a discrete uniform random variable taking values in $1, \ldots, N$. Its expectation is thus $\mathbb{E}R = (N + 1)/2$, and since there are m observations in the first group, we have an expected rank sum of $\mathbb{E}T = m\,\mathbb{E}R = m(N + 1)/2$.

Under the null hypothesis and for large n, the test statistic has approximately a normal distribution; see, for example, Wald and Wolfowitz (1944).

Example 11.3 (Rank Sum Test). The data given in Table 11.3 and depicted Fig. 11.1 was drawn from cdfs $F(x) = 1 - \exp(-x + 1), x \geq 1$ for Group 1 and $G(x) = 1 - \exp(-x), x \geq 0$ for Group 2.

Table 11.3 Data from (shifted) exponential distributions. Ranks are given below the observations

x	1.04	3.30	1.40	1.53	1.01	1.02	3.93	1.61	1.93	2.25
Rank	8	18	11	14	6	7	19	15	16	17

y	1.00	1.40	1.30	3.95	0.08	1.33	0.66	0.73	1.49	0.43
Rank	5	12	9	20	1	10	3	4	13	2

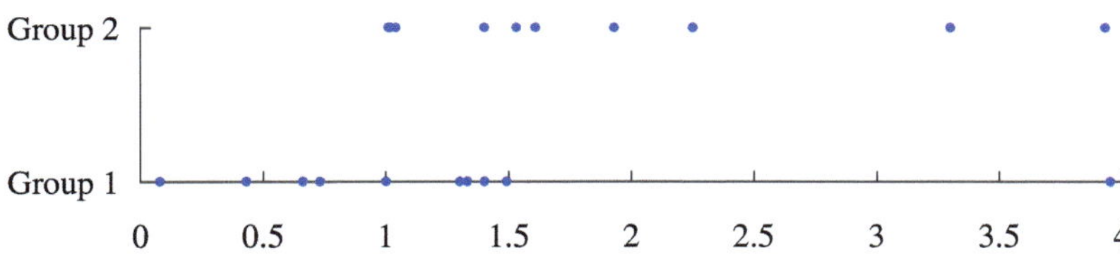

Fig. 11.1 Data from (shifted) exponential distributions

A two-sample t-test does not detect a difference between the two distribution, yielding a p-value of 0.166, as obtained via the following Julia program.

```
wilcox1.jl

using StatsBase, Distributions
x = [1.04,3.30,1.40,1.53,1.01,1.02,3.93,1.61,1.93,2.25]
y = [1.00,1.40,1.30,3.95,0.08,1.33,0.66,0.73,1.49,0.43]
m = length(x); n = length(y); N = m+n;


pooledV = ((m-1)var(x) + (n-1)var(y))/(N-2)
ttest = (mean(x) - mean(y))/sqrt(pooledV)/sqrt(1/m + 1/n)
p1 = 2*(1 - cdf(TDist(N-2), ttest))
print(p1)

0.1658502382402547
```

Let us investigate if the Wilcoxon rank sum test fairs better here, as the normality assumption is obviously violated. The smallest measurement is 0.08, so it gets rank 1 while the second smallest measurement is 0.43, and so on. There are no ties in this case. The null hypothesis is again that there is no difference between the distributions of the two groups and the alternative hypothesis is that there *is* a difference. The outcome of the test statistic is

$$t = 8 + 18 + 11 + 14 + 6 + 7 + 19 + 15 + 16 + 17 = 131\,.$$

We reject the null hypothesis for large and small values of the test statistic. For this two-sided test, the p-value is $2\,\mathbb{P}(T \geq 131)$. Using the normal approximation, with $\mathbb{E}T = 105$ and $\mathrm{Var}(T) = 175$, we obtain an approximate p-value of 0.0494, which gives reasonable evidence against the null hypothesis. The following code should be appended to the previous one to carry out the rank sum test.

```
wilcox1.jl
```

```
z = cat(x, y, dims=1)
ind = sortperm(z)
ranks = invperm(ind)
t = sum(ranks[1:10])

ET = m*(N+1)/2
sdT = sqrt(m*n*(N+1)/12)
p = 2*(1 - cdf(Normal(ET,sdT),t))
print(p)
```

```
0.0493661947519326
```

The exact p-value can be determined by enumerating over all $\binom{20}{10}$ binary vectors of length 20 with exactly 10 ones. Under the null hypothesis, each of these vectors has the same probability. We find a p-value of 0.052, which is close to the normal approximation. The following code, to be appended to the previous two, carries out the analysis.

```
wilcox2.jl
```

```
function pval(t)
    tot = 0
    a = 1:20
    for i = 0:2^20-1
        b = digits(i, base=2, pad=20)
        if sum(b)==10
            tot = tot + (sum(b .* a) >= t)
        end
    end
```

```
    return 2*tot / binomial(20,10)
end

print(pval(t))
```
```
0.05242590227110351
```

The **Mann–Whitney test** is closely related to the Wilcoxon rank sum test. Here, the test statistic is defined as

$$U = \sum_{i=1}^{m} \sum_{j=1}^{n} \mathbb{1}_{\{X_i > Y_j\}} \,.$$

Hence, U is the total number of times where a value in the first group is larger than a value in the second group. You may verify that the Mann–Whitney test static is related to the Wilcoxon rank sum test statistic T via

$$U = T - \frac{(m+1)m}{2} \,.$$

In fact, U is of the form (11.11), with $\alpha_r = r - (m+1)/2, r = 1, \ldots, N$, because

$$U = \sum_{r=1}^{N} r B_r - \frac{m+1}{2} \sum_{r=1}^{N} B_r = T - \frac{(m+1)m}{2} \,,$$

as $B_1 + \cdots + B_N = m$.

Finally, taking $\alpha_r = z_{(r)}, r = 1, \ldots, N$, we obtain a **randomization test**, also called a **permutation test**. In this case the test statistic T takes values $z_{i_1} + \cdots + z_{i_m}$ where $[i_1, \ldots, i_m]$ is any ordered arrangement of distinct elements in $\{1, \ldots, n\}$ of size m. There are $\binom{n}{m}$ of such arrangements, and under the null hypothesis all arrangements are equally likely. Note that the observed test statistic t is simply the sum of all observations in the first group, i.e., $t = x_1 + \cdots + x_m$. Using either full enumeration or Monte Carlo methods we can then assess how t compares with the sum of the variables in the first group after the observations are reshuffled.

Further information on nonparametric tests can be found in, for example, Kolassa (2020) and Pratt and Gibbons (1981).

11.3 Gram Matrix and Kernel Functions

For the linear model with $n \times m$ model matrix $\mathbf{X}$, with $n \geq m$, we saw in Sect. 9.2.1—leaving out the regularization—that by rewriting $\boldsymbol{\beta} = \mathbf{X}^\top \boldsymbol{\alpha}$, the minimization problem $\min_{\boldsymbol{\beta}} \|\boldsymbol{y} - \mathbf{X}\boldsymbol{\beta}\|^2$ leads to the alternative minimization problem

☞ 27

$$\min_{\boldsymbol{\alpha}} \|\boldsymbol{y} - \mathbf{K}\boldsymbol{\alpha}\|^2, \tag{11.12}$$

where $\mathbf{K}$ is the Gram matrix $\mathbf{X}\mathbf{X}^\top$. Because $\mathbf{K}$ is a singular matrix when $n > m$, solving the normal equations $\mathbf{K}^\top(\boldsymbol{y} - \mathbf{K}\boldsymbol{\alpha}) = \mathbf{0}$ does not lead to a unique solution; in fact, there is a subspace of dimension $n - m$ of possible solutions. However, each of these solutions $\boldsymbol{\alpha} = [\alpha_1, \ldots, \alpha_n]^\top$ gives the same value for $\mathbf{X}^\top\boldsymbol{\alpha} = \boldsymbol{\beta}$. The minimum-norm solution, that is, the solution $\widehat{\boldsymbol{\alpha}}$ to (11.12) such that $\|\widehat{\boldsymbol{\alpha}}\| \leq \|\widetilde{\boldsymbol{\alpha}}\|$ for any other solution $\widetilde{\boldsymbol{\alpha}}$, is given by $\widehat{\boldsymbol{\alpha}} = \mathbf{K}^+\boldsymbol{y}$, where $\mathbf{K}^+$ is the (Moore–Penrose) pseudo-inverse of $\mathbf{K}$.

Using any solution $\widehat{\boldsymbol{\alpha}}$ leads to the (unique) prediction function

$$g_\tau(\boldsymbol{x}) = \boldsymbol{x}^\top\boldsymbol{\beta} = \sum_{i=1}^n \widehat{\alpha}_i \langle \boldsymbol{x}, \boldsymbol{x}_i \rangle, \tag{11.13}$$

for training data $\tau = \{(\boldsymbol{x}_i, y_i)\}$. This reformulation may seem contrived, but in fact it opens up a whole new way of thinking about linear models. The key point is that the estimation procedure and the prediction function only depend on the inner products of the explanatory variables (feature vectors).

Suppose that instead of using the data $\{(\boldsymbol{x}_i, y_i)\}$, we transform the feature vectors via a function $\boldsymbol{\phi} : \mathbb{R}^m \to \mathbb{R}^p$, denoting $\boldsymbol{z}_i = \boldsymbol{\phi}(\boldsymbol{x}_i), i = 1, \ldots, n$. The inner products of the transformed features are

$$\langle \boldsymbol{z}_i, \boldsymbol{z}_j \rangle = \boldsymbol{z}_i^\top \boldsymbol{z}_j = (\boldsymbol{\phi}(\boldsymbol{x}_i))^\top \boldsymbol{\phi}(\boldsymbol{x}_j), \tag{11.14}$$

and the corresponding Gram matrix can be written as

$$\mathbf{K} = \boldsymbol{\Phi}\boldsymbol{\Phi}^\top,$$

where $\boldsymbol{\Phi}$ is the matrix whose j-th column is $\boldsymbol{\phi}(\boldsymbol{x}_j), j = 1, \ldots, n$. Note that any such matrix $\mathbf{K}$ is a *covariance matrix*. For instance, it is the covariance matrix of the random vector $\boldsymbol{X} = \boldsymbol{\Phi}\boldsymbol{U}$, where $\boldsymbol{U} \sim \mathcal{N}(\mathbf{0}, \mathbb{I}_n)$. As such, $\mathbf{K}$ is a

☞ 77   symmetric and positive semidefinite matrix.

Example 11.4 (Polynomial Regression). The polynomial regression
☞ 108 model in (4.10) can be viewed in the framework discussed above. Here, each original one-dimensional explanatory variable (feature) u is transformed into a $(d + 1)$-dimensional feature vector $\boldsymbol{x} = [1, u, \ldots, u^d]^\top$. The corresponding prediction function is a linear function of $\boldsymbol{x}$ and can also be written as a linear combination of the inner products $\langle \boldsymbol{x}, \boldsymbol{x}_i \rangle$, as in (11.13).

A powerful generalization of (11.13) and (11.14) is to associate with each feature $\boldsymbol{x} \in \mathcal{X}$ for some arbitrary set $\mathcal{X}$ (e.g., $\mathbb{R}$ or $\mathbb{R}^m$) a whole feature *function* $\kappa(\boldsymbol{x}, \cdot) : \mathcal{X} \to \mathbb{R}$ and define the inner product of $\kappa(\boldsymbol{x}, \cdot)$ and $\kappa(\boldsymbol{x}', \cdot)$ as $\kappa(\boldsymbol{x}, \boldsymbol{x}')$. This approach is only valid if the matrix $\mathbf{K} = [\kappa(\boldsymbol{x}_i, \boldsymbol{x}_j)]$ is a covariance matrix for every choice of $\boldsymbol{x}_i, i = 1, \ldots, n$ and n. Such a function κ is called a **covariance function** or **kernel function** on $\mathcal{X}$. To verify if a function κ is a kernel function, we need to establish that it is finite and symmetric (i.e., $-\infty < \kappa(\boldsymbol{x}, \boldsymbol{x}') = \kappa(\boldsymbol{x}', \boldsymbol{x}) < \infty$) and that

$$\boldsymbol{\alpha}^\top \mathbf{K} \boldsymbol{\alpha} \geq 0 \tag{11.15}$$

for every $\boldsymbol{\alpha} \in \mathbb{R}^n$ and every choice of $\{\boldsymbol{x}_i\}$ and n. The latter is equivalent to

$$\sum_{i=1}^n \sum_{j=1}^n \alpha_i \, \kappa(\boldsymbol{x}_i, \boldsymbol{x}_j) \, \alpha_j \geq 0 \tag{11.16}$$

for all $\{\boldsymbol{x}_i\}_{i=1}^n$ from $\mathcal{X}$ and real numbers $\{\alpha_i\}_{i=1}^n$. The prediction function in (11.13) is then generalized to

$$g_\tau(\boldsymbol{x}) = \sum_{i=1}^n \widehat{\alpha}_i \, \kappa(\boldsymbol{x}, \boldsymbol{x}_i), \tag{11.17}$$

for training data $\tau = \{(\boldsymbol{x}_i, y_i)\}$, with $\widehat{\boldsymbol{\alpha}} = \mathbf{K}^+ \boldsymbol{y}$.

The standard kernel function on $\mathcal{X} = \mathbb{R}^m$ is the **linear kernel**:

$$\kappa(\boldsymbol{x}, \boldsymbol{x}') = \boldsymbol{x}^\top \boldsymbol{x}'.$$

An example of a non-standard kernel is given next.

Example 11.5 (Wiener Kernel). The Wiener kernel on $\mathcal{X} = \mathbb{R}_+$ is defined as

$$\kappa(x, x') = \min\{x, x'\}, \quad x, x' \geq 0.$$

We will see in Sect. 11.5 that it is the covariance function of the **Wiener process** (standard Brownian motion). We can use this kernel to construct prediction functions of the form

$$g(x) = \sum_{i=1}^n \alpha_i \min\{x, x_i\}$$

from data $\{(x_i, y_i), i = 1, \ldots, n\}$. As a concrete example, suppose we wish to reconstruct the function $\sin(x), x \in [0, 2\pi]$ from the function values at the points $x_i = i - 1, i = 1, \ldots, 7$. The parameter vector $\boldsymbol{\alpha} = [\alpha_1, \ldots, \alpha_7]^\top$ is found from (11.12) with $\mathbf{K} = [\kappa(x_i, x_j)]$. The following Julia program computes the approximation.

```
wienerkernel.jl
```

```julia
using LinearAlgebra, Plots
x = (0:1:2*pi)'
n = length(x)
y = sin.(x)
```

```julia
k(x,u) = min(x,u) # kernel
K = zeros(n,n)
for i=1:n
    for j=1:n
        K[i,j] = k(x[i], x[j])
    end
end
alpha = pinv(K)*y'      # compute an optimal alpha
xx = 0:0.01:2*pi
N = length(xx); g = zeros(N);
Kx = zeros(n,N)
for i=1:n
    for j=1:N
        Kx[i,j] = k(x[i],xx[j])
    end
end
g =  Kx'*alpha;  # function values

plot(xx,sin.(xx),color=:black,linestyle=:dash)
plot!(xx,g,color=:blue)
scatter!(x,y,legend=false,color=:black)
```

Figure 11.2 shows that the approximating function in this case simply interpolates between the known values of the function.

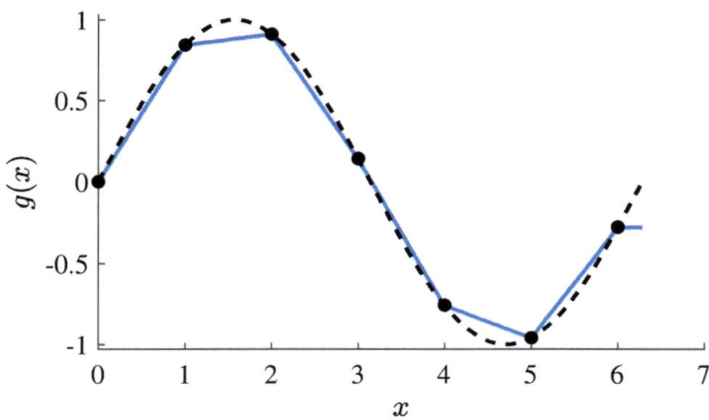

Fig. 11.2 Approximating the sine function using the Wiener kernel

Many different ways to build kernel functions may be found in Shawe-Taylor and Cristianini (2004). For example, the sum of two kernel functions is again a kernel function and so is their product; see also Problems 11.8–

11.11. A helpful way to produce kernel functions is to employ the following result, involving characteristic functions. ☞ 36

> **Theorem 11.1. (Kernels and Characteristic Functions).** Let X be a random variable with a pdf f that is symmetric around 0 (i.e., $f(x) = f(-x)$ for all $x \in \mathbb{R}$. Define
>
> $$\psi(r) = \mathbb{E}\mathrm{e}^{\mathrm{i}rX} = \int \mathrm{e}^{\mathrm{i}rx} f(x)\,\mathrm{d}x, \quad r \in \mathbb{R}$$
>
> to be its characteristic function. Then, $\kappa(x, x') = \psi(x - x')$ is a kernel function.

Proof. Note that $\psi(r)$ is real-valued, because the imaginary part of $\psi(r)$ is

$$\psi(r) = \mathbb{E}\sin(rX) = \int_{-\infty}^{\infty} \sin(rx)f(x)\,\mathrm{d}x = 0\,,$$

since $\sin(-rx)f(-x) = -\sin(rx)f(x)$ for all x. To verify (11.15), take any $n \geq 1$, $\alpha_1, \ldots, \alpha_n \in \mathbb{R}$, and $x_1, \ldots, x_n \in \mathbb{R}$. We have

$$\boldsymbol{\alpha}^\top \mathbf{K}\boldsymbol{\alpha} = \sum_{j=1}^{n}\sum_{\ell=1}^{n} \alpha_j \alpha_\ell \kappa(x_j, x_\ell) = \sum_{j=1}^{n}\sum_{\ell=1}^{n} \alpha_j \alpha_\ell \psi(x_j - x_\ell)$$

$$= \sum_{j=1}^{n}\sum_{\ell=1}^{n} \alpha_j \alpha_\ell \int \mathrm{e}^{\mathrm{i}x_j u}\mathrm{e}^{-\mathrm{i}x_\ell u} f(u)\,\mathrm{d}u = \int \left(\sum_{j=1}^{n} \alpha_j \mathrm{e}^{\mathrm{i}x_j u}\right)\overline{\left(\sum_{\ell=1}^{n} \alpha_\ell \mathrm{e}^{\mathrm{i}x_\ell u}\right)} f(u)\,\mathrm{d}u$$

$$= \int \left\|\sum_{j=1}^{n} \alpha_j \mathrm{e}^{\mathrm{i}x_j u}\right\|^2 f(u)\,\mathrm{d}u \geq 0\,,$$

where $\bar{z}$ denotes that complex conjugate of $z \in \mathbb{C}$. Since also $\kappa(x, x') = \psi(x - x') = \psi(x' - x) = \kappa(x', x)$, the function κ is a kernel function.

The same principle and proof carries over to the multidimensional case where $\boldsymbol{X}$ is a random vector in $\mathbb{R}^d$. The characteristic function is then defined as

$$\psi(\boldsymbol{r}) = \mathbb{E}\mathrm{e}^{\mathrm{i}\boldsymbol{r}^\top \boldsymbol{X}}, \quad \boldsymbol{r} \in \mathbb{R}^d.$$

The most important case is where $\boldsymbol{X} \sim \mathcal{N}(\boldsymbol{0}, b^2 \mathbb{I}_d)$, which has the characteristic function

$$\psi(\boldsymbol{r}) = \exp\left(-\frac{1}{2}\frac{\|\boldsymbol{r}\|^2}{b^2}\right), \quad \boldsymbol{r} \in \mathbb{R}^d.$$

Consequently, we obtain the **Gaussian kernel** on $\mathbb{R}^d$

$$\kappa(\boldsymbol{x}, \boldsymbol{x}') = \exp\left(-\frac{1}{2}\frac{\|\boldsymbol{x} - \boldsymbol{x}'\|^2}{b^2}\right). \tag{11.18}$$

The parameter b is sometimes called the **bandwidth**. Note that the kernel is of the form $\kappa(\boldsymbol{x}, \boldsymbol{x}') = f(\|\boldsymbol{x} - \boldsymbol{x}'\|)$ for some function $f : \mathbb{R} \to \mathbb{R}$. Such kernels are called **radial basis function (rbf)** kernels. By multiplying (11.18) with a positive number, we obtain another kernel function, which we call a *scaled* Gaussian kernel.

Prediction functions corresponding to (scaled) Gaussian kernels are therefore of the form

$$g(\boldsymbol{x}) = \sum_{i=1}^{n} \alpha_i \exp\left(-\frac{1}{2}\frac{\|\boldsymbol{x} - \boldsymbol{x}_i\|^2}{b^2}\right).$$

Think of each point $\boldsymbol{x}_i$ as having a feature $\kappa(\boldsymbol{x}_i, \cdot)$ that is a scaled multivariate Gaussian pdf centered at $\boldsymbol{x}_i$.

Example 11.6 (Gaussian Kernel). Figure 11.3 shows what happens if in Example 11.5 we replace the Wiener kernel with a Gaussian kernel, but otherwise keep the Julia code exactly the same.

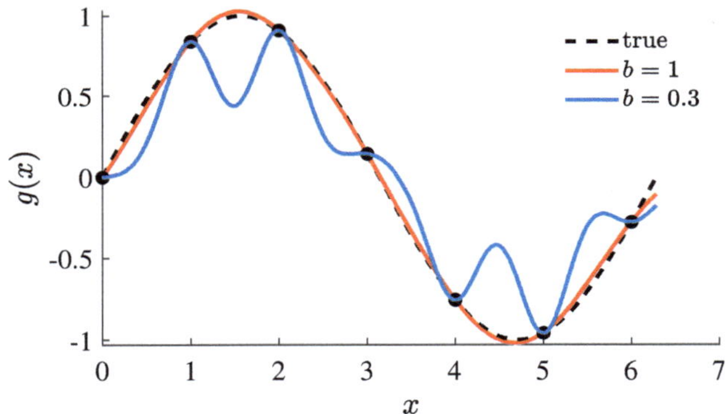

Fig. 11.3 Approximating the sine function using Gaussian kernels

For large bandwidths (e.g., $b \geq 1$), we obtain an excellent agreement with the true curve. However, for small bandwidths (e.g., $b = 0.3$), significant overfitting occurs.

11.4 Regression Splines and Smoothing Splines

☞ 101 In Chap. 4 we introduced a variety of nonlinear regression models, such as polynomial regression and log-linear models, to describe the nonlinear relationships between the response and explanatory variables. However, they are all parametric models in the sense that the user needs to specify a known functional form that maps the explanatory variables to the response. In many applications, we might not have sufficient domain knowledge to assume a particular functional form. In those cases, it is desirable to learn the nonlinear relationship from the data without imposing strong parametric assumptions.

In this section we consider piecewise polynomials and splines that are designed to flexibly capture local features of the data. To fix ideas, we focus on the case where there is a single explanatory variable x. A piecewise polynomial function $g(x)$ is constructed by first partitioning the domain of x into disjoint intervals. Then, in each interval, we obtain a separate polynomial function using only data that fall within the interval. Example 11.7 gives a simple illustration of approximating the sine function using a piecewise quadratic polynomial.

Example 11.7 (Piecewise Quadratic Polynomial). In this example we use a piecewise quadratic polynomial with a break-point or **knot** at ξ to approximate the sine function in Example 11.5. In particular, we construct a prediction function of the form

$$g(x) = \begin{cases} \beta_{01} + \beta_{11}x + \beta_{21}x^2, & x \leq \xi, \\ \beta_{02} + \beta_{12}x + \beta_{22}x^2, & x > \xi. \end{cases}$$

The parameters of $g(x)$ can be estimated by running two separate regressions using data $x \leq \xi$ and $x > \xi$, respectively. Figure 11.4 shows the estimated piecewise quadratic polynomial $g(x)$ with a knot at $\xi = 3$.

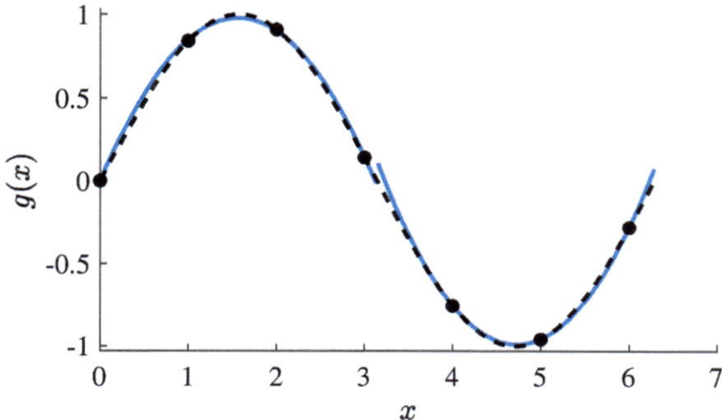

Fig. 11.4 Approximating the sine function using a piecewise quadratic polynomial

Note that the function $g(x)$ is discontinuous at ξ, which is often undesirable in many applications. To ensure that $g(x)$ is continuous at the knot ξ, one can impose the linear constraint $\beta_{01} + \beta_{11}\xi + \beta_{21}\xi^2 = \beta_{02} + \beta_{12}\xi + \beta_{22}\xi^2$ in the least squares estimation. Similar constraints can be imposed to ensure that higher-order derivatives are also continuous at the knot.

In general, constructing a piecewise polynomial that is continuous at the knots $\xi_1, \ldots, \xi_K$ amounts to solving a least squares problem subject to a system of linear constraints. The prototypical problem can be formulated as

$$\min_{\beta} \|\boldsymbol{y} - \mathbf{X}\boldsymbol{\beta}\|^2$$
$$\text{subject to } \mathbf{R}\boldsymbol{\beta} = \boldsymbol{r}\,, \tag{11.19}$$

where $\mathbf{R}$ is assumed to have full row rank (otherwise any redundant equations can be removed). This problem can be solved using Lagrange's method (see, e.g., Botev et al. (2025, Section B.2.2)), which amounts to finding a stationary point of

$$\|\boldsymbol{y} - \mathbf{X}\boldsymbol{\beta}\|^2 + \boldsymbol{\lambda}^{\top}(\mathbf{R}\boldsymbol{\beta} - \boldsymbol{r})$$

with respect to $\boldsymbol{\beta}$ and $\boldsymbol{\lambda}$, where $\boldsymbol{\lambda}$ is the vector of *Lagrange multipliers*. Since this is a convex optimization problem, we can take derivative with respect to $\boldsymbol{\beta}$ and $\boldsymbol{\lambda}$ and equate them to zero to find that the solution of the constrained least squares problem in (11.19) follows from solving

$$\begin{bmatrix} \mathbf{X}^{\top}\mathbf{X} & \mathbf{R}^{\top} \\ \mathbf{R} & \mathbf{O} \end{bmatrix} \begin{bmatrix} \boldsymbol{\beta} \\ \boldsymbol{\lambda} \end{bmatrix} = \begin{bmatrix} \mathbf{X}^{\top}\boldsymbol{y} \\ \boldsymbol{r} \end{bmatrix}. \tag{11.20}$$

To see that (11.20) is the set of optimality conditions for the constrained least squares problem in (11.19), suppose that $(\widehat{\boldsymbol{\beta}}, \widehat{\boldsymbol{\lambda}})$ satisfies (11.20) and $\boldsymbol{\beta}$ is any point that satisfies the linear constraints $\mathbf{R}\boldsymbol{\beta} = \boldsymbol{r}$. Then,

$$\begin{aligned}
\|\boldsymbol{y} - \mathbf{X}\boldsymbol{\beta}\|^2 &= \|\boldsymbol{y} - \mathbf{X}\widehat{\boldsymbol{\beta}} - \mathbf{X}(\boldsymbol{\beta} - \widehat{\boldsymbol{\beta}})\|^2 \\
&= \|\boldsymbol{y} - \mathbf{X}\widehat{\boldsymbol{\beta}}\|^2 + \|\mathbf{X}(\boldsymbol{\beta} - \widehat{\boldsymbol{\beta}})\|^2 - 2(\boldsymbol{\beta} - \widehat{\boldsymbol{\beta}})^{\top}\mathbf{X}^{\top}(\boldsymbol{y} - \mathbf{X}\widehat{\boldsymbol{\beta}}) \\
&= \|\boldsymbol{y} - \mathbf{X}\widehat{\boldsymbol{\beta}}\|^2 + \|\mathbf{X}(\boldsymbol{\beta} - \widehat{\boldsymbol{\beta}})\|^2 - 2(\boldsymbol{\beta} - \widehat{\boldsymbol{\beta}})^{\top}\mathbf{R}^{\top}\widehat{\boldsymbol{\lambda}} \\
&= \|\boldsymbol{y} - \mathbf{X}\widehat{\boldsymbol{\beta}}\|^2 + \|\mathbf{X}(\boldsymbol{\beta} - \widehat{\boldsymbol{\beta}})\|^2 \\
&\geq \|\boldsymbol{y} - \mathbf{X}\widehat{\boldsymbol{\beta}}\|^2\,,
\end{aligned}$$

where the third equality holds because of the optimality condition $\mathbf{X}^{\top}\boldsymbol{y} - \mathbf{X}^{\top}\mathbf{X}\widehat{\boldsymbol{\beta}} = \mathbf{R}^{\top}\widehat{\boldsymbol{\lambda}}$; the fourth equality holds because $\mathbf{R}\widehat{\boldsymbol{\beta}} = \mathbf{R}\boldsymbol{\beta} = \boldsymbol{r}$. Hence, $\widehat{\boldsymbol{\beta}}$ is a minimizer.

We have seen how one can construct a continuous piecewise polynomial with continuous higher-order derivatives by solving a linearly constrained least squares problem. Often, however, it is more convenient to use a different parameterization that incorporates the constraints directly. As an example, consider a function of the form

$$g(x) = \beta_0 + \beta_1 x + \beta_2 x^2 + \beta_3 x^3 + \beta_4 (x - \xi)_+^3\,,$$

where $(t)_+^3 = t^3$ for $t > 0$ and 0 otherwise. It can be shown that this function is a piecewise cubic polynomial that is continuous at the knot ξ, with continuous first and second derivatives at ξ; see Problem 11.17. This is an instant of a **cubic spline**. Estimation of the unknown parameters in $g(x)$ is easy: we can simply obtain the least squares estimates of a linear regression of y on an intercept, x, x^2, x^3 and $(x - \xi)_+^3$.

More generally, splines are a wide class of piecewise polynomial functions that are continuous and have continuous (higher-order) derivatives at the knots.

Definition 11.1. **(Spline).** A degree-N (or order $N + 1$) spline with knots $\xi_1, \ldots, \xi_K$ is a piecewise polynomial of degree N that has continuous derivatives up to order $N - 1$ at the knots.

The cubic spline example above is a degree-3 spline, and a continuous piecewise linear function is a degree-1 spline. While there are many ways to construct splines, a particularly convenient approach, at least theoretically, is based on the truncated-power basis. More specifically, let

$$g_j(x) = x^j, \quad j = 0, 1, \ldots, N,$$
$$g_{N+j}(x) = (x - \xi_j)_+^N, \quad j = 1, \ldots, K,$$

where $(\cdot)_+^N$ is the truncated power function with exponent N, i.e., $(t)_+^N = t^N$ for $t > 0$ and 0 otherwise. Then,

$$g(x) = \sum_{j=0}^{N+K} \beta_j \, g_j(x)$$

is a degree-N spline with knots $\xi_1, \ldots, \xi_K$.

The fit of a spline tends to be erratic near the boundary knots because of fewer data points at the extremes. As such, extrapolation beyond the boundaries can be wildly unreliable. One can ameliorate this problem by regularizing the spline outside the knots. An example is a **natural cubic spline**, which imposes additional restrictions that the function is linear beyond the boundary knots. This amounts to imposing four linear constraints on the coefficients $\beta_j, j = 0, 1, \ldots, 3 + K$. More specifically, starting from the cubic spline with knots at $\xi_1, \ldots, \xi_K$:

$$g(x) = \sum_{j=0}^{3} \beta_j \, x^j + \sum_{k=1}^{K} \beta_{3+k} \, (x - \xi_k)_+^3,$$

restricting that $g(x)$ is linear on $x < \xi_1$ and $x > \xi_K$ is equivalent (see Problem 11.18) to imposing the linear constraints:

$$\beta_2 = 0, \quad \beta_3 = 0, \quad \sum_{k=1}^{K} \beta_{3+k} = 0, \quad \sum_{k=1}^{K} \beta_{3+k} \, \xi_k = 0.$$

Note that for a natural cubic spline with K knots, there are K free parameters. Finally, the unknown parameters can be estimated by solving a linearly constrained least squares problem as formulated in (11.19).

Even though splines can be piecewise polynomials of any degree, in practice cubic splines are the most widely used. They tend to strike the right balance between flexibility and parsimony in most applications. The fitted curve typically also appears to be smooth to the naked eye.

In constructing a spline, we need to specify the number and the locations of the knots. Often domain knowledge about the application would help make these choices. If the relevant domain knowledge is unavailable, a standard practice is to select the number of knots using cross-validation. Since a spline function can be represented as a linear regression, its predicted residual sum ☞ 153 of squares can be computed easily (see Theorem 5.4). Then, given the number of knots, the locations can be set as the appropriate empirical percentiles of the data. For example, if the number of knots is chosen to be 3, typical choices of the locations are the 25-th, 50-th, and 75-th percentiles of x.

Example 11.8. In Example 5.18 we fitted various polynomial regression ☞ 154 functions for the data in Table 5.4 and found that a cubic polynomial had the best predictive performance. Here, we fit a cubic spline and a natural cubic spline using the same data. Given the relatively few observations of $n = 20$, we use $K = 3$ knots at the 25-th, 50-th, and 75-th percentiles of the data. To fit the cubic spline, we regress the response y on an intercept, x, x^2, x^3, $(x - \xi_1)_+^3$, $(x - \xi_2)_+^3$ and $(x - \xi_3)_+^3$, where $\xi_1, \xi_2,$ and ξ_3 are the knots. For the natural cubic spline, we impose four linear restrictions on the coefficients so that the splines are linear outside the boundary knots ξ_1 and ξ_3. In particular, the system of restrictions can be written as

$$
\underbrace{\begin{bmatrix} 0 & 0 & 1 & 0 & 0 & 0 & 0 \\ 0 & 0 & 0 & 1 & 0 & 0 & 0 \\ 0 & 0 & 0 & 0 & 1 & 1 & 1 \\ 0 & 0 & 0 & 0 & \xi_1 & \xi_2 & \xi_3 \end{bmatrix}}_{\mathbf{R}} \begin{bmatrix} \beta_1 \\ \beta_2 \\ \beta_3 \\ \beta_4 \\ \beta_5 \\ \beta_6 \\ \beta_7 \end{bmatrix} = \underbrace{\begin{bmatrix} 0 \\ 0 \\ 0 \\ 0 \end{bmatrix}}_{r} .
$$

Figure 11.5 plots the two estimated cubic splines together with the raw data. The cubic spline fits the data well and is very similar to the cubic polynomial regression function obtained using the least-squares method. In contrast, the natural cubic spline is much smoother than the other curves and it does not fit the data as closely. This is perhaps not surprising, given the moderate sample size of $n = 20$—the restriction that the natural cubic spline be linear outside the boundary knots has a relatively large impact on the shape of the curve.

The following Julia code implements the estimation of the two spline functions.

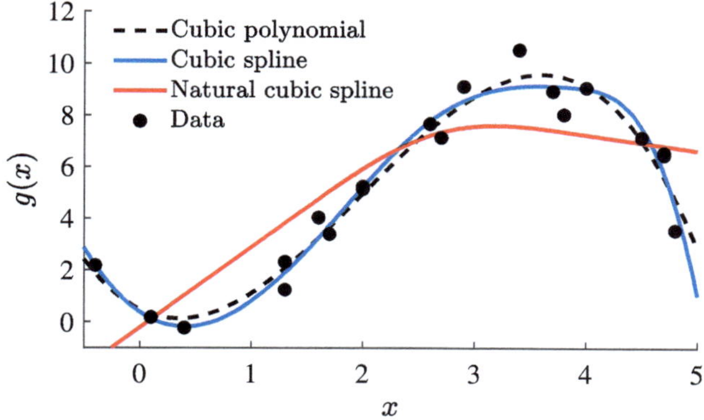

Fig. 11.5 The blue curve is the cubic spline function for the data in Table 5.4 (black dots), with three knots at the 25-th, 50-th, and 75-th percentiles of the data. The red curve is the natural cubic spline function. The dark dotted curve is the least-square cubic polynomial prediction function

```julia
spline.jl

using Plots, LinearAlgebra, StatsBase
x = [4.7,2,2.7,0.1,4.7,3.7,2,3.4,1.3,3.8,4.8,
    1.7,-0.4,4.5,1.3,0.4,2.6,4,2.9,1.6]
y = [6.57,5.15,7.15,0.18,6.48,8.95,5.24,10.54,1.24,8.05,3.56,
    3.4,2.18,7.16,2.32,-0.23,7.68,9.09,9.13,4.04]
n = length(x)
xi = quantile(x,[.25,.5,.75])   # knots
K = length(xi)

# cubic polynomial and cubic spline
X = hcat(ones(n),x,x.^2,x.^3)
beta_cp = (X'*X)(X'*y)
for k=1:K
    global X
    tmpX = (x .- xi[k]).^3;
    X = hcat(X,tmpX.*(tmpX.>0))
end
beta_cs = (X'*X)(X'*y)

# natural cubic spline
R = [0 0 1 0 0 0 0; 0 0 0 1 0 0 0; 0 0 0 0 1 1 1; 0 0 0 0 xi']
r = zeros(4)
A = vcat(hcat(X'*X,R'), hcat(R,zeros(4,4)))
```

```julia
beta_ns = A\vcat(X'*y,r)

xtilde = minimum(x):0.01:maximum(x)
ngrid = length(xtilde)
Xtilde = hcat(ones(ngrid),xtilde,xtilde.^2,xtilde.^3)
cp = Xtilde*beta_cp
for k=1:K
    global Xtilde
    tmp = (xtilde .- xi[k]).^3
    Xtilde = hcat(Xtilde,tmp.*(tmp.>0))
end
cspline = Xtilde*beta_cs
nspline = Xtilde*beta_ns[1:K+4]

plot(xtilde,cp,lw=2,color=:black,ls=:dash)
plot!(xtilde,cspline,lw=2,color=:blue,legend=false)
plot!(xtilde,nspline,lw=2,color=:red,legend=false)
scatter!(x,y,color=:black)
```

The previous approach of constructing a spline requires the specification of the number and the locations of the knots. The estimated spline is often sensitive to these choices, especially in applications with moderate sample sizes. An alternative approach avoids this specification problem by using a maximal set of knots: a knot is placed at every data point. Of course, this leads to overfitting, and regularization is used to control this overfitting problem.

More specifically, a **cubic smoothing spline** is defined as the minimizer of the penalized residual sum of squares

$$\widehat{g} = \underset{g}{\mathrm{argmin}} \sum_{i=1}^{n} (y_i - g(x_i))^2 + \lambda \int (g''(t))^2 \, \mathrm{d}t, \qquad (11.21)$$

where $\lambda \geq 0$ is a regularization parameter. It is clear that when $\lambda = 0$, a solution must satisfy $\widehat{g}(x_i) = y_i$, and this gives a perfect fit of the data with zero residual sum of squares. This is obviously undesirable—it is overfitting at its worst. Similar to the ridge regression defined in (9.7), the objective function also includes a penalty term that regularizes the solution and penalizes a more wiggly function with a large (absolute) second derivative. More specifically, it penalizes any function whose second derivative is not identically 0, i.e., any function that is not a line. In the limit $\lambda \to \infty$, the solution to the minimization problem in (11.21) coincides with the ordinary least squares regression line.

☞ 274

It is also possible to define a smoothing spline of any odd degree N by replacing the penalty term by $\lambda \int (g^{(N+1)/2}(t))^2 \, dt$. However, cubic smoothing splines with $N = 3$ are by far the most commonly used in applications.

For any finite $\lambda > 0$, (11.21) is an infinite-dimensional optimization problem over all functions g for the which the penalty term is defined. Remarkably, it can be shown that the minimizer is a *natural cubic spline* with knots at the data points $x_1, \ldots, x_n$; see, e.g., Green and Silverman (1993) and Hastie et al. (2009, Exercise 5.7).

Theorem 11.2. (Cubic Smoothing Spline). Given the data points $a < x_1 < \cdots < x_n < b$, if $g(x)$ is any twice differentiable function on $[a, b]$, then there exists a natural cubic spline $\widehat{g}$ with knots at $x_1, \ldots, x_n$ such that $\widehat{g}(x_i) = g(x_i), i = 1, \ldots, n$ and

$$\int_a^b (\widehat{g}''(t))^2 \, dt \leq \int_a^b (g''(t))^2 \, dt \, .$$

Proof. Since a natural cubic spline with n knots has n free parameters and its basis spans $\mathbb{R}^n$ for any n points $z_i = g(x_i), i = 1, \ldots, n$, we can find a natural cubic spline $\widehat{g}(x)$ with knots at $x_1, \ldots, x_n$ that satisfies $\widehat{g}(x_i) = z_i = g(x_i)$. This proves the first part of the theorem.

To prove the second part of the theorem, define $h(x) = g(x) - \widehat{g}(x)$. We claim that

$$\int_a^b \widehat{g}''(t) \, h''(t) \, dt = 0 \, . \tag{11.22}$$

Then, using $g''(x) = \widehat{g}''(x) + h''(x)$, we have

$$\int_a^b g''(t)^2 \, dt = \int_a^b \left(\widehat{g}''(t) + h''(t) \right)^2 \, dt$$

$$= \int_a^b \widehat{g}''(t)^2 \, dt + \int_a^b h''(t)^2 \, dt$$

$$\geq \int_a^b \widehat{g}''(t)^2 \, dt \, ,$$

where the second equality holds because of (11.22).

Finally, the claim (11.22) can be proved by using integration by parts:

$$\int_a^b \widehat{g}''(t)\, h''(t)\, \mathrm{d}t = \left[\widehat{g}''(t)\, h'(t)\right]_a^b - \int_a^b \widehat{g}^{(3)}(t)\, h'(t)\, \mathrm{d}t$$

$$= -\int_{x_1}^{x_n} \widehat{g}^{(3)}(t)\, h'(t)\, \mathrm{d}t$$

$$= -\sum_{i=1}^{n-1} \int_{x_i}^{x_{i+1}} \widehat{g}^{(3)}(t)\, h'(t)\, \mathrm{d}t$$

$$= -\sum_{i=1}^{n-1} \left\{ \left[\widehat{g}^{(3)}(t)\, h(t)\right]_{x_i}^{x_{i+1}} - \int_{x_i}^{x_{i+1}} \widehat{g}^{(4)}(t)\, h(t)\, \mathrm{d}t \right\}$$

$$= -\sum_{i=1}^{n-1} \widehat{g}^{(3)}(x_i^{+})(h(x_{i+1}) - h(x_i)) = 0 \,,$$

where the second equality holds because $\widehat{g}$ is a natural cubic spline that is linear outside the boundary knots x_1 and x_n; the fourth equality holds because $\widehat{g}^{(3)}$ is constant on (x_i, x_{i+1}) and $\widehat{g}^{(4)} = 0$; and the last equality follows from $h(x_i) = 0, i = 1, \ldots, n$.

An implication of Theorem 11.2 is that we can restrict our attention to the class of natural cubic splines with knots at the data points $x_1, \ldots, x_n$ in solving the functional optimization problem in (11.21). A natural cubic spline with n knots has n free parameters, and it can be represented as

$$\widehat{g}(x) = \sum_{j=1}^n \alpha_j\, g_j(x)$$

for some piecewise cubic polynomial functions $g_j, j = 1, \ldots, n$. Let $v_{ij} = g_j(x_i)$ and

$$k_{ij} = \int_a^b g_i''(t)\, g_j''(t)\, \mathrm{d}t \,,$$

and define $\mathbf{V} = [v_{ij}]$ and $\mathbf{K} = [k_{ij}]$. Then, the functional optimization problem in (11.21) reduces to the following finite-dimensional minimization problem

$$\widehat{\boldsymbol{\alpha}} = \operatorname*{argmin}_{\boldsymbol{\alpha}} \|\boldsymbol{y} - \mathbf{V}\boldsymbol{\alpha}\|^2 + \lambda \boldsymbol{\alpha}^\top \mathbf{K} \boldsymbol{\alpha} \,. \tag{11.23}$$

This is a slightly more general version of the ridge regression problem discussed in (9.7). It has an explicit solution (see Problem 11.19)

☞ 274

$$\widehat{\boldsymbol{\alpha}} = \left(\mathbf{V}^\top \mathbf{V} + \lambda \mathbf{K}\right)^{-1} \mathbf{V}^\top \boldsymbol{y} \,.$$

Therefore, the estimated prediction function has the form of a linear smoother

$$\widehat{g}(x) = \left[g_1(x) \ldots g_n(x)\right] \left(\mathbf{V}^\top \mathbf{V} + \lambda \mathbf{K}\right)^{-1} \mathbf{V}^\top \boldsymbol{y} \,,$$

where $g_j(x)$ is a function of x and the data $x_1, \ldots, x_n$.

A natural question is whether there exists a kernel function κ such that $\widehat{g}(x)$ can be represented as $\widehat{g}(x) = \sum_{j=1}^{n} \widehat{\alpha}_j \, \kappa(x, x_j)$ for some linear functions $\widehat{\alpha}_1, \ldots, \widehat{\alpha}_n$ of the responses $y_1, \ldots, y_n$. It turns out that the answer is true, with the kernel function (see, e.g., Kroese et al. (2019, Section 6.6)) given by

$$\kappa(x, u) = \frac{1}{2} \max\{x, u\} \min\{x, u\}^2 - \frac{1}{6} \min\{x, u\}^3 \, .$$

This thus shows that a cubic smoothing spline is equivalent to a kernel regression estimator.

11.5 Gaussian Process Regression

A Gaussian process can be thought of as a generalization of a multivariate Gaussian (i.e., normal) random vector, in the same way that the latter generalizes one-dimensional normal random variables.

Definition 11.2. (Gaussian Process). A **Gaussian process** on an index set $\mathcal{X} \subseteq \mathbb{R}^d$ is a stochastic process $Z = \{Z_{\boldsymbol{x}}, \boldsymbol{x} \in \mathcal{X}\}$ where, for any choice of indices $\boldsymbol{x}_1, \ldots, \boldsymbol{x}_n$ and n, the vector $[Z_{\boldsymbol{x}_1}, \ldots, Z_{\boldsymbol{x}_n}]^{\top}$ has a multivariate Gaussian distribution.

An alternative, but equivalent, definition is that any linear combination $\sum_{i=1}^{n} a_i Z_{\boldsymbol{x}_i}$ has a Gaussian distribution. The probability distribution of a Gaussian process Z is thus completely specified by its **expectation function**

$$\mu(\boldsymbol{x}) = \mathbb{E} Z_{\boldsymbol{x}}, \quad \boldsymbol{x} \in \mathcal{X}$$

and **covariance function**

$$\kappa(\boldsymbol{x}, \boldsymbol{x}') = \mathrm{Cov}(Z_{\boldsymbol{x}}, Z_{\boldsymbol{x}'}), \quad \boldsymbol{x}, \boldsymbol{x}' \in \mathcal{X} \, ,$$

in the same way that a multivariate normal distribution is completely determined by its mean vector and covariance matrix. We write $Z \sim \mathrm{GP}(\mu, \kappa)$. We already encountered covariance functions (kernel functions) in Sect. 11.3. A **zero-mean** Gaussian process is one for which $\mu(\boldsymbol{x}) = 0$ for all $\boldsymbol{x}$.

Example 11.9 (Two Gaussian Processes). Figure 11.6 displays five different paths of two Gaussian processes on the interval $[0, 1]$. The paths on the left correspond to the Wiener process; that is, the zero-mean Gaussian process with covariance function $\kappa(x, x') = \min\{x, x'\}$. The paths on the right are of a zero-mean Gaussian process with a Gaussian kernel (11.18), with $b = 0.2$. Note that in this case the paths are smooth, whereas the Wiener process has extremely ragged paths. In fact, the paths of the Wiener process are nowhere differentiable. Also, for the Wiener process $Z_x \sim \mathcal{N}(0, \kappa(x,x)) = \mathcal{N}(0,x)$, whereas for the second Gaussian process the distribution of each Z_x is $\mathcal{N}(0,1)$.

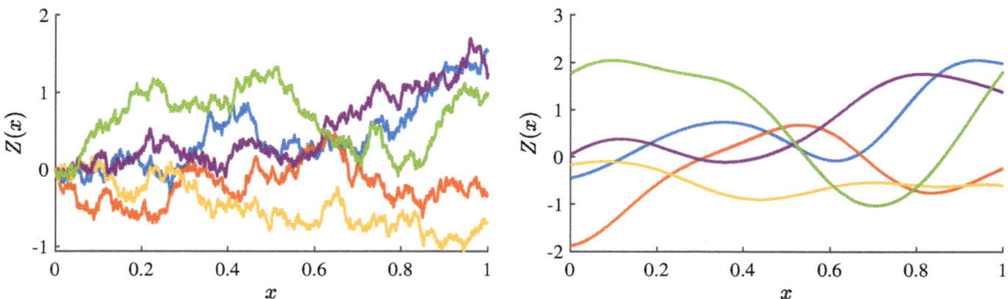

Fig. 11.6 Left: five realizations of the Wiener process. Right: five realizations of a Gaussian process with a Gaussian kernel, with bandwidth parameter $b = 0.2$

The following Julia code can be used to simulate the paths (uncomment the desired kernel function). To simulate a Gaussian random vector, we can use Algorithm 3.3, via a Cholesky factorization $\mathbf{K} = \mathbf{BB}^\top$ of the Gram matrix. To circumvent numerical issues with the Cholesky factorization, we establish a different factorization using a singular value decomposition $\mathbf{K} = \mathbf{USV}^\top$ and defining $\mathbf{B} = \mathbf{U}\sqrt{\mathbf{S}}$.

```julia
gp_wienkern.jl

using LinearAlgebra, Plots
xx = 0:0.001:1
kappa(x, u) = min(x, u)
# sigma = 0.2;
# kappa(x,u) = exp(-(x-u)^2/(2*sigma^2))
n = length(xx)
K = zeros(n, n)
for i = 1:n
    for j = 1:n
        K[i, j] = kappa(xx[i], xx[j])
    end
end
U, S, V = svd(K); # singular value decomposition
B = U * diagm(sqrt.(S));
g = plot()
for i = 1:5
    global g
    yy = B * randn(n)
    g = plot!(xx, yy, legend=false)
    display(g)
end
```

The idea of **Gaussian process regression** is to represent the regression function as a Gaussian process and to update its distribution using Bayesian principles.

Specifically, if g represents the regression function, then the prior information on g is modeled as

$$(g \mid b) \sim \mathrm{GP}(0, \kappa) \,, \tag{11.24}$$

where κ is a given covariance function, which may depend on one or more parameters b. For simplicity, we assume that κ is a scaled Gaussian kernel for some given bandwidth parameter b. For the likelihood of the data, we follow the standard regression model that the feature vectors $\boldsymbol{x}_1, \ldots, \boldsymbol{x}_n$ are fixed and the responses $y_1, \ldots, y_n$ are such that

$$(y_i \mid g, b, \sigma^2) = g(\boldsymbol{x}_i) + \varepsilon_i \,, \quad i = 1, \ldots, n \,, \tag{11.25}$$

where $\{\varepsilon_i\} \stackrel{\text{iid}}{\sim} \mathcal{N}(0, \sigma^2)$ and σ^2 is a known parameter. Observe that the conditional distribution of $\boldsymbol{y}$ given g is the same as the conditional distribution of $\boldsymbol{y}$ given only the vector of regression values $\boldsymbol{g} = [g(\boldsymbol{x}_1), \ldots, g(\boldsymbol{x}_n)]^{\top}$. This means that instead of using the prior (11.24) and likelihood (11.25), we may simplify our Bayesian model by considering only the prior and likelihood information on the random vectors $\boldsymbol{y} = [y_1, \ldots, y_n]^{\top}$ and $\boldsymbol{g}$. Firstly, the prior information on $\boldsymbol{g}$ follows directly from (11.24)

$$(\boldsymbol{g} \mid b) \sim \mathcal{N}(\boldsymbol{0}, \mathbf{K}) \,, \tag{11.26}$$

where $\mathbf{K} = [\kappa(\boldsymbol{x}_i, \boldsymbol{x}_j)]$ is the Gram matrix associated with the kernel κ. Secondly, from (11.25), the likelihood of $\boldsymbol{y}$ given $\boldsymbol{g}$ (and for a given b and σ^2) satisfies

$$(\boldsymbol{y} \mid \boldsymbol{g}, b, \sigma^2) \sim \mathcal{N}(\boldsymbol{g}, \sigma^2 \mathbb{I}_n) \,. \tag{11.27}$$

Solving this finite-dimensional Bayesian problem involves deriving the posterior distribution of $(\boldsymbol{g} \mid \boldsymbol{y}, b, \sigma^2)$. As both (11.26) and (11.27) involve multivariate normal distributions, and b and σ^2 are fixed, the joint distribution of $\boldsymbol{y}$ and $\boldsymbol{g}$ is again multivariate normal. Namely, let $\mathbf{B}$ be such that $\mathbf{K} = \mathbf{B}\mathbf{B}^{\top}$. From (11.26) and (11.27), we can write

$$\boldsymbol{g} = \mathbf{B}\boldsymbol{U},$$
$$\boldsymbol{y} = \boldsymbol{g} + \sigma\boldsymbol{V} = \mathbf{B}\boldsymbol{U} + \sigma\boldsymbol{V} \,,$$

where $\boldsymbol{U} \sim \mathcal{N}(\boldsymbol{0}, \mathbb{I}_n)$ and $\boldsymbol{V} \sim \mathcal{N}(\boldsymbol{0}, \mathbb{I}_n)$ are independent. Hence,

$$\begin{bmatrix} \boldsymbol{y} \\ \boldsymbol{g} \end{bmatrix} = \begin{bmatrix} \mathbf{B} & \sigma\,\mathbb{I}_n \\ \mathbf{B} & \mathbf{O} \end{bmatrix} \begin{bmatrix} \boldsymbol{U} \\ \boldsymbol{V} \end{bmatrix},$$

which shows that

$$\begin{bmatrix} \boldsymbol{y} \\ \boldsymbol{g} \end{bmatrix} \sim \mathcal{N}(\mathbf{0}, \mathbf{D}), \quad \mathbf{D} = \begin{bmatrix} \mathbf{B} & \sigma\,\mathbb{I}_n \\ \mathbf{B} & \mathbf{O} \end{bmatrix} \begin{bmatrix} \mathbf{B}^\top & \mathbf{B}^\top \\ \sigma\,\mathbb{I}_n & \mathbf{O} \end{bmatrix} = \begin{bmatrix} \mathbf{K} + \sigma^2\,\mathbb{I}_n & \mathbf{K} \\ \mathbf{K} & \mathbf{K} \end{bmatrix}. \tag{11.28}$$

In particular, the likelihood of $\boldsymbol{y}$ as a function of the bandwidth b and noise level σ is given by

$$f(\boldsymbol{y} \mid b, \sigma^2) = \frac{1}{\sqrt{(2\pi)^n |\mathbf{K} + \sigma^2\,\mathbb{I}_n|}} \exp\left(-\frac{1}{2} \boldsymbol{y}^\top (\mathbf{K} + \sigma^2\,\mathbb{I}_n)^2 \boldsymbol{y} \right). \tag{11.29}$$

☞ 86   Moreover, by Theorem 3.8, it follows that the posterior of $\boldsymbol{g}$ given the data $\boldsymbol{y}$ satisfies

$$(\boldsymbol{g} \mid \boldsymbol{y}, b, \sigma^2) \sim \mathcal{N}\left(\mathbf{K}(\mathbf{K} + \sigma^2\,\mathbb{I}_n)^{-1}\boldsymbol{y}, \ \mathbf{K} - \mathbf{K}(\mathbf{K} + \sigma^2\,\mathbb{I}_n)^{-1}\mathbf{K} \right). \tag{11.30}$$

The covariance matrix can be written more compactly as $\sigma^2\mathbf{K}(\mathbf{K} + \sigma^2\,\mathbb{I}_n)^{-1}$; see Problem 11.14.

More importantly, we can derive the posterior distribution of $g(\widetilde{\boldsymbol{x}})$ for a *new* input $\widetilde{\boldsymbol{x}}$. From the prior information, we know that the random vector $[\boldsymbol{g}^\top, g(\widetilde{\boldsymbol{x}})]^\top$ has a Gaussian distribution with zero mean and covariance matrix

$$\begin{bmatrix} \mathbf{K} & \boldsymbol{\kappa} \\ \boldsymbol{\kappa}^\top & \kappa(\widetilde{\boldsymbol{x}}, \widetilde{\boldsymbol{x}}) \end{bmatrix},$$

where $\boldsymbol{\kappa} = [\kappa(\boldsymbol{x}_1, \widetilde{\boldsymbol{x}}), \ldots, \kappa(\boldsymbol{x}_n, \widetilde{\boldsymbol{x}})]^\top$. Since $\boldsymbol{y} = \boldsymbol{g} + \sigma\boldsymbol{V}$, with $\boldsymbol{V} \sim \mathcal{N}(\mathbf{0}, \mathbb{I}_n)$, it follows that the random vector $[\boldsymbol{y}^\top, g(\widetilde{\boldsymbol{x}})]^\top$ has a $\mathcal{N}(\mathbf{0}, \mathbf{C})$ distribution with covariance matrix

$$\mathbf{C} = \begin{bmatrix} \mathbf{K} + \sigma^2\,\mathbb{I}_n & \boldsymbol{\kappa} \\ \boldsymbol{\kappa}^\top & \kappa(\widetilde{\boldsymbol{x}}, \widetilde{\boldsymbol{x}}) \end{bmatrix}. \tag{11.31}$$

Consequently, by Theorem 3.8, $(g(\widetilde{\boldsymbol{x}}) \mid \boldsymbol{y})$ has a normal distribution with mean and variance given respectively by

$$\mu(\widetilde{\boldsymbol{x}}) = \boldsymbol{\kappa}^\top (\mathbf{K} + \sigma^2\,\mathbb{I}_n)^{-1}\boldsymbol{y} \tag{11.32}$$

and

$$\sigma^2(\widetilde{\boldsymbol{x}}) = \kappa(\widetilde{\boldsymbol{x}}, \widetilde{\boldsymbol{x}}) - \boldsymbol{\kappa}^\top (\mathbf{K} + \sigma^2\,\mathbb{I}_n)^{-1}\boldsymbol{\kappa}. \tag{11.33}$$

These are the **predictive mean** and **predictive variance**. In particular, the predictive mean is equal to the expectation of a new response $\widetilde{y} \sim \mathcal{N}(g(\widetilde{\boldsymbol{x}}), \sigma^2)$ given the data; that is, $\mathbb{E}[\widetilde{y} \mid \boldsymbol{y}] = \mathbb{E}[g(\widetilde{\boldsymbol{x}}) \mid \boldsymbol{y}] = \mu(\widetilde{\boldsymbol{x}})$ in (11.32).

There remains the issue of how to choose the (hyper)parameters b and σ. A quick frequentist approach is to simply choose those as the maximum likelihood estimates of (11.29). This procedure is sometimes called **empirical Bayes**. Taking the logarithm, we thus need to solve

$$\max_{b>0,\sigma>0}\left\{-\frac{n}{2}\ln(2\pi)-\frac{1}{2}\ln|\mathbf{K}+\sigma^2\,\mathbb{I}_n|-\frac{1}{2}\boldsymbol{y}^\top(\mathbf{K}+\sigma^2\,\mathbb{I}_n)^{-1}\boldsymbol{y}\right\},\quad(11.34)$$

where we can ignore the constant first term.

Example 11.10 (GP Regression). In Example 5.18, we established that the best (in terms of predictive performance) polynomial regression function for the data in Table 5.4. is a cubic polynomial. In the current example, we wish to determine the GP regression function for these data. Figure 5.4 shows a dotplot of the data. The response data lie between -0.23 and 10.54, with a mean of $\overline{y}=5.394$. In our investigation we will use a mix of Bayesian and frequentist ideas. We take the Gaussian kernel (11.18) multiplied by 10, to better match the spread of the data. The bandwidth b and noise level σ are determined numerically from (11.34). Figure 11.7 shows the contour plot of the log-likelihood. The maximizer $(\widehat{\sigma},\widehat{b})$ of this function is found to be $(0.841,1.50)$.

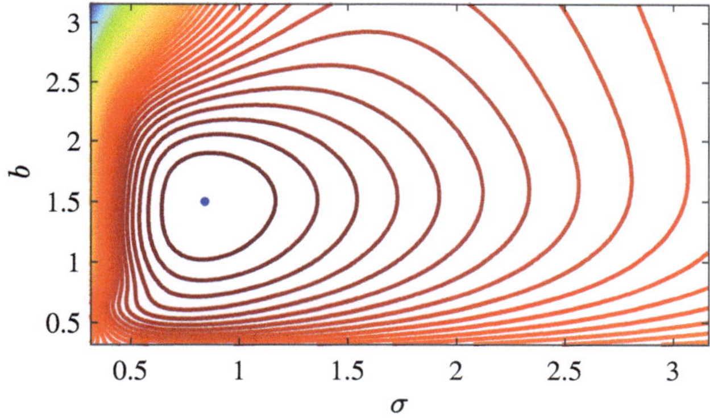

Fig. 11.7 Contour plot of the log-likelihood function as a function of the noise level σ and the bandwidth b. The maximizer is indicated by a blue dot

Figure 11.8 shows the GP regression function for the data in Table 5.4, using the above values for σ and b. We obtain a smooth curve that is quite close to the best cubic polynomial regression function that is estimated via the least-squares method. The Julia code follows.

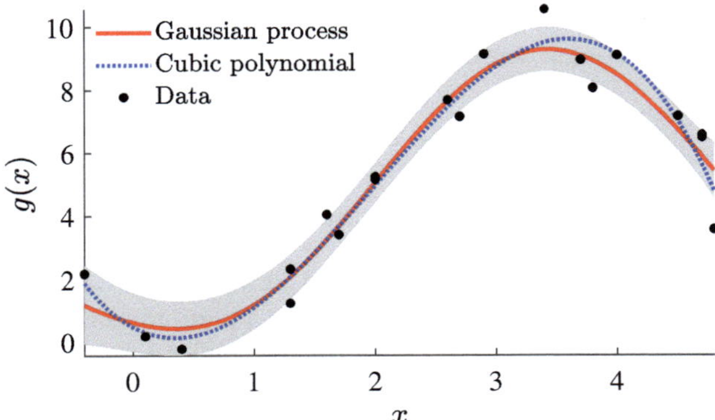

Fig. 11.8 The red curve is the GP regression function for the data in Table 5.4 (black dots), using a scaled Gaussian kernel with multiplication factor 10 and bandwidth $b = 1.50$. The noise level is $\sigma = 0.841$. The blue dotted curve is the least-square cubic polynomial prediction function. The shaded region is the 95% confidence band, corresponding to the predictive variance given in (11.33)

```julia
gpreg.jl

using Plots, LinearAlgebra, StatsBase
x = [4.7,2,2.7,0.1,4.7,3.7,2,3.4,1.3,3.8,4.8,
     1.7,-0.4,4.5,1.3,0.4,2.6,4,2.9,1.6]
y = [6.57,5.15,7.15,0.18,6.48,8.95,5.24,10.54,1.24,8.05,
     3.56,3.4,2.18,7.16,2.32,-0.23,7.68,9.09,9.13,4.04]
n = length(x)

# construct the optimal cubic regression polynomial
X = ones(n)
for k=1:3
    global X
    X = hcat(X, x.^k)    # make the design matrix
end
beta = X'*X(X'*y)   # optimal parameters
g(x,beta)=beta[1] .+ beta[2]*x .+ beta[3]*x.^2 .+ beta[4]*x.^3

b = 1.5; sigma = 0.841  # optimal hyperparameters
k(x,u,b) =  10*exp(-0.5*norm(x- u)^2/b^2) # scaled kernel

# function to construct the predictive mean and variance
function gp_pred(xtest, xtrain, ytrain, sigma, b, k)
    T = length(xtrain); N = length(xtest)
    K = zeros(T, T)
    mu = zeros(N); sigma_squared = zeros(N)
```

```
    for z = 1:N
        kappa = zeros(T)
        for i = 1:T
            kappa[i] = k(xtest[z], xtrain[i], b)
            for j = 1:T
                K[i, j] = k(xtrain[i], xtrain[j], b)
            end
        end
        mu[z] = kappa' * (K + sigma^2 * I)^(-1) * ytrain
        sigma_squared[z] = k(xtest[z], xtest[z], b) - kappa' *
            (K + sigma^2 * I)^(-1) * kappa
    end
    return mu, sigma_squared
end

xtilde = minimum(x):0.01:maximum(x)
mu,sigsquare = gp_pred(xtilde,x,y,sigma,b,k)
lo = mu -1.96*sqrt.(sigsquare); hi = mu+1.96*sqrt.(sigsquare);
plot(xtilde, mu,lw=2,color=:red,legend=false)
plot!(xtilde, mu, ribbon = (lo .- hi) ./ 2, fillalpha = 0.1,
    color=:black)
plot!(xtilde, mu,lw=2,color=:red)
plot!(xtilde,g(xtilde,beta),lw=2,color=:blue,ls=:dash)
scatter!(x,y,c=:black)
```

11.6 Problems

11.1. Let $X_1, \ldots, X_n \sim_{\text{iid}} \mathcal{U}(0, 1)$. Show that the r-th order statistic $X_{(r)}$ has a $\mathsf{Beta}(\alpha, \beta)$ distribution for some α and β, and identify the parameters. Derive the expectation of $X_{(r)}$ for $r = 1, \ldots, n$. ☞ 74

11.2. Let $X_1, \ldots, X_n \sim_{\text{iid}} \mathsf{Exp}(1)$. Show that conditional on $X_{(1)} = x$, the shifted order statistics $X_{(2)} - x, \ldots, X_{(n)} - x$ have the same joint distribution as $n - 1$ order statistics from the $\mathsf{Exp}(1)$ distribution. Use this to show that the moment generating function of the r-th order statistic is given by

$$\mathbb{E}e^{tX_{(r)}} = \prod_{k=r+1}^{n} \frac{k}{k-t}, \quad t < r+1.$$

11.3. In Sect. 11.2.1 we introduced Wilcoxon's positive-rank sum test statistic T^+, which sums the ranks of the absolute values for *positive* measurements. Similarly, we could sum the ranks of the absolute values for *negative* measurements, to give a test statistic T^-. The Wilcoxon **signed-rank test** statistic is

$T = T^+ - T^-$. That is, we first rank the absolute values of the measurements and then add them multiplied with the sign of the measurements.

Show that under the null hypothesis that the sampling distribution is symmetric around 0 the expectation and variance of T are given by

$$\mathbb{E}T = 0 \quad \text{and} \quad \operatorname{Var}(T) = \frac{1}{6}n(n+1)(2n+1).$$

11.4. Show that under the null hypothesis $H_0 : \mu = 0$ the rank sum test statistic T^+ in (11.9) has probability generating function

$$G(z) = \sum_{k=0}^{n(n+1)/2} z^k\, \mathbb{P}(T^+ = k) = 2^{-n} \prod_{r=1}^{n} (1 + z^r), \quad |z| \le 1.$$

For $n = 10$ use a symbolic computing package to expand $G(z)$ to find the exact probabilities $\mathbb{P}(T^+ = k)$ for $k = 0, \ldots, 55$. As a check, you should have $\mathbb{P}(T^+ = 31) = 39/1024$.

11.5. The data in Table 11.4, taken from Cox and Snell (1981), present the breaking loads of two types of yarns, from six different bobbins (spools). Ignoring the bobbin types, conduct a Wilcoxon ranked sum test to assess whether the two types of yarn have different breaking loads.

Table 11.4 Breaking loads (in ounce = 28.35 gram)

Bobbin	1	2	3	4	5	6
Yarn A	15.0	15.7	14.8	14.9	13.0	15.9
	17.0	15.6	15.8	14.2	16.2	15.6
	13.8	17.6	18.2	15.0	16.4	15.0
	15.5	17.1	16.0	12.8	14.8	15.5
Yarn B	18.2	17.2	15.2	15.6	19.2	16.2
	16.8	18.5	15.9	16.0	18.0	15.9
	18.1	15.0	14.5	15.2	17.0	14.9
	17.0	16.2	14.2	14.9	16.9	15.5

11.6. The **sinc kernel** on $\mathbb{R}$ is given by

$$\kappa(x, x') = \operatorname{sinc}(x - x'),$$

where $\operatorname{sinc}(z) = \sin(z)/z$ for $z \ne 0$ and $\operatorname{sinc}(0) = 1$. Show that κ is indeed a valid kernel function. Hint: consider the characteristic function of $X \sim \mathcal{U}[-1, 1]$.

11.7. Let $\psi(t) = \frac{1}{2}\mathbb{1}\{|t| \le 1\}$ be the pdf of a uniformly distributed random variable on the interval $[-1, 1]$. Show that the function $\kappa(x, x') = \psi(x - x')$

is not a kernel function. Hint: consider a matrix $\mathbf{K} = [\kappa(x_i, x_j), i, j = 1, 2, 3]$ for certain x_1, x_2, and x_3.

11.8. Let $\mathcal{X}$ be an arbitrary set. If κ is a kernel function on $\mathbb{R}^m$ and ϕ is a function from $\mathcal{X}$ to $\mathbb{R}^m$, then $\lambda(\boldsymbol{x}, \boldsymbol{x}') = \kappa(\phi(\boldsymbol{x}), \phi(\boldsymbol{x}'))$ defines a kernel function λ on $\mathcal{X}$. Prove this.

11.9. If κ is a kernel function on $\mathcal{X}$ and $f : \mathcal{X} \to \mathbb{R}_+$ is a function, then $\lambda(\boldsymbol{x}, \boldsymbol{x}') = f(\boldsymbol{x})\kappa(\boldsymbol{x}, \boldsymbol{x}')f(\boldsymbol{x}')$ defines a kernel function λ on $\mathcal{X}$. Prove this.

11.10. Show that if κ_1 and κ_2 are kernel functions on $\mathcal{X}$, then so is their sum $\kappa = \kappa_1 + \kappa_2$.

11.11. Let κ_1 and κ_2 be kernel functions on $\mathcal{X}$ of the form

$$\kappa(\boldsymbol{x}, \boldsymbol{x}') = \phi(\boldsymbol{x})^\top \phi(\boldsymbol{x}') = \sum_i \phi_i(\boldsymbol{x})\phi_i(\boldsymbol{x}') \tag{11.35}$$

determined by some finite- or infinite-dimensional feature function $\phi(\boldsymbol{x}) = [\phi_1(\boldsymbol{x}), \phi_2(\boldsymbol{x}), \ldots]^\top$, $\boldsymbol{x} \in \mathcal{X}$. Show that their product $\lambda = \kappa_1 \kappa_2$ is again a kernel function on $\mathcal{X}$ and is also of the form (11.35).

11.12. Let κ be a kernel function on $\mathcal{X}$ and let p be a positive integer. Using Problems 11.10 and 11.11, prove that the function

$$\lambda(\boldsymbol{x}, \boldsymbol{x}') = (1 + \kappa(\boldsymbol{x}, \boldsymbol{x}'))^p, \quad \boldsymbol{x} \in \mathcal{X}$$

is a kernel function on $\mathcal{X}$. Such a kernel function is said to be a **polynomial** kernel function.

For the special case $\kappa(x, x') = xx', x \in \mathbb{R}$, show that λ is of the form

$$\lambda(x, x') = \phi(x)^\top \phi(x'),$$

where $\phi(x)$ is a feature vector of dimension $p+1$ that involves the polynomials $1, x, \ldots, x^{p+1}$.

11.13. Let κ be a kernel function on $\mathcal{X}$ and let $\{q_j, j = 1, \ldots, m\}$ be real-valued functions on $\mathcal{X}$. Generalizing (11.13) and (11.17), consider prediction functions of the form

$$g(\boldsymbol{x}) = \sum_{i=1}^{n} \alpha_i \, \kappa(\boldsymbol{x}_i, \boldsymbol{x}) + \sum_{j=1}^{m} \eta_j \, q_j(\boldsymbol{x}), \tag{11.36}$$

where the optimal parameters $\boldsymbol{\alpha} = [\alpha_1, \ldots, \alpha_n]^\top$ and $\boldsymbol{\eta} = [\eta_1, \ldots, \eta_m]^\top$ are found from the regularized optimization problem:

$$\min_{\boldsymbol{\alpha}, \boldsymbol{\eta}} \| \boldsymbol{y} - (\mathbf{K}\boldsymbol{\alpha} + \mathbf{Q}\boldsymbol{\eta}) \|^2 + \gamma \, \boldsymbol{\alpha}^\top \mathbf{K}\boldsymbol{\alpha}, \tag{11.37}$$

where $\gamma > 0$ is a regularization parameter, $\mathbf{K}$ is the $n \times n$ Gram matrix, and $\mathbf{Q}$ is the $n \times m$ matrix with entries $[q_j(\boldsymbol{x}_i), i = 1, \ldots, n, \; j = 1, \ldots, m]$. This is a convex optimization problem, and its solution can be found by differentiating the function to minimize in (11.37) with respect to $\boldsymbol{\alpha}$ and $\boldsymbol{\eta}$ and equating the result to the zero vector. Find the corresponding system of $(n+m)$ linear equations.

11.14. Assuming that $\mathbf{K}$ is invertible, derive (11.30) directly from Theorem 8.1 and show that

$$\mathbf{K} - \mathbf{K}(\mathbf{K} + \sigma^2 \, \mathbb{I}_n)^{-1}\mathbf{K} = \sigma^2 \, \mathbf{K} \, (\mathbf{K} + \sigma^2 \, \mathbb{I}_n)^{-1} \, .$$

Hint: use the following matrix identity for symmetric invertible matrices:

$$\mathbf{A}^{-1} + \mathbf{B}^{-1} = \mathbf{B}(\mathbf{A} + \mathbf{B})^{-1}\mathbf{A} = \mathbf{A}(\mathbf{A} + \mathbf{B})^{-1}\mathbf{B} \, . \qquad (11.38)$$

11.15. In the GP regression model in Sect. 11.5, we have taken the mean function for the prior distribution of g to be identically zero. If instead we have a general mean function m and replace the prior (11.26) with

$$(\boldsymbol{g} \mid b) \sim \mathcal{N}(\boldsymbol{m}, \mathbf{K}) \, , \qquad (11.39)$$

for some mean vector $\boldsymbol{m} = [m(\boldsymbol{x}_1), \ldots, m(\boldsymbol{x}_n)]^{\top}$, what do the predictive mean (11.32) and variance (11.33) change to?

11.16. Consider again the GP regression model in Sect. 11.5, but now with a prior on σ^2, while the bandwidth b remains a constant.

  a. Assuming $\mathbf{K}$ is invertible, show that the prior $f(\sigma^2) = 1/\sigma^2$ yields

$$(\sigma^2 \mid \boldsymbol{y}, \boldsymbol{g}, b) \sim \mathsf{InvGamma}\left(\frac{n}{2}, \frac{1}{2}\|\boldsymbol{y} - \boldsymbol{g}\|^2\right) \, . \qquad (11.40)$$

  b. Since we already derived the distribution of $(\boldsymbol{g} \mid \boldsymbol{y}, \sigma^2, b)$ in (11.30), we can simulate from the joint posterior of $\boldsymbol{g}$ and σ^2. Modify the Julia program in Example 11.10 to simulate from posterior pdf of $\boldsymbol{g}$ and σ^2 and determine the posterior expectation of σ. Use a bandwidth of $b = 1.5$.

11.17. Consider a function of the form

$$g(x) = \beta_0 + \beta_1 x + \beta_2 x^2 + \beta_3 x^3 + \beta_4 (x - \xi)_+^3 \, ,$$

where $(t)_+^3 = t^3$ if $t > 0$ and 0 otherwise. Show that $g(x)$ is a piecewise cubic polynomial, continuous at ξ, and has continuous first and second derivatives at ξ.

11.18. Starting from the cubic spline with knots at $\xi_1, \ldots, \xi_K$:

$$g(x) = \sum_{j=0}^{3} \beta_j x^j + \sum_{k=1}^{K} \beta_{3+k}(x - \xi_k)_+^3 \,,$$

show that restricting $g(x)$ to be linear on $x < \xi_1$ and $x > \xi_K$ is equivalent to imposing the linear constraints:

$$\beta_2 = 0, \quad \beta_3 = 0, \quad \sum_{k=1}^{K} \beta_{3+k} = 0, \quad \sum_{k=1}^{K} \beta_{3+k}\xi_k = 0 \,.$$

11.19. Show that the generalized ridge regression problem

$$\widehat{\alpha} = \operatorname*{argmin}_{\alpha} \|y - V\alpha\|^2 + \lambda \alpha^\top K\alpha$$

has an explicit solution given by

$$\widehat{\alpha} = \left(V^\top V + \lambda K\right)^{-1} V^\top y \,.$$

Chapter 12
Dependent Data Models

In the models considered so far the responses $Y_1, \ldots, Y_n$ have been assumed to be independent given the model parameters. Though convenient, this independence assumption is implausible in two common situations. First, in the case of **time series**—observations measured over time—the responses typically exhibit strong serial dependence. For example, high unemployment tends to last for a long period of time; given a high unemployment rate in this period, one would expect that the unemployment rates in the next few periods would also be high.

The other situation in which observations are likely to be dependent is when they are measurements on the same or related subjects. For example, learning outcomes of children in the same school tend to be more similar—because they share the same academic environment and come from families of similar socioeconomic backgrounds—than those of other children in a different school.

In this chapter we introduce models that relax the usual independence assumption and are suitable for modeling data that arise in the two aforementioned situations.

12.1 Autoregressive and Moving Average Models

In this section we introduce a widely popular class of simple time series models called **autoregressive moving average** (ARMA) models. We begin our study of ARMA models with purely autoregressive specifications.

J. C. C. Chan, D. P. Kroese, *Statistical Modeling and Computation*, Springer Texts in Statistics, https://doi.org/10.1007/978-1-0716-4132-3_12

12.1.1 Autoregressive Models

Example 12.1 (Sales and Ads). In this motivating example, we consider a linear regression model in a time series context. Specifically, suppose a company has collected data on its quarterly sales and advertisement expenditures for the last 30 quarters. The data are given in Table 12.1.

Table 12.1 Sales and advertisement expenditures

Time	Sales	Ads	Time	Sales	Ads	Time	Sales	Ads
1	23.45	5.41	11	24.92	4.59	21	21.42	2.61
2	26.03	6.30	12	25.58	5.04	22	30.99	6.59
3	21.73	4.21	13	28.74	5.87	23	20.79	2.65
4	23.66	4.50	14	24.69	3.73	24	22.99	4.43
5	26.54	5.63	15	29.39	6.02	25	23.56	5.18
6	26.62	5.67	16	28.47	5.60	26	23.36	5.27
7	23.59	4.33	17	28.66	5.50	27	19.03	3.52
8	20.05	3.54	18	25.49	4.39	28	24.53	5.76
9	20.67	3.86	19	28.57	5.68	29	19.56	4.30
10	25.97	5.66	20	28.23	6.05	30	20.90	4.45

The marketing manager wonders how the two figures are correlated. To address this question, she considers the following linear regression model:

$$Y_t = \beta_0 + \beta_1 x_t + \varepsilon_t , \quad t = 1, \ldots, 30, \quad \{\varepsilon_t\} \overset{\text{iid}}{\sim} \mathcal{N}(0, \sigma^2) ,$$

where Y_t is the sales at quarter t and x_t is the corresponding advertisement expenditure. Given the outcomes $y_t, t = 1, \ldots, 30$, the maximum likelihood estimates of the model parameters, $\widehat{\beta}_0$, $\widehat{\beta}_1$, and $\widehat{\sigma^2}$, can be readily computed; see Example 5.5.

As a model diagnostic check, we can compute and plot the *residuals*

$$u_t = y_t - \widehat{\beta}_0 - \widehat{\beta}_1 x_t, \quad t = 1, \ldots, 30 .$$

The residuals $\{u_t\}$ are our best guess for the (unknown) error terms $\{\varepsilon_t\}$. If the model is correct, the residuals should be approximately iid and normally distributed, because the true error terms behave in this way. A plot of the residuals is given in Fig. 12.1. As the graph shows, the residuals exhibit systemic patterns across time. In particular, they tend to cluster together, indicating that the assumption of serially independent errors might not hold.

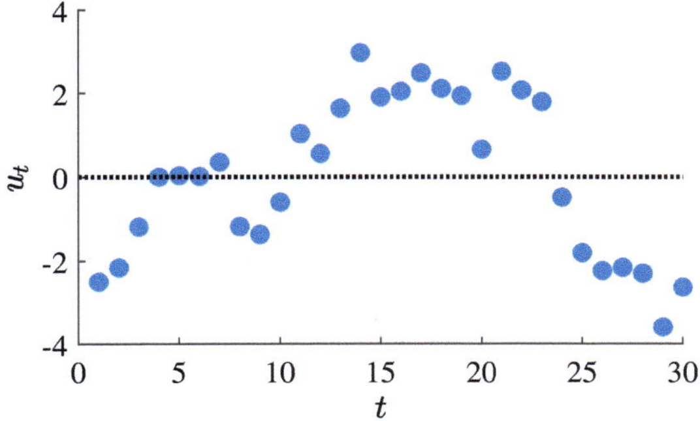

Fig. 12.1 A plot of the residuals of the linear regression model

Instead of the model $\{\varepsilon_t\} \sim_{\text{iid}} \mathcal{N}(0, \sigma^2)$ for the errors, one could consider the model where the current error depends on the past errors in a linear way; for example, as in

$$\varepsilon_t = \varrho\,\varepsilon_{t-1} + U_t \,, \quad \{U_t\} \sim_{\text{iid}} \mathcal{N}(0, \sigma^2) \,, \tag{12.1}$$

where and ϱ and σ^2 are fixed model parameters.

The model for the errors in (12.1) is an example of an autoregressive model.

Definition 12.1. (Autoregressive Model). In the **p-th-order autoregressive** (AR(p)) model, the observation at time t depends linearly on the previous p observations $Y_{t-1}, \ldots, Y_{t-p}$:

$$Y_t = \varrho_0 + \varrho_1 Y_{t-1} + \cdots + \varrho_p Y_{t-p} + \varepsilon_t \,, \tag{12.2}$$

$t = 1, \ldots, T$, where $\{\varepsilon_t\} \sim_{\text{iid}} \mathcal{N}(0, \sigma^2)$.

To complete the model, one needs to specify the **initial conditions**, that is, the probability distribution of the first p observations: $Y_{-p+1}, \ldots, Y_0$. For simplicity it is often assumed that these values are known. An alternative approach is to assume that (12.2) holds for every $t \in \mathbb{Z} = \{\ldots, -2, -1, 0, 1, 2, \ldots\}$ and that the time series is **stationary**, meaning that the distribution of $Y_1, Y_2, \ldots$ is the same as that of $Y_{n+1}, Y_{n+2}, \ldots$ for any $n \in \mathbb{Z}$. In particular, the distribution of Y_t does not depend on t (is the same for all t), and the joint distribution of (Y_t, Y_{t+s}) does not depend on t. Stationary AR processes only exist under certain conditions on the $\{\varrho_i\}$.

Example 12.2 (Autocorrelations of AR(1)). Consider an AR(1) time series on $\mathbb{Z}$, governed by

$$Y_t = \varrho Y_{t-1} + \varepsilon_t, \quad t \in \mathbb{Z},$$

where $\{\varepsilon_t\} \sim_{\text{iid}} \mathcal{N}(0, \sigma^2)$. By repeated substitution, we have

$$Y_t = \varepsilon_t + \varrho\varepsilon_{t-1} + \varrho^2\varepsilon_{t-2} + \varrho^3\varepsilon_{t-3} + \cdots. \tag{12.3}$$

Since the $\{\varepsilon_t\}$ are independent by assumption, the variance of Y_t is finite if $|\varrho| < 1$:

$$\begin{aligned}
\mathrm{Var}(Y_t) &= \mathrm{Var}(\varepsilon_t + \varrho\varepsilon_{t-1} + \varrho^2\varepsilon_{t-2} + \varrho^3\varepsilon_{t-3} + \cdots) \\
&= \sigma^2 + \varrho^2\sigma^2 + \varrho^4\sigma^2 + \varrho^6\sigma^2 + \cdots \\
&= \frac{\sigma^2}{1 - \varrho^2}.
\end{aligned}$$

It is worth noting that the variance of Y_t is a constant and does not depend on the time index t. In fact, using the representation (12.3), it is not difficult to see that the time series $\{Y_t\}$ is *stationary* and that each Y_t has a $\mathcal{N}(0, \sigma^2/(1 - \varrho^2))$ distribution.

Next, we compute the covariance $\mathrm{Cov}(Y_t, Y_{t-1})$, or the so-called (first-order) **autocovariance**:

$$\mathrm{Cov}(Y_t, Y_{t-1}) = \mathrm{Cov}(\varrho Y_{t-1} + \varepsilon_t, Y_{t-1}) = \mathrm{Cov}(\varrho Y_{t-1}, Y_{t-1})$$

$$= \varrho\,\mathrm{Var}(Y_{t-1}) = \varrho\frac{\sigma^2}{1 - \varrho^2},$$

where the second equality holds because Y_{t-1} is a function of $\varepsilon_s, s \leq t - 1$, and is therefore uncorrelated with ε_t. Using a similar argument, one can show that in general the autocovariance of **lag** s is given by

$$R(s) = \mathrm{Cov}(Y_t, Y_{t-s}) = \varrho^s \frac{\sigma^2}{1 - \varrho^2}.$$

Dividing by $\mathrm{Var}(Y_t) = \sigma^2/(1 - \varrho^2)$ gives the **autocorrelation** function:

$$\mathrm{Corr}(Y_t, Y_{t-s}) = \varrho^s, \quad s = 0, 1, 2, \ldots.$$

In other words, under the assumption $|\varrho| < 1$ the autocorrelations of the AR(1) model decrease geometrically. If ϱ is positive, the autocorrelations monotonously decrease; if ϱ is negative, they alternate in sign. In Fig. 12.2 we plot the autocorrelations of the AR(1) for four different values of ϱ.

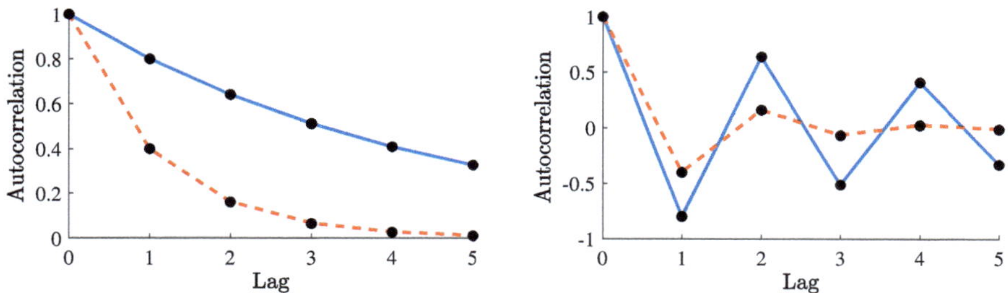

Fig. 12.2 Autocorrelations for the AR(1) model. Left: $\varrho = 0.8$ (solid) and $\varrho = 0.4$ (dashed). Right: $\varrho = -0.8$ (solid) and $\varrho = -0.4$ (dashed)

Remark 12.1 (Estimating Autocovariances). Suppose that $X_1, X_2, \ldots,$ X_T is a *stationary* time series with autocovariance function $R(s) = \mathrm{Cov}(X_t, X_{t+s})$. Note that $R(0) = \mathrm{Var}(X_t)$. The autocovariances can be estimated via their (unbiased) sample averages:

$$\widehat{R}(s) = \frac{1}{T - s - 1} \sum_{t=1}^{T-s} (X_t - \overline{X})(X_{t+s} - \overline{X}), \quad s = 0, 1, \ldots, T . \qquad (12.4)$$

In order to obtain a meaningful estimate, the lag s should be significantly smaller than T. If the time series is not stationary, it is customary to delete the first K, say, samples, similar to the *burn-in period* for Markov chain Monte Carlo, and view the remaining samples as stationary.   ☞ 22●

We now turn to the estimation of the model parameters. Under the AR(p) model past observations feed into the current value of the series, where their effects are determined by the vector of AR coefficients $\boldsymbol{\varrho} = [\varrho_0, \varrho_1, \ldots, \varrho_p]^\top$. One main appeal of the AR(p) model is that it is in the form of a normal linear model, and as such, estimation of the model parameters $\boldsymbol{\theta} = [\boldsymbol{\varrho}^\top, \sigma^2]^\top$ is easy. To proceed, let $\boldsymbol{y} = [y_1, \ldots, y_T]^\top$ be the observed data and denote the initial observations by $\boldsymbol{Y}_0 = [Y_{-p+1}, \ldots, Y_0]^\top$. Recall that the AR($p$) model determines the conditional pdf of the data given the initial conditions, that is, $f_{\boldsymbol{Y}|\boldsymbol{Y}_0}(\boldsymbol{y} \,|\, \boldsymbol{y}_0 ; \boldsymbol{\theta})$. The likelihood function of $\boldsymbol{\theta}$ for the observed data $\boldsymbol{y}$ is thus given by

$$L(\boldsymbol{\theta}; \boldsymbol{y}) = f_{\boldsymbol{Y}|\boldsymbol{Y}_0}(\boldsymbol{y} \,|\, \boldsymbol{y}_0 ; \boldsymbol{\theta}) f_{\boldsymbol{Y}_0}(\boldsymbol{y}_0) .$$

As mentioned before, there are two ways to deal with the initial observations. The first is to assume that the time series is *stationary*, and from this assumption, we derive the distributions of $\boldsymbol{Y}_0$ and $\boldsymbol{Y}$. An easier approach, which we will follow here, is to simply assume that $\boldsymbol{Y}_0 = \boldsymbol{y}_0$ is given and specify the likelihood function as

$$L(\boldsymbol{\theta}; \boldsymbol{y}, \boldsymbol{y}_0) = f_{\boldsymbol{Y}|\boldsymbol{Y}_0}(\boldsymbol{y} \,|\, \boldsymbol{y}_0; \boldsymbol{\theta}) .$$

In typical situations where T is much greater than p, it makes little difference for parameter estimation whether or not the initial conditions are explicitly modeled.

☞ 115　　Using the results of the normal linear model in Sect. 4.5, we can easily derive the joint density $f_{\boldsymbol{Y}|\boldsymbol{Y}_0}(\boldsymbol{y}\,|\,\boldsymbol{y}_0\,;\,\boldsymbol{\theta})$ and hence the likelihood function. To that end, write the $\mathrm{AR}(p)$ model in matrix notation:

$$\boldsymbol{Y} = \mathbf{X}\boldsymbol{\varrho} + \boldsymbol{\varepsilon}, \quad \boldsymbol{\varepsilon} \sim \mathcal{N}(\mathbf{0}, \sigma^2 \mathbb{I}_T)\,,$$

where

$$\mathbf{X} = \begin{bmatrix} 1 & Y_0 & Y_{-1} & \cdots & Y_{-p+1} \\ 1 & Y_1 & Y_0 & \cdots & Y_{-p+2} \\ \vdots & \vdots & \vdots & \ddots & \vdots \\ 1 & Y_{T-1} & Y_{T-2} & \cdots & Y_{T-p} \end{bmatrix}.$$

Thus, conditional on $\boldsymbol{Y}_0 = \boldsymbol{y}_0$ the random vector $\boldsymbol{Z} = \boldsymbol{Y} - \mathbf{X}\boldsymbol{\varrho}$ (with Y_k in matrix $\mathbf{X}$ replaced by y_k for $k = 0, -1, \ldots, -p+1$) has a $\mathcal{N}(\mathbf{0}, \sigma^2 \mathbb{I}_T)$ distribution with density function

$$f_Z(\boldsymbol{z}) = (2\pi\sigma^2)^{-\frac{T}{2}} \mathrm{e}^{-\frac{1}{2\sigma^2}\boldsymbol{z}^\top \boldsymbol{z}}\,.$$

Now, given the outcome $\boldsymbol{Y} = \boldsymbol{y}$ and initial conditions $\boldsymbol{Y}_0 = \boldsymbol{y}_0$, we have $\boldsymbol{z} = \boldsymbol{y} - \mathbf{X}\boldsymbol{\varrho}$ (with Y_k in matrix $\mathbf{X}$ replaced by y_k for $k = -p+1, \ldots, T$), and the likelihood function is given by

$$L(\boldsymbol{\theta}; \boldsymbol{y}, \boldsymbol{y}_0) = (2\pi\sigma^2)^{-\frac{T}{2}} \mathrm{e}^{-\frac{1}{2\sigma^2}(\boldsymbol{y}-\mathbf{X}\boldsymbol{\varrho})^\top (\boldsymbol{y}-\mathbf{X}\boldsymbol{\varrho})}\,.$$

The maximum likelihood estimators of $\boldsymbol{\varrho}$ and σ^2 are given by

$$\widehat{\boldsymbol{\varrho}} = (\mathbf{X}^\top \mathbf{X})^{-1}\mathbf{X}^\top \boldsymbol{Y} \qquad \text{and} \qquad \widehat{\sigma^2} = \frac{1}{T}(\boldsymbol{Y} - \mathbf{X}\widehat{\boldsymbol{\varrho}})^\top (\boldsymbol{Y} - \mathbf{X}\widehat{\boldsymbol{\varrho}})\,.$$

☞ 243　　Finally, Bayesian inference in the $\mathrm{AR}(p)$ model can proceed as in Sect. 8.2.2.

Example 12.3 (Modeling Unemployment with AR Models). In this example, we use autoregressive models with different lags to model US quarterly unemployment rates from the first quarter in 2002 to the last quarter in 2011—a total of 40 observations. The data are given in Table 12.2.

We fit two autoregressive models with one and two lags respectively. To that end, we divide the data into two subsets: the first two observations are reserved as the initial conditions, y_{-1} and y_0, and we explicitly model the remaining 38 observations $y_1, \ldots, y_{38}$. First we fit the following AR(1) model:

$$Y_t = \varrho_0 + \varrho_1 Y_{t-1} + \varepsilon_t\,,$$

where $\varepsilon_t \sim_{\text{iid}} \mathcal{N}(0, \sigma^2)$ for $t = 1, \ldots, 38$. By defining the design matrix $\mathbf{X}$ appropriately, the maximum likelihood estimates of ϱ_0, ϱ_1, and σ^2 can be computed easily; see the following Julia code.

```julia
urate_ar.jl

using Plots
urate = [5.7, 5.8, 5.7, 5.9, 5.9, 6.1, 6.1, 5.8, 5.7,
5.6, 5.4, 5.4, 5.3, 5.1, 5.0, 5.0, 4.7, 4.6, 4.6, 4.4,
4.5, 4.5, 4.7, 4.8, 5.0, 5.3, 6.0, 6.9, 8.3, 9.3, 9.6,
9.9, 9.8, 9.6, 9.5, 9.6, 9.0, 9.0,  9.1, 8.7]
y = urate[3:end]
T = length(y)
X = [ones(T,1) urate[2:end-1]]
rhohat = (X'*X)(X'*y)
yhat1 = X*rhohat                  # fitted values
uhat = y-yhat1                    # residuals
sig2hat = uhat'*uhat/T


t = 2002.5:.25:2011.75
plot(t,X*rhohat)
plot!(t,y)
```

To assess the model fit, we also computed the fitted values under the AR(1) model, as well as the residuals. The fitted values of the AR(1) are plotted in Fig. 12.3 (left panel).

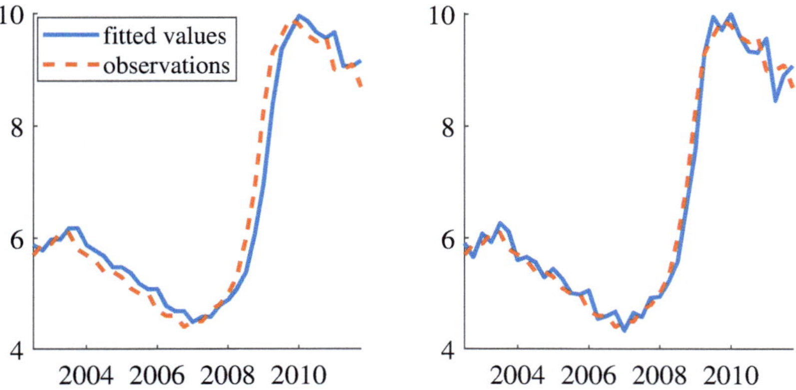

Fig. 12.3 The fitted values of the AR(1) (left panel) and the AR(2) (right panel)

It can be seen from the graph that the fitted values appear to be quite close to the actual observations. However, the AR(1) model seems to systematically

Table 12.2 US quarterly unemployment rates from 2002 Q1 to 2011 Q4

Year	Unemploy- ment rate	Year	Unemploy- ment rate	Year	Unemploy- ment rate
2002 Q1	5.7	2006 Q1	4.7	2009 Q1	8.3
Q2	5.8	Q2	4.6	Q2	9.3
Q3	5.7	Q3	4.6	Q3	9.6
Q4	5.9	Q4	4.4	Q4	9.9
2003 Q1	5.9	2007 Q1	4.5	2010 Q1	9.8
Q2	6.1	Q2	4.5	Q2	9.6
Q3	6.1	Q3	4.7	Q3	9.5
Q4	5.8	Q4	4.8	Q4	9.6
2004 Q1	5.7	2008 Q1	5.0	2011 Q1	9.0
Q2	5.6	Q2	5.3	Q2	9.0
Q3	5.4	Q3	6.0	Q3	9.1
Q4	5.4	Q4	6.9	Q4	8.7
2005 Q1	5.3				
Q2	5.1				
Q3	5.5				
Q4	5.5				

underestimate the unemployment rate before 2007 and then overestimate it after 2007. To check whether the residuals have any serial correlation, we can estimate the autocovariance function via (12.4). In Julia we can do this, for example, via the following function.

```julia
function acov(x,s)  # make sure StatsBase is used
return sum((x[1:end-s] .- mean(x)).*(x[s+1:end] .- mean(x)
        ))/(length(x) - s - 1);
end
```

We find the autocorrelation at lag 1 via `acov(uhat,1)/acov(uhat,0)`, which turns out to be 0.7028. Similarly, for lags 2 and 3 we find the autocorrelations 0.5580 and 0.4421, respectively. This indicates that the model assumption of serially independent errors might not be valid, since the autocorrelations of the residuals remain substantial.

Next, we investigate if we can improve the model fit by using the AR(2): model:

$$Y_t = \phi_0 + \phi_1 y_{t-1} + \phi_2 y_{t-2} + \varepsilon_t \,,$$

where $\varepsilon_t \sim_{\text{iid}} \mathcal{N}(0, \sigma^2)$ for $t = 1, \ldots, 38$. By defining the design matrix appropriately, the maximum likelihood estimates for the model parameters and the corresponding fitted values can be obtained easily. The fitted values of the AR(2) are plotted in Fig. 12.3 (right panel), which appear to fit the actual observations better. In this case the lag-1 and lag-2 autocorrelations of the residuals are respectively -0.12 and -0.001.

We now return to the modeling situation of Example 12.1, using a more ☞ 35 general setting. In particular, we consider a linear regression model

$$\boldsymbol{Y} = \mathbf{X}\boldsymbol{\beta} + \boldsymbol{\varepsilon} \; ,$$

where the errors $\{\varepsilon_t\}$ follow an AR(p) model (with $\varrho_0 = 0$):

$$\varepsilon_t = \varrho_1 \varepsilon_{t-1} + \cdots + \varrho_p \varepsilon_{t-p} + U_t \; , \tag{12.5}$$

where $\{U_t\} \sim_{\text{iid}} \mathcal{N}(0, \sigma^2)$ and $\varepsilon_{1-p} = \cdots = \varepsilon_0 = 0$. To keep the discussion concrete, we let $p = 1$ and define $\varrho_1 = \varrho$; higher-order AR models can be estimated similarly. Now, rewrite (12.5) in matrix notation

$$\mathbf{H}\boldsymbol{\varepsilon} = \boldsymbol{U} \; ,$$

where $\boldsymbol{\varepsilon} = [\varepsilon_1, \ldots, \varepsilon_T]^\top$, $\boldsymbol{U} = [U_1, \ldots, U_T]^\top \sim \mathcal{N}(\boldsymbol{0}, \sigma^2 \mathbb{I}_T)$, and

$$\mathbf{H} = \begin{bmatrix} 1 & 0 & 0 & \cdots & 0 \\ -\varrho & 1 & 0 & \cdots & 0 \\ 0 & -\varrho & 1 & \cdots & 0 \\ \vdots & & & \ddots & \vdots \\ 0 & 0 & \cdots & -\varrho & 1 \end{bmatrix}$$

is a lower-triangular $T \times T$ matrix with ones on the main diagonal. Note that $\mathbf{H}$ is **sparse**, i.e., it contains only a small proportion of nonzero elements. Now, since its determinant is 1, $\mathbf{H}$ is invertible for any ϱ. By a simple change of variables, we have

$$\boldsymbol{Y} - \mathbf{X}\boldsymbol{\beta} = \mathbf{H}^{-1}\boldsymbol{U} \sim \mathcal{N}(\boldsymbol{0}, \sigma^2 (\mathbf{H}^\top \mathbf{H})^{-1}) \; .$$

Noting that the determinant of $\mathbf{H}$ is 1, the log-likelihood function is given by

$$l(\boldsymbol{\beta}, \varrho, \sigma^2; \boldsymbol{y}) = -\frac{T}{2} \ln(2\pi\sigma^2) - \frac{1}{2\sigma^2} (\boldsymbol{y} - \mathbf{X}\boldsymbol{\beta})^\top \mathbf{H}^\top \mathbf{H} (\boldsymbol{y} - \mathbf{X}\boldsymbol{\beta}) \; . \tag{12.6}$$

If the number of parameters is small, the maximum likelihood estimates can be obtained by numerically maximizing the log-likelihood function in (12.6). But when the dimension of the maximization is large, this approach is time-consuming and sometimes even infeasible.

Here we introduce a method to reduce the dimension of the numerical optimization; see also Example 6.14. First note that if ϱ is known, the maximum ☞ 17 likelihood estimates of $\boldsymbol{\beta}$ and σ^2 are available analytically (see Problem 12.6):

$$\widehat{\boldsymbol{\beta}} = (\mathbf{X}^\top \mathbf{H}^\top \mathbf{H} \mathbf{X})^{-1} \mathbf{X}^\top \mathbf{H}^\top \mathbf{H} \boldsymbol{y}, \quad \widehat{\sigma^2} = \frac{1}{T}(\boldsymbol{y} - \mathbf{X}\widehat{\boldsymbol{\beta}})^\top \mathbf{H}^\top \mathbf{H}(\boldsymbol{y} - \mathbf{X}\widehat{\boldsymbol{\beta}}) \; . \tag{12.7}$$

Now, we plug the maximum likelihood estimators of $\boldsymbol{\beta}$ and $\widehat{\sigma^2}$ back into the log-likelihood function to obtain the *profile log-likelihood*, also called the **concentrated log-likelihood**

$$\widetilde{l}(\varrho; \boldsymbol{y}) = l(\widehat{\boldsymbol{\beta}}, \varrho, \widehat{\sigma^2}; \boldsymbol{y}) \,,$$

which is a function of ϱ only. Thus, we can maximize numerically the profile log-likelihood function to obtain the maximum likelihood estimate $\widehat{\varrho}$. Finally, given $\widehat{\varrho}$, we can use (12.7) to obtain $\widehat{\boldsymbol{\beta}}$ and $\widehat{\sigma^2}$ analytically.

Example 12.4 (Sales and Ads Continued). Consider the model for the sales data in Example 12.1

$$Y_t = \beta_0 + \beta_1 x_t + \varepsilon_t \,,$$
$$\varepsilon_t = \varrho \varepsilon_{t-1} + U_t \,,$$

where Y_t is the sales in quarter t, x_t is the corresponding ads expenditure, $\varepsilon_0 = 0$, and $\{U_t\} \sim_{\text{iid}} \mathcal{N}(0, \sigma^2)$. We wish to compute the maximum likelihood estimates for $\boldsymbol{\beta}$, σ^2, and ϱ. Note that throughout we will use the matrix notation introduced earlier.

To that end, we first write a Julia function to evaluate the profile log-likelihood $\widetilde{l}(\varrho; \boldsymbol{y}) = l(\widehat{\boldsymbol{\beta}}, \varrho, \widehat{\sigma^2}; \boldsymbol{y})$.

```julia
function AR1_loglike(rho,y,X)
  T = length(y);
  H = sparse(I,T,T)  .- rho*sparse(2:T,1:T-1,ones(T-1),T,T);
  HH = H'*H;
  betahat = (X'*HH*X)(X'*HH*y);
  e = y-X*betahat;
  sigma2hat = e'*HH*e/T;
  l = -T/2*log(2*pi*sigma2hat) - .5/sigma2hat*e'*HH*e;
return l, betahat,sigma2hat
end
```

In the above code, note that the matrix $\mathbf{H}$ is constructed by writing

$$\mathbf{H} = \begin{bmatrix} 1 & 0 & 0 & \cdots & 0 \\ -\varrho & 1 & 0 & \cdots & 0 \\ 0 & -\varrho & 1 & \cdots & 0 \\ \vdots & & & \ddots & \vdots \\ 0 & 0 & \cdots & -\varrho & 1 \end{bmatrix} = \begin{bmatrix} 1 & 0 & 0 & \cdots & 0 \\ 0 & 1 & 0 & \cdots & 0 \\ 0 & 0 & 1 & \cdots & 0 \\ \vdots & & & \ddots & \vdots \\ 0 & 0 & \cdots & 0 & 1 \end{bmatrix} - \varrho \begin{bmatrix} 0 & 0 & 0 & \cdots & 0 \\ 1 & 0 & 0 & \cdots & 0 \\ 0 & 1 & 0 & \cdots & 0 \\ \vdots & & & \ddots & \vdots \\ 0 & 0 & \cdots & 1 & 0 \end{bmatrix} \,.$$

Then, in the main script, we define the function $f(\varrho) = -\widetilde{l}(\varrho; \boldsymbol{y})$ and use the built-in minimization function **optimize** to minimize f to obtain the maximum likelihood estimate $\widehat{\varrho}$. Finally, given $\widehat{\varrho}$, we use (12.7) to compute $\widehat{\boldsymbol{\beta}}$ and $\widehat{\sigma^2}$ analytically.

```
sales.jl
```

```julia
using SparseArrays, LinearAlgebra, Optim, Plots,
    DelimitedFiles
ads = readdlm("ads.csv",',')
y = ads[:,1]
T = length(y)
X = [ones(T,1) ads[:,2]]
f(rho)   = -(AR1_loglike(rho,y,X)[1])

res = optimize(f,0.1,1)
rhohat = res.minimizer
l, betahat, sigma2hat = AR1_loglike(rhohat,y,X)
```

The maximum likelihood estimate of $\widehat{\varrho}$ is 0.95, indicating very strong first-order serial correlation in the error terms $\{\varepsilon_t\}$. The maximum likelihood estimates of $\widehat{\boldsymbol{\beta}}$ and $\widehat{\sigma^2}$ are, respectively, $[11.03, 2.32]^\top$ and 0.81.

To assess the appropriateness of the model assumption $\{U_t\} \sim_{\text{iid}} \mathcal{N}(0, \sigma^2)$, we compute the residuals $\{u_t\}$, which are our best guess for the (unknown) $\{U_t\}$. Recall that under the model we have $\mathbf{H}\boldsymbol{\varepsilon} = \boldsymbol{U}$. Hence, we can obtain the residuals using

$$\boldsymbol{u} = \widehat{\mathbf{H}}(\boldsymbol{y} - \mathbf{X}\widehat{\boldsymbol{\beta}}) \,,$$

where $\widehat{\mathbf{H}}$ is the same as $\mathbf{H}$ but with ϱ replaced by its estimate $\widehat{\varrho}$. This is implemented in Julia as follows:

```julia
e = y - X*betahat
H = sparse(I,T,T) .- rhohat*sparse(2:T,1:T-1,ones(T-1),T,T);
u = H*e;
scatter(u)
```

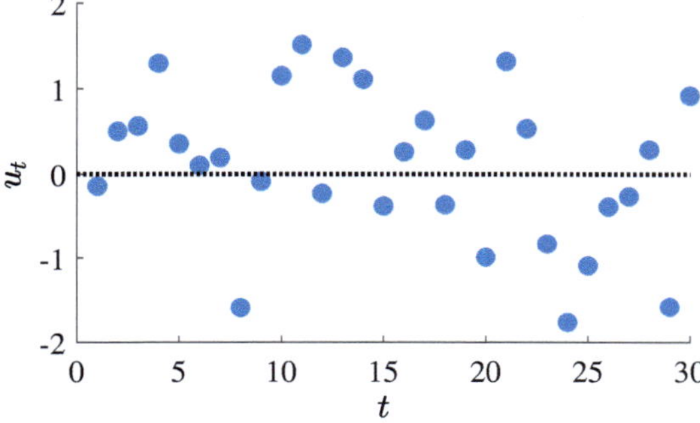

Fig. 12.4 A plot of the residuals of the linear regression model with AR(1) errors

A plot of the residuals is given in Fig. 12.4. As the graph shows, the residuals now do not seem to have any systematic patterns across time, indicating no evidence of invalidating the assumption that $\{U_t\}$ are serially independent; see also Problem 12.4.

12.1.2 Moving Average Models

In an AR model, dependence of the responses is constructed by defining the current response in terms of a linear combination of previous responses. In contrast, in a moving average (MA) model the current response Y_t depends on a linear combination of past error terms.

Definition 12.2. (Moving Average Model). In the **q-th-order moving average** (MA(q)) model the observation at time t depends linearly on the previous q error terms:

$$Y_t = \varepsilon_t + \psi_1 \varepsilon_{t-1} + \cdots + \psi_q \varepsilon_{t-q} , \tag{12.8}$$

where $\{\varepsilon_t\} \sim_{\text{iid}} \mathcal{N}(0, \sigma^2)$.

A standard way to treat the initial conditions is to assume $\varepsilon_0 = \varepsilon_{-1} = \cdots = \varepsilon_{1-q} = 0$, although relaxing this assumption is straightforward (see Problem 12.3)

Under the MA(q) model, past shocks feed into the current value of the series, where their effects are determined by the signs and magnitudes of the MA coefficients $\psi_1, \ldots, \psi_q$. Unlike the AR(p) model each response always has a finite variance, as the following example shows.

Example 12.5 (Autocorrelations of MA(q)). We investigate the autocorrelation structure implied by the MA(q) model. First, we compute the variance of Y_t for $t > q$

$$\begin{aligned}
\mathrm{Var}(Y_t) &= \mathrm{Var}(\varepsilon_t + \psi_1 \varepsilon_{t-1} + \cdots + \psi_q \varepsilon_{t-q}) \\
&= \mathrm{Var}(\varepsilon_t) + \psi_1^2 \mathrm{Var}(\varepsilon_{t-1}) + \cdots + \psi_q^2 \mathrm{Var}(\varepsilon_{t-q}) \\
&= \sigma^2 (1 + \psi_1^2 + \cdots + \psi_q^2) ,
\end{aligned}$$

which is finite and independent of the time index t for $t > q$. Next, we compute the autocovariance at lag 1 as

$$\mathrm{Cov}(Y_t, Y_{t-1}) = \mathrm{Cov}(\varepsilon_t + \cdots + \psi_q \varepsilon_{t-q}, \varepsilon_{t-1} + \cdots + \psi_q \varepsilon_{t-q-1})$$
$$= \psi_1 \mathrm{Cov}(\varepsilon_{t-1}, \varepsilon_{t-1}) + \psi_2 \psi_1 \mathrm{Cov}(\varepsilon_{t-2}, \varepsilon_{t-2}) + \cdots +$$
$$\psi_q \psi_{q-1} \mathrm{Cov}(\varepsilon_{t-q}, \varepsilon_{t-q})$$
$$= (\psi_1 + \psi_2 \psi_1 + \cdots + \psi_q \psi_{q-1}) \sigma^2 .$$

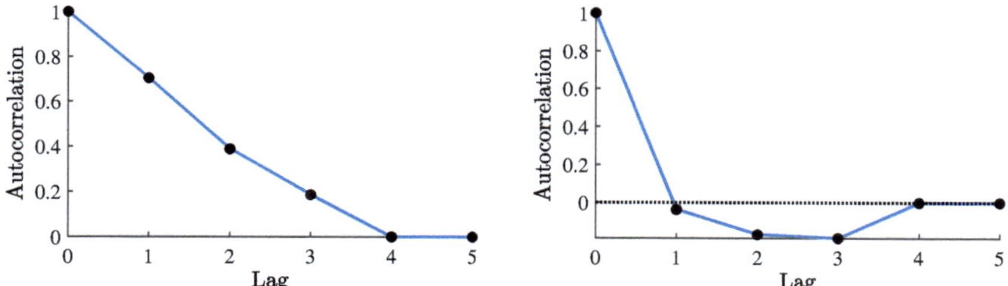

Fig. 12.5 The autocorrelations for the MA(3) with $\psi_1 = 0.8, \psi_2 = 0.6$ and $\psi_3 = 0.4$ (left panel), and $\psi_1 = -0.8, \psi_2 = -0.6$ and $\psi_3 = -0.4$ (right panel)

More generally, it can be shown that (see Problem 12.2)

$$\mathrm{Cov}(Y_t, Y_{t-j}) = \begin{cases} \sigma^2 \sum_{i=0}^{q-j} \psi_{i+j} \psi_i, & j = 0, \ldots, q, \\ 0, & j > q, \end{cases} \qquad (12.9)$$

where $\psi_0 = 1$. Hence, the autocorrelations are

$$\mathrm{Corr}(Y_t, Y_{t-j}) = \frac{\sum_{i=0}^{q-j} \psi_{i+j} \psi_i}{1 + \psi_1^2 + \cdots + \psi_q^2}$$

for $j = 0, \ldots, q$ and $\mathrm{Corr}(Y_t, Y_{t-j}) = 0$ for $j > q$. In contrast to the AR case where the autocorrelation declines geometrically, those of the MA drop to zero after only q lags. As an illustration, in Fig. 12.5 we plot the autocorrelations of two MA(3) models.

We now turn to estimation of the model parameters. Recall that under the MA(q) model, the responses $Y_1, \ldots, Y_T$ are a linear combination of T normal random variables $\varepsilon_1, \ldots, \varepsilon_T$. Therefore, $\boldsymbol{Y} = [Y_1, \ldots, Y_T]^\top$ has a multivariate normal distribution, and evaluating the log-likelihood should be simple. In practice, however, this approach requires manipulating large matrices, which is often time-consuming. The key to make this approach feasible is to realize that, as in the AR(p) case, the matrices involved in the MA(q) model are sparse, which makes the computation quick.

☞ 83

To keep the discussion concrete, consider evaluating the log-likelihood of the MA(1) model

$$Y_t = \varepsilon_t + \psi \varepsilon_{t-1}, \quad t = 1, \ldots T, \quad \varepsilon_0 = 0 .$$

First, we write this model in matrix form

$$\boldsymbol{Y} = \mathbf{H}\boldsymbol{\varepsilon}, \tag{12.10}$$

where $\boldsymbol{\varepsilon} = [\varepsilon_1, \ldots, \varepsilon_T]^\top \sim \mathcal{N}(\mathbf{0}, \sigma^2 \mathbb{I}_T)$, and

$$\mathbf{H} = \begin{bmatrix} 1 & 0 & 0 & \cdots & 0 \\ \psi & 1 & 0 & \cdots & 0 \\ 0 & \psi & 1 & \cdots & 0 \\ \vdots & & & \ddots & \vdots \\ 0 & 0 & \cdots & \psi & 1 \end{bmatrix}$$

is a sparse $T \times T$ matrix that contains only $2T-1$ nonzero elements. It follows that

$$\boldsymbol{Y} \sim \mathcal{N}(\mathbf{0}, \sigma^2 \mathbf{H}\mathbf{H}^\top) \, .$$

Noting that the determinant of $\mathbf{H}$ is 1, the log-likelihood function is given by

$$l(\psi, \sigma^2; \boldsymbol{y}) = -\frac{T}{2} \ln(2\pi\sigma^2) - \frac{1}{2\sigma^2} \boldsymbol{y}^\top (\mathbf{H}\mathbf{H}^\top)^{-1} \boldsymbol{y} \, . \tag{12.11}$$

It is important to note that one need not compute the inverse $(\mathbf{H}\mathbf{H}^\top)^{-1}$ in order to evaluate the log-likelihood—it is a time-consuming operation. Instead, one only needs to obtain the product $(\mathbf{H}\mathbf{H}^\top)^{-1}\boldsymbol{y}$, which can be quickly computed by solving the linear equation

$$\mathbf{H}\mathbf{H}^\top \boldsymbol{z} = \boldsymbol{y}$$

for $\boldsymbol{z}$. In Julia it can be done by using the backslash ($\backslash$) command. The latter operation is much quicker, especially because $\mathbf{H}\mathbf{H}^\top$ is a sparse matrix.

Hence, one can evaluate the log-likelihood function $l(\psi, \sigma^2; \boldsymbol{y})$ quickly without inverting any large matrices. Then, the MLE for ψ and σ^2 can be obtained numerically. To evaluate the log-likelihood function for a general MA(q) model, one only needs to redefine the matrix $\mathbf{H}$ appropriately, and everything else follows directly as in the MA(1) case.

Given the method to quickly evaluate the log-likelihood function described above, the maximum likelihood estimate can be computed readily by numerical methods. For Bayesian inference, posterior draws of the parameters can be obtained using the Metropolis–Hastings algorithm.

Example 12.6 (Modeling U.S. Inflation with MA(1)). In this example, we model the dynamics of US quarterly inflation rate—computed from the consumer price index (CPI)—using a variant of the MA(1) model. Specifically, given the CPI z_t at time t, we compute the (annualized) inflation rate as $y_t = 400 \ln(z_t/z_{t-1})$. The CPI inflation rate from the second quarter of 1947 to the second quarter of 2011 is plotted in Fig. 12.6. A prominent feature of the CPI inflation is that it exhibits high persistence, in the sense that high (or low) inflation in the past tends to continue into the future. For instance, inflation tends to stay high (and variable) in the late 1970s and early 1980s, but it has become much lower (and less variable) since the mid-1980 until the global financial crisis in 2008.

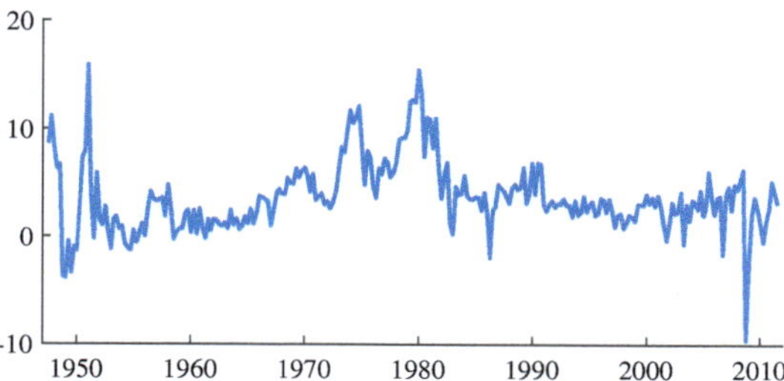

Fig. 12.6 US CPI inflation rate from 1947Q2 to 2011Q2

There are various reasons why one might want to model the past inflation and accurately forecast future inflation. For example, the prices of many financial and real assets—such as bonds, properties, precious metals, etc.—depend on future inflation. Another example is for conducting monetary policy: many central banks have explicit inflation targets, and in order to manage future inflation, it is important to be able to forecast it accurately.

In this example we consider the following model:

$$Y_t = Y_{t-1} + \varepsilon_t + \psi\, \varepsilon_{t-1}\,,$$

where $\varepsilon_1, \ldots, \varepsilon_T \sim_{\text{iid}} \mathcal{N}(0, \sigma^2)$ and $\varepsilon_0 = 0$.

This is a variation of the MA(1) model, sometimes called the **first-order integrated moving average** model. Instead of using the inflation rate as our dependent variable to fit the MA(1) model, we use its first difference $\Delta Y_t = Y_t - Y_{t-1}$. Estimation proceeds the same way as in the MA(1) model, with the minor modification of using ΔY_t as the dependent variable.

To obtain the maximum likelihood estimates for σ^2 and ψ, we first need the following function to evaluate the log-likelihood for the MA(1) model as given in (12.11):

```
function loglike_MA1(theta,y)
   # the log-likelihood function for MA(1)
   # input: theta = [psi sigma2]; y = data
   psi = theta[1]; sigma2 = theta[2];
   T = length(y);
   H = sparse(I,T,T) .+ psi*sparse(2:T,1:T-1,ones(T-1),T,T);
   HH = H*H';
   l = -T/2*log(2*pi*sigma2) - .5/sigma2*y'*(HH\y);
   return l
end
```

Then, in the main script, we use the function `loglike_MA1` to compute the maximum likelihood estimates numerically. Specifically, we first construct the function `f` that evaluates the negative log-likelihood for the MA(1) model. (Recall that in `Optim` all optimization routines are framed in terms of minimization.) Then, we minimize `f` using the numerical minimization function `optimize` with starting values 0 for ψ and the sample variance of Δy_t for σ^2.

```
CPI_MA.jl

using SparseArrays, LinearAlgebra, Optim, StatsBase,Plots,
    DelimitedFiles
USCPI= readdlm("USCPI.csv")
y0 = USCPI[1]
y = USCPI[2:end]
Dely = y - [y0; y[1:end-1]]; # define the dependent variable
T = length(Dely)
theta0 = [0 ,var(Dely)]
f = theta -> -loglike_MA1(theta,Dely)
res = optimize(f,theta0)
thetahat = res.minimizer
psihat = thetahat[1]
l = loglike_MA1(thetahat,Dely)
```

The maximum likelihood estimates for ψ and σ^2 are, respectively, -0.402 and 5.245, and the corresponding maximized log-likelihood value is -577.74. To assess model fit, we compute the fitted value $\widehat{y}_t$

$$\widehat{y}_t = y_{t-1} + \widehat{\psi}\,\widehat{u}_{t-1}\,,$$

where $\widehat{\psi}$ is the maximum likelihood estimate of ψ and $\widehat{u}_{t-1}$ is the residual for period $t-1$. Note that the residuals can be computed easily by

```
Hhat = sparse(I,T,T) .+ psihat*sparse(2:T,1:T-1,ones(T-1),T,T)
uhat = Hhat\Dely
```

Finally, we plot the fitted vs. the observed values of the inflation rates in Fig. 12.7

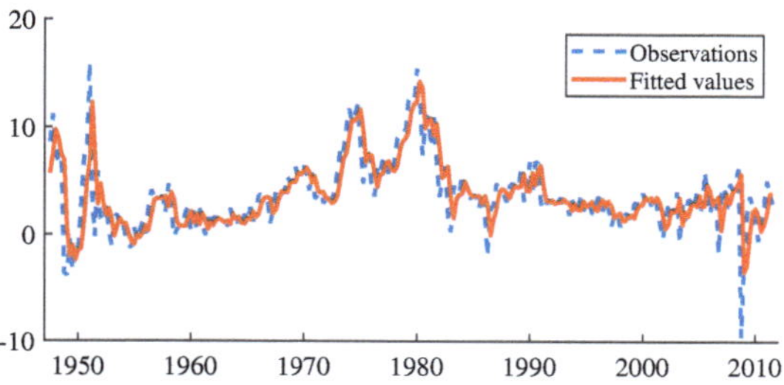

Fig. 12.7 The fitted values for the MA(1) model

12.1.3 Autoregressive Moving Average Models

Of course, we can combine autoregressive and moving average models to have more complex autocorrelation patterns.

> **Definition 12.3. (Autoregressive Moving Average Model).** In the (p, q)-th-order autoregressive moving average (ARMA(p, q)) model the observation at time t depends linearly on the previous p observations as well as the previous q error terms
>
> $$Y_t = \varrho_0 + \varrho_1 Y_{t-1} + \cdots + \varrho_p Y_{t-p} + \varepsilon_t + \psi_1 \varepsilon_{t-1} + \cdots + \psi_q \varepsilon_{t-q} \,, \quad (12.12)$$
>
> where $\{\varepsilon_t\} \overset{\text{iid}}{\sim} \mathcal{N}(0, \sigma^2)$ for $t = 1, \ldots, T$, and $\varepsilon_0 = \cdots = \varepsilon_{1-q} = 0$.

In matrix notation, we can write the system (12.12) as

$$\mathbf{Y} = \mathbf{X}\boldsymbol{\varrho} + \mathbf{H}\boldsymbol{\varepsilon} \,,$$

where $\boldsymbol{\varepsilon} = [\varepsilon_1, \ldots, \varepsilon_T]^\top \sim \mathcal{N}(\mathbf{0}, \sigma^2 \mathbb{I}_T)$, $\boldsymbol{\varrho} = [\varrho_0, \varrho_1, \ldots, \varrho_p]^\top$,

$$\mathbf{X} = \begin{bmatrix} 1 & Y_0 & Y_{-1} & \cdots & Y_{-p+1} \\ 1 & Y_1 & Y_0 & \cdots & Y_{-p+2} \\ \vdots & \vdots & \vdots & \ddots & \vdots \\ 1 & Y_{T-1} & Y_{T-2} & \cdots & Y_{T-p} \end{bmatrix} \,,$$

and $\mathbf{H}$ is a lower triangular matrix with ones on the main diagonal, ψ_1 on the first diagonal below the main diagonal, ψ_2 on the second diagonal below the main diagonal, and so on. We define $\boldsymbol{\psi} = [\psi_1, \ldots, \psi_q]^\top$. Similar to the AR and MA models, we have

$$\mathbf{Y} - \mathbf{X}\boldsymbol{\varrho} \sim \mathcal{N}(\mathbf{0}, \sigma^2 \mathbf{H}\mathbf{H}^\top) \,,$$

and the log-likelihood function $l(\boldsymbol{\varrho}, \boldsymbol{\psi}, \sigma^2; \boldsymbol{y}, \boldsymbol{y}_0)$ is given by (with Y_k in matrix $\mathbf{X}$ replaced by y_k for $k = -p + 1, \ldots, T$):

$$l(\boldsymbol{\varrho}, \boldsymbol{\psi}, \sigma^2; \boldsymbol{y}, \boldsymbol{y}_0) = -\frac{T}{2}\ln(2\pi\sigma^2)$$
$$-\frac{1}{2\sigma^2}(\boldsymbol{y} - \mathbf{X}\boldsymbol{\varrho})^\top (\mathbf{HH}^\top)^{-1}(\boldsymbol{y} - \mathbf{X}\boldsymbol{\varrho}) . \tag{12.13}$$

In principle we can numerically maximize $l(\boldsymbol{\varrho}, \boldsymbol{\psi}, \sigma^2; \boldsymbol{y}, \boldsymbol{y}_0)$ to find the maximum likelihood estimates of the parameters. But this approach is time-consuming in this context as the dimension of the parameter vector is typically large. Instead, as discussed earlier, we reduce the dimension of the numerical maximization by first obtaining the *profile log-likelihood*

$$\widetilde{l}(\boldsymbol{\psi}; \boldsymbol{y}) = l(\widehat{\boldsymbol{\varrho}}, \boldsymbol{\psi}, \widehat{\sigma^2}; \boldsymbol{y}, \boldsymbol{y}_0) ,$$

where the maximum likelihood estimates of $\boldsymbol{\varrho}$ and σ^2 are available analytically (see Problem 12.6)

$$\widehat{\boldsymbol{\varrho}} = (\mathbf{X}^\top \Sigma^{-1} \mathbf{X})^{-1} \mathbf{X}^\top \Sigma^{-1} \boldsymbol{y}, \quad \widehat{\sigma^2} = \frac{1}{T}(\boldsymbol{y} - \mathbf{X}\widehat{\boldsymbol{\varrho}})^\top \Sigma^{-1}(\boldsymbol{y} - \mathbf{X}\widehat{\boldsymbol{\varrho}}) , \tag{12.14}$$

where $\Sigma = \mathbf{HH}^\top$. We then maximize numerically the profile log-likelihood—which is a function of $\boldsymbol{\psi}$ only—to obtain the maximum likelihood estimate $\widehat{\boldsymbol{\psi}}$. Finally, given $\widehat{\boldsymbol{\psi}}$, we use (12.14) to obtain $\widehat{\boldsymbol{\varrho}}$ and $\widehat{\sigma^2}$ analytically.

Example 12.7 (Modeling US Inflation with ARMA(1,1)). In Example 12.6 we fitted the US inflation data with an integrated MA(1) model. In this example we consider a slight generalization by including an intercept and allowing a first-order AR coefficient

$$Y_t = \varrho_0 + \varrho_1 Y_{t-1} + \varepsilon_t + \psi \varepsilon_{t-1} ,$$

where $\varepsilon_1, \ldots, \varepsilon_T \sim_{\text{iid}} \mathcal{N}(0, \sigma^2)$ and $\varepsilon_0 = 0$. Hence, given the data, the design matrix $\mathbf{X}$ is

$$\mathbf{X} = \begin{bmatrix} 1 & y_0 \\ 1 & y_1 \\ \vdots & \vdots \\ 1 & y_{T-1} \end{bmatrix} .$$

In this example, we compute the maximum likelihood estimates of the model parameters; for a Bayesian treatment of the model, see Problem 12.7.

The Julia function `loglike_ARMA11` takes the design matrix $\mathbf{X}$ and the outcomes $\boldsymbol{y}$ and evaluates the profile log-likelihood function at ψ. Note that the function also reports the maximum likelihood estimates of $\boldsymbol{\varrho} = [\varrho_0, \varrho_1]^\top$ and $\widehat{\sigma^2}$ given the value of ψ.

```julia
function loglike_ARMA11(psi,X,y)
   T = length(y)
   H = sparse(I,T,T) + psi*sparse(2:T,1:T-1,ones(T-1),T,T)
   HH = H*H'
   rhohat = (X'*(HH\X))(X'*(HH\y))
   uhat = y-X*rhohat
   sigma2hat = uhat'*(HH\uhat)/T
   l = -T/2*log(2*pi*sigma2hat) - .5/sigma2hat*uhat'*(HH\uhat)
   return l, rhohat, sigma2hat
end
```

Then, in the main script, we numerically minimize the negative of the function `loglike_ARMA11` with respect to ψ. Given the maximum likelihood estimate $\widehat{\psi}$, which is calculated as -0.277, we use `loglike_ARMA11` again to compute the maximum likelihood estimates of ϱ and σ^2, which are, respectively, $[0.536, 0.849]^\top$ and 4.91. The corresponding maximized log-likelihood value is -569.15.

CPI_ARMA.jl

```julia
using  SparseArrays, LinearAlgebra, Optim, StatsBase,
    DelimitedFiles
USCPI= readdlm("USCPI.csv")
y0 = USCPI[1]
y = USCPI[2:end]
T = length(y)
X = [ones(T,1) [y0; y[1:end-1]]]
f = psi ->  -loglike_ARMA11(psi,X,y)[1]
res = optimize(f,-1,1)
psihat = res.minimizer
l, rhohat, sigma2hat = loglike_ARMA11(psihat,X,y)
```

Compared with the integrated MA(1) model in Example 12.6, it is not obvious that the ARMA(1,1) is a better model. Although it does fit the data better—its maximized log-likelihood value is -569.15 compared to -577.74, the corresponding value for the integrated MA(1) model—it is also more complex and has more parameters.

To compare these two models while taking into account both goodness-of-fit and model complexity, we make use of two popular information criteria: **Akaike information criterion** (AIC) and the **Bayesian information criterion** (BIC); see Problem 12.4. The AIC and BIC for the integrated MA(1) model are, respectively, -1159.5 and -1166.6, whereas the corresponding values for the ARMA(1,1) model are -1146.3 and -1160.5. Hence, both information criteria suggest that ARMA(1,1) is a better model for the inflation data.

☞ 38

12.2 Gaussian Models

As discussed in the introduction, an important case where observations are
likely to be dependent is when there are measurements on related subjects.
One convenient class of models for dependent data are *Gaussian models*,
where the data, say, $Y_1, \ldots, Y_n$, are distributed according to a multivariate
normal (i.e., Gaussian) distribution:

$$\boldsymbol{Y} = [Y_1, \ldots, Y_n]^\top \sim \mathcal{N}(\boldsymbol{\mu}, \boldsymbol{\Sigma})$$

for some known or unknown mean vector $\boldsymbol{\mu}$ and covariance matrix $\boldsymbol{\Sigma}$. In order
for the model to be meaningful for statistical analysis, one usually needs to
impose extra structure on the parameters $\boldsymbol{\mu}$ and $\boldsymbol{\Sigma}$.

As a first illustration, consider an extension of the two-sample normal model in Example 4.3, where in addition to measuring the heights
of men whose mothers smoked (group 1) and did not smoke (group 2),
we also measure the weights. The data can then be described by a vec-
tor $\boldsymbol{Y} = [X_1, V_1, \ldots X_{60}, V_{60}, Y_1, W_1, \ldots, Y_{140}, W_{140}]^\top$, where (X_i, V_i) is the
(height,weight) of person i in group 1 and (Y_i, W_i) the (height,weight) of
person i in group 2. The vector $\boldsymbol{Y}$ can be modeled with a $\mathcal{N}(\boldsymbol{\mu}, \boldsymbol{\Sigma})$ distribution, where $\boldsymbol{\mu} = [\mu_{11}, \mu_{12}, \ldots, \mu_{11}, \mu_{12}, \mu_{21}, \mu_{22}, \ldots, \mu_{21}, \mu_{22}]^\top$ (60 pairs
μ_{11}, μ_{12} followed by 140 pairs μ_{21}, μ_{22}), and the covariance matrix $\boldsymbol{\Sigma}$ is block-
diagonal with 2×2 blocks. The first 60 blocks on the diagonal (all the same)
correspond to the covariance matrix of the height X and weight W of a person from the first group, which are clearly not independent. Similarly the
remaining 140 diagonal blocks (all the same) correspond to the covariance
matrix of the height Y and weight W of a person from the second group. This
Gaussian model has only 10 parameters, as opposed to the possibly 80600
parameters of the general multivariate Gaussian model; see also Problem 4.4.

Recall from Sect. 3.6 some important properties of the multivariate normal
distribution. Let $\boldsymbol{X} = [X_1, \ldots, X_n]^\top \sim \mathcal{N}(\boldsymbol{\mu}, \boldsymbol{\Sigma})$.

1. All the marginal distributions are Gaussian.
2. Conditional distributions are Gaussian.
3. Any affine combination $b_0 + \sum_{i=1}^{n} b_i X_i$ has a normal distribution.
4. To simulate $\boldsymbol{X}$:

    a. Derive the *Cholesky decomposition* $\boldsymbol{\Sigma} = \mathbf{A}\mathbf{A}^\top$.
    b. Generate $Z_1, \ldots, Z_n \sim_{\text{iid}} \mathcal{N}(0, 1)$. Let $\boldsymbol{Z} = [Z_1, \ldots, Z_n]^\top$.
    c. Return $\boldsymbol{X} = \boldsymbol{\mu} + \mathbf{A}\boldsymbol{Z}$.

12.2.1 Gaussian Graphical Model

Since a Gaussian distribution is fully characterized by the mean vector $\boldsymbol{\mu}$ and
the covariance matrix $\boldsymbol{\Sigma}$, it suffices to specify these two quantities to construct
a Gaussian model. It is often convenient to represent the covariance structure

of a Gaussian model via a graph: a **Gaussian graphical model**. This graph
is similar to a Bayesian network in Sect. 8.3, but is *undirected*.

☞ 25

The purpose of a Gaussian graphical model is to summarize the conditional independence properties of the variables. In particular, in a Gaussian
graphical model of a random vector $\boldsymbol{X} = [X_1, \ldots, X_n]^\top \sim \mathcal{N}(\boldsymbol{\mu}, \boldsymbol{\Sigma})$, the
nodes represent the components $X_1, \ldots, X_n$. Two nodes are connected by an
undirected edge if and only if the corresponding variables are *conditionally
dependent given all the other values*. Recall that X_i and X_j are conditionally
independent if (using Bayesian notation for simplicity)

$$f(x_i, x_j \mid x_k, k \neq i, j) = f(x_i \mid x_k, k \neq i, j)\, f(x_j \mid x_k, k \neq i, j)\,.$$

Because $\boldsymbol{X}$ is Gaussian, its pdf is given by

$$f(\boldsymbol{x}) = (2\pi)^{-n/2}\sqrt{\det(\boldsymbol{\Lambda})}\,\mathrm{e}^{-\frac{1}{2}(\boldsymbol{x}-\boldsymbol{\mu})^\top \boldsymbol{\Lambda}(\boldsymbol{x}-\boldsymbol{\mu})}\,,$$

where $\boldsymbol{\Lambda} = (\lambda_{ij})$ is the inverse of the covariance matrix $\boldsymbol{\Sigma}$, called the **precision matrix**. Therefore, the conditional joint pdf of X_i and X_j is

$$f(x_i, x_j \mid x_k, k \neq i, j) \propto \exp\left(-\frac{1}{2}(\lambda_{ii}x_i^2 + 2x_i\,a + \lambda_{ij}x_ix_j + \lambda_{jj}x_j^2 + 2x_j\,b)\right),$$

where a and b may depend on $x_k, k \neq i, j$. This shows that X_i and X_j
are conditionally independent given $\{X_k, k \neq i, j\}$, if and only if $\lambda_{ij} = 0$.
Consequently, (i, j) is an edge in the graphical model if and only if $\lambda_{ij} \neq 0$.
In typical applications (e.g., in image analysis) each vertex in the graphical
model only has a small number of adjacent vertices. In such cases the precision
matrix is thus sparse, and the Gaussian vector can be generated efficiently
using, for example, sparse Cholesky factorization.

For a sparse precision matrix the following algorithm is more efficient than
Algorithm 3.3 for generating independent samples.

☞ 84

**Algorithm 12.1. (Multivariate Normal Vector Generation Us-
ing the Precision Matrix).** To generate N independent draws from
a $\mathcal{N}(\boldsymbol{\mu}, \boldsymbol{\Lambda}^{-1})$ distribution of dimension n carry out the following steps:

1. Determine the lower Cholesky factorization $\boldsymbol{\Lambda} = \mathbf{D}\mathbf{D}^\top$.
2. Generate $\boldsymbol{Z} = [Z_1, \ldots, Z_n]^\top$, with $Z_1, \ldots, Z_n \sim_{\mathrm{iid}} \mathcal{N}(0, 1)$.
3. Solve $\boldsymbol{Y}$ from $\boldsymbol{Z} = \mathbf{D}^\top\boldsymbol{Y}$.
4. Output $\boldsymbol{X} = \boldsymbol{\mu} + \boldsymbol{Y}$.
5. Repeat Steps 2–4 independently N times.

Example 12.8 (Gaussian Graphical Model). In Fig. 12.8 a Gaussian
graphical model is depicted for $n = 8$ normal random variables, divided into

three groups. Variables in different groups are independent of each other. The first group contains only X_1, which is independent of all the other variables. In the second group, X_2, X_3, and X_4, each variable is conditionally dependent of the other two. In the last group, $X_5, \ldots, X_8$, each variable is conditionally dependent on one or two variables, while conditionally independent of the rest. For example, X_6 is conditionally independent of X_8 given X_7.

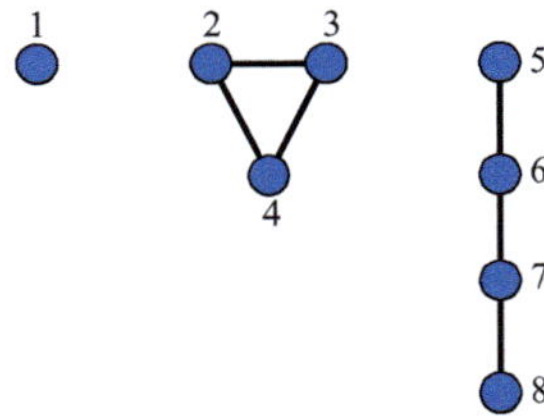

Fig. 12.8 An example of a Gaussian graphical model

The covariance and precision matrices have the following structure:

$$
\Sigma =
\begin{bmatrix}
\boxed{*} & & \\
 & \begin{matrix} * & * & * \\ * & * & * \\ * & * & * \end{matrix} & \\
 & & \begin{matrix} * & * & * & * \\ * & * & * & * \\ * & * & * & * \\ * & * & * & * \end{matrix}
\end{bmatrix}
, \qquad
\Lambda =
\begin{bmatrix}
\boxed{*} & & \\
 & \begin{matrix} * & * & * \\ * & * & * \\ * & * & * \end{matrix} & \\
 & & \begin{matrix} * & * & 0 & 0 \\ * & * & * & 0 \\ 0 & * & * & * \\ 0 & 0 & * & * \end{matrix}
\end{bmatrix} .
$$

Namely, the (i,j)-th element of the covariance matrix Σ is the covariance between X_i and X_j. Hence, Σ consists of three diagonal blocks, each corresponding to the covariances among the variables within each group. The precision matrix has nonzero entries λ_{ij} precisely when (i,j) is an edge in the graph. Notice that here the precision matrix is sparser than the covariance matrix.

12.2.2 Random Effects

In the ANOVA models introduced in Chap. 4, it was assumed that the "effects" of the factors—that is, the parameters μ, α_j, β_k, etc.—are *fixed* (deterministic). In a variety of situations, it is more appropriate to assume that certain model parameters are *random*. The following example illustrates the idea.

Example 12.9 (One-factor Random Effects ANOVA Model). To investigate whether geographical location is important in the effectiveness of a new type of herbicide, a researcher selects ten locations from a large number of possible locations within a country. At each location the herbicide is applied to three similar test plots. Each test plot is divided in half. One half (randomly selected) receives the herbicide, and the other half is left untreated. The difference in crop yield for each plot is measured, giving 30 measurements (response variables) in total. The experimental design is here *hierarchical* in structure: first the locations are chosen, and then the measurements are taken. The selection of the location could be modeled via independent random variables

$$\mu_1, \ldots, \mu_{10} \overset{\text{iid}}{\sim} \mathcal{N}(\mu, \sigma_\mu^2) \,,$$

representing the expected difference in crop yields at the ten locations, where μ and σ_μ^2 are fixed parameters. Given the $\{\mu_i\}$, the actual difference in crop yield for the k-th crop at location i could be modeled as

$$(Y_{ik} \mid \mu_i) \sim \mathcal{N}(\mu_i, \sigma^2), \text{ independently for } i = 1, \ldots, 10 \,,$$

where σ^2 is fixed.

For this designed experiment, the researcher is not interested *per se* in statements about the ten selected locations, but rather in conclusions pertaining to *all* possible geographical locations—in particular, regarding the parameters μ and σ_μ^2. For example, is the treatment effective across the country ($\mu > 0$)? Is geographical location much more important than measurement error in explaining the variability in the measurements (σ_μ^2 is much greater than σ^2)?

We summarize the one-factor random effects ANOVA model as follows.

Definition 12.4. (One-factor Random Effects ANOVA Model).
Let Y_{ik} be the response for the k-th replication at level i. Then

$$Y_{ik} = \mu_i + \varepsilon_{ik} \,, \quad k = 1, \ldots, n_i \,, \ i = 1, \ldots, d \,, \tag{12.15}$$

where

$$\mu_1, \ldots, \mu_d \overset{\text{iid}}{\sim} \mathcal{N}(\mu, \sigma_\mu^2) \,,$$

independent of $\{\varepsilon_{ik}\} \sim_{\text{iid}} \mathcal{N}(0, \sigma^2)$.

The model is again Gaussian, but, due to the hierarchical formulation, the $\{Y_{ik}\}$ are no longer independent within the i-th level. By the model assumptions in (12.15), the responses $Y_{i1}, \ldots, Y_{in_i}$ are independent conditional on the random effect μ_i. However, marginalized over μ_i, the covariance between, say, Y_{ij} and $Y_{ik}, j \neq k$, is nonzero:

$$\mathrm{Cov}(Y_{ij}, Y_{ik}) = \mathrm{Cov}(\mu_i + \varepsilon_{ij}, \mu_i + \varepsilon_{ik}) = \sigma_\mu^2 \, .$$

If we define $\boldsymbol{Y}_i = (Y_{i1}, \ldots, Y_{in_i})^\top$, then, each $\boldsymbol{Y}_i$ is independent but not identically distributed (denoted by "ind" below) as

$$\boldsymbol{Y}_i \overset{\text{ind}}{\sim} \mathcal{N}(\mu \boldsymbol{1}_{n_i}, \sigma^2 I_{n_i} + \sigma_\mu^2 \boldsymbol{1}_{n_i} \boldsymbol{1}_{n_i}^\top), \quad i = 1, \ldots, d \, ,$$

where $\boldsymbol{1}_{n_i}$ is an $n_i \times 1$ column of ones and I_{n_i} is the n_i-dimensional identity matrix. To see this, first note that, by definition,

$$\boldsymbol{Y}_i = \mu_i \boldsymbol{1}_{n_i} + \boldsymbol{\varepsilon}_i \, ,$$

where $\boldsymbol{\varepsilon}_i = [\varepsilon_1, \ldots, \varepsilon_{n_i}]^\top \sim \mathcal{N}(\boldsymbol{0}, \sigma^2 \mathbb{I}_{n_i})$. In other words, $\boldsymbol{Y}_i$ is a linear combination of normal random variables and therefore has a normal distribution. In addition, it is easy to check that its expectation is $\mathbb{E}\boldsymbol{Y}_i = \mu \boldsymbol{1}_{n_i}$, and its covariance matrix is

$$\mathrm{Cov}(\boldsymbol{Y}_i) = \mathrm{Var}(\mu_i)\boldsymbol{1}_{n_i}\boldsymbol{1}_{n_i}^\top + \mathrm{Cov}(\boldsymbol{\varepsilon}_i) = \sigma_\mu^2 \boldsymbol{1}_{n_i}\boldsymbol{1}_{n_i}^\top + \sigma^2 \mathbb{I}_{n_i} \, .$$

Hence, the claim follows.

From the above discussion, we have also derived the log-likelihood function for the one-factor random effects model in (12.15). More specifically, given the outcomes $\boldsymbol{Y}_1 = \boldsymbol{y}_1, \ldots, \boldsymbol{Y}_d = \boldsymbol{y}_d$, the log-likelihood function is given by

$$
\begin{aligned}
l(\mu, \sigma_\mu^2, \sigma^2; \boldsymbol{y}) = &- \frac{n}{2} \ln(2\pi) - \frac{1}{2} \sum_{i=1}^d \ln |\boldsymbol{\Sigma}_i| \\
&- \frac{1}{2} \sum_{i=1}^d (\boldsymbol{y}_i - \mu \boldsymbol{1}_{n_i})^\top \boldsymbol{\Sigma}_i^{-1} (\boldsymbol{y}_i - \mu \boldsymbol{1}_{n_i}) \, ,
\end{aligned}
\tag{12.16}
$$

where $\boldsymbol{y} = [\boldsymbol{y}_1^\top, \ldots, \boldsymbol{y}_d^\top]^\top$ and $\boldsymbol{\Sigma}_i = \sigma_\mu^2 \boldsymbol{1}_{n_i} \boldsymbol{1}_{n_i}^\top + \sigma^2 \mathbb{I}_{n_i}$.

Since the log-likelihood function is of low dimension, the maximum likelihood estimates of μ, σ_μ^2, and σ^2 can be obtained quickly by numerically maximizing the log-likelihood. For a Bayesian analysis of the one-factor random effect model, see Problem 12.11.

Example 12.10 (One-factor Random Effects ANOVA Model Continued). Consider again Example 12.9 in which we investigate if geographical location is important in the effectiveness of a new type of herbicide. Suppose the researcher has carried out the experiments and collected data from ten randomly selected locations. Specifically, at each location the differences in crop yield (kg) for three test plots are measured. The results are reported in Table 12.3.

Table 12.3 Differences in crop yield (kg)

Location	Difference in Crop Yield			Location	Difference in Crop Yield		
1	22.6	20.5	20.8	6	14.5	10.5	12.3
2	22.6	21.2	20.5	7	20.8	19.1	21.3
3	17.3	16.2	16.6	8	17.4	18.6	18.6
4	21.4	23.7	23.2	9	25.1	24.8	24.9
5	20.9	22.2	22.6	10	14.9	16.3	16.6

To compute the maximum likelihood estimates of μ, σ_μ^2, and σ^2, we first write a Julia function to evaluate the log-likelihood function $l(\mu, \sigma_\mu^2, \sigma^2; \boldsymbol{y})$. Note that in the code below the outcomes are stored as a matrix, where each row contains the experimental results in one of the randomly selected locations.

```julia
function sfran_loglike(mu,sigma2_mu,sigma2,y)
    d, ni = size(y)
    Sigmai = sigma2*diagm(ones(ni)) .+ sigma2_mu*ones(ni,ni)
    l = -(ni*d)/2*log(2*pi) - d/2*log(det(Sigmai))
    for i=1:d
      yi = y[i,:];
      l = l - .5*(yi .- mu)'*(Sigmai(yi .- mu))
    end
    return l
end
```

Next, in the main script, we load the data and define a trivariate function that is the negative of the log-likelihood function `sfran_loglike`. The new function is then passed to the built-in minimization routine `fminsearch` to compute the minimizer. For the starting values for μ, σ_μ^2, and σ^2, we use

$$\bar{y} = \frac{1}{d}\sum_{i=1}^{d}\bar{y}_i, \quad s^2 = \frac{1}{d-1}\sum_{i=1}^{d}(\bar{y}_i - \bar{y})^2, \quad \bar{s}^2 = \frac{1}{d}\sum_{i=1}^{d}s_i^2,$$

where $\bar{y}_i$ and s_i^2 are, respectively, the sample mean and sample variance of the outcomes in location i.

```julia
sfran.jl

using LinearAlgebra, StatsBase, Optim
y = [ 22.6 20.5 20.8; 22.6 21.2 20.5; 17.3 16.2 16.6;
      21.4 23.7 23.2; 20.9 22.2 22.6; 14.5 10.5 12.3;
      20.8 19.1 21.3; 17.4 18.6 18.6; 25.1 24.8 24.9;
```

```
      14.9 16.3 16.6];
f =  theta -> -sfran_loglike(theta[1],theta[2],theta[3],y)
ybar = mean(y,dims=2)
theta0 = [mean(ybar) var(ybar) mean(var(y,dims=2))]
res = optimize(f,theta0);
thetahat = res.minimizer
```

The maximum likelihood estimates of μ, σ_μ^2, and σ^2 are 19.6, 12.19, and 1.167, respectively. For this example the herbicide seems to be quite effective.

The two-factor random effects ANOVA model can be defined similarly. Below we use the "factor effects" representation.

☞ 114

Definition 12.5. (Two-factor Random Effects ANOVA Model). Let Y_{ijk} be the response for the k-th replication at cell (i, j). Then

$$Y_{ijk} = \mu + \alpha_i + \beta_j + \gamma_{ij} + \varepsilon_{ijk} \,,$$
$$k = 1, \ldots, n_{ij} \,, \ i = 1, \ldots, d_1 \,, \ j = 1, \ldots, d_2 \,, \tag{12.17}$$

where μ is a fixed constant and the following random variables are independent of each other:

$$\{\alpha_i\} \stackrel{\text{iid}}{\sim} \mathcal{N}(0, \sigma_\alpha^2) \,, \qquad \{\beta_j\} \stackrel{\text{iid}}{\sim} \mathcal{N}(0, \sigma_\beta^2),$$
$$\{\gamma_{ij}\} \stackrel{\text{iid}}{\sim} \mathcal{N}(0, \sigma_\gamma^2), \qquad \{\varepsilon_{ijk}\} \stackrel{\text{iid}}{\sim} \mathcal{N}(0, \sigma^2).$$

Note that there are much fewer parameters than for the corresponding fixed effects model. Also, there are no restrictions such as $\sum_i \alpha_i = 0$ on the parameters.

To derive the likelihood function, we first rewrite (12.17) in matrix form. To that end, let $\boldsymbol{\alpha} = [\alpha_1, \ldots, \alpha_{d_1}]^\top$, $\boldsymbol{\beta} = [\beta_1, \ldots, \beta_{d_2}]^\top$, and $\boldsymbol{\gamma} = [\gamma_{11}, \ldots, \gamma_{d_1 d_2}]^\top$. Arrange the responses $\{Y_{ijk}\}$ and errors $\{\varepsilon_{ijk}\}$ as $\boldsymbol{Y} = [Y_1, \ldots, Y_n]^\top$ and $\boldsymbol{\varepsilon} = [\varepsilon_1, \ldots, \varepsilon_n]^\top$, where $n = \sum_{i,j} n_{ij}$. Then,

$$\boldsymbol{Y} = \mu\mathbf{1} + \mathbf{X}_\alpha \boldsymbol{\alpha} + \mathbf{X}_\beta \boldsymbol{\beta} + \mathbf{X}_\gamma \boldsymbol{\gamma} + \boldsymbol{\varepsilon} \,, \tag{12.18}$$

where $\mathbf{1}$ an n-dimensional vector of 1s and the design matrices $\mathbf{X}_\alpha, \mathbf{X}_\beta$, and $\mathbf{X}_\gamma$ are appropriately defined. Again, $\boldsymbol{Y}$ is an affine transformation of normal random variables and therefore has a multivariate normal distribution. Its mean is $\mathbb{E}\boldsymbol{Y} = \mu\mathbf{1}$, and its covariance matrix is given by

$$\boldsymbol{\Sigma} = \sigma_\alpha^2 \mathbf{X}_\alpha \mathbf{X}_\alpha^\top + \sigma_\beta^2 \mathbf{X}_\beta \mathbf{X}_\beta^\top + \sigma_\gamma^2 \mathbf{X}_\gamma \mathbf{X}_\gamma^\top + \sigma^2 \mathbb{I}_n \,.$$

Hence, given the outcomes $\boldsymbol{Y} = \boldsymbol{y}$, the log-likelihood function for the two-factor ANOVA model is

$$
\begin{aligned}
l(\mu, \sigma_\alpha^2, \sigma_\beta^2, \sigma_\gamma^2, \sigma^2; \boldsymbol{y}) = & -\frac{n}{2}\ln(2\pi) - \frac{1}{2}\ln|\boldsymbol{\Sigma}| \\
& -\frac{1}{2}(\boldsymbol{y} - \mu\mathbf{1})^\top \boldsymbol{\Sigma}^{-1}(\boldsymbol{y} - \mu\mathbf{1}) \, .
\end{aligned}
\tag{12.19}
$$

Calculation of the maximum likelihood estimates involves a five-dimensional maximization problem, which may be time-consuming, but can still be done numerically. There are two computational issues that are worth mentioning. First, note that evaluation of the log-likelihood function (12.19) involves calculating the log determinant $\ln|\boldsymbol{\Sigma}|$. When the dimension n is large, computing the determinant $|\boldsymbol{\Sigma}|$ first and then taking the log might lead to substantial rounding error. Instead, consider the following equivalent calculations: obtain the Cholesky factor $\mathbf{C}$ of $\boldsymbol{\Sigma}$. Since $\mathbf{C}$ is a lower triangular matrix, its determinant is equal to the product of the diagonal elements, say, $c_{11}, \ldots, c_{nn}$. It follows then that

$$
\ln|\boldsymbol{\Sigma}| = 2\ln|\mathbf{C}| = 2\sum_{i=1}^{n}\ln c_{ii} \, .
$$

The second issue concerns the restrictions on the variance parameters σ_α^2, σ_β^2, σ_γ^2, and σ^2—since they represent variances, they have to be positive. In other words, computing their maximum likelihood estimates is in fact a constrained maximization problem, and ignoring the restrictions might lead to numerical errors. One solution to this problem is to reparameterize in terms of

$$
\eta_\alpha = \ln(\sigma_\alpha^2), \quad \eta_\beta = \ln(\sigma_\beta^2), \quad \eta_\gamma = \ln(\sigma_\gamma^2), \quad \eta = \ln(\sigma^2) \, ,
$$

and maximize the log-likelihood (12.19)

$$
l(\mu, \sigma_\alpha^2, \sigma_\beta^2, \sigma_\gamma^2, \sigma^2; \boldsymbol{y}) = l(\mu, \mathrm{e}^{\eta_\alpha}, \mathrm{e}^{\eta_\beta}, \mathrm{e}^{\eta_\gamma}, \mathrm{e}^{\eta}; \boldsymbol{y})
$$

with respect to μ, η_α, η_β, η_γ, and η. Once the maximum likelihood estimates of the new parameters are obtained, those for the original parameterization can be computed easily. The following example illustrates these points.

Example 12.11 (Two-factor Random Effects ANOVA Model). In this example we investigate the breeding value of a set of five sires in raising pigs. Each sire is mated to a random group of dams, and the mating produces a litter of pigs whose characteristics are measured. In particular, the average daily gain of two piglets in each litter (in pounds) over a given period of time is recorded. The outcomes are reported in Table 12.4.

The model we consider is

$$
Y_{ijk} = \mu + \alpha_i + \gamma_{ij} + \varepsilon_{ijk} \, ,
$$

Table 12.4 Average daily gain of two piglets in each litter (in pounds)

Sire	Dam	Gain		Sire	Dam	Gain
1	1	1.39		3	2	0.95
1	1	1.29		3	2	0.96
1	2	1.12		4	1	0.82
1	2	1.16		4	1	0.92
2	1	1.52		4	2	1.18
2	1	1.62		4	2	1.20
2	2	1.88		5	1	1.47
2	2	1.87		5	1	1.41
3	1	1.24		5	2	1.57
3	1	1.18		5	2	1.65

where α_i is the random effect associated with the i-th sire and γ_{ij} is the random effect associated with the i-th sire and j-th dam. To write the model in matrix form, let $\boldsymbol{Y} = [Y_{111}, Y_{112}, Y_{121}, Y_{122}, \ldots, Y_{521}, Y_{522}]^{\top}$, $\boldsymbol{\alpha} = [\alpha_1, \ldots, \alpha_5]^{\top}$, and $\boldsymbol{\gamma} = [\gamma_{11}, \gamma_{12}, \ldots, \gamma_{51}, \gamma_{52}]^{\top}$. Then,

$$\boldsymbol{Y} = \mu \mathbf{1}_{20} + \mathbf{X}_{\alpha} \boldsymbol{\alpha} + \mathbf{X}_{\gamma} \boldsymbol{\gamma} + \boldsymbol{\varepsilon} \,,$$

where $\mathbf{X}_{\alpha} = \mathbb{I}_5 \otimes \mathbf{1}_4$, $\mathbf{X}_{\gamma} = \mathbb{I}_{10} \otimes \mathbf{1}_2$, $\otimes$ is the Kronecker product, $\mathbf{1}_p$ is a $p \times 1$ vector of ones, and $\mathbb{I}_q$ is the q-dimensional identity matrix.

As in the previous example, we first write a Julia function to evaluate the log-likelihood function parameterized in terms of μ, $\eta_{\alpha} = \ln(\sigma_{\alpha}^2)$, $\eta_{\gamma} = \ln(\sigma_{\gamma}^2)$, and $\eta = \ln(\sigma^2)$.

```julia
function sfran2_loglike(mu,eta_alpha,eta_gamma,eta,y,Xalpha,
    Xgamma)
  sigma2_alpha = exp.(eta_alpha)
  sigma2_gamma = exp.(eta_gamma)
  sigma2 = exp.(eta)
  n = length(y)
  Sigma = sigma2*diagm(ones(n)) .+ sigma2_alpha*(Xalpha*
      Xalpha') .+
      sigma2_gamma*(Xgamma*Xgamma')
  l = -n/2*log(2*pi) - sum(log.(diag(cholesky(Sigma).L))) -
      0.5*(y .- mu)'*(Sigma(y .- mu));
end
```

Then, in the main script, we maximize the log-likelihood function numerically with respect to μ, η_{α}, η_{γ}, and η. The maximizer is then transformed to get the maximum likelihood estimates of the original parameters. The estimates of μ, σ_{α}^2, σ_{γ}^2, and σ^2 are, respectively, 1.32, 0.0537, 0.0318, and 0.023.

For this dataset, the sires seem to be the most important factor in explaining the variation in the average daily gain of the piglets.

```
sfran2.jl
```

```julia
using Kronecker, LinearAlgebra, StatsBase, Optim
y = [1.39, 1.29, 1.12, 1.16, 1.52, 1.62, 1.88, 1.87, 1.24,
   1.18,0.95, 0.96, 0.82, 0.92, 1.18, 1.20, 1.47, 1.41,
   1.57, 1.65]
Xalpha = kronecker(diagm(ones(5)),ones(4,1))
Xgamma = kronecker(diagm(ones(10)),ones(2,1))
yhat = mean(reshape(y,4,5),dims=2)
theta0 = [mean(y),log(var(yhat)),log(var(y)/3),log(var(y)/3)]
f(theta) = -sfran2_loglike(theta[1],theta[2],theta[3],
                           theta[4],y,Xalpha,Xgamma)
res = optimize(f,theta0);
thetahat = res.minimizer
```

12.2.3 Gaussian Linear Mixed Models

It is also possible to combine fixed and random factors. This leads to the so-called **mixed models**. A general formulation for such models is given below. We first discuss an example.

Example 12.12 (Two-Factor Mixed ANOVA Model). Suppose the experiment in Example 12.9 is modified in the following way. Each of the 30 test plots is subjected to three different treatments of herbicide: (1) the new herbicide, (2) a standard herbicide, and (3) no herbicide. Specifically, each test plot is divided into three subplots, and the three treatments are assigned in a random (and uniform) way to the subplots. The crop yield is recorded for each of the subplots. For each of the ten plots, there are thus nine measurements—three for each treatment. There are now two factors to consider: herbicide and location. The first is a *fixed* factor; the second is a *random* factor. Denoting by Y_{ijk} the k-th crop yield at location j, with treatment i, we obtain the two-factor mixed ANOVA model

$$Y_{ijk} = \mu + \alpha_i + \beta_j + \gamma_{ij} + \varepsilon_{ijk} \,,$$
$$i = 1,2,3, \quad j = 1,2,\ldots,10, \quad k = 1,2,3 \,,$$

where μ is a constant, $\alpha_1,\ldots,\alpha_3$ are the fixed incremental effects of the herbicide, and $\beta_1,\ldots,\beta_{10}$ are the random incremental effects due to location. As in the fixed ANOVA case, we impose the restriction $\sum_i \alpha_i = 0$. The random incremental effects are modeled via $\{\beta_j\} \sim_{\text{iid}} \mathcal{N}(0, \sigma_\beta^2)$. The measurement errors $\{\varepsilon_{ijk}\}$ are assumed to be independent of each other and of the $\{\beta_j\}$ and are all $\mathcal{N}(0, \sigma_\varepsilon^2)$-distributed, for some fixed σ_ε^2. Finally, for the terms γ_{ij} there are two common model choices. The simplest one is to assume that $\{\gamma_{ij}\} \sim_{\text{iid}} \mathcal{N}(0, \sigma_\gamma^2)$. However, this introduces a subtle problem regarding the interpretation of α_i as an "incremental effect" due to treatment i. To circumvent this difficulty, one often imposes the restriction

$$\sum_i \gamma_{ij} = 0 \quad \text{for all } j \ .$$

The latter is called a **restricted** mixed ANOVA model, as opposed to the former **unrestricted** model.

Here we give a general formulation for the linear mixed models.

Definition 12.6. (Gaussian Linear Mixed Model). Let $\boldsymbol{Y}$ be an $n \times 1$ vector of responses, then

$$\boldsymbol{Y} = \mathbf{X}\boldsymbol{\beta} + \mathbf{Z}\boldsymbol{U} + \boldsymbol{\varepsilon} \ , \tag{12.20}$$

where $\boldsymbol{\beta}$ is a $p \times 1$ vector of fixed effects, $\mathbf{X}$ is an $n \times p$ design matrix for the fixed effects, and $\mathbf{Z}$ is an $n \times q$ design matrix for the random effects. In addition, $\boldsymbol{U}$ and $\boldsymbol{\varepsilon}$ are independent of each other, and

$$\boldsymbol{U} \sim \mathcal{N}(\mathbf{0}, \boldsymbol{\Sigma}_U) \ , \quad \boldsymbol{\varepsilon} \sim \mathcal{N}(\mathbf{0}, \sigma^2 \mathbb{I}_n) \ .$$

The covariance matrix of $\boldsymbol{Y}$ is $\boldsymbol{\Sigma} = \sigma^2 \mathbb{I}_n + \mathbf{Z}\, \boldsymbol{\Sigma}_U\, \mathbf{Z}^\top$. Hence, given the outcome $\boldsymbol{Y} = \boldsymbol{y}$, the log-likelihood function is

$$l(\boldsymbol{\beta}, \sigma^2, \boldsymbol{\Sigma}_U; \boldsymbol{y}) = -\frac{n}{2}\ln(2\pi) - \frac{1}{2}\ln|\boldsymbol{\Sigma}| - \frac{1}{2}(\boldsymbol{y} - \mathbf{X}\boldsymbol{\beta})^\top \boldsymbol{\Sigma}^{-1}(\boldsymbol{y} - \mathbf{X}\boldsymbol{\beta}) \ . \tag{12.21}$$

Unless the dimension of the log-likelihood function is low, direct maximization could be time-consuming. Instead, dimension reduction techniques such as using the profile likelihood can be applied to speed up the estimation. Alternatively, the linear mixed model can be estimated using the Gibbs sampler, as the following example illustrates.

Example 12.13 (Gaussian Linear Mixed Model). In an experiment concerning the growth rate of rats, 30 different rats are weighed at five different points in time — 8, 15, 22, 29, and 36 days since birth. Using Bayesian notation, let y_{ik} denote the weight of the i-th rat at the k-th measurement, and let x_{ik} denote the corresponding age of the rat. Then,

$$x_{i1} = 8 \ , \quad x_{i2} = 15 \ , \quad x_{i3} = 22 \ , \quad x_{i4} = 29 \ , \quad x_{i5} = 36$$

for $i = 1, \ldots, 30$. The data are taken from Gelfand et al. (1990), and the growth curves are depicted in Fig. 12.9.

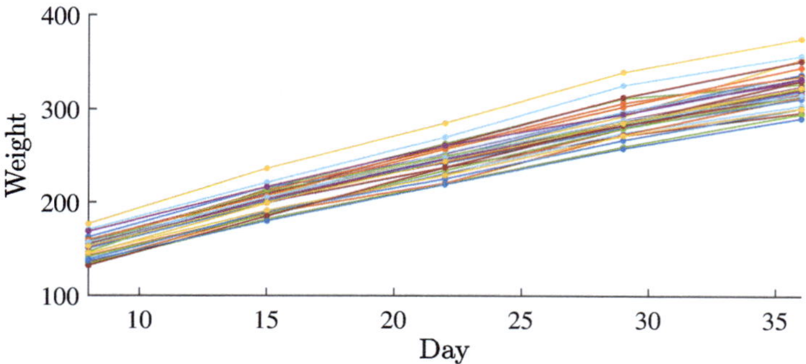

Fig. 12.9 Growth curves for 30 rats

In the model, we allow for individual-specific variation in the initial birth weight but assume the same growth rate

$$y_{ik} = \beta_0 + \beta_1 x_{ik} + \alpha_i + \varepsilon_{ik} \, ,$$

where $\{\alpha_i\} \sim_{\text{iid}} \mathcal{N}(0, \sigma_\alpha^2)$ and $\{\varepsilon_{ik}\} \sim_{\text{iid}} \mathcal{N}(0, \sigma^2)$ are independent, $i = 1, \ldots,$ 30, $k = 1, \ldots, 5$.

To write the model in the form in (12.20), let

$$\boldsymbol{y} = [y_{11}, \ldots, y_{15}, y_{21}, \ldots, y_{25}, \ldots, y_{30,1}, \ldots, y_{30,5}]^\top,$$

and define $\boldsymbol{\varepsilon}$ similarly. Further, let $\boldsymbol{\beta} = [\beta_0, \beta_1]^\top$, $\boldsymbol{\alpha} = [\alpha_1, \ldots, \alpha_{30}]^\top$, $\mathbf{Z} = \mathbb{I}_{30} \otimes \mathbf{1}_5$, $\mathbf{X} = \mathbf{1}_{30} \otimes [\mathbf{1}_5, \boldsymbol{x}_i]$, $\boldsymbol{x}_i = [x_{i1}, \ldots, x_{i5}]^\top$, and let $\mathbf{1}_m$ be an $m \times 1$ vector of ones. Then,

$$\boldsymbol{y} = \mathbf{X}\boldsymbol{\beta} + \mathbf{Z}\boldsymbol{\alpha} + \boldsymbol{\varepsilon} \, ,$$

where $\boldsymbol{\alpha} \sim \mathcal{N}(\mathbf{0}, \sigma_\alpha^2 \mathbb{I}_{30})$ and $\boldsymbol{\varepsilon} \sim \mathcal{N}(\mathbf{0}, \sigma^2 \mathbb{I}_{150})$ are independent. The actual outcomes of the experiment are reported in Table 12.5.

To perform a Bayesian analysis, consider the following independent priors:

$$\boldsymbol{\beta} \sim \mathcal{N}(\boldsymbol{\beta}_0, 100\,\mathbb{I}_2), \quad \sigma_\alpha^2 \sim \mathsf{InvGamma}(3, 100), \quad \sigma^2 \sim \mathsf{InvGamma}(3, 100) \, ,$$

where $\boldsymbol{\beta}_0 = [100, 10]^\top$. The degree of freedom parameters for the inverse-gamma distributions are chosen to be small so that the prior variances are large. Since $\boldsymbol{\alpha}$ and $\boldsymbol{\beta}$ enter the likelihood additively, we sample them in one block to improve efficiency. Specifically, we consider the three-block Gibbs sampler: (1) simulate from $f(\boldsymbol{\alpha}, \boldsymbol{\beta} \,|\, y, \sigma^2, \sigma_\alpha^2)$, (2) simulate from $f(\sigma^2 \,|\, \boldsymbol{y}, \boldsymbol{\alpha}, \boldsymbol{\beta}, \sigma_\alpha^2)$, and (3) simulate from $f(\sigma_\alpha^2 \,|\, \boldsymbol{y}, \boldsymbol{\alpha}, \boldsymbol{\beta}, \sigma^2)$. Steps 2 and 3 are straightforward as the two conditional distributions are both inverse-gamma

Table 12.5 Weight measurements of rats

Rat i	y_{i1}	y_{i2}	y_{i3}	y_{i4}	y_{i5}	Rat i	y_{i1}	y_{i2}	y_{i3}	y_{i4}	y_{i5}
1	151	199	246	283	320	16	160	207	248	288	324
2	145	199	249	293	354	17	142	187	234	280	316
3	147	214	263	312	328	18	156	203	243	283	317
4	155	200	237	272	297	19	157	212	259	307	336
5	135	188	230	280	323	20	152	203	246	286	321
6	159	210	252	298	331	21	154	205	253	298	334
7	141	189	231	275	305	22	139	190	225	267	302
8	159	201	248	297	338	23	146	191	229	272	302
9	177	236	285	340	376	24	157	211	250	285	323
10	134	182	220	260	296	25	132	185	237	286	331
11	160	208	261	313	352	26	160	207	257	303	345
12	143	188	220	273	314	27	169	216	261	295	333
13	154	200	244	289	325	28	157	205	248	289	316
14	171	221	270	326	358	29	137	180	219	258	291
15	163	216	242	281	312	30	153	200	244	286	324

☞ 245 (see Theorem 8.1):

$$(\sigma^2 \mid \boldsymbol{y}, \boldsymbol{\alpha}, \boldsymbol{\beta}, \sigma_\alpha^2) \sim \mathsf{InvGamma}(78, \lambda),$$

$$(\sigma_\alpha^2 \mid \boldsymbol{y}, \boldsymbol{\alpha}, \boldsymbol{\beta}, \sigma^2) \sim \mathsf{InvGamma}(18, \lambda_\alpha) \,,$$

where $\lambda = 100 + (\boldsymbol{y} - \mathbf{X}\boldsymbol{\beta} - \mathbf{Z}\boldsymbol{\alpha})^\top (\boldsymbol{y} - \mathbf{X}\boldsymbol{\beta} - \mathbf{Z}\boldsymbol{\alpha})/2$ and $\lambda_\alpha = 100 + \boldsymbol{\alpha}^\top \boldsymbol{\alpha}/2$. For Step 1, let $\boldsymbol{\gamma} = [\boldsymbol{\beta}^\top, \boldsymbol{\alpha}^\top]^\top$. Then, the prior for $\boldsymbol{\gamma}$ is $\mathcal{N}(\boldsymbol{\gamma}_0, \mathbf{V}_{\boldsymbol{\gamma}})$, where

$$\boldsymbol{\gamma}_0 = \begin{bmatrix} \boldsymbol{\beta}_0 \\ \mathbf{0} \end{bmatrix}, \quad \mathbf{V}_{\boldsymbol{\gamma}} = \begin{bmatrix} 100\, \mathbb{I}_2 & 0 \\ 0 & \sigma_\alpha^2\, \mathbb{I}_{30} \end{bmatrix}.$$

Note that the covariance matrix $\mathbf{V}_{\boldsymbol{\gamma}}$ is in fact diagonal. In addition, the linear mixed model can be written as

$$\boldsymbol{y} = \mathbf{W}\boldsymbol{\gamma} + \boldsymbol{\varepsilon} \,,$$

☞ 245 where $\mathbf{W} = [\mathbf{X}, \mathbf{Z}]$. Hence, using Theorem 8.1, we have

$$(\boldsymbol{\gamma} \mid \boldsymbol{y}, \sigma^2, \sigma_\alpha^2) \sim \mathcal{N}(\widehat{\boldsymbol{\gamma}}, \mathbf{K}_{\boldsymbol{\gamma}}^{-1}) \,,$$

where

$$\mathbf{K}_{\boldsymbol{\gamma}} = \mathbf{W}^\top \mathbf{W}/\sigma^2 + \mathbf{V}_{\boldsymbol{\gamma}}^{-1} \,, \quad \widehat{\boldsymbol{\gamma}} = \mathbf{K}_{\boldsymbol{\gamma}}^{-1}(\mathbf{V}_{\boldsymbol{\gamma}}^{-1}\boldsymbol{\gamma}_0 + \mathbf{W}^\top \boldsymbol{y}/\sigma^2).$$

It is important to realize that although $\boldsymbol{\gamma}$ is high-dimensional, sampling from its conditional distribution is quick if we use sparse matrix routines and avoid
☞ 371 inverting the large precision matrix; see Algorithm 12.1.

The following Julia code implements the Gibbs sampler discussed above to fit the experimental data.

```julia
linmix.jl

using DelimitedFiles, Kronecker, SparseArrays, Distributions,
    LinearAlgebra
rats = readdlm("rats.csv",',')
d, ni = size(rats)
n = d*ni
y = reshape(rats',n,1);
nloop = 11000
burnin = 1000
    # storage
store_beta = zeros(nloop-burnin,2)
store_alpha = zeros(nloop-burnin,d)
store_var = zeros(nloop-burnin,2)
    # priors
beta0 = [100 10]'
invVbeta = [1/100 1/100]
gamma0 = [beta0; spzeros(d,1)]
nu_alpha = 3; lam_alpha = 100
nu = 3; lam = 100;
    # initialize the Markov chain
sigma2 = 100
sigma2_alpha = 100
    # compute a few things before the loop
Z = sparse(kronecker(diagm(ones(d)), ones(ni,1)))
xi = [8 15 22 29 36]'
X = kronecker(ones(d,1),[ones(ni,1) xi])
W = [X Z]
WW = W'*W
Wy = W'*y
newnu_alpha = d/2 + nu_alpha;
newnu = n/2 + nu;
for loop=1:nloop
    global sigma2_alpha, sigma2
        # sample alpha and beta
    invVgamma = sparse(1:d+2,1:d+2, vec([invVbeta 1/
        sigma2_alpha*ones(1,d)]))
    invDgamma = invVgamma + WW/sigma2
    gammahat = invDgamma(invVgamma*gamma0 + Wy/sigma2)
    gamma = gammahat + cholesky(invDgamma).L'\randn(d+2,1)
    beta = gamma[1:2]
    alpha = gamma[3:end]
        # sample sigma2_alpha
```

```
    newlam_alpha = lam_alpha + sum(alpha.^2)/2
    sigma2_alpha = 1/rand(Gamma(newnu_alpha, 1/newlam_alpha));
        # sample sigma2
    newlam = lam + sum((y-W*gamma).^2)/2
    sigma2 = 1/rand(Gamma(newnu, 1/newlam))
        # storage
    if loop>burnin
        i = loop-burnin;
        store_beta[i,:] = beta';
        store_alpha[i,:] = alpha';
        store_var[i,:] = [sigma2 sigma2_alpha];
    end
end
betahat = mean(store_beta,dims=1)
alphahat = mean(store_alpha,dims=1)
varhat = mean(store_var,dims=1)
```

In Table 12.6 we report the posterior means, standard deviations, and quantiles for selected parameters. The results indicate that there is substantial variation in initial birth weight—the posterior mean of σ_α^2 is about three times the estimate corresponding to the measurement error σ^2. Inference on individual random effects can also be easily carried out. For example, the birth weight of the 14-th rat is estimated to be between 19.90 and 34.73 above average with probability 80%.

Table 12.6 Posterior means, standard deviations, and quantiles for selected parameters

Parameter	Post. mean	Post. std.	Post. 0.1 quantile	Post. 0.9 quantile
β_0	106.10	2.73	102.82	112.58
β_1	6.19	0.07	6.11	6.35
σ^2	63.97	8.16	54.38	85.90
σ_α^2	170.89	46.62	119.98	313.66
α_{14}	25.01	4.19	19.90	34.73

12.3 Problems

12.1. Calculate the lag-1, 2, and 3 autocorrelations of the residuals in Example 12.1.

12.2. Prove Eq. 12.9; that is, show that under the MA(q) model, the autoco-variances of the responses are given by

$$\mathrm{Cov}(Y_t, Y_{t-j}) = \begin{cases} \sigma^2 \sum_{i=0}^{q-j} \psi_{i+j}\psi_i, & j = 0, \ldots, q , \\ 0, & j > q , \end{cases}$$

where $\psi_0 = 1$.

12.3. Consider again the MA(q) model:

$$Y_t = \varepsilon_t + \psi\varepsilon_{t-1} + \cdots + \psi_q\varepsilon_{t-q} .$$

In this exercise we relax the standard assumption that $\varepsilon_0 = \varepsilon_{-1} = \cdots = \varepsilon_{1-q} = 0$. Instead, we assume $\{\varepsilon_t\} \sim_{\mathrm{iid}} \mathcal{N}(0, \sigma^2)$ for $t = 1 - q, \ldots, T$. Derive the likelihood function for the outcome $\boldsymbol{Y} = \boldsymbol{y}$, where $\boldsymbol{Y} = [Y_1, \ldots, Y_T]^\top$ and $\boldsymbol{y} = [y_t, \ldots, y_T]^\top$.

12.4. In many situations, the data can be described by several competing models, and the question then is which model is "the best." Complex models tend to fit the data better, but they run the risk of overfitting. Hence, we want a measure that awards goodness-of-fit while penalizing model complexity. Two popular selection criteria that explicitly take this trade-off into account are the **Akaike information criterion** (AIC) and the **Bayesian information criterion** (BIC); see, for example, Bishop (2006) for a detailed introduction. Given a model defined by the log-likelihood function $l(\boldsymbol{\theta}; \boldsymbol{y})$, where $\boldsymbol{\theta}$ is a $p \times 1$ vector of model parameters and $\boldsymbol{y}$ is a $n \times 1$ vector of outcomes, the two information criteria are defined as follows:

$$\mathrm{AIC} = 2l(\boldsymbol{\theta}; \boldsymbol{y}) - 2p ,$$
$$\mathrm{BIC} = 2l(\boldsymbol{\theta}; \boldsymbol{y}) - p \ln n .$$

The only difference between the two information criteria is the penalty term: BIC tends to penalize complex model more heavily when $n \geq 8$. Given a set of competing models, the preferred model is the one with the maximum AIC/BIC value.

Use the two information criteria to compare the linear regression models in Examples 12.1 and 12.4.

12.5. Show that the log-likelihood function of the ARMA(p, q) model in (12.12) is given by (12.13). That is,

$$l(\boldsymbol{\varrho}, \boldsymbol{\psi}, \sigma^2; \boldsymbol{y}, \boldsymbol{y}_0) = -\frac{T}{2} \ln(2\pi\sigma^2) - \frac{1}{2\sigma^2}(\boldsymbol{y} - \mathbf{X}\boldsymbol{\varrho})^\top (\mathbf{H}\mathbf{H}^\top)^{-1}(\boldsymbol{y} - \mathbf{X}\boldsymbol{\varrho}) .$$

12.6. Consider the linear regression model with general covariance matrix $\sigma^2\boldsymbol{\Sigma}$:

$$\boldsymbol{Y} = \mathbf{X}\boldsymbol{\beta} + \boldsymbol{\varepsilon} , \qquad \boldsymbol{\varepsilon} \sim \mathcal{N}(\boldsymbol{0}, \sigma^2\boldsymbol{\Sigma}) .$$

Suppose $\boldsymbol{\Sigma}$ is a symmetric invertible constant matrix. Show that the maximum likelihood estimators of $\boldsymbol{\beta}$ and σ^2 are

$$\widehat{\boldsymbol{\beta}} = (\mathbf{X}^\top \boldsymbol{\Sigma}^{-1} \mathbf{X})^{-1} \mathbf{X}^\top \boldsymbol{\Sigma}^{-1} \boldsymbol{y}, \quad \widehat{\sigma^2} = \frac{1}{T}(\boldsymbol{y} - \mathbf{X}\widehat{\boldsymbol{\beta}})^\top \boldsymbol{\Sigma}^{-1}(\boldsymbol{y} - \mathbf{X}\widehat{\boldsymbol{\beta}}) \,.$$

12.7. We revisit Example 12.7 on fitting the inflation data with an ARMA(1,1) model

$$Y_t = \varrho_0 + \varrho_1 y_{t-1} + \varepsilon_t + \psi \varepsilon_{t-1} \,,$$

where $\varepsilon_1, \ldots, \varepsilon_T \sim_{\text{iid}} \mathcal{N}(0, \sigma^2)$ and $\varepsilon_0 = 0$. Specifically, we consider a Bayesian analysis of the model using the following independent priors:

$$\boldsymbol{\varrho} \sim \mathcal{N}(\boldsymbol{0}, 10\,\mathbb{I}_2), \quad \psi \sim \mathcal{U}(-1, 1), \quad \sigma^2 \sim \mathsf{InvGamma}(3, 1) \,,$$

where $\boldsymbol{\varrho} = [\varrho_0, \varrho_1]^\top$.

a. Derive the posterior conditional densities $f(\boldsymbol{\varrho} \,|\, \boldsymbol{y}, \psi, \sigma^2)$, $f(\psi \,|\, \boldsymbol{y}, \boldsymbol{\varrho}, \sigma^2)$, and $f(\sigma^2 \,|\, \boldsymbol{y}, \boldsymbol{\varrho}, \psi)$.
b. Fit the model using the dataset `USCPI.csv`.
c. Compute the posterior means of $\boldsymbol{\varrho}, \psi$, and σ^2, and compare them with their corresponding maximum likelihood estimates.

12.8. What is the "factor effects" representation of the one-factor random effects model in (12.15)?

12.9. Write the two-factor mixed ANOVA model in Example 12.12 as a Gaussian model. That is, arrange $\{Y_{ijk}\}$ as $\boldsymbol{Y} = [Y_1, \ldots, Y_n]^\top \sim \mathcal{N}(\boldsymbol{\mu}, \boldsymbol{\Sigma})$, and determine $\boldsymbol{\mu}$ and $\boldsymbol{\Sigma}$.

12.10. Determine the Gaussian graphical model for each of the following situations.

a. For the random variables $Y_1, \ldots, Y_6$, Y_2 depends only on Y_1, and Y_t depends only on Y_{t-1} and Y_{t-2}, $t = 3, \ldots, 6$.
b. A one-factor ANOVA model with $d = 3$, $n_1 = 2, n_2 = 3$, and $n_3 = 4$.
c. A two-factor ANOVA model with $d_1 = 2$, $d_2 = 3$, and $n_{ij} = 1, i = 1, 2$, $j = 1, 2, 3$.

12.11. We wish to design a Gibbs sampler for estimating the one-factor random effects model. To that end, consider the following independent priors:

$$\mu \sim \mathcal{N}(\mu_0, V_\mu), \quad \sigma_\mu^2 \sim \mathsf{InvGamma}(\alpha_\mu, \lambda_\mu), \quad \sigma^2 \sim \mathsf{InvGamma}(\alpha, \lambda) \,.$$

Let $\boldsymbol{\mu} = [\mu_1, \ldots, \mu_d]^\top$. Derive the following conditional distributions:

a. $f(\boldsymbol{\mu} \,|\, \boldsymbol{y}, \mu, \sigma_\mu^2, \sigma^2) = \prod_{i=1}^d f(\mu_i \,|\, \boldsymbol{y}, \mu, \sigma_\mu^2, \sigma^2)$;
b. $f(\mu \,|\, \boldsymbol{y}, \boldsymbol{\mu}, \sigma_\mu^2, \sigma^2) = f(\mu \,|\, \boldsymbol{\mu}, \sigma_\mu^2)$;

c. $f(\sigma_\mu^2 \mid \boldsymbol{y}, \boldsymbol{\mu}, \mu, \sigma^2) = f(\sigma_\mu^2 \mid \boldsymbol{\mu}, \mu)$;
d. $f(\sigma^2 \mid \boldsymbol{y}, \boldsymbol{\mu}, \mu, \sigma_\mu^2) = f(\sigma^2 \mid \boldsymbol{y}, \boldsymbol{\mu})$.

12.12. Implement the Gibbs sampler developed in Problem 12.11 for the one-factor random effects model to fit the crop yield data in Example 12.10. Use the following independent priors:

$$\mu \sim \mathcal{N}(0, 100), \quad \sigma_\mu^2 \sim \mathsf{InvGamma}(3, 1), \quad \sigma^2 \sim \mathsf{InvGamma}(3, 1) \,.$$

Estimate the posterior means $\mathbb{E}(\mu \mid \boldsymbol{y})$, $\mathbb{E}(\sigma_\mu^2 \mid \boldsymbol{y})$, and $\mathbb{E}(\sigma^2 \mid \boldsymbol{y})$. What is the posterior probability that $\sigma_\mu^2 > 5\sigma^2$?

12.13. Show that the two-factor random effects model in (12.18) is a special case of the linear mixed model by writing the former in the form (12.20).

Chapter 13
State Space Models

In this chapter we discuss versatile generalizations of the basic time series models in Sect. 12.1, collectively known under the name **state space models**. These models not only can capture the *serial dependence* of the observations (i.e., the dependence across time) but also can describe the *persistence* and *volatility* of the measurements. That is, they can model continued periods of high or low measurements and time-varying amounts of random fluctuation. In contrast, the AR(p) model, for example, cannot capture these features, as the model parameters do not depend on time. Throughout this chapter we shall use *Bayesian* notation when specifying (conditional) densities, even when working in a non-Bayesian setting.

A state space model typically consists of two modeling levels: in the first level, observations are related to the latent or unobserved variables called **states** according to the **observation** or **measurement equation**. In the second level, the evolution of the states is modeled via the **state** or **transition equation.**

> **Definition 13.1. (State Space Model).** In a **state space model**, the **observations** $y_t, t = 1, 2, \ldots$ are drawn from a conditional pdf $f(y_t \mid x_t, y_{t-1}, \ldots, y_1, \boldsymbol{\theta})$, where x_t is the hidden **state** at time t. The states $x_t, t = 1, 2, \ldots$ evolve according to a Markov chain with transition density $f(x_t \mid x_{t-1}, \boldsymbol{\theta})$. Here, $\boldsymbol{\theta}$ denotes the vector of model parameters.

Typically one assumes that each observation y_t only depends on the latent state x_t and not on previous states or observations. In that case the state space model can be viewed as a *hidden Markov model*; see Problem 8.14. Note that the $\{x_t\}$ and $\{y_t\}$ may be vector-valued.

© The Author(s), under exclusive license to Springer Science+Business Media, LLC, part of Springer Nature 2025
J. C. C. Chan, D. P. Kroese, *Statistical Modeling and Computation*,
Springer Texts in Statistics, https://doi.org/10.1007/978-1-0716-4132-3_13

Example 13.1 (Kalman Filter). State space models originate from the analysis of *dynamical systems*. One of the most fundamental examples is the **linear Gaussian discrete-time state space model**

$$
\begin{aligned}
\boldsymbol{x}_t &= \mathbf{A}\,\boldsymbol{x}_{t-1} + \boldsymbol{\delta}_t \\
\boldsymbol{y}_t &= \mathbf{B}\,\boldsymbol{x}_t + \boldsymbol{\varepsilon}_t\,, \qquad t = 1, 2, \ldots,
\end{aligned}
\tag{13.1}
$$

where $\boldsymbol{x}_t$ is an n-dimensional (hidden) **state** vector and $\boldsymbol{y}_t$ an m-dimensional **output** vector. $\mathbf{A}$ and $\mathbf{B}$ are fixed matrices, and $\boldsymbol{\delta}_t$ and $\boldsymbol{\varepsilon}_t$ are zero-mean normal random vectors with covariance matrices $\mathbf{D}$ and $\mathbf{E}$, respectively. All $\{\boldsymbol{\delta}_t\}$ and $\{\boldsymbol{\varepsilon}_t\}$ are independent. The initial state $\boldsymbol{x}_0$ is assumed to be $\mathcal{N}(\boldsymbol{\mu}_0, \boldsymbol{\Sigma}_0)$ distributed.

Define $\boldsymbol{y}_{1:t} = [\boldsymbol{y}_1^\top, \ldots, \boldsymbol{y}_t^\top]^\top$. Assuming the model parameters are known, two main objectives are to obtain the:

- **predictive distribution**; that is, the conditional distribution of $\boldsymbol{x}_t$ given $\boldsymbol{y}_{1:t-1}$ (the observations *before* time t), and the
- **filtering distribution**; that is, the conditional distribution of $\boldsymbol{x}_t$ given $\boldsymbol{y}_{1:t}$ (the observations *up to* time t).

Since we are dealing only with affine transformations of Gaussian vectors, we have by Theorem 3.6 that $(\boldsymbol{x}_t \mid \boldsymbol{y}_{1:t}) \sim \mathcal{N}(\boldsymbol{\mu}_t, \boldsymbol{\Sigma}_t)$ for some mean vector $\boldsymbol{\mu}_t$ and covariance matrix $\boldsymbol{\Sigma}_t$. Similarly, $(\boldsymbol{x}_t \mid \boldsymbol{y}_{1:t-1}) \sim \mathcal{N}(\widetilde{\boldsymbol{\mu}}_t, \widetilde{\boldsymbol{\Sigma}}_t)$ for some mean vector $\widetilde{\boldsymbol{\mu}}_t$ and covariance matrix $\widetilde{\boldsymbol{\Sigma}}_t$. These mean vectors and covariance matrices can be computed sequentially. First, since $\boldsymbol{x}_t = \mathbf{A}\,\boldsymbol{x}_{t-1} + \boldsymbol{\delta}_t$ and $(\boldsymbol{x}_{t-1} \mid \boldsymbol{y}_{1:t-1}) \sim \mathcal{N}(\boldsymbol{\mu}_{t-1}, \boldsymbol{\Sigma}_{t-1})$, we have

$$
(\boldsymbol{x}_t \mid \boldsymbol{y}_{1:t-1}) \sim \mathcal{N}(\mathbf{A}\,\boldsymbol{\mu}_{t-1},\ \mathbf{A}\boldsymbol{\Sigma}_{t-1}\mathbf{A}^\top + \mathbf{D})\,.
$$

Thus, the updating formulas for the predictive distribution are

$$
\begin{aligned}
\widetilde{\boldsymbol{\mu}}_t &= \mathbf{A}\,\boldsymbol{\mu}_{t-1}\,, \\
\widetilde{\boldsymbol{\Sigma}}_t &= \mathbf{A}\boldsymbol{\Sigma}_{t-1}\mathbf{A}^\top + \mathbf{D}\,.
\end{aligned}
\tag{13.2}
$$

Next, we determine the joint pdf of $\boldsymbol{x}_t$ and $\boldsymbol{y}_t$, given $\boldsymbol{y}_{1:t-1}$. Decomposing $\widetilde{\boldsymbol{\Sigma}}_t$ and $\mathbf{E}$ as $\widetilde{\boldsymbol{\Sigma}}_t = \mathbf{R}\mathbf{R}^\top$ and $\mathbf{E} = \mathbf{Q}\mathbf{Q}^\top$, respectively, we can write (using Definition 3.10 of the multivariate normal distribution)

$$
\left(\begin{matrix} \boldsymbol{x}_t \\ \boldsymbol{y}_t \end{matrix} \,\middle|\, \boldsymbol{y}_{1:t-1} \right) = \begin{bmatrix} \widetilde{\boldsymbol{\mu}}_t \\ \mathbf{B}\widetilde{\boldsymbol{\mu}}_t \end{bmatrix} + \begin{bmatrix} \mathbf{R} & \mathbf{O} \\ \mathbf{B}\mathbf{R} & \mathbf{Q} \end{bmatrix} \begin{bmatrix} \boldsymbol{u} \\ \boldsymbol{v} \end{bmatrix},
$$

where, conditional on $\boldsymbol{y}_{1:t-1}$, $\boldsymbol{u}$ and $\boldsymbol{v}$ are independent standard normal random vectors. The corresponding covariance matrix is

$$
\begin{bmatrix} \mathbf{R} & \mathbf{O} \\ \mathbf{B}\mathbf{R} & \mathbf{Q} \end{bmatrix} \begin{bmatrix} \mathbf{R}^\top & \mathbf{R}^\top\mathbf{B}^\top \\ \mathbf{O} & \mathbf{Q}^\top \end{bmatrix} = \begin{bmatrix} \mathbf{R}\mathbf{R}^\top & \mathbf{R}\mathbf{R}^\top\mathbf{B}^\top \\ \mathbf{B}\mathbf{R}\mathbf{R}^\top & \mathbf{B}\mathbf{R}\mathbf{R}^\top\mathbf{B}^\top + \mathbf{Q}\mathbf{Q}^\top \end{bmatrix},
$$

so that we have

$$\left(\begin{matrix} \boldsymbol{x}_t \\ \boldsymbol{y}_t \end{matrix} \,\middle|\, \boldsymbol{y}_{1:t-1}\right) \sim \mathcal{N}\left(\begin{bmatrix} \widetilde{\boldsymbol{\mu}}_t \\ \mathbf{B}\widetilde{\boldsymbol{\mu}}_t \end{bmatrix}, \begin{bmatrix} \widetilde{\boldsymbol{\Sigma}}_t & \widetilde{\boldsymbol{\Sigma}}_t\mathbf{B}^\top \\ \mathbf{B}\widetilde{\boldsymbol{\Sigma}}_t & \mathbf{B}\widetilde{\boldsymbol{\Sigma}}_t\mathbf{B}^\top + \mathbf{E} \end{bmatrix}\right). \tag{13.3}$$

A direct application of Theorem 3.8 yields that $\boldsymbol{x}_t$ given $\boldsymbol{y}_{1:t}$ has a $\mathcal{N}(\boldsymbol{\mu}_t, \boldsymbol{\Sigma}_t)$ ☞ 86
distribution with

$$\begin{aligned} \boldsymbol{\mu}_t &= \widetilde{\boldsymbol{\mu}}_t + \widetilde{\boldsymbol{\Sigma}}_t\mathbf{B}^\top(\mathbf{B}\widetilde{\boldsymbol{\Sigma}}_t\mathbf{B}^\top + \mathbf{E})^{-1}(\boldsymbol{y}_t - \mathbf{B}\widetilde{\boldsymbol{\mu}}_t)\,, \\ \boldsymbol{\Sigma}_t &= \widetilde{\boldsymbol{\Sigma}}_t - \widetilde{\boldsymbol{\Sigma}}_t\mathbf{B}^\top(\mathbf{B}\widetilde{\boldsymbol{\Sigma}}_t\mathbf{B}^\top + \mathbf{E})^{-1}\mathbf{B}\widetilde{\boldsymbol{\Sigma}}_t\,. \end{aligned} \tag{13.4}$$

We leave the details as an exercise; see Problem 13.1. Updating formulas (13.2) and (13.4) form the (discrete-time) **Kalman filter**. Starting with some known $\boldsymbol{\mu}_0$ and $\boldsymbol{\Sigma}_0$, one determines $\widetilde{\boldsymbol{\mu}}_1$ and $\widetilde{\boldsymbol{\Sigma}}_1$, then $\boldsymbol{\mu}_1$ and $\boldsymbol{\Sigma}_1$, and so on. Notice that $\widetilde{\boldsymbol{\Sigma}}_t$ and $\boldsymbol{\Sigma}_t$ do not depend on the observations $\boldsymbol{y}_1, \boldsymbol{y}_2, \dots$ and can therefore be determined *off-line*.

In the remainder of this chapter, we will discuss various popular state space models that fall within the framework defined above. From the definition it is obvious that state space models are high-dimensional, often with more latent variables and parameters than observations. Instead of using generalizations of the Kalman filter, we will discuss the precision-based approach of Chan and Jeliazkov (2009), McCausland et al. (2011), and Chan (2013) to estimating state space models, which builds upon earlier work by Rue (2001) on Gaussian Markov random fields. Due to its simple and transparent derivation as well as computational efficiency, the precision-based approach is increasingly used in a wide range of empirical applications.

13.1 Unobserved Components Model

An important state space model is the **unobserved components model** pioneered by Harvey (1985) and Watson (1986). In the first level, the (real-valued) observable y_t at time t is modeled to depend on the state or **unobserved component** τ_t as follows:

$$y_t = \tau_t + \varepsilon_t\,, \tag{13.5}$$

where $\{\varepsilon_t\} \sim_{\mathrm{iid}} \mathcal{N}(0, \sigma^2)$. That is, the observable y_t is modeled as the sum of the unobserved component τ_t and the error term ε_t. As we shall see shortly, this is a popular specification for modeling the evolution of univariate time series such as inflation rate. For example, in the context of inflation modeling the unobserved component τ_t can be interpreted as the stochastic trend or underlying inflation.

Since for every y_t we have an associated latent variable τ_t, there are more latent variables and parameters (i.e., $\boldsymbol{\tau} = [\tau_1, \ldots, \tau_T]^\top$ and σ^2) than the number of observations. As such, if we have the measurement equation only, the maximum likelihood estimator for $(\boldsymbol{\tau}, \sigma^2)$ is not defined. Specifically, the likelihood function is unbounded in $(\boldsymbol{\tau}, \sigma^2)$, and therefore the maximum does not exist (see Problem 13.3).

The fundamental problem is that if the unobserved components are unrestricted, then we have the extreme situation where we can fit the data perfectly (e.g., by choosing $\tau_t = y_t$). One way to get around this problem is to impose some structure on the model to make estimation feasible. Since we are dealing with time series data, it seems reasonable to assume that the unobserved component evolves gradually over time. In the inflation example, consecutive inflation trends are likely to be "close." More precisely, consider the following **random walk** specification

$$\tau_t = \tau_{t-1} + u_t , \tag{13.6}$$

for $t = 2, \ldots, T$, where $\{u_t\} \sim_{\text{iid}} \mathcal{N}(0, \omega^2)$. That is, the conditional distribution of τ_t given τ_{t-1} and ω^2 is $\mathcal{N}(\tau_{t-1}, \omega^2)$: the current state τ_t centers around the previous one τ_{t-1}, while ω^2 controls how close the two terms are on average.

The smoothness parameter ω^2 can either be fixed in advance to some "reasonable value" or treated as a parameter to be estimated from the data. Should it be fixed as a constant, its choice should reflect the desired smoothness of the evolution of the states: large values for ω^2 allow τ_t to evolve quickly, whereas for small values the transition of τ_t becomes more gradual. In a Bayesian framework, one often assumes a hierarchical prior distribution for ω^2 that reflects the desired smoothness of the transition equation.

Note that (13.6) does not explicitly provide a distribution for τ_1. To complete the model specification, one typically assumes that the process is initialized with $\tau_1 \sim \mathcal{N}(\tau_0, \omega_0^2)$ for some known constants τ_0 and ω_0^2. This is referred to as the **initial condition**.

We summarize the unobserved components model as follows:

Definition 13.2. (Unobserved Components Model). In the **unobserved components model**, the measurement equation is given by

$$y_t = \tau_t + \varepsilon_t ,$$

where $\{\varepsilon_t\} \sim_{\text{iid}} \mathcal{N}(0, \sigma^2)$. The states, in turn, are initialized with $\tau_1 \sim \mathcal{N}(\tau_0, \omega_0^2)$ for some known constants τ_0 and ω_0^2, and evolve according to the transition equation

$$\tau_t = \tau_{t-1} + u_t ,$$

for $t = 2, \ldots, T$, where $\{u_t\} \sim_{\text{iid}} \mathcal{N}(0, \omega^2)$.

It is obvious that the unobserved components model falls within the family of state space models. In fact, in the notation of Definition 13.1, the state x_t in this case is the univariate unobserved component τ_t and $\boldsymbol{\theta} = [\sigma^2, \omega^2]$. The conditional distribution of y_t given τ_t is $\mathcal{N}(\tau_t, \sigma^2)$, whereas the transition density $f(\tau_t \mid \tau_{t-1}, \boldsymbol{\theta})$ corresponds to the pdf of the $\mathcal{N}(\tau_{t-1}, \omega^2)$ distribution. Furthermore, since both the measurement and transition equations are linear in the states with Gaussian errors, the unobserved components model is an example of the linear Gaussian state space model discussed in Example 13.1.

13.1.1 Frequentist Inference

Let $\boldsymbol{y} = [y_1, \ldots, y_T]^\top$ and $\boldsymbol{\tau} = [\tau_1, \ldots, \tau_T]^\top$ be the vector of observations and latent variables, respectively. Throughout this section, we fix ω^2, and the only *parameter* in the model is σ^2. To obtain the maximum likelihood estimate for σ^2, which we denote as $\widehat{\sigma^2}$, in principle we can maximize the likelihood function

$$L(\sigma^2; \boldsymbol{y}) = \int f(\boldsymbol{y} \mid \boldsymbol{\tau}, \sigma^2) f(\boldsymbol{\tau} \mid \omega^2)\, \mathrm{d}\boldsymbol{\tau} \qquad (13.7)$$

with respect to σ^2, where the densities $f(\boldsymbol{y} \mid \boldsymbol{\tau}, \sigma^2)$ and $f(\boldsymbol{\tau} \mid \omega^2)$ follow from (13.5) and (13.6), respectively (their exact expressions are given below). In practice, however, evaluating the above integral directly is often time-consuming as it involves a high-dimensional integration. Conventionally, Kalman filter is used to evaluate the integral, as discussed in Harvey (1990) (see also Problem 13.5 for an alternative method).

Instead, we will obtain $\widehat{\sigma^2}$ using the EM algorithm introduced in Chap. 6.6. To this end we first write the system (13.5)–(13.6) in matrix form and derive explicit expressions for $\ln f(\boldsymbol{y} \mid \boldsymbol{\tau}, \sigma^2)$ and $\ln f(\boldsymbol{\tau} \mid \omega^2)$.

Defining $\boldsymbol{\varepsilon} = [\varepsilon_1, \ldots, \varepsilon_T]^\top$, we can rewrite (13.5) as

$$\boldsymbol{y} = \boldsymbol{\tau} + \boldsymbol{\varepsilon}, \quad \boldsymbol{\varepsilon} \sim \mathcal{N}(\boldsymbol{0}, \sigma^2 \mathbb{I}_T), \qquad (13.8)$$

where $\boldsymbol{0}$ is a $T \times 1$ column of zeros and $\mathbb{I}_T$ is the $T \times T$ identity matrix. From (13.8), we see that

$$\ln f(\boldsymbol{y} \mid \boldsymbol{\tau}, \sigma^2) = -\frac{T}{2} \ln(2\pi\sigma^2) - \frac{1}{2\sigma^2} (\boldsymbol{y} - \boldsymbol{\tau})^\top (\boldsymbol{y} - \boldsymbol{\tau}). \qquad (13.9)$$

Next, we derive an expression for $\ln f(\boldsymbol{\tau} \mid \omega^2)$. For simplicity, we assume $\tau_0 = 0$; the general case follows similarly (see Problem 13.7). Note that we can rewrite the transition equation (13.6) as

$$\underbrace{\begin{bmatrix} 1 & 0 & 0 & \cdots & 0 \\ -1 & 1 & 0 & \cdots & 0 \\ 0 & -1 & 1 & \cdots & 0 \\ \vdots & & & \ddots & \vdots \\ 0 & 0 & \cdots & -1 & 1 \end{bmatrix}}_{\mathbf{H}} \begin{bmatrix} \tau_1 \\ \tau_2 \\ \tau_3 \\ \vdots \\ \tau_T \end{bmatrix} = \begin{bmatrix} u_1 \\ u_2 \\ u_3 \\ \vdots \\ u_T \end{bmatrix} , \qquad (13.10)$$

i.e., $\mathbf{H}\boldsymbol{\tau} = \boldsymbol{u}$, $\boldsymbol{u} \sim \mathcal{N}(\mathbf{0}, \boldsymbol{\Omega})$, where $\boldsymbol{\Omega} = \mathrm{diag}(\omega_0^2, \omega^2, \ldots, \omega^2)$ is a diagonal matrix. Noting that $|\mathbf{H}| \overset{\mathrm{def}}{=} |\det(\mathbf{H})| = 1$ and hence $\mathbf{H}$ is invertible, we have

$$\boldsymbol{\tau} = \mathbf{H}^{-1}\boldsymbol{u} \sim \mathcal{N}(\mathbf{0}, (\mathbf{H}^\top \boldsymbol{\Omega}^{-1}\mathbf{H})^{-1}) ,$$

where $\boldsymbol{\Omega}^{-1} = \mathrm{diag}(\omega_0^{-2}, \omega^{-2}, \ldots, \omega^{-2})$ is again a diagonal matrix. It follows that

$$\ln f(\boldsymbol{\tau} \,|\, \omega^2) = -\frac{1}{2}\ln((2\pi)^T|(\mathbf{H}^\top \boldsymbol{\Omega}^{-1}\mathbf{H})^{-1}|) - \frac{1}{2}\boldsymbol{\tau}^\top(\mathbf{H}^\top \boldsymbol{\Omega}^{-1}\mathbf{H})\boldsymbol{\tau}$$

$$= -\frac{T}{2}\ln(2\pi) - \frac{1}{2}\ln\omega_0^2 - \frac{T-1}{2}\ln\omega^2 - \frac{1}{2}\boldsymbol{\tau}^\top(\mathbf{H}^\top \boldsymbol{\Omega}^{-1}\mathbf{H})\boldsymbol{\tau} . \qquad (13.11)$$

To implement the *E-step*, we need to derive the conditional density of the states given the data

$$g_i(\boldsymbol{\tau}) = f(\boldsymbol{\tau} \,|\, \boldsymbol{y}, \sigma_{i-1}^2, \omega^2) ,$$

where σ_{i-1}^2 is the current value for σ^2 in iteration i. We first show that $(\boldsymbol{\tau} \,|\, \boldsymbol{y}, \sigma_{i-1}^2, \omega^2)$ has a multivariate normal density of dimension T. Then we discuss how one can evaluate this typically high-dimensional density efficiently.

Using (13.9) and (13.11), while ignoring constant terms not involving $\boldsymbol{\tau}$, we have

$$\begin{aligned} \ln f(\boldsymbol{\tau} \,|\, \boldsymbol{y}, \sigma_{i-1}^2, \omega^2) &= \ln f(\boldsymbol{y}, \boldsymbol{\tau} \,|\, \sigma_{i-1}^2, \omega^2) + \mathrm{const} \\ &= \ln f(\boldsymbol{y} \,|\, \boldsymbol{\tau}, \sigma_{i-1}^2) + \ln f(\boldsymbol{\tau} \,|\, \omega^2) + \mathrm{const} \\ &= -\frac{1}{2}\left(\frac{(\boldsymbol{y} - \boldsymbol{\tau})^\top(\boldsymbol{y} - \boldsymbol{\tau})}{\sigma_{i-1}^2} + \boldsymbol{\tau}^\top(\mathbf{H}^\top \boldsymbol{\Omega}^{-1}\mathbf{H})\boldsymbol{\tau} \right) + \mathrm{const} \\ &= -\frac{1}{2}\left(\boldsymbol{\tau}^\top \mathbf{K}_i \boldsymbol{\tau} - \frac{2}{\sigma_{i-1}^2}\boldsymbol{y}^\top \boldsymbol{\tau} \right) + \mathrm{const} , \end{aligned}$$

where $\mathbf{K}_i = \mathbf{H}^\top \boldsymbol{\Omega}^{-1}\mathbf{H} + \sigma_{i-1}^{-2}\,\mathbb{I}_T$. Note that the expression above defines the pdf of a normal distribution, and we only need to determine the mean vector and the covariance matrix. By *completing the squares* as in Theorem 8.1, we see that

☞ 245

$$(\boldsymbol{\tau} \,|\, \boldsymbol{y}, \sigma_{i-1}^2, \omega^2) \sim \mathcal{N}(\widehat{\boldsymbol{\tau}}_i, \mathbf{K}_i^{-1}) , \qquad (13.12)$$

where $\widehat{\boldsymbol{\tau}}_i = \sigma_{i-1}^{-2}\mathbf{K}_i^{-1}\boldsymbol{y}.$

Next, we compute the expectation

$$Q_i(\sigma^2) = \mathbb{E}_{g_i} \ln f(\boldsymbol{y}, \boldsymbol{\tau} \mid \sigma^2, \omega^2) \,.$$

To simplify the computation, we ignore all the terms not involving σ^2, as they will eventually drop out when we maximize $Q_i(\sigma^2)$ with respect to σ^2. Hence, we have, from (13.9),

$$\begin{aligned}
Q_i(\sigma^2) &= \mathbb{E}_{g_i} \ln f(\boldsymbol{y} \mid \boldsymbol{\tau}, \sigma^2) + \text{const} \\
&= -\frac{T}{2} \ln(2\pi\sigma^2) - \frac{1}{2\sigma^2} \mathbb{E}_{g_i} (\boldsymbol{y} - \boldsymbol{\tau})^\top (\boldsymbol{y} - \boldsymbol{\tau}) + \text{const} \\
&= -\frac{T}{2} \ln(2\pi\sigma^2) - \frac{1}{2\sigma^2} \left[\text{tr}(\mathbf{K}_i^{-1}) + (\boldsymbol{y} - \widehat{\boldsymbol{\tau}}_i)^\top (\boldsymbol{y} - \widehat{\boldsymbol{\tau}}_i) \right] + \text{const} \,.
\end{aligned}$$

Note that we used the fact that for any random vector $\boldsymbol{x}$ with mean vector $\boldsymbol{\mu}$ and covariance matrix $\boldsymbol{\Sigma}$, we have $\mathbb{E}(\boldsymbol{x}^\top \boldsymbol{x}) = \text{tr}(\boldsymbol{\Sigma}) + \boldsymbol{\mu}^\top \boldsymbol{\mu}$ (see Problem 13.2).

Finally, to implement the *M-step*, we differentiate $Q_i(\sigma^2)$ with respect to σ^2 and solve for the maximizer:

$$\sigma_i^2 = \underset{\sigma^2}{\text{argmax}}\, Q_i(\sigma^2) = \frac{1}{T} \left[\text{tr}(\mathbf{K}_i^{-1}) + (\boldsymbol{y} - \widehat{\boldsymbol{\tau}}_i)^\top (\boldsymbol{y} - \widehat{\boldsymbol{\tau}}_i) \right] \,. \tag{13.13}$$

We summarize the EM algorithm as follows: given a starting value σ_0^2, iterate the following steps until convergence:

- **E-Step.** Given the current value σ_{i-1}^2, compute

$$\mathbf{K}_i = \mathbf{H}^\top \boldsymbol{\Omega}^{-1} \mathbf{H} + \sigma_{i-1}^{-2} \mathbb{I}_T \qquad \text{and} \qquad \widehat{\boldsymbol{\tau}}_i = \mathbf{K}_i^{-1} \boldsymbol{y} / \sigma_{i-1}^2 \,.$$

- **M-Step.** Given $\mathbf{K}_i$ and $\widehat{\boldsymbol{\tau}}_i$ from the E-step, update the value for σ^2 using (13.13).

Although the estimation procedures presented above are relatively straightforward, one thing to notice is that the computations involve various large matrices. For example, $\mathbf{K}_i^{-1}$ is a full $T \times T$ matrix. In typical applications the sample size T could be as large as several hundred or a few thousand, and computing the inverse $\mathbf{K}_i^{-1}$ is very time-consuming. However, note that the matrix $\mathbf{K}_i$, as well as $\mathbf{H}$ and $\boldsymbol{\Omega}^{-1}$, are *sparse* and computations involving sparse matrices (multiplication, Cholesky decomposition, etc.) are generally very fast. See also Appendix A for some useful Julia built-in routines for handling sparse matrices.

Also, for computing $\widehat{\boldsymbol{\tau}}_i = \mathbf{K}_i^{-1} \boldsymbol{y} / \sigma_{i-1}^2$, one need not obtain the inverse $\mathbf{K}_i^{-1}$, which is a time-consuming matrix operation. Instead, we solve the linear system $\mathbf{K}_i \boldsymbol{x} = \boldsymbol{y}$ for $\boldsymbol{x}$, the solution of which is $\mathbf{K}_i^{-1} \boldsymbol{y}$. In contrast to inverting large matrices, the latter operation can be done much more quickly and accurately.

Finally, to compute $\mathrm{tr}(\mathbf{K}_i^{-1})$ in (13.13) without obtaining the inverse $\mathbf{K}_i^{-1}$, we use the following result:

$$\mathrm{tr}(\mathbf{K}_i^{-1}) = \sum_{j=1}^{T} \lambda_j^{-1} \,,$$

where $\lambda_1, \ldots, \lambda_T$ are the eigenvalues of the sparse matrix $\mathbf{K}_i$. At the end of the EM iterations, we obtain the estimate $\widehat{\sigma^2}$. However, it is typically not the quantity of interest in the analysis—what we are really after is the expected value of the underlying inflation, $\mathbb{E}(\boldsymbol{\tau} \mid \boldsymbol{y}, \sigma^2, \omega^2)$. We can estimate this quantity using the "plug-in" estimate $\mathbb{E}(\boldsymbol{\tau} \mid \boldsymbol{y}, \sigma^2 = \widehat{\sigma^2}, \omega^2)$, which is $\widehat{\mathbf{K}}^{-1}\boldsymbol{y}/\widehat{\sigma^2}$, where $\widehat{\mathbf{K}}$ is the $\mathbf{K}_i$ matrix evaluated at the final iteration of the EM algorithm.

We illustrate the EM algorithm using the following empirical example that involves fitting the US inflation with the unobserved components model.

Example 13.2 (Modeling Inflation with Unobserved Components Model).   In Example 12.6, we first modeled the US inflation data with an integrated MA(1) model. Later we continued our analysis with a more general ARMA(1,1) model in Example 12.7. In this empirical example, we consider the unobserved components model for the same data. The unobserved components model may be viewed as a convenient way to allow for a stochastic trend (see Problem 13.4). As such, it is highly flexible and is capable of modeling a variety of features. In addition, using the state space framework makes it easy to consider further extensions with richer dynamics (e.g., see Problem 13.8).

☞ 364

☞ 368

Recall that the quarterly inflation rate is computed from the consumer price index (CPI). Specifically, given z_t, the CPI at time t, we compute the (annualized) inflation rate as $y_t = 400 \ln(z_t/z_{t-1})$.

In what follows, we fit the unobserved components model (13.5)–(13.6) with the U.S. CPI inflation data. In order to proceed, we first need to set the values for ω_0^2 and ω^2. Recall that ω_0^2 is the variance of the initial condition (i.e., $\tau_1 \sim \mathcal{N}(0, \omega_0^2)$). We set $\omega_0^2 = 9$. What this means is that the initial τ_1 is between -6 to 6 with a probability approximately equal to 95%. As for the smoothness parameter ω^2, we consider two cases: $\omega^2 = 1^2$ and $\omega^2 = 0.5^2$. The value for ω^2 reflects the desired smoothness of the transition for τ_t. For example, if $\omega^2 = 0.5^2$, then with high probability the difference between consecutive unobserved components, $\tau_t - \tau_{t-1}$, is between -1 and 1.

Recall that the estimation consists of two steps. First, given the prefixed values for ω_0^2 and ω^2, we iterate the E- and M-steps until the sequence of σ_t^2 converges. Then, given the maximum likelihood estimate $\widehat{\sigma^2}$, we once again use the E-step to obtain $\mathbb{E}(\boldsymbol{\tau} \mid \sigma^2 = \widehat{\sigma^2}, \omega^2)$. The following Julia script performs these two tasks.

```
UC_EM.jl

using SparseArrays, LinearAlgebra, StatsBase,Plots,
    DelimitedFiles
y = readdlm("USCPI.csv")
T = length(y)
omega2_0 = 9        # initial condition
omega = .5^2        # fix omega
H = sparse(I,T,T) - sparse(2:T,1:(T-1),ones(T-1),T,T)
invOmega = sparse(1:T,1:T,vcat(1/omega2_0, 1/omega*ones(T-1)),
    T,T)
HinvOmegaH = H'*invOmega*H
sigma2t = var(y)   # initial guess
err = 1
while err> 10^(-4)
        # E-step
    Kt = HinvOmegaH + sparse(I,T,T)/sigma2t
    taut = Kt(y/sigma2t)
        # M-step
    lam =  eigvals(Matrix(Kt))
    newsigma2t = (sum(1 ./ lam) .+ only((y-taut)'*(y-taut)))/T
        # update
    err = abs(sigma2t-newsigma2t)
    sigma2t = newsigma2t
end
Kt = HinvOmegaH + sparse(I,T,T)/sigma2t
taut = Kt(y/sigma2t)
plot(y)
plot!(taut)
```

We used the above code to obtain the maximum likelihood estimates for σ^2 with $\omega^2 = 1^2$ and $\omega^2 = 0.5^2$. The plug-in estimates for $\boldsymbol{\tau}$ are plotted in Fig. 13.1. It can be seen that both curves fit the data reasonably well, without fitting the observed series too closely (otherwise we might run into overfitting problems). In particular, both seem to be able to capture the high inflation periods in the 1970s and 1980s, whereas the estimated trend remains low and stable since the 1990s until the last credit crisis. But as expected, when ω^2 is larger, the estimated $\boldsymbol{\tau}$ fit the data better. But we emphasize that if one sets ω^2 to be too large, one might run into over-fitting problems.

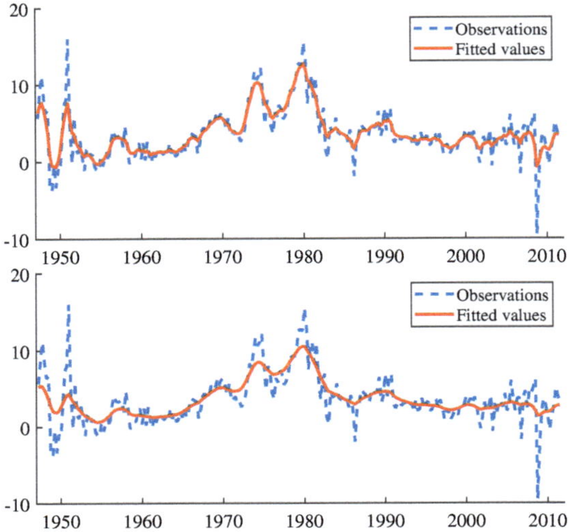

Fig. 13.1 Fitted values for τ under the unobserved components model with $\omega^2 = 1^2$ (top panel) and $\omega^2 = 0.5^2$ (bottom panel)

13.1.2 Bayesian Estimation

The unobserved components model, and state space models in general, may be viewed as a Bayesian hierarchical model, where the measurement equation provides the likelihood function and the transition equation specifies a prior for the states. For the remaining parameters, namely, σ^2 and ω^2 (note that ω^2 can be estimated if we specify a proper prior for ω^2), we assume the independent priors

$$\sigma^2 \sim \mathsf{InvGamma}(\alpha_{\sigma^2}, \lambda_{\sigma^2}), \quad \omega^2 \sim \mathsf{InvGamma}(\alpha_{\omega^2}, \lambda_{\omega^2}) , \qquad (13.14)$$

where $\alpha_{\sigma^2}, \lambda_{\sigma^2}, \alpha_{\omega^2}$, are λ_{ω^2} constants specified by the user. Typically we set the shape parameters α_{σ^2} and α_{ω^2} to be some small numbers, so that the priors are relatively noninformative. We then choose the rate parameters λ_{σ^2} and λ_{ω^2} such that the prior means for σ^2 and ω^2 have the desired values.

Given the measurement and state equations (13.5)–(13.6), as well as the prior for σ^2 and ω^2 in (13.14), we have the following joint posterior density:

$$f(\boldsymbol{\tau}, \sigma^2, \omega^2 \,|\, \boldsymbol{y}) \propto f(\boldsymbol{y} \,|\, \boldsymbol{\tau}, \sigma^2) f(\boldsymbol{\tau} \,|\, \omega^2) f(\sigma^2) f(\omega^2) , \qquad (13.15)$$

where $f(\sigma^2)$ and $f(\omega^2)$ are the inverse-gamma priors. We can then obtain posterior draws via the following two-step Gibbs sampler: alternatively draw from $f(\boldsymbol{\tau} \,|\, \boldsymbol{y}, \sigma^2, \omega^2)$ and $f(\sigma^2, \omega^2 \,|\, \boldsymbol{y}, \boldsymbol{\tau})$.

Sampling from the high-dimensional density $f(\boldsymbol{\tau} \mid \boldsymbol{y}, \sigma^2, \omega^2)$ is conventionally done using Kalman filter based methods, such as in Carter and Kohn (1994) and Durbin and Koopman (2002). In contrast, we implement a conceptually simpler and computationally more efficient approach based on fast band matrix routines, as proposed in Chan and Jeliazkov (2009). More specifically, we first show that $f(\boldsymbol{\tau} \mid \boldsymbol{y}, \sigma^2, \omega^2)$ is a normal density, and then discuss how one can sample from it efficiently. To this end, note that from (13.15) we have,

$$
\begin{aligned}
\ln f(\boldsymbol{\tau} \mid \boldsymbol{y}, \sigma^2, \omega^2) &= \ln f(\boldsymbol{\tau}, \sigma^2, \omega^2 \mid \boldsymbol{y}) + \text{const} \\
&= \ln f(\boldsymbol{y} \mid \boldsymbol{\tau}, \sigma^2) + \ln f(\boldsymbol{\tau} \mid \omega^2) + \text{const} \\
&= -\frac{1}{2}\left(\frac{(\boldsymbol{y} - \boldsymbol{\tau})^\top (\boldsymbol{y} - \boldsymbol{\tau})}{\sigma^2} + \boldsymbol{\tau}^\top (\mathbf{H}^\top \boldsymbol{\Omega}^{-1} \mathbf{H})\boldsymbol{\tau}\right) + \text{const} \\
&= -\frac{1}{2}\left(\boldsymbol{\tau}^\top \mathbf{K}\boldsymbol{\tau} - \frac{2}{\sigma^2}\boldsymbol{y}^\top \boldsymbol{\tau}\right) + \text{const}.
\end{aligned}
$$

It follows, similar to the derivation of (13.12), that

$$
(\boldsymbol{\tau} \mid \boldsymbol{y}, \sigma^2, \omega^2) \sim \mathcal{N}(\widehat{\boldsymbol{\tau}}, \mathbf{K}^{-1}),
$$

where $\mathbf{K} = \mathbf{H}^\top \boldsymbol{\Omega}^{-1} \mathbf{H} + \sigma^{-2}\mathbb{I}_T$, and $\widehat{\boldsymbol{\tau}} = \sigma^{-2}\mathbf{K}^{-1}\boldsymbol{y}$.

Since the covariance matrix $\mathbf{K}^{-1}$ is a full matrix and is typically of very high-dimension, drawing $\mathcal{N}(\widehat{\boldsymbol{\tau}}, \mathbf{K}^{-1})$ the usual way (that is, via Algorithm 3.3) is time-consuming. Instead, we exploit the special structure of the *precision* matrix $\mathbf{K}$, namely, that it is sparse (see the discussion on page 395). As such, a Cholesky decomposition of the precision matrix $\mathbf{K} = \mathbf{C}\mathbf{C}^\top$ can be obtained quickly. Then, we can use Algorithm 12.1 to quickly sample from $\mathcal{N}(\widehat{\boldsymbol{\tau}}, \mathbf{K}^{-1})$. Specifically, if we let $\boldsymbol{x} = (\mathbf{C}^\top)^{-1}\boldsymbol{z}$, where $\boldsymbol{z} \sim \mathcal{N}(\mathbf{0}, \mathbb{I}_T)$, then $\boldsymbol{x} \sim \mathcal{N}(\mathbf{0}, \mathbf{K}^{-1})$. Recall that one can obtain $\widehat{\boldsymbol{\tau}}$ efficiently by solving $\mathbf{K}\widehat{\boldsymbol{\tau}} = \sigma^{-2}\boldsymbol{y}$. Finally, $\boldsymbol{\tau} = \widehat{\boldsymbol{\tau}} + (\mathbf{C}^\top)^{-1}\boldsymbol{z}$ has the desired distribution.

Next, we derive the conditional density $f(\sigma^2, \omega^2 \mid \boldsymbol{y}, \boldsymbol{\tau})$. From (13.15) we have

$$
\begin{aligned}
f(\sigma^2, \omega^2 \mid \boldsymbol{y}, \boldsymbol{\tau}) &\propto f(\boldsymbol{\tau}, \sigma^2, \omega^2 \mid \boldsymbol{y}) \\
&\propto f(\boldsymbol{y} \mid \boldsymbol{\tau}, \sigma^2)f(\sigma^2) \times f(\boldsymbol{\tau} \mid \omega^2)f(\omega^2).
\end{aligned}
$$

In other words, σ^2 and ω^2 are conditionally independent given $\boldsymbol{y}$ and $\boldsymbol{\tau}$, with

$$
f(\sigma^2 \mid \boldsymbol{y}, \boldsymbol{\tau}) \propto f(\boldsymbol{y} \mid \boldsymbol{\tau}, \sigma^2)f(\sigma^2) \qquad \text{and} \qquad f(\omega^2 \mid \boldsymbol{y}, \boldsymbol{\tau}) \propto f(\boldsymbol{\tau} \mid \omega^2)f(\omega^2).
$$

In fact, one can show that both conditional densities are inverse-gamma densities. Namely, by (13.9) and the prior pdf of σ^2 we have (up to a constant)

$$
\ln f(\sigma^2 \mid \boldsymbol{y}, \boldsymbol{\tau}) = \frac{T}{2}\ln(\frac{1}{\sigma^2}) - \frac{1}{2\sigma^2}(\boldsymbol{y} - \boldsymbol{\tau})^\top (\boldsymbol{y} - \boldsymbol{\tau}) + (1 + \alpha_{\sigma^2})\ln(\frac{1}{\sigma^2}) - \frac{\lambda_{\sigma^2}}{\sigma^2},
$$

☞ 240 which shows that

$$(\sigma^2 \mid \boldsymbol{y}, \boldsymbol{\tau}) \sim \mathsf{InvGamma}\left(\alpha_{\sigma^2} + \frac{T}{2}, \ \lambda_{\sigma^2} + \frac{1}{2}(\boldsymbol{y} - \boldsymbol{\tau})^\top(\boldsymbol{y} - \boldsymbol{\tau})\right). \tag{13.16}$$

Using a similar reasoning, we find

$$(\omega^2 \mid \boldsymbol{y}, \boldsymbol{\tau}) \sim \mathsf{InvGamma}\left(\alpha_{\omega^2} + \frac{T-1}{2}, \ \lambda_{\omega^2} + \frac{1}{2}\sum_{t=2}^{T}(\tau_t - \tau_{t-1})^2\right). \tag{13.17}$$

13.2 Time-Varying Parameter Model

The unobserved components model discussed in the last section may be viewed as a linear regression model with only an intercept, where the intercept is allowed to change over time. More generally, one can consider linear regression models where all the regression coefficients are time-varying. As discussed in the introduction, this is motivated by the empirical findings that typical macroeconomic and financial variables exhibit time-varying persistence and dynamics. In this section we discuss a particular type of time-varying parameter models, called **time-varying parameter autoregressive models**. Consider again the autoregressive model introduced in Definition 12.1. Instead of assuming constant autoregressive coefficients, we allow them to evolve over time.

Definition 13.3. (Time-Varying Parameter Autoregressive Model). In the **p-th-order time-varying parameter autoregressive model**, or time-varying parameter AR(p), the measurement equation is given by:

$$y_t = \beta_{0t} + \beta_{1t}y_{t-1} + \cdots + \beta_{pt}y_{t-p} + \varepsilon_t , \tag{13.18}$$

for $t = 1, \ldots, T$, where $\{\varepsilon_t\} \sim_{\mathrm{iid}} \mathcal{N}(0, \sigma^2)$, and $y_0, \ldots, y_{1-p}$ are initial observations. The autoregressive coefficients $\boldsymbol{\beta}_t = [\beta_{0t}, \beta_{1t}, \ldots, \beta_{pt}]^\top$ in turn evolve according to the following transition equation:

$$\boldsymbol{\beta}_t = \boldsymbol{\beta}_{t-1} + \boldsymbol{u}_t , \tag{13.19}$$

for $t = 2, \ldots, T$, where $\{\boldsymbol{u}_t\} \sim_{\mathrm{iid}} \mathcal{N}(\boldsymbol{0}, \boldsymbol{\Omega})$, and the transition equation is initialized with $\boldsymbol{\beta}_1 \sim \mathcal{N}(\boldsymbol{\beta}_0, \boldsymbol{\Omega}_0)$.

In the above definition, we treat the initial observations $y_0, \ldots, y_{1-p}$ as given, and we do not model them separately. For T much greater than p this has little influence on estimation and inference.

13.2.1 Bayesian Estimation

We begin by writing (13.18) in matrix notation:

$$y_t = \boldsymbol{x}_t^\top \boldsymbol{\beta}_t + \varepsilon_t \,,$$

where $\boldsymbol{x}_t^\top = [1, y_{t-1}, \ldots, y_{t-p}]$, $\boldsymbol{\beta}_t = [\beta_{0t}, \beta_{1t}, \ldots, \beta_{pt}]^\top$, and $\varepsilon_t \sim \mathcal{N}(0, \sigma^2)$. Now, stack the observations over all times t:

$$\boldsymbol{y} = \mathbf{X}\boldsymbol{\beta} + \boldsymbol{\varepsilon} \,, \tag{13.20}$$

where $\boldsymbol{y} = [y_1, \ldots, y_T]^\top$, $\boldsymbol{\beta} = [\boldsymbol{\beta}_1^\top, \ldots, \boldsymbol{\beta}_T^\top]^\top$, $\boldsymbol{\varepsilon} = [\varepsilon_1, \ldots, \varepsilon_T]^\top \sim \mathcal{N}(\mathbf{0}, \sigma^2 \mathbb{I}_T)$, and

$$\mathbf{X} = \begin{bmatrix} \boldsymbol{x}_1^\top & 0 & \ldots & 0 \\ 0 & \boldsymbol{x}_2^\top & \ldots & 0 \\ \vdots & \vdots & \ddots & \vdots \\ 0 & 0 & \ldots & \boldsymbol{x}_T^\top \end{bmatrix}.$$

Thus, the joint density of $\boldsymbol{y}$ is given by (suppressing the dependence on the initial observations $y_0, \ldots, y_{1-p}$):

$$\ln f(\boldsymbol{y} \,|\, \boldsymbol{\beta}, \sigma^2) = -\frac{T}{2} \ln \sigma^2 - \frac{1}{2\sigma^2}(\boldsymbol{y} - \mathbf{X}\boldsymbol{\beta})^\top (\boldsymbol{y} - \mathbf{X}\boldsymbol{\beta}) + \text{const}. \tag{13.21}$$

Next, we stack the transition equation (13.19) over t. For simplicity we set $\boldsymbol{\beta}_0 = \mathbf{0}$ (the general case follows similarly). The transition equations can be written in matrix form as

$$\mathbf{H}\boldsymbol{\beta} = \boldsymbol{u} \,,$$

where $\boldsymbol{u} \sim \mathcal{N}(\mathbf{0}, \mathbf{S})$, $\boldsymbol{u} = [\boldsymbol{u}_1^\top, \ldots, \boldsymbol{u}_T^\top]^\top$, with

$$\mathbf{H} = \begin{bmatrix} \mathbb{I}_{p+1} & 0 & \ldots & 0 & 0 \\ -\mathbb{I}_{p+1} & \mathbb{I}_{p+1} & \ldots & 0 & 0 \\ \vdots & \vdots & \ddots & \vdots & \vdots \\ 0 & 0 & \ldots & -\mathbb{I}_{p+1} & \mathbb{I}_{p+1} \end{bmatrix} \quad \text{and} \quad \mathbf{S} = \begin{bmatrix} \boldsymbol{\Omega}_0 & 0 & \ldots & 0 \\ 0 & \boldsymbol{\Omega} & \ldots & 0 \\ \vdots & \vdots & \ddots & \vdots \\ 0 & 0 & \ldots & \boldsymbol{\Omega} \end{bmatrix}.$$

Note that $|\mathbf{H}| = 1$ and $|\mathbf{S}| = |\boldsymbol{\Omega}_0| \, |\boldsymbol{\Omega}|^{T-1}$. It follows that the joint density of $\boldsymbol{\beta}$ satisfies

$$\ln f(\boldsymbol{\beta} \,|\, \boldsymbol{\Omega}) = -\frac{T-1}{2} \ln |\boldsymbol{\Omega}| - \frac{1}{2} \boldsymbol{\beta}^\top \mathbf{H}^\top \mathbf{S}^{-1} \mathbf{H} \boldsymbol{\beta} + \text{const}. \tag{13.22}$$

Since $\mathbf{\Omega}$ is a $(p+1) \times (p+1)$ symmetric matrix, it contains $(p+1)(p+2)/2$ distinct parameters. Even when p is small, say, $p = 4$, there are 15 distinct parameters. In typical empirical applications one cannot accurately estimate these many parameters. We can reduce the number of parameters by assuming that $\mathbf{\Omega}$ is diagonal. We adopt this approach and let $\boldsymbol{\omega}^2 = [\omega_0^2, \omega_1^2, \ldots, \omega_p^2]^\top$ denote the vector of diagonal elements of $\mathbf{\Omega}$.

To derive the posterior density, it remains to specify the prior for σ^2 and $\boldsymbol{\omega}^2$ (note that $\boldsymbol{\omega}^2$ can be estimated from the data rather than fixed as a vector of constants if a proper prior is adopted). We assume an independent prior $f(\sigma^2, \boldsymbol{\omega}^2) = f(\sigma^2)f(\boldsymbol{\omega}^2)$, where

$$\sigma^2 \sim \mathsf{InvGamma}(\alpha_{\sigma^2}, \lambda_{\sigma^2}), \quad \omega_i^2 \sim \mathsf{InvGamma}(\alpha_{\omega_i^2}, \lambda_{\omega_i^2}), \tag{13.23}$$

and $\alpha_{\sigma^2}, \lambda_{\sigma^2}, \alpha_{\omega_i^2}$, and $\lambda_{\omega_i^2}, i = 0, \ldots, p$, are constants specified by the user.

Finally, the posterior density is given by

$$f(\boldsymbol{\beta}, \sigma^2, \boldsymbol{\omega}^2 \,|\, \boldsymbol{y}) \propto f(\boldsymbol{y} \,|\, \boldsymbol{\beta}, \sigma^2)f(\boldsymbol{\beta} \,|\, \boldsymbol{\omega}^2)f(\sigma^2)f(\boldsymbol{\omega}^2), \tag{13.24}$$

where $f(\boldsymbol{y} \,|\, \boldsymbol{\beta}, \sigma^2)$ and $f(\boldsymbol{\beta} \,|\, \mathbf{\Omega}) = f(\boldsymbol{\beta} \,|\, \boldsymbol{\omega}^2)$ are provided in (13.21) and (13.22), respectively. Posterior draws can be obtained using the Gibbs sampler. Specifically, we sequentially draw from $f(\boldsymbol{\beta} \,|\, \boldsymbol{y}, \sigma^2, \boldsymbol{\omega}^2)$ followed by a draw from $f(\sigma^2, \boldsymbol{\omega}^2 \,|\, \boldsymbol{y}, \boldsymbol{\beta})$.

For the first step, we note that $f(\boldsymbol{\beta} \,|\, \boldsymbol{y}, \sigma^2, \boldsymbol{\omega}^2)$ is again a normal density. Hence, once we determine the mean vector and the precision matrix, we can apply Algorithm 12.1 to obtain a draw from it efficiently. Using (13.21) and (13.22), we have,

$$\begin{aligned}
\ln f(\boldsymbol{\beta} \,|\, \boldsymbol{y}, \sigma^2, \boldsymbol{\omega}^2) &= \ln f(\boldsymbol{y} \,|\, \boldsymbol{\beta}, \sigma^2) + \ln f(\boldsymbol{\beta} \,|\, \boldsymbol{\omega}^2) + \mathrm{const} \\
&= -\frac{1}{2\sigma^2}(\boldsymbol{y} - \mathbf{X}\boldsymbol{\beta})^\top(\boldsymbol{y} - \mathbf{X}\boldsymbol{\beta}) - \frac{1}{2}\boldsymbol{\beta}^\top \mathbf{H}^\top \mathbf{S}^{-1}\mathbf{H}\boldsymbol{\beta} + \mathrm{const} \\
&= -\frac{1}{2}(\boldsymbol{\beta} - \widehat{\boldsymbol{\beta}})^\top \mathbf{K}_{\boldsymbol{\beta}}(\boldsymbol{\beta} - \widehat{\boldsymbol{\beta}}) + \mathrm{const},
\end{aligned}$$

where

$$\mathbf{K}_{\boldsymbol{\beta}} = \frac{1}{\sigma^2}\mathbf{X}^\top\mathbf{X} + \mathbf{H}^\top\mathbf{S}^{-1}\mathbf{H} \qquad \text{and} \qquad \widehat{\boldsymbol{\beta}} = \mathbf{K}_{\boldsymbol{\beta}}^{-1}\left(\frac{1}{\sigma^2}\mathbf{X}^\top\boldsymbol{y}\right).$$

In other words, $(\boldsymbol{\beta} \,|\, \boldsymbol{y}, \sigma^2, \boldsymbol{\omega}^2) \sim \mathcal{N}(\widehat{\boldsymbol{\beta}}, \mathbf{K}_{\boldsymbol{\beta}}^{-1})$.

Next, note that σ^2 and $\boldsymbol{\omega}^2$ are conditionally independent given $\boldsymbol{y}$ and $\boldsymbol{\beta}$. Namely, from (13.24) we have

$$f(\sigma^2 \,|\, \boldsymbol{y}, \boldsymbol{\beta}) \propto f(\boldsymbol{y} \,|\, \boldsymbol{\beta}, \sigma^2)f(\sigma^2) \qquad \text{and} \qquad f(\boldsymbol{\omega}^2 \,|\, \boldsymbol{y}, \boldsymbol{\beta}) \propto f(\boldsymbol{\beta} \,|\, \boldsymbol{\omega}^2)f(\boldsymbol{\omega}^2).$$

Similar to (13.16) it follows from (13.21) and the prior $f(\sigma^2)$ that

☞ 371

$$(\sigma^2 \mid \boldsymbol{y}, \boldsymbol{\beta}) \sim \mathsf{InvGamma}\left(\alpha_{\sigma^2} + \frac{T}{2}, \lambda_{\sigma^2} + \frac{1}{2}(\boldsymbol{y} - \mathbf{X}\boldsymbol{\beta})^{\top}(\boldsymbol{y} - \mathbf{X}\boldsymbol{\beta})\right).$$

To find the distribution of $(\boldsymbol{\omega}^2 \mid \boldsymbol{y}, \boldsymbol{\beta})$, we use (13.22) and the assumption that $\boldsymbol{\Omega} = \mathrm{diag}(\boldsymbol{\omega}^2)$, to find

$$\ln f(\boldsymbol{\omega}^2 \mid \boldsymbol{y}, \boldsymbol{\beta}) = -\frac{T-1}{2}\sum_{i=0}^{p} \ln \omega_i^2 - \frac{1}{2}\sum_{i=0}^{p}\frac{1}{\omega_i^2}\sum_{t=2}^{T}(\beta_{it} - \beta_{i,t-1})^2 + \mathrm{const}.$$

From this we can deduce that conditional on $\boldsymbol{y}$ and $\boldsymbol{\beta}$ the components of $\boldsymbol{\omega}^2$ are independent of each other and each has an inverse-gamma distribution:

$$(\omega_i^2 \mid \boldsymbol{y}, \boldsymbol{\beta}) \overset{\text{ind}}{\sim} \mathsf{InvGamma}\left(\alpha_{\omega_i^2} + \frac{T-1}{2}, \lambda_{\omega_i^2} + \frac{1}{2}\sum_{t=2}^{T}(\beta_{it} - \beta_{i,t-1})^2\right)$$

for $i = 0, \ldots, p$.

Example 13.3 (Modeling Inflation with Time-Varying Parameter AR Model). In Example 13.2 we used the unobserved components model to fit the U.S. quarterly CPI inflation rate from 1947 to 2011. Here we illustrate Bayesian estimation in the more general time-varying parameter AR model. Specifically, we fit the time-varying parameter AR model in (13.18)–(13.19) using the inverse-gamma priors in (13.23). For simplicity, we fix p, the number of lags, to be 2. As for the hyperparameters in the prior, we choose relatively small values for the shape parameters so that the prior is relatively noninformative (e.g., large prior variances): $\alpha_{\sigma^2} = \alpha_{\omega_i^2} = 5, i = 0, \ldots, p$. Next, we set $\lambda_{\sigma^2} = (\alpha_{\sigma^2} - 1)$, $\lambda_{\omega_0^2} = 0.5^2(\alpha_{\omega_0^2} - 1)$, and $\lambda_{\omega_i^2} = 0.1^2(\alpha_{\omega_i^2} - 1)$ for $i = 1, \ldots, p$. These values imply $\mathbb{E}\sigma^2 = 1$, $\mathbb{E}\omega_0^2 = 0.5^2$ and $\mathbb{E}\omega_i^2 = 0.1^2$ for $i = 1, \ldots, p$. The covariance matrix $\boldsymbol{\Omega}_0$ is set to be diagonal with diagonal elements 5.

Before we discuss the main Gibbs sampler, we need a fast routine to build an appropriate sparse matrix. Recall that we want to write the measurement equation in matrix notation $\boldsymbol{y} = \mathbf{X}\boldsymbol{\beta} + \boldsymbol{\varepsilon}$ (see (13.20)).

The following function `SURform` takes the $T \times (p+1)$ matrix

$$\begin{bmatrix} \boldsymbol{x}_1^{\top} \\ \boldsymbol{x}_2^{\top} \\ \vdots \\ \boldsymbol{x}_T^{\top} \end{bmatrix},$$

and produces the sparse matrix $\mathbf{X}$, which is of dimension $T \times T(p+1)$.

```julia
function SURform(X)
   r, c = size(X);
   idi = vec(Int64.(kronecker(1:r,ones(c))))
   idj = 1:r*c
   return sparse(idi,idj,X'[:])
end
```

It is also convenient to use the following function to sample from a Gamma distribution for multiple scale parameters.

```julia
function gamrnd(a,c) # c is scale not rate
  n = length(c)
  x = zeros(n)
  for i=1:n
   x[i]  = rand(Gamma(a,c[i]))
  end
  return x
end
```

The script that implements the Gibbs sampler is given below. The number of iterations in the main Gibbs run is 1000. We ignore the burn-in.

```julia
TVPAR.jl

using SparseArrays, Kronecker,LinearAlgebra, Distributions
using StatsBase,Plots,DelimitedFiles
USCPI= readdlm("USCPI.csv")
nloop = 10000
p = 2    # number of lags
y0 = USCPI[1:p];   y = USCPI[p+1:end]
T = length(y)
q = p+1; Tq = T*q    # dimensions
    # priors
asigma2 = 5
lsigma2 = 1*(asigma2-1)
aomega2 = 5
lomega2 = (aomega2-1)*[0.5^2; 0.1^2*ones(p,1)]
invOmega0 = ones(q)/5
   # initialize
omega2 = .1*ones(q)
sigma2 = 1
store_omega2 = zeros(nloop,q)
store_sigma2 = zeros(nloop)
store_beta = zeros(Tq)
```

```
    # construct/compute a few things
X = [ones(T,1) [y0[end]; y[1:end-1]] [y0; y[1:end-2]]]
bigX = SURform(X)
H = sparse(I,Tq,Tq) - sparse(q+1:Tq,1:(T-1)*q, ones((T-1)*q),
    Tq,Tq)
newaomega2 = aomega2 + T - 1
newasigma2 = asigma2 + T
for loop = 1:nloop
    global omega2,sigma2,store_beta,betahat
        # sample beta
    invS = sparse(1:Tq,1:Tq,vec([invOmega0' repeat(1 ./ omega2
        ',1,T-1)]))
    K = H'*invS*H + bigX'*bigX/sigma2
    R = cholesky(K)  # sparse Cholesky
    P = sparse(1:Tq,R.p,ones(Tq))
    C = P'*sparse(R.L) # C*C' = K
    betahat = K(bigX'*y/sigma2)
    beta = betahat + C'\ randn(Tq)
        # sample omega2
    erromega2 = reshape(H*beta,q,T)
    newlomega2 = lomega2 + sum(erromega2[:,2:end].^2,dims=2)/2
    omega2 = 1 ./ gamrnd(newaomega2, 1 ./ newlomega2)
        # sample sigma2
    newlsigma2 = lsigma2 + sum((y-bigX*beta).^2)/2
    sigma2 = 1/rand(Gamma(newasigma2,1/newlsigma2))
        # store
    store_beta = store_beta + beta
    store_omega2[loop,:] = omega2'
    store_sigma2[loop] = sigma2
end
betahat = store_beta/nloop
sigma2hat = mean(store_sigma2)
omega2hat = mean(store_omega2,dims=1)
t = 1947.25:.25:2011.5
p1 = plot(t[3:end],betahat[1:3:end]);
p2 = plot(t[3:end],betahat[2:3:end]);
p3 = plot(t[3:end],betahat[3:3:end]);
plot(p1,p2,p3,layout=(1,3))
```

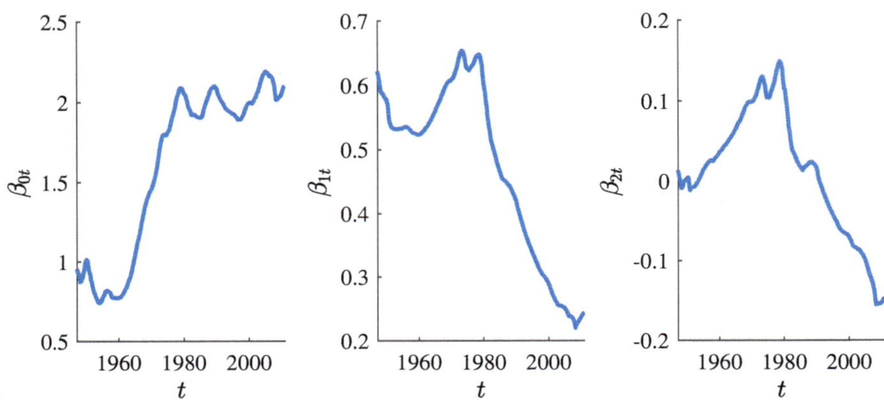

Fig. 13.2 Estimated posterior means for $\boldsymbol{\beta}_t$

The estimated posterior means for $\boldsymbol{\beta}_t = [\beta_{0t}, \beta_{1t}, \beta_{2t}]^\top$ are reported in Fig. 13.2. It is evident from the plots that there is a lot of time variation in the regression coefficients, which suggests that a time-invariant autoregressive model might not be appropriate. For instance, the intercept β_{0t} is estimated to be about 1% in the 1960s, while the estimate jumps to around 2% in the 1980s. Moreover, the estimate for the lag-1 coefficient β_{1t} increases from around 0.5 in 1960 to about 0.65 in the 1980s, which then decreases gradually in the following two decades and reaches a small value of 0.2 in 2010. Taken together, the hyperinflation in the 1970s–1980s may be viewed as a combination of a large shift in the level of the underlying inflation, together with an increase in persistence. After the 1980s, however, the underlying inflation stays at around 2%, but since the persistence decreases substantially, the inflation rate remains at a relatively low level.

13.3 Stochastic Volatility Model

A prominent feature of many time series, particularly macroeconomic and financial data, is the so-called **volatility clustering**—the phenomenon that large changes in observations tend to be followed by large changes and small changes followed by small changes. For example, large movements in asset returns tend to cluster together (e.g., during crisis), whereas there might be little variation over long stretches of "normal periods." Models with constant variance obviously do not allow the volatility of the observations to change over time and hence cannot model volatility clustering. In this section we introduce a class of state space models that can accommodate time-varying volatility. To focus our discussion on modeling the variance of the time series, we assume for the moment that the observations $\{y_t\}$ have zero mean; one could add a suitable conditional mean process such as an $\mathrm{AR}(p)$ component later on.

> **Definition 13.4. (Stochastic Volatility Model).** In the **stochastic volatility** model the observation at time t is given by
>
> $$y_t = \mathrm{e}^{h_t/2} \varepsilon_t, \qquad (13.25)$$
>
> where $\{\varepsilon_t\} \sim_{\mathrm{iid}} \mathcal{N}(0,1)$. Consequently, the **volatility** of y_t is $\mathrm{Var}(y_t) = \mathrm{e}^{h_t}$. The states are initialized with $h_1 \sim \mathcal{N}(h_0, \sigma_0^2)$ for some known constants h_0 and σ_0^2 and evolve according to a random walk
>
> $$h_t = h_{t-1} + v_t, \quad t = 2, \ldots, T, \qquad (13.26)$$
>
> where $\{v_t\} \sim_{\mathrm{iid}} \mathcal{N}(0, \omega^2)$. The state h_t is called the **log-volatility**.

The stochastic volatility model is an example of a *nonlinear* state space model where the measurement equation (13.25) is not linear in the state. One challenge of fitting this nonlinear model is that the joint conditional density of the states $\boldsymbol{h} = [h_1, \ldots, h_T]^\top$ given $\boldsymbol{y}$ is nonstandard (in contrast to previous examples where the conditional densities of the states are all Gaussian). As such, Bayesian estimation using MCMC and frequentist estimation via EM both become more difficult.

13.3.1 Auxiliary Mixture Sampling Approach

A popular method for estimating the stochastic volatility model is **auxiliary mixture sampling**. The basic idea underlying this approach is as follows. First, we transform the observation y_t so that the measurement equation becomes linear in h_t. Specifically, we square both sides of the measurement equation (13.25) and take the (natural) logarithm

$$y_t^* = h_t + \varepsilon_t^*, \qquad (13.27)$$

where $y_t^* = \ln y_t^2$ and $\varepsilon_t^* = \ln \varepsilon_t^2$. In practice, it is often recommended to set $y_t^* = \ln(y_t^2 + c)$ for some small constant c, say, $c = 0.0001$, to avoid numerical problems when y_t is close to zero. Now, after the transformation, (13.27) and (13.26) define a linear state space model. However, the error ε_t^* no longer has a Gaussian distribution (in fact, it has a log-χ_1^2 distribution), and the estimation techniques for linear Gaussian state space models discussed earlier cannot be directly applied.

In view of this difficulty, the second ingredient of the auxiliary mixture sampling approach is to find a suitable Gaussian mixture that approximates the pdf of ε_t^*

$$f(\varepsilon_t^*) \approx \sum_{i=1}^{n} p_i \, \varphi(\varepsilon_t^* ; \mu_i, \sigma_i^2) \,, \tag{13.28}$$

where $\varphi(x ; \mu, \sigma^2)$ is the Gaussian density with mean μ and variance σ^2, p_i is the mixture probability for the i-th component, and n is the number of components. The idea is to approximate the nonlinear stochastic volatility model using a mixture of linear Gaussian models, where the estimation of the latter models is standard. We can equivalently write (13.28) in terms of an auxiliary random variable $s_t \in \{1, \ldots, n\}$ that serves as the mixture component indicator (hence, the name of the approach):

$$(\varepsilon_t^* \mid s_t = i) \sim \mathcal{N}(\mu_i, \sigma_i^2) \,, \tag{13.29}$$

$$\mathbb{P}(s_t = i) = p_i \,. \tag{13.30}$$

Now, conditional on the component indicator s_t, we have a linear Gaussian model and the machinery for estimating such models can be applied.

It remains to select a suitable Gaussian mixture. By matching the moments of the log-χ_1^2 distribution, Kim et al. (1998) propose a seven-component Gaussian mixture

$$f(x) = \sum_{i=1}^{7} p_i \, \varphi(x ; \mu_i - 1.2704, \sigma_i^2) \,,$$

where the values of the parameters are given in Table 13.1. It is important to note that since the log-χ_1^2 distribution does not involve any unknown parameters, neither does this Gaussian mixture. In fact, all the parameter values of the approximating density are known.

Table 13.1 A seven-component Gaussian mixture for approximating the log-χ_1^2 distribution

comp.	p_i	μ_i	σ_i^2
1	0.00730	-10.12999	5.79596
2	0.10556	-3.97281	2.61369
3	0.00002	-8.56686	5.17950
4	0.04395	2.77786	0.16735
5	0.34001	0.61942	0.64009
6	0.24566	1.79518	0.34023
7	0.25750	-1.08819	1.26261

To summarize the model, define $\boldsymbol{s} = [s_1, \ldots, s_T]^{\top}$, $\boldsymbol{y}^* = [y_1^*, \ldots, y_T^*]^{\top}$, $\boldsymbol{h} = [h_1, \ldots, h_T]^{\top}$, $\boldsymbol{v} = [v_1, \ldots, v_T]^{\top}$, and $\boldsymbol{\varepsilon}^* = [\varepsilon_1^*, \ldots, \varepsilon_T^*]^{\top}$. Let $\mathbf{H}$ be the same matrix as in (13.10). By (13.27) we can write

$$\boldsymbol{y}^* = \boldsymbol{h} + \boldsymbol{\varepsilon}^* \,,$$

where $(\varepsilon^* \,|\, \boldsymbol{s}) \sim \mathcal{N}(\boldsymbol{d}, \boldsymbol{\Sigma}_{\boldsymbol{y}^*})$, with $\boldsymbol{d} = [\mu_{s_1} - 1.2704, \ldots, \mu_{s_T} - 1.2704]^\top$ and $\boldsymbol{\Sigma}_{\boldsymbol{y}^*} = \mathrm{diag}(\sigma_{s_1}^2, \ldots, \sigma_{s_T}^2)$. The (fixed) $\{\mu_i\}$ and $\{\sigma_i^2\}$ are given in Table 13.1. Consequently,

$$(\boldsymbol{y}^* \,|\, \boldsymbol{s}, \boldsymbol{h}) \sim \mathcal{N}(\boldsymbol{h} + \boldsymbol{d}, \boldsymbol{\Sigma}_{\boldsymbol{y}^*}) \,. \tag{13.31}$$

Using an inverse-gamma prior for ω^2, the hierarchical Bayesian model is thus as follows:

1. $(\boldsymbol{y}^* \,|\, \boldsymbol{s}, \boldsymbol{h}) \sim \mathcal{N}(\boldsymbol{h} + \boldsymbol{d},\, \boldsymbol{\Sigma}_{\boldsymbol{y}^*})$,
2. It follows from (13.26) that the random vector $\boldsymbol{h}$ is of the form $\boldsymbol{h} = \mathbf{H}^{-1}\boldsymbol{v}$, where $\boldsymbol{v} \sim \mathcal{N}(\mathbf{0}, \boldsymbol{\Omega}_{\boldsymbol{v}})$, with $\boldsymbol{\Omega}_{\boldsymbol{v}} = \mathrm{diag}(\omega_0^2, \omega^2, \ldots, \omega^2)$,
3. The components $s_1, \ldots, s_t$ of $\boldsymbol{s}$ are independent, with $\mathbb{P}(s_t = i) = p_i, \quad i = 1, \ldots, T$,
4. $\omega^2 \sim \mathsf{InvGamma}(\alpha_{\omega^2}, \lambda_{\omega^2})$.

In order to perform a Bayesian analysis, we need to be able to sample from the posterior pdf $f(\boldsymbol{h}, \boldsymbol{s}, \omega^2 \,|\, \boldsymbol{y})$. Due to the augmentation of the mixture component indicators $\boldsymbol{s}$, it becomes more cumbersome to implement a standard Gibbs sampler that sequentially samples from all the full conditional distributions. For example, $f(\omega^2 \,|\, \boldsymbol{y}, \boldsymbol{h}, \boldsymbol{s})$ is a nonstandard pdf. Instead, we follow Del Negro and Primiceri (2015) and implement a collapsed Gibbs sampler, by sequentially sampling from (1) $f(\boldsymbol{s}, \omega^2 \,|\, \boldsymbol{y}^*, \boldsymbol{h})$, which is done by sampling from (1a) $f(\omega^2 \,|\, \boldsymbol{y}^*, \boldsymbol{h})$ and (1b) $f(\boldsymbol{s} \,|\, \boldsymbol{y}^*, \boldsymbol{h}, \omega^2)$; and (2) $f(\boldsymbol{h} \,|\, \boldsymbol{y}^*, \boldsymbol{s}, \omega^2)$. More generally, for models with more blocks of parameters to sample, the main thing to remember is that $\boldsymbol{h}$ should be sampled immediately after $\boldsymbol{s}$.

First, implementation of (1a) is similar to the derivation in (13.17). In particular, given $\boldsymbol{y}$ and $\boldsymbol{h}$, ω^2 has again an inverse-gamma distribution:

$$(\omega^2 \,|\, \boldsymbol{y}, \boldsymbol{h}) \sim \mathsf{InvGamma}\left(\alpha_{\omega^2} + \frac{T-1}{2}, \ \lambda_{\omega^2} + \frac{1}{2}\sum_{t=2}^{T}(h_t - h_{t-1})^2\right).$$

To implement (1b), note that $f(\boldsymbol{s} \,|\, \boldsymbol{y}^*, \boldsymbol{h}) = \prod_{t=1}^{T} f(s_t \,|\, y_t^*, h_t)$, and therefore we can draw each s_t independently. Since s_t is a discrete random variable that follows a seven-point distribution, it can be easily sampled as long as we can compute $\mathbb{P}(s_t = i \,|\, y_t^*, h_t)$ for $i = 1, \ldots, 7$. In fact, we have

$$\mathbb{P}(s_t = i \,|\, y_t^*, h_t) = \frac{1}{c_t} p_i\, \varphi(y_t^* \,;\, \mu_i - 1.2704 + h_t, \sigma_i^2) \,,$$

where $c_t = \sum_{j=1}^{7} p_j\, \varphi(y_t^* \,;\, \mu_j - 1.2704 + h_t, \sigma_j^2)$ is the normalization constant. Finally, to implement (2), we write

$$\ln f(\boldsymbol{h} \,|\, \boldsymbol{y}^*, \boldsymbol{s}, \omega^2) = \ln f(\boldsymbol{y}^* \,|\, \boldsymbol{s}, \boldsymbol{h}) + \ln f(\boldsymbol{h} \,|\, \omega^2) + \mathrm{const} \,,$$

where $f(\boldsymbol{y}^* \,|\, \boldsymbol{s}, \boldsymbol{h})$ follows from (13.31) and $f(\boldsymbol{h} \,|\, \omega^2)$ follows from

$$(\boldsymbol{h} \,|\, \omega^2) \sim \mathcal{N}(\mathbf{0}, (\mathbf{H}^\top \boldsymbol{\Omega}_{\boldsymbol{v}}^{-1} \mathbf{H})^{-1}) \,.$$

Using a similar reasoning as in Sect. 13.1.2, we find

$$(\boldsymbol{h} \mid \boldsymbol{y}^*, \boldsymbol{s}, \omega^2) \sim \mathcal{N}(\widehat{\boldsymbol{h}}, \mathbf{K}_{\boldsymbol{h}}^{-1}) \,,$$

where

$$\mathbf{K}_{\boldsymbol{h}} = \boldsymbol{\Sigma}_{\boldsymbol{y}^*}^{-1} + \mathbf{H}^{\top} \boldsymbol{\Omega}_v^{-1} \mathbf{H} \qquad \text{and} \qquad \widehat{\boldsymbol{h}} = \mathbf{K}_{\boldsymbol{h}}^{-1} \boldsymbol{\Sigma}_{\boldsymbol{y}^*}^{-1} (\boldsymbol{y}^* - \boldsymbol{d}) \,.$$

A draw from the above Gaussian distribution can be efficiently obtained using
☞ 371   Algorithm 12.1.

Example 13.4 (Modeling Inflation with Unobserved Components Stochastic Volatility Model). We have considered in Example 13.2 an unobserved components model with constant variance for modeling the US quarterly CPI inflation. In this example, we extend the constant variance to include stochastic volatility in the measurement equation. This model is a simplified version of the unobserved components model in Stock and Watson (2007) that features stochastic volatility in both the measurement and state equations. Specifically, consider

$$
\begin{aligned}
y_t &= \tau_t + \mathrm{e}^{h_t/2} \varepsilon_t \,, \\
\tau_t &= \tau_{t-1} + u_t \,, \\
h_t &= h_{t-1} + v_t \,,
\end{aligned}
$$

where $\{\varepsilon_t\} \sim_{\mathrm{iid}} \mathcal{N}(0,1)$, $\{u_t\} \sim_{\mathrm{iid}} \mathcal{N}(0,\omega_\tau^2)$, and $\{v_t\} \sim_{\mathrm{iid}} \mathcal{N}(0,\omega_h^2)$. The state equations are initialized with $\tau_1 \sim \mathcal{N}(\tau_0, V_\tau)$ and $h_1 \sim \mathcal{N}(h_0, V_h)$, where $\tau_0 = h_0 = 0$ and $V_\tau = V_h = 9$. Again we assume independent inverse-gamma priors for ω_τ^2 and ω_h^2

$$\omega_\tau^2 \sim \mathsf{InvGamma}(\alpha_\tau, \lambda_\tau) \qquad \text{and} \qquad \omega_h^2 \sim \mathsf{InvGamma}(\alpha_h, \lambda_h) \,,$$

where we set $\alpha_\tau = \alpha_h = 10$, $\lambda_\tau = 0.25^2(\alpha_\tau - 1)$, and $\lambda_h = 0.2^2(\alpha_h - 1)$. These values imply $\mathbb{E}\omega_\tau^2 = 0.25^2$ and $\mathbb{E}\omega_h^2 = 0.2^2$. By defining y_t^* appropriately, the results derived earlier in this section can be applied to construct a suitable Gibbs sampler. More precisely, let

$$y_t^* = \ln((y_t - \tau_t)^2 + 0.0001) \,.$$

Then, by using the auxiliary mixture sampling approach, we sequentially draw from

(1) $f(\boldsymbol{s} \mid \boldsymbol{y}, \boldsymbol{\tau}, \boldsymbol{h}, \omega_\tau^2, \omega_h^2) = f(\boldsymbol{s} \mid \boldsymbol{y}^*, \boldsymbol{\tau}, \boldsymbol{h})$;
(2) $f(\boldsymbol{h} \mid \boldsymbol{y}, \boldsymbol{\tau}, \boldsymbol{s}, \omega_\tau^2, \omega_h^2) = f(\boldsymbol{h} \mid \boldsymbol{y}^*, \boldsymbol{\tau}, \boldsymbol{s}, \omega_h^2)$;
(3) $f(\boldsymbol{\tau} \mid \boldsymbol{y}, \boldsymbol{h}, \omega_\tau^2, \omega_h^2) = f(\boldsymbol{\tau} \mid \boldsymbol{y}, \boldsymbol{h}, \omega_\tau^2)$; and
(4) $f(\omega_\tau^2, \omega_h^2 \mid \boldsymbol{y}, \boldsymbol{\tau}, \boldsymbol{h}) = f(\omega_\tau^2, \omega_h^2 \mid \boldsymbol{\tau}, \boldsymbol{h})$.

For Steps (1) and (2), we can use the following Julia function `SVRW` to draw from the full conditional densities for $\boldsymbol{s}$ and $\boldsymbol{h}$:

```julia
function SVRW(ystar, h, omega2h, Vh)
  T = length(h)
  # parameters for the Gaussian mixture
  pi = [0.0073 0.10556 0.00002 0.04395 0.34001 0.24566 0.2575]
  mui = [-10.12999 -3.97281 -8.56686 2.77786 0.61942 1.79518
      -1.08819]
  sig2i = [5.79596 2.61369 5.17950 0.16735 0.64009 0.34023
      1.26261]
  sigi = sqrt.(sig2i)
  s = zeros(Int64, T)
  for t = 1:T
    q = zeros(7)
    for i = 1:7
      q[i] = pi[i]*pdf(Normal(mui[i]-1.2704+h[t],sigi[i]),
          ystar[t])
    end
    q = q ./ sum(q)
    s[t] = minimum(findall(cumsum(q) .> rand()))
  end
  H = sparse(I, T, T) - sparse(2:T,1:(T-1),ones(T - 1), T, T)
  invOmegah = spdiagm(vec([1/Vh; 1/omega2h*ones(T - 1, 1)]))
  d = mui[s]
  invSigystar = spdiagm(vec(1 ./ sig2i[s]))
  Kh = H' * invOmegah * H + invSigystar
  R = cholesky(Kh)
  P = sparse(1:T, R.p, ones(T))
  Ch = P' * sparse(R.L)
  hhat = Kh \ (invSigystar * (ystar - d))
  h = hhat + Ch' \ randn(T, 1)
  return h, s
end
```

Next, using a similar derivation as on Page 398, one can show that

$$(\boldsymbol{\tau} \mid \boldsymbol{y}, \boldsymbol{h}, \omega_\tau^2) \sim \mathcal{N}(\widehat{\boldsymbol{\tau}}, \mathbf{K}_\tau^{-1}) \,,$$

where $\boldsymbol{\Sigma}_{\boldsymbol{y}}^{-1} = \mathrm{diag}(\mathrm{e}^{-h_1}, \ldots, \mathrm{e}^{-h_T})$,

$$\mathbf{K}_\tau = \mathbf{H}^\top \boldsymbol{\Omega}_\tau^{-1} \mathbf{H} + \boldsymbol{\Sigma}_{\boldsymbol{y}}^{-1} \qquad \text{and} \qquad \widehat{\boldsymbol{\tau}} = \mathbf{K}_\tau^{-1} \boldsymbol{\Sigma}_{\boldsymbol{y}}^{-1} \boldsymbol{y} \,.$$

Hence, Step 3 can be implemented easily. Lastly, to complete Step 4, note that ω_τ^2 and ω_h^2 are conditionally independent given the states. Moreover,

$$(\omega_\tau^2 \mid \boldsymbol{\tau}, \boldsymbol{h}) \sim \mathsf{InvGamma}\left(\alpha_\tau + \frac{T-1}{2}, \, \lambda_\tau + \frac{1}{2}\sum_{t=2}^{T}(\tau_t - \tau_{t-1})^2\right) \,,$$

$$(\omega_h^2 \,|\, \boldsymbol{\tau}, \boldsymbol{h}) \sim \mathsf{InvGamma}\left(\alpha_h + \frac{T-1}{2},\ \lambda_h + \frac{1}{2}\sum_{t=2}^{T}(h_t - h_{t-1})^2\right).$$

The main script below fits the unobserved components model with stochastic volatility using the auxiliary mixture sampling approach.

```julia
UCSV.jl

using SparseArrays, Kronecker,LinearAlgebra, Distributions
using StatsBase,Plots,DelimitedFiles
y = readdlm("USCPI.csv")
T = length(y)
nloop = 10000
Vtau = 9
Vh = 9
atau = 10
ltau = .25^2*(atau-1)
ah = 10
lh = .2^2*(ah-1)
  # initialize the Markov chain
omega2tau = .25^2
omega2h = .2^2
h = log(var(y)*.8)*ones(T)
H = sparse(I,T,T) - sparse(2:T,1:(T-1),ones(T-1),T,T)
  # initialize for storage
store_omega2tau = zeros(nloop)
store_omega2h = zeros(nloop)
store_tau = zeros(nloop,T)
store_h = zeros(nloop,T)
 #  compute a few things
newatau = (T-1)/2 + atau
newah = (T-1)/2 + ah

for loop = 1:nloop
  global h, omega2tau, omega2h,tauhat
  invOmegatau = sparse(1:T, 1:T,
        vec([1 / Vtau 1 / omega2tau * ones(1, T - 1)]))
  invSigy = sparse(1:T, 1:T, vec(exp.(-h)))
  Ktau = H' * invOmegatau * H + invSigy
  R = cholesky(Ktau) # sparse Cholesky )
  P = sparse(1:T, R.p, ones(T))
  Ctau = P' * sparse(R.L) # Ctau*Ctau' = K
  tauhat = Ktau \ (invSigy * y)
  tau = tauhat + Ctau' \ randn(T)
  ystar = log.((y - tau) .^ 2 .+ 0.0001)
```

```julia
    h, s = SVRW(ystar, h, omega2h, Vh)
    # sample omega2tau
    newltau = ltau + sum((tau[2:end] - tau[1:end-1]) .^ 2) / 2
    omega2tau = 1 / rand(Gamma(newatau, 1 / newltau))
    # sample omega2h
    newlh = lh + sum((h[2:end] - h[1:end-1]) .^ 2) / 2
    omega2h = 1 / rand(Gamma(newah, 1 / newlh))
    store_tau[loop, :] = tau'
    store_h[loop, :] = h'
    store_omega2tau[loop] = omega2tau
    store_omega2h[loop] = omega2h
end

tauhat = mean(store_tau,dims=1)'
hhat = mean(store_h,dims=1)'

t = 1947.25:.25:2011.5
p1 = plot(t,tauhat);
p2 = plot(t,hhat);
plot(p1,p2)
```

We use the above code to obtain 10000 posterior, ignoring the burn-in. We present in Fig. 13.3 the estimated posterior means for the underlying inflation τ and the log-volatilities h.

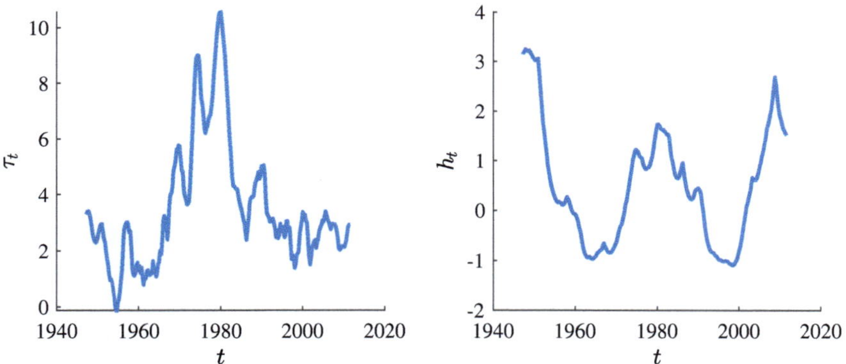

Fig. 13.3 Estimated posterior means for τ (left panel) and h (right panel)

Compared to the results obtained under the constant variance unobserved components model, the estimated underlying inflation exhibits a similar pattern, but is seemingly more variable. In addition, the estimated log-volatilities show that there is substantial time variation in the variance in the measurement equation, highlighting the relevance of the stochastic volatility model.

13.4 Problems

13.1. Prove the updating formulas in (13.4) by using the joint distribution in (13.3) and Theorem 3.8.

13.2. The **trace** of a square matrix $\mathbf{A} = (a_{ij})$ is the sum of the diagonal elements: $\mathrm{tr}(\mathbf{A}) = \sum_i a_{ii}$.

a. Let $\mathbf{A}$ and $\mathbf{B}$ be matrices (not necessarily square) such that $\mathbf{AB}$ and $\mathbf{BA}$ are square matrices (not necessarily of the same dimension). Show that $\mathrm{tr}(\mathbf{AB}) = \mathrm{tr}(\mathbf{BA})$.
b. Let $\mathbf{A}$ be a square matrix and let $\boldsymbol{x}$ be a random vector with mean $\boldsymbol{\mu}$ and covariance matrix $\boldsymbol{\Sigma}$. Using (a) and the fact that $\mathrm{tr}(\mathbb{E}\mathbf{Z}) = \mathbb{E}\,\mathrm{tr}(\mathbf{Z})$ for a random square matrix $\mathbf{Z}$, show that

$$\mathbb{E}(\boldsymbol{x}^{\top}\mathbf{A}\boldsymbol{x}) = \mathrm{tr}(\mathbf{A}\boldsymbol{\Sigma}) + \boldsymbol{\mu}^{\top}\mathbf{A}\boldsymbol{\mu} .$$

13.3. Show that for the measurement equation in (13.5), if one fixes $\tau_t = y_t$, then the function

$$g(\sigma^2) = \ln f(\boldsymbol{y} \,|\, \boldsymbol{\tau}, \sigma^2)$$

is unbounded in σ^2.

13.4. Another interpretation of the unobserved components model is to view it as a way to specify *stochastic trends*. Using the transition equation (13.6) and recursive substitution, show that

$$\mathrm{Var}(\tau_t \,|\, \tau_1) = (t - 1)\omega^2 ,$$

i.e., the stochastic trend τ_t has variance that is increasing with time, which implies that τ_t can wander over an increasing range of values as time increases.

13.5. For the unobserved components model (and more generally linear Gaussian state space models), it is possible to evaluate the likelihood function $L(\sigma^2; \boldsymbol{y})$ without computing the high-dimensional integral in (13.7). More specifically, by Bayes' theorem, the likelihood function can be written as (recall that ω^2 is a fixed constant)

$$L(\sigma^2; \boldsymbol{y}) = f(\boldsymbol{y} \,|\, \sigma^2, \omega^2) = \frac{f(\boldsymbol{y} \,|\, \boldsymbol{\tau}, \sigma^2) f(\boldsymbol{\tau} \,|\, \omega^2)}{f(\boldsymbol{\tau} \,|\, \boldsymbol{y}, \sigma^2, \omega^2)} ,$$

where the densities $f(\boldsymbol{y} \mid \boldsymbol{\tau}, \sigma^2), f(\boldsymbol{\tau} \mid \omega^2)$, and $f(\boldsymbol{\tau} \mid \boldsymbol{y}, \sigma^2, \omega^2)$ are all normal and can be evaluated quickly. Since the second equality holds for all $\boldsymbol{\tau}$, one can simply choose some convenient values, say, $\boldsymbol{\tau} = \boldsymbol{0}$.

Redo Example 13.2 by directly maximizing the log-likelihood function $l(\sigma^2; \boldsymbol{y})$. Specifically, plot $l(\sigma^2; \boldsymbol{y})$ as a function of σ^2. Moreover, find the maximum likelihood estimate for σ^2.

13.6. In this exercise we generalize the unobserved components model to allow for an additional channel for persistence. Specifically, consider

$$y_t = \tau_t + \beta(y_{t-1} - \tau_{t-1}) + \varepsilon_t \,,$$
$$\tau_t = \tau_{t-1} + u_t \,,$$

where $\{\varepsilon_t\} \sim_{\text{iid}} \mathcal{N}(0, \sigma^2)$, $\{u_t\} \sim_{\text{iid}} \mathcal{N}(0, \omega^2)$, and $\omega^2 = 1$. The underlying trend is initialized with $\tau_1 \sim \mathcal{N}(0, 5)$ and $\tau_0 = 0$. It is obvious that if $\beta = 0$, it reduces to the standard unobserved components model.

a. Derive the log-density $\ln f(\boldsymbol{y} \mid y_0, \boldsymbol{\tau}, \beta, \sigma^2)$.
b. Show that the conditional density $f(\boldsymbol{\tau} \mid \boldsymbol{y}, y_0, \beta, \sigma^2, \omega^2)$ is normal, and derive its parameters.
c. Describe how one can estimate the model parameters using frequentist and Bayesian methods.

13.7. Under the unobserved components model, suppose the state equation is given by

$$\tau_t = \beta\tau_{t-1} + u_t, \quad u_t \sim \mathcal{N}(0, \omega^2)$$

for $t = 2, \ldots, T$, with $\tau_1 \sim \mathcal{N}(\tau_0, \omega_0^2)$. Derive the joint density $f(\boldsymbol{\tau} \mid \beta, \omega^2)$.

13.8. Consider the following unobserved components model with AR(1) transition equation:

$$y_t = \tau_t + \varepsilon_t \,,$$
$$\tau_t = \beta\tau_{t-1} + u_t \,,$$

where $\{\varepsilon_t\} \sim_{\text{iid}} \mathcal{N}(0, \sigma^2)$, $\{u_t\} \sim_{\text{iid}} \mathcal{N}(0, \omega^2)$, and the underlying trend is initialized with $\tau_1 \sim \mathcal{N}(0, 5)$. Suppose we assume the priors: $\beta \sim \mathcal{N}(0, 1)$, $\sigma_\tau^2 \sim \mathsf{InvGamma}(10, 9)$, and $\omega^2 \sim \mathsf{InvGamma}(10, 9)$. Derive all the full conditional distributions. Fit this model with the US CPI data. In particular, use the **kde.m** program to plot a kernel density estimate of posterior distribution of β.

Solutions

Selected Problems of Chap. 1

1.1 (a) $\Omega = \{1,2,3,4,5,6\}$; (b) $\Omega = \mathbb{R}_+$; (c) $\Omega = \{0,1,\dots\}$; (d) $\Omega = \{0,1,\dots,50\}$; (e) $\Omega = \{(x_1,\dots,x_{10}) : x_i \geq 0, i = 1,\dots,10\} = \mathbb{R}_+^{10}$.

1.4 (a) $1/5$; (b) $5/36$.

1.5 (a) Ω is the set of all $6!$ permutations of $(1,\dots,6)$; (b) $\mathbb{P}(A) = |A|/720$; (c) $15/720$.

1.8 (a) $\Omega = \{(1,2,3),\dots,(52,51,50)\}$. Each elementary event is equally likely; (b) $\frac{4\times3\times2}{52\times51\times50} = \frac{3}{16575}$; (c) $\frac{6\times4^4}{52\times51\times50} = 64/5525$; (d) $\frac{36\times35\times34}{52\times51\times50} = \frac{1071}{3315}$.

1.9 $\frac{\binom{17}{7}}{\binom{20}{10}} = \frac{2}{19}$.

1.10 (a) $\frac{1}{6}$; (b) $\frac{1}{3}$.

1.13 $\frac{1}{365^2}$.

1.14 $\binom{10}{4} \times 0.4^4 \times 0.6^6 = 0.2508$.

1.15 (a) 0.0791; (b) 0.1239.

1.17 $1/96$.

1.19 (a) $\frac{1}{36} \times \left(\frac{35}{36}\right)^9 = 0.0216$; (b) $1 - (35/36)^{100} = 0.94022$.

1.21 `ceil.(6*rand(100))`.

J. C. C. Chan, D. P. Kroese, *Statistical Modeling and Computation,* Springer Texts in Statistics, https://doi.org/10.1007/978-1-0716-4132-3

Selected Problems of Chap. 2

2.1 (a)

x	1	2	3	4	5	6
$f(x)$	$\frac{11}{36}$	$\frac{9}{36}$	$\frac{7}{36}$	$\frac{5}{36}$	$\frac{3}{36}$	$\frac{1}{36}$

(b) $\frac{4}{9}$; (c) $\mathbb{E}M = \frac{91}{36}$, $\mathrm{Var}(M) = \frac{2555}{1296}$.

2.2 (b): (i) 4/5; (ii) 3/5; (iii) 3/5; (iv) 19/20.

2.6 $X \sim \mathrm{Bin}(100, 0.12)$; $\mathbb{P}(X \le 7) = \sum_{k=0}^{7} \binom{100}{k} 0.12^k (1 - 0.12)^{100-k} = 0.0761$.

2.8 $M(s) = \frac{e^{bs} - e^{as}}{s(b-a)}$, $s \in \mathbb{R}$.

2.11 (a) $1 - e^{-2}$; (b) e^{-8}; (c) e^{-4}; (d) $1/2$.

2.12 (a) The expectation does not exist ($\infty - \infty$ is ill-defined); (b) the expectation is ∞.

2.16 In the first model $X \sim \mathrm{Exp}(1/3)$ and $\mathbb{P}(X > 4.5 \mid X > 4) = 0.8465$. In the second model $X \sim \mathcal{N}(3, 9)$ and $\mathbb{P}(X > 4.5 \mid X > 4) = 0.8351$.

2.18 (b): (i) $\Phi(-1/3)$, (ii) $1 - \Phi(0) = 1/2$, (iii) $\Phi(1/3) - \Phi(-5/3)$; (c) 9; (d) 25.

2.20 (a) `2+rand()`; (b)`3+3*randn()`; (c) `-log(rand())/4`; (d) `sum(rand(10) .< 0.5)`; (e) `ceil(log(rand())/(1-1/6))`.

2.21 Use `X = sqrt.(-log.(rand(1000)));` `histogram(X)`.

Selected Problems of Chap. 3

3.1

	y			
x		-2	0	2
	-1	0	$\frac{1}{2}$	0	$\frac{1}{2}$
	1	$\frac{1}{4}$	0	$\frac{1}{4}$	$\frac{1}{2}$
		$\frac{1}{4}$	$\frac{1}{2}$	$\frac{1}{4}$	1

X and Y are not independent since, for example, $\mathbb{P}(X = -1, Y = -2) = 0 \neq \frac{1}{2} \times \frac{1}{4} = \mathbb{P}(X = -1)\mathbb{P}(Y = -2)$.

3.3 (a) $f_X(x) = \frac{1}{3}$ for $x = 1, 2, 3$; (b) $f_{Y|X}(y \mid 1) = \frac{1}{2}$ for $y = 0, 1$, $f_{Y|X}(y \mid 2) = \frac{4 - 3(y-1)^2}{6}$ for $y = 0, 1, 2$, $f_{Y|X}(y \mid 3) = \frac{1}{2}$ for $y = 1, 2$;

(c)

x	y = 0	1	2	
1	$\frac{1}{6}$	$\frac{1}{6}$	0	$\frac{1}{3}$
2	$\frac{1}{18}$	$\frac{2}{9}$	$\frac{1}{18}$	$\frac{1}{3}$
3	0	$\frac{1}{6}$	$\frac{1}{6}$	$\frac{1}{3}$
	$\frac{2}{9}$	$\frac{5}{9}$	$\frac{2}{9}$	1

; (d) $f_Y(0) = f_Y(2) = 2/9$ and $f_Y(1) = 5/9$; (e) $f_{X|Y}(x\,|\,0) = \begin{cases} \frac{3}{4}, & x = 1 \\ \frac{1}{4}, & x = 2, \end{cases}$ $f_{X|Y}(x\,|\,1) = \begin{cases} \frac{3}{10}, & x = 1 \\ \frac{2}{5}, & x = 2 \\ \frac{3}{10}, & x = 3, \end{cases}$ $f_{X|Y}(x\,|\,2) = \begin{cases} \frac{1}{4}, & x = 2 \\ \frac{3}{4}, & x = 3 \end{cases}$.

3.4 $f_{X|Y}(x\,|\,1) = \frac{1/(6x)}{147/360} = \frac{60}{147x}$ for $x = 1, \ldots, 6$, and $\mathbb{E}[X\,|\,Y = 1] = \sum_{x=1}^{6} x \times \frac{60}{147x} = \frac{360}{147}$.

3.6 (a) $f(x, y) = f_X(x) f_Y(y) = e^{-y}$ for $0 \le x \le 1$, and $y \ge 0$; (b) $1 - e^{-1}$; (c) e^{-1}.

3.8 (a) $f(x, y) = f_X(x) f_{Y|X}(y\,|\,x) = e^{-x} \times x e^{-xy} = x e^{-x(y+1)}$ for $x > 0, y > 0$; (b) $f_Y(y) = \frac{1}{(y+1)^2}, y \ge 0$.

3.9 Since $X \sim \mathcal{U}[-\pi/2, \pi/2]$, $f_X(x) = 1/\pi$, $x \in (-\pi/2, \pi/2)$. Let $Y = \tan(X)$. Then, the inverse transformation is $g^{-1}(y) = \arctan(x)$, and the associated matrix of Jacobi is $\mathbf{J}_{g^{-1}}(y) = 1/(1 + y^2)$. Hence, $f_Y(y) = \frac{1}{\pi(1+y^2)}$, which is the pdf of the Cauchy distribution.

3.11 (a) $f_{S_2}(x) = x$ for $0 \le x \le 1$, $f_{S_2}(x) = 2 - x$ for $1 < x \le 2$, and 0 otherwise; (b) $\mathcal{N}(10, 5/3)$; (c) 0.0607.

3.12 (a) $\mathbb{E}T = 5, \mathrm{Var}(T) = \frac{5}{2}$; (b) 0.2635; (c) $T \sim \mathsf{Gamma}(10, 2)$.

3.15 (a) $\left(\frac{7}{8}\right)^6$; (b) $1 - \left(\frac{7}{8}\right)^6$.

3.18 (b) $\frac{(n-1)}{n}\sigma^2$.

3.20 W is the sum of the weights of six randomly chosen people and has a $\mathcal{N}(600, 600)$ distribution. $6X_1$ is 6 times the weight of the first chosen person, and has a $\mathcal{N}(600, 3600)$ distribution.

3.21 Recall that if $Z \sim \chi_\nu^2$, then its moment generating function is $M_Z(s) = 1/(1 - 2s)^{\nu/2} = (1 - 2s)^{-\nu/2}$. Now, $M_{X+Y}(s) = \mathbb{E}e^{s(X+Y)} = \mathbb{E}e^{sX}\mathbb{E}e^{sY} = (1-2s)^{-m/2}(1-2s)^{-n/2} = (1-2s)^{-(m+n)/2}$, which is the moment generating function of χ_{m+n}^2.

3.23 0.9867.

3.24 (a) 1.0524; (b) 0.0838.

Selected Problems of Chap. 4

4.1

(a) $X_1, \ldots, X_9 \sim_{\text{iid}} \mathcal{N}(\mu, \sigma^2)$, where X_i is the volume of paint in the i-th tin. The primary interest is to determine if μ is less than 20.

(b) $X_1, \ldots, X_{12} \sim_{\text{iid}} \mathcal{N}(\mu_1, \sigma_1^2)$ and $Y_1, \ldots, Y_{12} \sim_{\text{iid}} \mathcal{N}(\mu_2, \sigma_2^2)$ independently. Here, X_i (Y_i) is the time of completion for the i-th man (woman). The primary interest is to determine if $\mu_1 - \mu_2$ is significantly different from 0 or not.

(c) $Z_1, \ldots, Z_{12} \sim_{\text{iid}} \mathcal{N}(\mu, \sigma^2)$, where Z_i is the difference in marks for the i-th exam as marked by lecturers A and B. The primary interest is to determine if μ is significantly different from 0 or not.

(d) $X_1, \ldots, X_{500} \sim_{\text{iid}} \mathsf{Ber}(p)$, where $X_i = 1$ if the i-th coin toss is Heads and $X_i = 0$ otherwise. The primary interest is to determine if p equals $1/2$.

4.2 (a) Let X_i be the *average* weight of five randomly selected packets from the packaging line at hour i, $i = 1, \ldots, 24$. A possible model is to assume that the $\{X_i\}$ are independent and that each $X_i \sim \mathcal{N}(\mu_i, \sigma_i^2)$ for some unknown μ_i and σ_i^2. Typical questions of interest are whether the $\{\mu_i\}$ and $\{\sigma_i^2\}$ lie within an acceptable range.

4.7

(a) If one expects that shipping cost is a linear or quadratic function in distance, then a possible model is $Y_i = \beta_0 + \beta_1 x_i + \beta_2 x_i^2 + \varepsilon_i$, $\{\varepsilon_i\} \sim_{\text{iid}} \mathcal{N}(0, \sigma^2)$, $i = 1, \ldots, 9$, where Y_i is the shipping cost of the i-th air freight and x_i the corresponding distance traveled.

(b) Single-factor ANOVA model $Y_{ik} = \mu_i + \varepsilon_{ik}$, $\{\varepsilon_{ik}\} \sim_{\text{iid}} \mathcal{N}(0, \sigma^2)$, $k = 1, \ldots, 20$, $i = 1, 2, 3$, where Y_{ik} is the average fuel consumption for the k-th car of brand i, $k = 1, \ldots, 20$, $i = 1, 2, 3$.

(d) Simple linear regression model $Y_i = \beta_0 + \beta_1 x_i + \varepsilon_i$, $\{\varepsilon_i\} \sim_{\text{iid}} \mathcal{N}(0, \sigma^2)$, $i = 1, \ldots, 10$, where Y_i is the military expenditure of the country in year i and x_i is the gross national product in that year.

4.9 The $n \times 6$ design matrix is given by

$$\begin{bmatrix} 1 & x_{11} & x_{21} & x_{11}^2 & x_{21}^2 & x_{11}x_{21} \\ 1 & x_{12} & x_{22} & x_{12}^2 & x_{22}^2 & x_{12}x_{22} \\ \vdots & \vdots & \vdots & \vdots & \vdots & \vdots \\ 1 & x_{1n} & x_{2n} & x_{1n}^2 & x_{2n}^2 & x_{1n}x_{2n} \end{bmatrix}.$$

4.11 The following Julia script generates realizations from the linear regression model.

```julia
using Printf
beta= [-1 0 1]; # 2 free parameters
alpha = [-2 2]; # 1 free parameter
mu = 6; # 1 parameter
gamma = [
0.2 -1 0.8; -0.2 1 -0.8]; # 2 free parameters
eps = 0.1*randn(2,3,3);
y = zeros(2,3,3)
for i=1:2
  for j=1:3
    y[i,j,:] = mu .+ alpha[i] .+ beta[j] .+ gamma[i,j] .+ eps[
        i,j,:];
  end
end
for i=1:2
   for j=1:3
      for k=1:3
          @printf("%3.2f  ",y[i,j,k])
      end
   end
   @printf("\n");
end
```

Selected Problems of Chap. 5

5.1 For $\mathsf{Geom}(p)$, $\widehat{p} = 1/\overline{x}$; for $\mathsf{Poi}(\lambda)$, $\widehat{\lambda} = \overline{x}$; for $\mathsf{Gamma}(\alpha, \lambda)$, $\widehat{\alpha} = \overline{x}^2/v^2$ and $\widehat{\lambda} = \overline{x}/v^2$, where $v^2 = n^{-1} \sum_{i=1}^{n} (x_i - \overline{x})^2$.

5.5 (a) $\widehat{\lambda} = \overline{X}$; (b) From the central limit theorem, $\overline{X}$ has approximately a normal distribution with expectation $\mathbb{E}\overline{X} = 1/\lambda$ and variance $\mathrm{Var}(\overline{X}) = 1/(\lambda^2 n)$, so that

$$\mathbb{P}\left(\frac{1 - z_{1-\alpha/2}/\sqrt{n}}{\overline{X}} \leq \lambda \leq \frac{1 + z_{1-\alpha/2}/\sqrt{n}}{\overline{X}} \right) \approx 1 - \alpha \,,$$

from which the $1 - \alpha$ approximate confidence interval for λ follows.

5.7 $(0.045, 0.055)$ ml.

5.8 The confidence interval $(1.015, 1.810)$ does not contain the value 1, so there is reasonable evidence to suspect that the claim on the packet is not true.

5.10 Evaluating $\widehat{\boldsymbol{\beta}} = (\mathbf{X}^\top \mathbf{X})^{-1}\mathbf{X}^\top \boldsymbol{Y}$ gives

$$
\begin{aligned}
\widehat{\boldsymbol{\beta}} &= \begin{bmatrix} n & \sum_{i=1}^n x_i \\ \sum_{i=1}^n x_i & \sum_{i=1}^n x_i^2 \end{bmatrix}^{-1} \begin{bmatrix} \sum_{i=1}^n Y_i \\ \sum_{i=1}^n x_i Y_i \end{bmatrix} \\
&= \frac{1}{n\sum_{i=1}^n x_i^2 - n^2\overline{x}^2} \begin{bmatrix} \sum_{i=1}^n x_i^2 & -n\overline{x} \\ -n\overline{x} & n \end{bmatrix} \begin{bmatrix} n\overline{Y} \\ \sum_{i=1}^n x_i Y_i \end{bmatrix} \\
&= \frac{1}{nS_{xx}} \begin{bmatrix} \sum_{i=1}^n x_i^2 n\overline{Y} - n\overline{x}\sum_{i=1}^n x_i Y_i \\ -n^2\overline{x}\,\overline{Y} + n\sum_{i=1}^n x_i Y_i \end{bmatrix} \\
&= \frac{1}{S_{xx}} \begin{bmatrix} \sum_{i=1}^n x_i^2 \overline{Y} - \overline{x}\sum_{i=1}^n x_i Y_i \\ S_{xY} \end{bmatrix} \\
&= \frac{1}{S_{xx}} \begin{bmatrix} \overline{Y}(\sum_{i=1}^n x_i^2 - n\overline{x}^2) + \overline{x}(\overline{Y}n\overline{x} - \sum_{i=1} x_i Y_i) \\ S_{xY} \end{bmatrix} \\
&= \begin{bmatrix} \overline{Y} - \overline{x}S_{xY}/S_{xx} \\ S_{xY}/S_{xx} \end{bmatrix}.
\end{aligned}
$$

5.12 Model: $Y_i = a\sqrt{h_i} + \varepsilon_i$, $i = 1,\ldots,4$, where the $\{\varepsilon_i\}$ are iid and $\mathcal{N}(0,\sigma^2)$ distributed. The least-square estimate of a is $\widehat{a} = 0.452$.

5.13 Let X be the number of low fat milk sales out of 1500. The model is $X \sim \mathsf{Bin}(1500,p)$ for some unknown p. We wish to test $H_0 : p = 0.3$ versus $H_1 : p < 0.3$. The outcome of X is $x = 400$. The corresponding p-value is $\mathbb{P}_{H_0}(X \leq 400) \approx 0.00243$. There is thus very strong evidence that the true proportion p is less than 0.3, indicating a move toward low fat milk.

5.17 Let $X_1,\ldots,X_n \sim_{\mathrm{iid}} \mathcal{N}(\mu, 16)$ be the PFC amounts.

(a) The average PFC is $\overline{X}$, which has a $\mathcal{N}(\mu, 16/n) = \mathcal{N}(\mu, 4)$ distribution.
(b) $\mathbb{P}_{\mu=38.5}(\overline{X} < 39) = \Phi(0.025) = 0.51$.
(c) Find n such that $\mathbb{P}_{\mu=38}(\overline{X} < 39) \geq 0.9$. The smallest such n is 27.

5.23 Let Y_{ik} be the walking age of the k-th baby in group $i = 1,2,3,4$ (corresponding to A,B,C,D). Consider the 1-factor ANOVA model

$$ Y_{ik} = \mu + \alpha_i + \varepsilon_{ik}, \quad i = 1,\ldots,4, \quad k = 1,\ldots,6, $$

with $\{\varepsilon_{ik}\} \sim_{\mathrm{iid}} \mathcal{N}(0,\sigma^2)$ and $\sum_{i=1}^4 \alpha_i = 0$. To test the hypothesis $\alpha_1 = \ldots = \alpha_4 = 0$, we use the test statistic $T = \frac{\mathrm{MS_{treatment}}}{\mathrm{MS_{error}}}$, which under H_0 has an F(3, 20) distribution. By changing the data matrix yy in the first Julia program in Example 5.17 , we find the outcome 2.1370 for the test statistic, which gives a p-value of 0.1275. Since this is not very small, we accept the null hypothesis that there is no difference in expected walking age between the groups.

  To compute the 95% confidence intervals for the expected walking ages $\mu_i = \mu + \alpha_i$, $i = 1,\ldots,4$, we apply Theorem 5.3 using specific vectors $\boldsymbol{a}$. For example, to find a confidence interval for μ_1, take $\boldsymbol{a} = [1,1,0,0]^\top$.

☞ 148
☞ 142

Similarly, for μ_4, take $\boldsymbol{a} = [1, -1, -1, -1]^\top$. By modifying the Julia program `linregestconf.jl` in Example 5.12, as in,

```
tquant = quantile(TDist(n-m),0.975) # 0.975 quantile
a = [1, 1, 0, 0]
ucl = a'*betahat + tquant*norm(y - X*betahat)*sqrt(a'*inv(X'*X
    )*a)/sqrt(n-m)
lcl = a'*betahat .- tquant*norm(y - X*betahat)*sqrt(a'*inv(X'*
    X)*a)/sqrt(n-m)
[lcl ucl]
```

we find the following 95% numerical confidence intervals, $(8.85, 11.39)$, $(10.10, 12.64)$, $(10.44, 12.97)$, and $(10.94, 13.48)$, which clearly overlap, corroborating our finding that there is no evidence for a difference in expected walking age.

Selected Problems of Chap. 6

6.2 The derivative of the log-likelihood for θ is $\frac{\mathrm{d}l}{\mathrm{d}\theta} = -\frac{n}{2\theta} + \frac{1}{2\theta^2}\sum_{i=1}^n x_i^2 - \frac{n}{2}$. Solving the likelihood equation $\frac{\mathrm{d}l}{\mathrm{d}\theta} = 0$, one obtains the maximum likelihood estimate $\widehat{\theta} = -\frac{1}{2} + \frac{1}{2}\sqrt{1 + \frac{4}{n}\sum_{i=1}^n x_i^2}$. Substitute X_i for x_i to obtain the estimator.

6.5 (a) $\widehat{\theta}_{\mathrm{M}} = (2\overline{X} - 1)/(1 - \overline{X})$; (b) $\widehat{\theta} = -1 - n/\sum_{i=1}^n \ln X_i$.

6.6 $\mathbb{P}(X > 68.5) = \mathbb{P}((X - \mu)/\sigma > (68.5 - \mu)/\sigma) = 1 - \Phi((68.5 - \mu)/\sigma)$. Hence, by Theorem 6.6, the MLE is $1 - \Phi((68.5 - 56.3)/7.6) = 0.0542$.   ☞ 18

6.9 $l(\lambda; \boldsymbol{x}) = n\ln(\lambda/2) - \lambda\sum_{i=1}^n |x_i|$. Setting $l'(\lambda; \boldsymbol{x}) = 0$ gives $\widehat{\lambda} = n/\sum_{i=1}^n |x_i| = 0.5893$.

6.12 $l(p; \boldsymbol{x}) = \ln p \sum_{i=1}^n x_i + \ln(1 - p)\sum_{i=1}^n (k - x_i) + \text{const}$, so that $l'(p; \boldsymbol{X}) = \sum_{i=1}^n X_i/p - \sum_{i=1}^n (k - X_i)/(1 - p)$. Setting $l'(p; \boldsymbol{X}) = 0$ gives the maximum likelihood estimator $\widehat{p} = \overline{X}/k$. The information number $I(p)$ is, by Theorem 6.4, equal to $n\mathring{I}(p)$, where $\mathring{I}(p)$ is the information number for   ☞ 17 $X \sim \mathrm{Bin}(k, p)$. By (6.11) $\mathring{I}(p) = k/(p(1 - p))$. Also, $\mathrm{Var}(\widehat{p}) = \mathrm{Var}(\overline{X}/k) = \mathrm{Var}(X_1)/(nk^2) = kp(1 - p)/(nk^2) = p(1 - p)/(nk) = I^{-1}(p)$. Hence, $\widehat{p}$ attains the Cramér–Rao lower bound.

6.14

(a) The log-likelihood corresponding to $X \sim \mathrm{Exp}(1/v)$ is $\mathring{l}(v; x) = -\ln(v) - x/v$, with score function $\mathring{S}(v; x) = -1/v + x/v^2$. The score function corresponding to $X_1, \ldots, X_n \sim_{\text{iid}} \mathrm{Exp}(1/v)$ is $S(v; \boldsymbol{x}) = \sum_{i=1}^n \mathring{S}(v; x_i) = -n/v + \sum_{i=1}^n x_i/v^2$.

(b) The Fisher information for $X \sim \mathsf{Exp}(1/v)$ is $\mathring{I}(v) = \mathrm{Var}(\mathring{S}(v, \boldsymbol{X})) = \mathrm{Var}(X)/v^4 = v^2/v^4 = 1/v^2$. The Fisher information corresponding to $X_1, \ldots, X_n \sim_{\text{iid}} \mathsf{Exp}(1/v)$ is $I(v) = n\mathring{I}(v) = n/v^2$.

(c) Setting $S(v; \boldsymbol{X}) = 0$, we find the MLE $\widehat{v} = \overline{X}$.

(d) $\widehat{\sin(v)} = \sin(\widehat{v}) = \sin(\overline{X})$.

(e) $\mathrm{Var}(\widehat{v}) = \mathrm{Var}(\overline{X}) = \mathrm{Var}(X_1)/n = v^2/n = I^{-1}(v)$.

6.18 The score function is $n/\theta - \sum_{i=1}^{n} X_i$, and the Fisher information is $n\mathrm{Var}(\theta - X_1) = n/\theta^2$. The $1 - \alpha$ stochastic confidence set is thus

$$
\left\{ \theta : -z_{1-\alpha/2} < \frac{n/\theta - \sum_{i=1}^{n} X_i}{\sqrt{n/\theta^2}} < z_{1-\alpha/2} \right\}
$$
$$
= \left\{ \frac{n - z_{1-\alpha/2}\sqrt{n}}{\sum_{i=1}^{n} X_i} < \theta < \frac{n + z_{1-\alpha/2}\sqrt{n}}{\sum_{i=1}^{n} X_i} \right\},
$$

which is an interval. Taking $z_{1-\alpha/2} = z_{0.95} = 1.645$, we find the numeric 90% confidence interval $(0.480, 1.520)$.

6.19 Let $\boldsymbol{X} = [X_1, \ldots, X_n]$ be an iid sample from $\mathsf{Exp}(\lambda)$ and $\boldsymbol{Y} = [Y_1, \ldots, Y_n]$ an iid sample from $\mathsf{Exp}(\mu)$.

(a) The MLEs of λ and μ are, respectively, $\widehat{\lambda} = 1/\overline{X}$ and $1/\overline{Y}$.

(b) Under H_0, the MLE of θ is $\widehat{\theta} = \dfrac{2n}{\sum_{i=1}^{n} X_i + \sum_{i=1}^{n} Y_i}$.

(c) The likelihood ratio is given by

$$
\Lambda = \frac{(2n)^{2n}}{\left(\sum_{i=1}^{n} x_i + \sum_{i=1}^{n} y_i\right)^{2n}} \times \frac{\left(\sum_{i=1}^{n} x_i\right)^n \left(\sum_{i=1}^{n} y_i\right)^n}{n^{2n}}
$$
$$
= \frac{2^{2n}}{\left(1 + \frac{\sum_{i=1}^{n} y_i}{\sum_{i=1}^{n} x_i}\right)^{2n}} \times \left(\frac{\sum_{i=1}^{n} y_i}{\sum_{i=1}^{n} x_i}\right)^n
$$
$$
= 2^{2n}(1 + T)^{-2n} T^n = 2^{2n} \left(\frac{T}{(1 + T)^2}\right)^n.
$$

Hence, we can use $T/(1 + T)^2$ as a test statistic, and we reject H_0 when the likelihood ratio is "too small," i.e., when $\frac{T}{(1+T)^2} < \alpha$ for some critical value α.

(d) T has approximately a $\mathcal{N}(\lambda/\mu, \sigma^2/n)$ distribution, with

$$
\sigma^2 = \mathbf{J}\boldsymbol{\Sigma}\mathbf{J}^\top = \left(-\frac{\lambda^2}{\mu}, \lambda\right) \begin{bmatrix} \lambda^{-2} & 0 \\ 0 & \mu^{-2} \end{bmatrix} \begin{bmatrix} -\frac{\lambda^2}{\mu} \\ \lambda \end{bmatrix} = \frac{2\lambda^2}{\mu^2}.
$$

6.24 Initial guesses for α and λ are obtained via the method of moments: $\alpha_0 = \frac{\overline{x}^2}{s^2}$, $\lambda_0 = \frac{\overline{x}}{s^2}$.

The following Julia program implements the Newton–Raphson scheme to find the MLE for α and λ, which are estimated to be $\widehat{\alpha} = 3.9853$ and $\widehat{\lambda} = 0.0696$.

```julia
using StatsBase, SpecialFunctions
x = [
29.7679, 12.8406, 105.3225, 46.6101, 75.7135, 72.0340,
64.1004, 33.9008, 35.2510,  50.9201, 29.8086, 32.6963,
131.5229, 65.3381, 29.1369, 61.8774, 31.0650, 54.4877,
103.6889, 68.0230, 89.6879, 30.1994, 48.3140, 54.4447,
29.2253, 27.0242, 102.5929, 63.7344, 43.0354, 96.5552];
n = length(x);
sumlogx = sum(log.(x)); sumx = sum(x);
alpt = mean(x)^2/var(x); lamt = mean(x)/var(x); # intl. guess
thetat = [alpt, lamt]
for i=1:5 # just repeat the NR step 5 times
  global lamt, alpt, thetat
    S = [ n*(log(lamt) - digamma(alpt)) + sumlogx; n*alpt/lamt
        - sumx ];
    I = n * [trigamma(alpt) -1/lamt; -1/lamt alpt/lamt^2 ];
    thetat = thetat + inv(I)*S # using inv is OK (dim =2)
    alpt = thetat[1]; lamt = thetat[2];
end
print(thetat)
```

```
[3.9853256640599644, 0.06955520473406741]
```

Selected Problems of Chap. 7

7.1

(a) The distribution of T does not depend on σ.
(b) Define $Y_i = X_i/\sigma$ for $i = 1,\ldots,n$. Then $Y_1,\ldots,Y_n \sim_{\text{iid}} \mathcal{N}(0,1)$ under H_0, and $T = \sqrt{n}\overline{X}/S_X = \sqrt{n}\overline{Y}/S_Y$, which is exactly of the form (5.17). ☞ 13
The true p-value is therefore 0.0197 (using `cdf(TDist(3),-3.5)` and the `Distributions` package in Julia).
(c) The following code uses vectorization and is much faster.

```julia
using StatsBase
# @time begin  # uncomment begin ... end for timing
xbar_obs = -0.7; s_obs = 0.4; t_obs = 2*xbar_obs/s_obs;
N = 10^5;
```

```julia
x = randn(4,N);
xbar = mean(x,dims=1);
s = std(x,dims=1);
t = 2*xbar./s;
count = sum(t .<= t_obs);
phat = count/N # estimated p-value
# end
```

7.3 X takes values $x_1,\ldots,x_N$ with probability $1/N$, so the expectation is $\mathbb{E}X = x_1/N + x_2/N + \cdots + x_N/N = \overline{x}$, and the second moment is $\mathbb{E}X^2 = N^{-1}\sum_{i=1}^{N} x_i^2$. The variance is therefore $\mathrm{Var}(X) = \mathbb{E}X^2 - (\mathbb{E}X)^2 = N^{-1}\sum_{i=1}^{N} x_i^2 - \overline{x}^2 = N^{-1}\sum_{i=1}^{N}(x_i - \overline{x})^2$.

7.4

(a) By the product rule, the joint pdf of X and J is given by $f_{X,J}(x,j) = f_J(j)f_{X|J}(x\,|\,j) = w_j f_j(x)$ and the marginal pdf of X is found as $f(x) = \sum_{j=1}^{k} f_{X,J}(x,j) = \sum_{j=1}^{k} w_j f_j(x)$.

(b) First, draw $J \in \{1,\ldots,k\}$ with probabilities $w_1,\ldots,w_k$. Then, given $J = j$, draw X from the pdf f_j.

(c) $\mathbb{E}X = \sum_{j=1}^{k} w_j \mu_j$ and $\mathrm{Var}(X) = \sum_{j=1}^{k} w_j(\sigma_j^2 + \mu_j^2) - (\sum_{j=1}^{k} w_j \mu_j)^2$.

7.8

(a) Solving $\mathbb{P}(X \geq m) = \mathrm{e}^{-\lambda m} = 1/2$ gives $m = \ln(2)/\lambda$.

(b) The sample median is $\widetilde{x} = 1.4073$. Hence, the estimate is $\widetilde{\lambda} = \ln(2)/\widetilde{x} = 0.4925$. The maximum likelihood estimate is $1/\overline{x} = 0.2773$.

(c) The following code produces Fig. 13.4. The pdf of the "median" estimator (solid line) is bimodal and much more spread out than the pdf of the maximum likelihood estimator. Because the resampled data is discrete, the automatic bandwidth selection in **kde** will produce highly spiked KDEs, unless the **res=true** flag is set.

```julia
include("ThetaKDE.jl")
using .ThetaKDE, Plots, StatsBase
xorg = [1.4066, 1.2917, 1.408, 4.2801, 1.2136, 2.7461,
11.1076, 0.9247, 5.8833, 10.2513, 3.8285, 3.2116,
0.5451, 0.9896, 1.1602, 7.7723, 0.1702, 0.8907,
0.2276,3.1197, 11.4909,0.6475, 11.2279, 0.7639]
n = length(xorg);
est1org = log(2)/median(xorg)
est2org = 1/mean(xorg)
K= 10000;
est1 = zeros(K); est2 = zeros(K);
```

```
for i=1:K
    ind = ceil.(Int64,n*rand(n)); # draw random indices
    x = xorg[ind]; # resampled data
    est1[i] =log(2)/median(x);
    est2[i] =1/mean(x);
end
kde(est1,plt=true,res=true)
xmesh,density,bw = kde(est2,res=true)
plot!(xmesh,density)
```

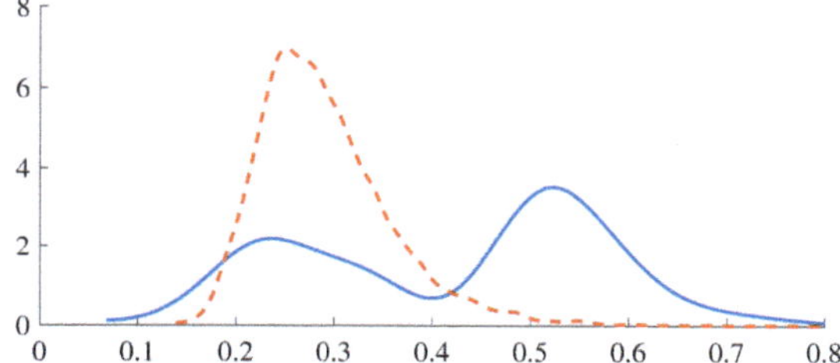

Fig. 13.4 KDEs for the pdfs of $\ln(2)/\widetilde{X}$ (solid line) and $1/\overline{X}$ (dashed line)

7.11 All the $x_1, \dots, x_n$ are smaller than θ, and so are the $M_i^*, k = i, \dots, K$. Hence, θ is not contained in any $1 - \alpha$ bootstrap confidence interval.

7.13

(a) With positive probability, it is possible to reach each state from another state, in at most four steps. So the chain is irreducible. However, to return to a starting state, it always requires a multiple of two steps. Hence, the chain is periodic with period 2.

(b) The local balance equations hold, because the system is reversible. By symmetry $f(1) = f(2) = f(5) = f(6)$ and $f(3) = f(4)$. By local balance, $f(1)/2 = f(3)/3$. Hence, $4f(1) + 3f(1) = 1$, so that $f(1) = 1/7$ and $f(3) = 3/14$.

(c) For example, for odd t the probability $\mathbb{P}(X_t = 1) = 0$, because, starting from 1 at time 0, it requires an even number of steps to return to 1. On the other hand, the probability $\mathbb{P}(X_{2t} = 1)$ converges to $2/7$ as $t \to \infty$. Hence, the sequence $\mathbb{P}(X_t = 1), t = 0, 1, 2, \dots$ does not converge. In this case the *stationary* probability is not equal to the *limiting* probability.

7.16 $Z = -\ln U_1$ has an $\mathsf{Exp}(1)$ distribution, by the inverse-transform method and $R = 2\mathbb{1}_{\{U_2 \leq 1/2\}} - 1$ takes values -1 and 1 with equal probability. Hence, X is obtained by first generating Z and then flipping its sign with probability $1/2$. The cdf of X is therefore given by

$$\mathbb{P}(X \le x) = \begin{cases} 1 - \mathbb{P}(X > x) = 1 - \mathbb{P}(Z > x)/2 = 1 - \mathrm{e}^{-x}/2 & \text{for } x \ge 0 \\ \mathbb{P}(Z > -x)/2 = \mathrm{e}^{x}/2 & \text{for } x \le 0 \,. \end{cases}$$

By differentiating the cdf, we obtain the pdf $g(x) = \mathrm{e}^{-|x|}/2$ for all x.

Selected Problems of Chap. 8

8.2

(a) The posterior pdf is given by $f(\lambda \,|\, \boldsymbol{x}) \propto f(\lambda) \times f(\boldsymbol{x} \,|\, \lambda) = (1/\lambda) \times \lambda^5 \exp(-\lambda \sum_{i=1}^{5} x_i)$. This is the pdf of the $\mathsf{Gamma}(5, \sum_{i=1}^{5} x_i)$ distribution, where $\sum_{i=1}^{5} x_i = 15.7487$.

(b) The expectation is $5/\sum_{i=1}^{5} x_i = 0.317487$.

8.3 The posterior pdf is $f(\lambda \,|\, x) \propto f(\lambda) \times f(x \,|\, \lambda) \propto \lambda^{a-1} \exp(-b\lambda) \times \lambda^x \exp(-\lambda) = \lambda^{a+x-1} \exp(-\lambda(1+b))$. This is the pdf of the $\mathsf{Gamma}(a+x, b+1)$ distribution.

8.6 Let $Y_1, \ldots, Y_{m+1}$ with $Y_i \sim \mathsf{Gamma}(\alpha_i, 1), i = 1, \ldots, m+1$ be independent random variables. By Theorem 8.2, $Z_i = Y_i/(Y_i + Y)$, with $Y = \sum_{j \ne i} Y_j$, has the same distribution as the i-th coordinate of $\boldsymbol{Z} = (Z_1, \ldots, Z_m) \sim \mathsf{Dirichlet}(\alpha_1, \ldots, \alpha_{m+1})$. Moreover, Y_i and Y are independent, and $Y \sim \mathsf{Gamma}(\sum_{j \ne i} \alpha_j, 1)$, because its moment generating function is $(1/(1-s))^{\sum_{j \ne i} \alpha_j}$. Hence, again by Theorem 8.2, $Z_i \sim \mathsf{Dirichlet}(\alpha_i, \sum_{j \ne i} \alpha_j)$.

☞ 247

8.7

(a) The prior pdf is $f(p \,|\, x) \propto f(x \,|\, p) = p(1-p)^{x-1}$, which is a $\mathsf{Beta}(2, x)$ distribution.

(b) The posterior mode is $1/x$; see Problem 8.6.

(c) The posterior expectation is $2/(2+x)$; see Problem 8.6.

8.13 We have $f(x_{i+1} \,|\, x_i) = f(x_i, x_{i+1})/f(x_i) = f(x_i \,|\, x_{i+1})f(x_{i+1})/f(x_i)$. Hence,

$$f(x_1, \ldots, x_n) = f(x_1)f(x_2 \,|\, x_1) \cdots f(x_n \,|\, x_{n-1})$$
$$= f(x_1)f(x_1 \,|\, x_2)\frac{f(x_2)}{f(x_1)} f(x_2 \,|\, x_3)\frac{f(x_3)}{f(x_2)} \cdots f(x_{n-1} \,|\, x_n)\frac{f(x_n)}{f(x_{n-1})}$$
$$= f(x_n)f(x_{n-1} \,|\, x_n) \cdots f(x_1 \,|\, x_2) \,.$$

8.14

☞ 16

(a) By the law of total probability $f(x_t, \boldsymbol{y}_{1:t}) = \sum_{x_{t-1}} f(x_t, x_{t-1}, y_t, \boldsymbol{y}_{1:t-1})$. Conditioning $f(x_t, x_{t-1}, y_t, \boldsymbol{y}_{1:t-1})$ on x_{t-1} and $\boldsymbol{y}_{1:t-1}$ gives $f(x_t, \boldsymbol{y}_{1:t}) = \sum_{x_{t-1}} f(x_t, y_t \,|\, x_{t-1}, \boldsymbol{y}_{1:t-1})f(x_{t-1}, \boldsymbol{y}_{1:t-1})$.

(b) $f(x_t, y_t \,|\, x_{t-1}, \boldsymbol{y}_{1:t-1}) = f(x_t \,|\, x_{t-1}, \boldsymbol{y}_{1:t-1}) f(y_t \,|\, x_t, x_{t-1}, \boldsymbol{y}_{1:t-1})$. Because of the structure of the Bayesian network, x_t given x_{t-1} is independent of $\boldsymbol{y}_{1:t-1}$, and y_t given x_t is independent of x_{t-1} and $\boldsymbol{y}_{1:t-1}$. Hence, $f(x_t \,|\, x_{t-1}, \boldsymbol{y}_{1:t-1}) = f(x_t \,|\, x_{t-1})$ and $f(y_t \,|\, x_t, x_{t-1}, \boldsymbol{y}_{1:t-1}) = f(y_t \,|\, x_t)$.

(c) $f(x_1, y_1) = f(y_1 \,|\, x_1) f(x_1)$, where both $f(x_1)$ and $f(y_1 \,|\, x_1)$ are known. Hence, $f(x_1, y_1)$ can be evaluated. Next, $f(x_2 \,|\, y_1, y_2)$ can be evaluated via (8.32) because both factors in the sum are known. The first one is known via (8.33) and the second as part of the recursion for $t = 1$. Repeating this, we see that $f(x_t, \boldsymbol{y}_{1:t})$ can be evaluated for any t. The posterior pdf $f(x_t \,|\, \boldsymbol{y}_{1:t}) \propto f(x_t, \boldsymbol{y}_{1:t})$ follows simply by normalization.

8.18

(a) The Bayesian network is given in Fig. 13.5.

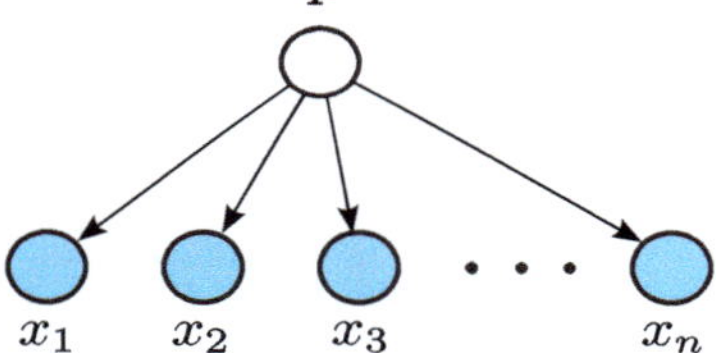

Fig. 13.5 The Bayesian network for the bag-of-words model

(b) The posterior pdf is

$$f(p \,|\, \boldsymbol{x}) \propto \exp\left(-\frac{1}{2} \sum_{i=1}^{n} \frac{(x_i - \mu_{pi})^2}{\sigma^2}\right) = \exp\left(-\frac{1}{2} \frac{\|\boldsymbol{x} - \boldsymbol{\mu}_p\|^2}{\sigma^2}\right).$$

This is maximal when $\|\boldsymbol{x} - \boldsymbol{\mu}_p\|$ is minimal. Thus p^* maximizes the posterior pdf.

(c) The posterior pdf is

$$f(p \,|\, \boldsymbol{x}) \propto (\sigma_{p1} \cdots \sigma_{pn})^{-1} \exp\left(-\frac{1}{2} \sum_{i=1}^{n} \frac{(x_i - \mu_{pi})^2}{\sigma_{pi}^2}\right).$$

The (unscaled) values for $f(p), p = 1, \ldots, 4$ are 53, 0.24, 8.36, and 3.5×10^{-6}. Hence the object should be classified as 1. The following code was used.

```
x = [1.67,2,4.23]
mu = [1.6 2.4 4.3; 1.5 2.9 6.1;
      1.8 2.5 4.2; 1.1 3.1 5.6];
sig = [0.1 0.5 0.2; 0.2 0.6 0.9;
       0.3 0.3 0.3; 0.2 0.7 0.3];
```

```
f(p) = prod(sig[p,:]).^(-1) .*
       exp(-0.5*sum((x-mu[p,:]).^2 ./ sig[p,:].^2));
f(1), f(2), f(3), f(4)
```

Selected Problems of Chap. 9

9.1 We use the fact that if $Z \sim \mathsf{InvGamma}(a,b)$, then $\mathbb{E}Z = b/(a-1)$ for $a > 1$. We know that $\{X_i\} \sim_{\text{iid}} \mathcal{N}(\alpha, 1 + \tau^2)$. From Theorem 5.1, it follows that

$$Z = \frac{\sum_{i=1}^{N}(X_i - \overline{X})^2}{1 + \tau^2} \sim \chi^2_{N-1} = \mathsf{Gamma}(a,b),$$

with $a = (N-1)/2$ and $b = 1/2$, so that $\mathbb{E}[1/Z] = b/(a-1) = 1/(N-3)$ for $N > 3$. Consequently,

$$\mathbb{E}\left[1 - \frac{N-3}{\sum_{i=1}^{N}(X_i - \overline{X})^2}\right] = 1 - \frac{1}{1+\tau^2} = \tau^2/(\tau^2 + 1) = \sigma^2.$$

Selected Problems of Chap. 10

10.4 We are interested in the pdf of $\Phi(\boldsymbol{x}^\top \boldsymbol{\beta})$, where $\boldsymbol{\beta}$ is distributed according to the posterior pdf and $\boldsymbol{x}^\top = [1, 1, 10, 1, 0, 16, 1]$. The following Julia script uses the posterior draws for $\boldsymbol{\beta}$ (stored in **store_beta**) to draw from the corresponding posterior pdf.

```
N = size(store_beta)[1];
store_prob = zeros(N);
x = [1 1 10 1 0 16 1];
for loop=1:N
store_prob[loop] = cdf.(Normal(0,1),x*store_beta[loop,:])[1]
end
include("ThetaKDE.jl")
using .ThetaKDE
kde(store_prob,plt=true)
```

The expected value of the posterior probability is estimated to be 0.324. A KDE of the posterior probability is plotted in Fig. 13.6.

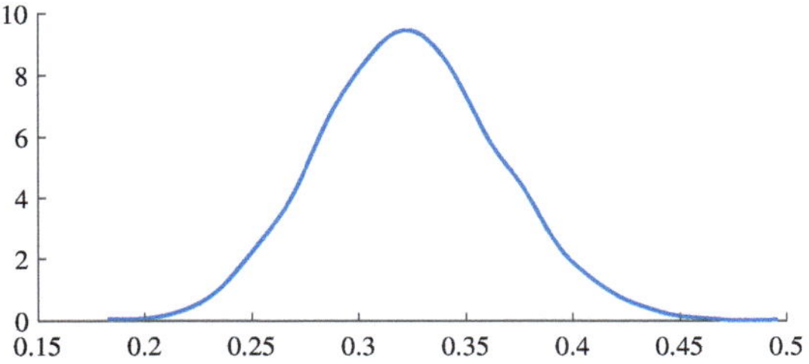

Fig. 13.6 A KDE of the posterior probability that a subject with certain characteristics will have an extramarital affair

10.6 (c) $1/(\nu - 2)$.

10.8 First recall that $Q_t(\boldsymbol{\beta}) = -\frac{1}{2}\sum_{i=1}^{n}\left\{(\boldsymbol{x}_i^\top\boldsymbol{\beta})^2 - 2\,v_i\,\boldsymbol{x}_i^\top\boldsymbol{\beta}\right\} + \text{const}$. Noting that $(\boldsymbol{x}_i^\top\boldsymbol{\beta})^2 = \boldsymbol{\beta}^\top\boldsymbol{x}_i\boldsymbol{x}_i^\top\boldsymbol{\beta}$ and using the formulas for multivariate differentiation in Appendix B.1, we have

$$\nabla Q_t(\boldsymbol{\beta}) = -\frac{1}{2}\sum_{i=1}^{n}\left(2\boldsymbol{x}_i\boldsymbol{x}_i^\top\boldsymbol{\beta} - 2\,v_i\,\boldsymbol{x}_i\right).$$

Now solve $\nabla Q_t(\boldsymbol{\beta}) = \boldsymbol{0}$ for $\boldsymbol{\beta}$ to find $\sum_{i=1}^{n}\boldsymbol{x}_i\boldsymbol{x}_i^\top\boldsymbol{\beta} = \sum_{i=1}^{n}v_i\,\boldsymbol{x}_i$.

Selected Problems of Chap. 11

11.3 Note that $T^+ + T^- = n(n+1)/2$ (the sum of all ranks). Hence,

$$T = 2T^+ - n(n+1)/2.$$

It follows then from (11.10), that $\mathbb{E}T = 2\mathbb{E}T^+ - n(n+1)/2 = 0$ and $\mathrm{Var}(T) = 4\mathrm{Var}(T^+) = n(n+1)(2n+1)/6$.

11.6 The characteristic function ψ of a $\mathcal{U}[-1,1]$ random variable is real-valued, as the distribution is symmetric around 0. Hence, for $r \neq 0$:

$$\psi(r) = \int_{-1}^{1}\frac{1}{2}\cos(rx)\,\mathrm{d}x = \frac{\sin(x)}{x}$$

and for $r = 0$, $\psi(r) = 1$, trivially. Since $\psi(r) = \mathrm{sinc}(r)$, it follows from Theorem 11.1. that $\kappa(x, x') = \mathrm{sinc}(x - x')$ is a valid kernel.

11.10 Take an arbitrary collection $\{\boldsymbol{x}_i\}_{i=1}^{n}$ from $\mathcal{X}$ and real numbers $\{\alpha_i\}_{i=1}^{n}$. Then,

$$\sum_{i=1}^{n}\sum_{j=1}^{n}\alpha_i\,\kappa(\boldsymbol{x}_i,\boldsymbol{x}_j)\,\alpha_j = \sum_{i=1}^{n}\sum_{j=1}^{n}\alpha_i\left[\kappa_1(\boldsymbol{x}_i,\boldsymbol{x}_j)+\kappa_2(\boldsymbol{x}_i,\boldsymbol{x}_j)\right]\alpha_j$$

$$= \sum_{i=1}^{n}\sum_{j=1}^{n}\alpha_i\,\kappa_1(\boldsymbol{x}_i,\boldsymbol{x}_j)\,\alpha_j + \sum_{i=1}^{n}\sum_{j=1}^{n}\alpha_i\,\kappa_2(\boldsymbol{x}_i,\boldsymbol{x}_j)\,\alpha_j \geq 0,$$

because κ_1 and κ_2 are kernel functions on $\mathcal{X}$. Symmetry and finiteness follow directly from those properties of κ_1 and κ_2.

11.14 We apply Theorem 8.1 with $\boldsymbol{g}$ taking the role of $\boldsymbol{\beta}$, $\boldsymbol{\Sigma}_0 = \mathbf{K}$, $\boldsymbol{\beta}_0 = \mathbf{0}$, and $\mathbf{X} = \mathbb{I}_n$. Thus, $(\boldsymbol{g}\,|\,\sigma^2,\boldsymbol{y}) \sim \mathcal{N}(\boldsymbol{\mu},\mathbf{D})$, with

$$\mathbf{D} = (\sigma^{-2}\,\mathbb{I}_n + \mathbf{K}^{-1})^{-1}$$

and

$$\boldsymbol{\mu} = \mathbf{D}\boldsymbol{y}/\sigma^2.$$

To verify that the mean vector and covariance matrix are indeed of the form (11.30), we can use the matrix identity (11.38), which gives

$$\mathbf{D} = \sigma^2\,\mathbf{K}\,(\mathbf{K}+\sigma^2\,\mathbb{I}_n)^{-1} = \sigma^2(\mathbf{K}+\sigma^2\,\mathbb{I})^{-1}\,\mathbf{K},$$

so that indeed

$$\boldsymbol{\mu} = \mathbf{K}\,(\mathbf{K}+\sigma^2\,\mathbb{I}_n)^{-1}\boldsymbol{y}.$$

Moreover, the following shows that $\mathbf{D} = \mathbf{K} - \mathbf{K}(\mathbf{K}+\sigma^2\,\mathbb{I}_n)^{-1}\mathbf{K}$:

$$(\mathbf{K} - \mathbf{K}(\mathbf{K}+\sigma^2\,\mathbb{I}_n)^{-1}\mathbf{K})\,\mathbf{D}^{-1}$$
$$= (\mathbf{K} - \mathbf{K}(\mathbf{K}+\sigma^2\,\mathbb{I}_n)^{-1}\mathbf{K})\,\mathbf{K}^{-1}(\mathbf{K}+\sigma^2\,\mathbb{I}_n)\,\sigma^{-2}$$
$$= \sigma^{-2}\,\mathbf{K} + \mathbb{I}_n - \sigma^{-2}\,\mathbf{K} = \mathbb{I}_n.$$

Selected Problems of Chap. 12

12.1 The lag-1, 2, and 3 autocorrelations are, respectively, 0.830, 0.618, and 0.448.

12.3 Let $\boldsymbol{\varepsilon} = [\varepsilon_{1-q},\ldots,\varepsilon_T]^{\top}$ be the vector of error terms, and let $\boldsymbol{\psi} = [\psi_1,\ldots,\psi_q]^{\top}$ denote the vector of MA coefficients. Then we can write the MA(q) model as

$$\boldsymbol{Y} = \mathbf{H}\boldsymbol{\varepsilon}\,.$$

where $\mathbf{H}$ is a $T \times (T+q)$ **circulant** matrix, where each row vector is rotated one element to the right relative to the previous row vector. In particular, the first row is $[\psi_q, \psi_{q-1},\ldots,\psi_1,0,\ldots,0]$. Since $\boldsymbol{\varepsilon} \sim \mathcal{N}(\mathbf{0},\sigma^2\,\mathbb{I}_{T+q})$, the log-likelihood function is given by

$$l(\psi, \sigma^2; \boldsymbol{y}) = -\frac{T}{2}\ln(2\pi\sigma^2) - \frac{1}{2}|\mathbf{HH}^\top| - \frac{1}{2\sigma^2}\boldsymbol{y}^\top(\mathbf{HH}^\top)^{-1}\boldsymbol{y}\ .$$

12.7 (a) To derive the full conditional distribution, we first write the ARMA(1,1) as

$$\boldsymbol{y} = \mathbf{X}\boldsymbol{\varrho} + \mathbf{H}\boldsymbol{\varepsilon}\ ,$$

where $\boldsymbol{\varepsilon} = [\varepsilon_1, \ldots, \varepsilon_T]^\top \sim \mathcal{N}(\mathbf{0}, \sigma^2\,\mathbb{I}_T)$, $\boldsymbol{\varrho} = [\varrho_0, \varrho_1]^\top$,

$$\mathbf{X} = \begin{bmatrix} 1 & y_0 \\ 1 & y_1 \\ \vdots & \vdots \\ 1 & y_{T-1} \end{bmatrix}, \qquad \mathbf{H} = \begin{bmatrix} 1 & 0 & 0 & \cdots & 0 \\ \psi & 1 & 0 & \cdots & 0 \\ 0 & \psi & 1 & \cdots & 0 \\ \vdots & & & \ddots & \vdots \\ 0 & 0 & \cdots & \psi & 1 \end{bmatrix}.$$

The likelihood function is given by

$$f(\boldsymbol{y} \mid \boldsymbol{\varrho}, \psi, \sigma^2) = (2\pi\sigma^2)^{-\frac{T}{2}} e^{-\frac{1}{2\sigma^2}(\boldsymbol{y}-\mathbf{X}\boldsymbol{\varrho})^\top(\mathbf{HH}^\top)^{-1}(\boldsymbol{y}-\mathbf{X}\boldsymbol{\varrho})}\ .$$

Since this has the form of a linear regression model with covariance matrix $\sigma^2\mathbf{HH}^\top$, it follows from Corollary 8.1 that ☞ 24

$$(\boldsymbol{\varrho} \mid \boldsymbol{y}, \psi, \sigma^2) \sim \mathcal{N}(\widehat{\boldsymbol{\varrho}}, \mathbf{D}_{\boldsymbol{\varrho}})\ ,$$

where

$$\mathbf{D}_{\boldsymbol{\varrho}} = \left(\frac{1}{10}I + \frac{1}{\sigma^2}\mathbf{X}^\top(\mathbf{HH}^\top)^{-1}\mathbf{X}\right)^{-1}, \qquad \widehat{\boldsymbol{\varrho}} = \mathbf{D}_{\boldsymbol{\varrho}}\left(\frac{1}{\sigma^2}\mathbf{X}^\top(\mathbf{HH}^\top)^{-1}\boldsymbol{y}\right).$$

Next, using the likelihood function given above, it can be easily checked that

$$(\sigma^2 \mid \boldsymbol{y}, \boldsymbol{\varrho}, \psi) \sim \mathsf{InvGamma}\left(3 + \frac{T}{2}, \lambda\right),$$

where $\lambda = 1 + (\boldsymbol{y} - \mathbf{X}\boldsymbol{\varrho})^\top(\mathbf{HH}^\top)^{-1}(\boldsymbol{y} - \mathbf{X}\boldsymbol{\varrho})/2$.

Lastly, given the uniform prior $\psi \sim \mathcal{U}[-1, 1]$, the full conditional posterior distribution for ψ is simply

$$f(\psi \mid \boldsymbol{y}, \boldsymbol{\varrho}, \sigma^2) \propto f(\boldsymbol{y}, \boldsymbol{\varrho}, \psi, \sigma^2) \propto e^{-\frac{1}{2\sigma^2}(\boldsymbol{y}-\mathbf{X}\boldsymbol{\varrho})^\top(\mathbf{HH}^\top)^{-1}(\boldsymbol{y}-\mathbf{X}\boldsymbol{\varrho})}$$

for $-1 < \psi < 1$ and 0 otherwise.

12.9 We first write the two-factor mixed model in matrix form. To that end, let

$$\boldsymbol{Y} = [Y_{111}, Y_{112}, Y_{113}, Y_{121}, Y_{122}, Y_{123}, \ldots, Y_{3,10,1}, Y_{3,10,2}, Y_{3,10,3}]^\top,$$

and define $\boldsymbol{\varepsilon}$ accordingly. Also, stack $\boldsymbol{\alpha} = [\alpha_1, \alpha_2, \alpha_3]^\top$, $\boldsymbol{\beta} = [\beta_1, \ldots, \beta_{10}]^\top$, and $\boldsymbol{\gamma} = [\gamma_{11}, \gamma_{12}, \ldots, \gamma_{39}, \gamma_{3,10}]^\top$. Then,

$$\boldsymbol{Y} = \mu \mathbf{1}_{90} + \mathbf{X}_{\boldsymbol{\alpha}}\boldsymbol{\alpha} + \mathbf{X}_{\boldsymbol{\beta}}\boldsymbol{\beta} + \mathbf{X}_{\boldsymbol{\gamma}}\boldsymbol{\gamma} + \boldsymbol{\varepsilon} \, ,$$

where $\mathbf{X}_{\boldsymbol{\alpha}} = \mathbb{I}_3 \otimes \mathbf{1}_{30}$, $\mathbf{X}_{\boldsymbol{\beta}} = \mathbf{1}_3 \otimes \mathbf{A}$, $\mathbf{A} = \mathbb{I}_{10} \otimes \mathbf{1}_3$, $\mathbf{X}_{\boldsymbol{\gamma}} = \mathbb{I}_{30} \otimes \mathbf{1}_3$, $\otimes$ is the Kronecker product, $\mathbf{1}_p$ is a $p \times 1$ vector of ones, and $\mathbb{I}_q$ is the q-dimensional identity matrix.

Since $\boldsymbol{Y}$ is an affine transformation of normal random variables, it has a normal distribution. Its expected value is $\mathbb{E}\boldsymbol{Y} = \mu \mathbf{1}_{90}$, and its covariance matrix is given by

$$\boldsymbol{\Sigma} = \sigma_{\boldsymbol{\alpha}}^2 \mathbf{X}_{\boldsymbol{\alpha}}\mathbf{X}_{\boldsymbol{\alpha}}^\top + \sigma_{\boldsymbol{\beta}}^2 \mathbf{X}_{\boldsymbol{\beta}}\mathbf{X}_{\boldsymbol{\beta}}^\top + \sigma_{\boldsymbol{\gamma}}^2 \mathbf{X}_{\boldsymbol{\gamma}}\mathbf{X}_{\boldsymbol{\gamma}}^\top + \sigma^2 \mathbb{I}_{90} \, .$$

12.11 In deriving the full conditional distributions, we will repeatedly make use Theorem 8.1. First, the one-factor random effects model can be written as

$$\boldsymbol{Y}_i = \mu_i \mathbf{1}_{n_i} + \boldsymbol{\varepsilon}_i \, ,$$

where $\boldsymbol{\varepsilon}_i = [\varepsilon_1, \ldots, \varepsilon_{n_i}]^\top \sim_{\text{ind}} \mathcal{N}(\mathbf{0}, \sigma^2 \mathbb{I}_{n_i})$. From this and the assumption $\{\mu_i\} \sim_{\text{iid}} \mathcal{N}(\mu, \sigma_\mu^2)$, the random effects $\mu_1, \ldots, \mu_d$ are conditionally independent given $\boldsymbol{y}$, μ, σ_μ^2, and σ^2. In fact, using Theorem 8.1, we have

$$(\mu_i \,|\, \boldsymbol{y}, \mu, \sigma_\mu^2, \sigma^2) \stackrel{\text{ind}}{\sim} \mathcal{N}(\widehat{\mu}_i, D_{\mu_i}) \, ,$$

where $D_{\mu_i} = (1/\sigma_\mu^2 + n_i/\sigma^2)^{-1}$ and $\widehat{\mu}_i = D_{\mu_i}(\mu/\sigma_\mu^2 + \mathbf{1}_{n_i}^\top \boldsymbol{y}_i/\sigma^2)$.

Next, to derive $f(\mu \,|\, \boldsymbol{y}, \boldsymbol{\mu}, \sigma_\mu^2, \sigma^2)$, the relevant distributions are the prior for μ and $\{\mu_i\} \sim_{\text{iid}} \mathcal{N}(\mu, \sigma_\mu^2)$. It is then clear that given $\boldsymbol{\mu}$ and σ_μ^2, μ is conditionally independent of $\boldsymbol{y}$ and σ^2. Again, using Theorem 8.1,

$$(\mu \,|\, \boldsymbol{\mu}, \sigma_\mu^2) \sim \mathcal{N}(\widehat{\mu}, D_\mu) \, ,$$

where $D_\mu = (1/V_\mu + d/\sigma_\mu^2)^{-1}$ and $\widehat{\mu} = D_\mu(\mu_0/V_\mu + \sum_{i=1}^d \mu_i/\sigma_\mu^2)$.

Similarly, σ_μ^2 is conditionally independent of $\boldsymbol{y}$ and σ^2 given $\boldsymbol{\mu}$ and μ. In fact, using Theorem 8.1, we have

$$(\sigma_\mu^2 \,|\, \boldsymbol{\mu}, \mu) \sim \mathsf{InvGamma}\left(\alpha_\mu + \frac{d}{2}, \lambda_\mu + \frac{\sum_{i=1}^d (\mu_i - \mu)^2}{2}\right) \, .$$

Finally, following a similar reasoning,

$$(\sigma^2 \,|\, \boldsymbol{y}, \boldsymbol{\mu}) \sim \mathsf{InvGamma}\left(\alpha + \frac{n}{2}, \lambda + \frac{\sum_{i=1}^d (\boldsymbol{y}_i - \mu_i \mathbf{1}_{n_i})^\top (\boldsymbol{y}_i - \mu_i \mathbf{1}_{n_i})}{2}\right) \, .$$

Selected Problems of Chap. 13

13.3 Recall that the log-density $\ln f(\boldsymbol{y} \mid \boldsymbol{\tau}, \sigma^2)$ is given by

$$\ln f(\boldsymbol{y} \mid \boldsymbol{\tau}, \sigma^2) = -\frac{T}{2} \ln(2\pi\sigma^2) - \frac{1}{2\sigma^2}(\boldsymbol{y} - \boldsymbol{\tau})^\top (\boldsymbol{y} - \boldsymbol{\tau}) \,.$$

Hence, setting $\boldsymbol{\tau} = \boldsymbol{y}$, we obtain $\ln f(\boldsymbol{y} \mid \boldsymbol{\tau} = \boldsymbol{y}, \sigma^2) = -\frac{T}{2}\ln(2\pi\sigma^2)$, which approaches infinity as σ^2 approaches 0.

13.4 By recursive substitution using the transition equation, we have $\tau_t = \tau_1 + \sum_{s=2}^{t} u_s$. Hence,

$$\mathrm{Var}(\tau_t \mid \tau_1) = \mathrm{Var}\left(\sum_{s=2}^{t} u_s\right) = \sum_{s=2}^{t} \mathrm{Var}(u_s) = (t-1)\omega^2 \,.$$

13.5 We first write a Julia function to evaluate the log-likelihood function via

$$l(\sigma^2; \boldsymbol{y}) = \ln f(\boldsymbol{y} \mid \boldsymbol{\tau}, \sigma^2) + \ln f(\boldsymbol{\tau} \mid \omega^2) - \ln f(\boldsymbol{\tau} \mid \boldsymbol{y}, \sigma^2, \omega^2) \,.$$

Since the equality holds for any $\boldsymbol{\tau}$, we choose $\boldsymbol{\tau} = \boldsymbol{0}$ to reduce the number of computations involved.

```julia
function loglike_UC(sigma2,omega2,omega2_0,y)
    T = length(y)
    H = sparse(I,T,T) - sparse(2:T,1:(T-1),ones(T-1),T,T)
    invOmega = sparse(1:T,1:T, vec([1/omega2_0 1/omega2*ones(1,
        T-1)]),T,T)
    HinvOmegaH = H'*invOmega*H
    K = HinvOmegaH + sparse(I,T,T)/sigma2
    tauhat = K\y/sigma2
    C = cholesky(Matrix(K)).L # not sparse, so C is triangular
    logfy = -T/2*log(2*pi*sigma2) - only(.5/sigma2*(y'*y))
    logftau_pri = -T/2*log(2*pi) - .5*log(omega2_0) - (T-1)/2*
        log(omega2)
    logftau_post = -T/2*log(2*pi) + sum(log.(diag(C))) - only
        (.5*tauhat'*K*tauhat)
    return  logfy + logftau_pri - logftau_post;
end
```

Note that evaluating the log-density $\ln f(\boldsymbol{\tau} \mid \boldsymbol{y}, \sigma^2, \omega^2)$ involves the term $-\frac{1}{2}\ln|\mathbf{K}^{-1}|$, where $\mathbf{K} = \mathbf{H}\boldsymbol{\Omega}^{-1}\mathbf{H} + \mathbb{I}_T/\sigma^2$. To speed up computation, we use the fact that if $\mathbf{C}$ is the Cholesky factor of $\mathbf{K}$ such that $\mathbf{K} = \mathbf{C}\mathbf{C}^\top$, then

$$-\frac{1}{2}\ln|\mathbf{K}^{-1}| = \frac{1}{2}\ln|\mathbf{K}| = \ln|\mathbf{C}| = \sum_{i}\ln c_{ii}\,,$$

where c_{ii} is the i-th diagonal element of $\mathbf{C}$. The last equality holds because $\mathbf{C}$ is lower triangular.

Next, in the main script, we build a grid, and use the function `loglike_UC` to evaluate the log-likelihood function at every point on the grid. A plot of $l(\sigma^2; \boldsymbol{y})$ is given in Fig. 13.7. The maximum likelihood estimate of σ^2 computed using this grid search is about 4.401, compared to the value 4.405 obtained by the numerical maximization.

Q11_8.jl

```julia
using SparseArrays, LinearAlgebra, Distributions
using StatsBase,Plots,DelimitedFiles
y = readdlm("USCPI.csv")
T = length(y)
omega2_0 = 9
# initial condition
omega2 = .5^2
# fix omega2
ngrid = 300
# # of grid points
sigma2grid = range(1,10,length=ngrid)
l = zeros(ngrid)
for i=1:ngrid
    l[i] = loglike_UC(sigma2grid[i],omega2,omega2_0,y);
end
plot(sigma2grid,l)
maxl, maxid = findmax(l)
sigma2hat = sigma2grid[maxid]
```

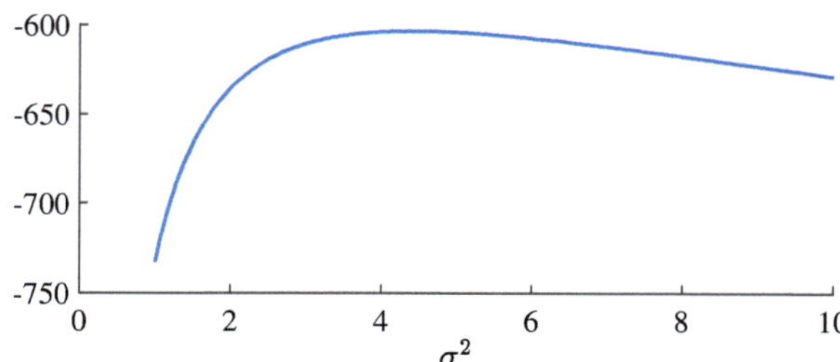

Fig. 13.7 The log-likelihood function $l(\sigma^2; \boldsymbol{y})$ under the unobserved components model

13.6

(a) First write the model in matrix form: $\mathbf{H}_\beta \mathbf{y} = \mathbf{H}_\beta \boldsymbol{\tau} + \tilde{\boldsymbol{\alpha}} + \boldsymbol{\varepsilon}$, where $\mathbf{y} = [y_1, \ldots, y_T]^\top$, $\boldsymbol{\varepsilon} = [\varepsilon_1, \ldots, \varepsilon_T]^\top$, $\tilde{\boldsymbol{\alpha}} = [\beta y_0, 0, \ldots, 0]^\top$, and

$$
\mathbf{H}_\beta = \begin{bmatrix} 1 & 0 & 0 & \cdots & 0 \\ -\beta & 1 & 0 & \cdots & 0 \\ 0 & -\beta & 1 & \cdots & 0 \\ \vdots & & & \ddots & \vdots \\ 0 & 0 & \cdots & -\beta & 1 \end{bmatrix} .
$$

Since the determinant of $\mathbf{H}_\beta$ is 1 for any β, $\mathbf{H}_\beta$ is invertible. Then, $\mathbf{y} = \boldsymbol{\tau} + \boldsymbol{\alpha} + \mathbf{H}_\beta^{-1}\boldsymbol{\varepsilon}$, where $\boldsymbol{\alpha} = \mathbf{H}_\beta^{-1}\tilde{\boldsymbol{\alpha}}$. In other words,

$$
(\mathbf{y} \mid y_0, \boldsymbol{\tau}, \beta, \sigma^2) \sim \mathcal{N}(\boldsymbol{\tau} + \boldsymbol{\alpha}, \sigma^2 (\mathbf{H}_\beta^\top \mathbf{H}_\beta)^{-1}) ,
$$

and the joint log-density of $\mathbf{y}$ is

$$
\ln f(\mathbf{y} \mid y_0, \boldsymbol{\tau}, \beta, \sigma^2) = -\frac{T}{2}\ln(2\pi\sigma^2)
$$
$$
- \frac{1}{2\sigma^2}(\mathbf{y} - \boldsymbol{\tau} - \boldsymbol{\alpha})^\top \mathbf{H}_\beta^\top \mathbf{H}_\beta (\mathbf{y} - \boldsymbol{\tau} - \boldsymbol{\alpha}) .
$$

(b) The derivation of $f(\boldsymbol{\tau} \mid \mathbf{y}, y_0, \beta, \sigma^2, \omega^2)$ follows closely the discussion in Sect. 13.1.2. More specifically, since the transition equation is exactly the same as before, we have ☞ 39

$$
\ln f(\boldsymbol{\tau} \mid \omega^2) = -\frac{T}{2}\ln(2\pi) - \frac{1}{2}\ln\omega_0^2 - \frac{T-1}{2}\ln\omega^2 - \frac{1}{2}\boldsymbol{\tau}^\top (\mathbf{H}^\top \boldsymbol{\Omega}^{-1} \mathbf{H})\boldsymbol{\tau} ,
$$

where $\mathbf{H}$ is the usual first difference matrix, $\boldsymbol{\Omega} = \operatorname{diag}(\omega_0^2, \omega^2, \ldots, \omega^2)$, and $\omega_0^2 = 5$. Then, using the expression for $\ln f(\mathbf{y} \mid y_0, \boldsymbol{\tau}, \beta, \sigma^2)$ given above, we "complete the squares" to obtain ☞ 24

$$
(\boldsymbol{\tau} \mid \mathbf{y}, y_0, \beta, \sigma^2, \omega^2) \sim \mathcal{N}(\hat{\boldsymbol{\tau}}, \mathbf{K}^{-1}) ,
$$

where $\mathbf{K} = \mathbf{H}^\top \boldsymbol{\Omega}^{-1} \mathbf{H} + \mathbf{H}_\beta^\top \mathbf{H}_\beta / \sigma^2$ and $\hat{\boldsymbol{\tau}} = \mathbf{K}^{-1}\mathbf{H}_\beta^\top \mathbf{H}_\beta (\mathbf{y} - \boldsymbol{\alpha})/\sigma^2$.

(c) For classical estimation, we can maximize the log-likelihood function numerically using the method of direct likelihood evaluation described in Problem 13.5. Since the number of parameters is only two (β and σ^2), this approach is computationally feasible.

For Bayesian estimation, if we assume conjugate priors for β and σ^2, we can implement a 3-block Gibbs sampler for posterior analysis. The full conditional distribution for $\boldsymbol{\tau}$ is normal as given above. The full conditional distributions for β and σ^2 are normal and inverse-gamma, respectively, which can be sampled from easily.

Appendix A
Julia Primer

The purpose of this appendix is to give the reader a basic introduction to the Julia programming language. Julia's style and syntax are similar to MATLAB, R, and Python. As such, Julia provides the same ease of use and flexibility of these *interpreted* languages. On the other hand, Julia is a *compiled* language, making it almost as fast as C and Fortran.

A.1 Getting Started

Julia can be installed from

$$https://julialang.org/.$$

Here you will find full documentation, examples, tools, and more.

Julia comes with an interactive command-line executable, called the REPL (read-eval-print-loop), which allows for a line-by-line evaluation of Julia statements. Simply click the Julia executable or type `julia` from a system command line. For example, entering the following statement in the REPL:

```julia
print("Hello World!")
```

produces the output:

```
Hello World!
```

Or we can use the REPL as a calculator (note that # is used to comment the code):

© The Author(s), under exclusive license to Springer Science+Business Media, LLC, part of Springer Nature 2025
J. C. C. Chan, D. P. Kroese, *Statistical Modeling and Computation*,
Springer Texts in Statistics, https://doi.org/10.1007/978-1-0716-4132-3

```
x = 1.234;   # the semicolon suppresses output
y = sin(x)*sqrt(x^2)/x
```
```
0.9438182093746337
```

Julia uses the modern software paradigm where a *base* (i.e., built-in) library of code can be supplemented by loading additional *packages*. For example, the sine function **sin** is part of the in-built library of functions.

To use a package, two steps need to be taken. First, the package needs to be installed. Second, to use an installed package in a Julia program, the package needs to be loaded. The first step only has to be performed once, as Julia will remember which packages have been installed at any time. The second step needs to be repeated for every program that wants to use the particular package. Installing packages can be carried out via Julia's package manager, as in

```
import Pkg
Pkg.add("NameOfPackage")
```

Table A.1 lists a number of useful Julia packages, some of which are already built into the base library.

Table A.1 A few useful Julia packages.

Plots	Main plotting library
LinearAlgebra	Built-in library for linear algebra
IJulia	Package to interface with Jupyter notebooks
Random	Built-in library for random number generation
Distributions	Collection of probability distributions
Statistics	Built-in statistics library
StatsBase	Basic functionality for statistics
DelimitedFiles	Reading and writing delimited files
Downloads	Provides download functionality
NaNStatistics	Fast statistic with missing data
FFTW	Fast Fourier transforms
Optim	Optimization package
SparseArrays	Functionality for sparse arrays

You can check which additional packages have been installed with

```
import Pkg
Pkg.status()
```

Once a package has been installed, it can be included in the code by preceding the package name with **using** or **import**. For example, the following code uses the built-in random generator to generate a billion random numbers and stores them in a vector `x`. The macro `@time` reports the run time as well as the memory storage.

```julia
using Random
@time x = rand(10^9);
```
```
1.603207 seconds (2 allocations: 7.451 GiB, 15.27% gc time)
```

A Julia program or *script* is a collection of statements that can be run by the julia executable. Its file extension is `.jl`. A Julia script `mycode.jl`, say, can be executed in various ways. One way is to run the Julia executable in a system shell, as in

```
julia mycode.jl
```

It is then important that either Julia is started in the correct working directory or that the path to the file is specified completely. Another way is to execute the file from within the REPL, via

```julia
include("mycode.jl")
```

But the most convenient way to develop and execute Julia programs is to use an integrated development environment such as Visual Studio Code (VSCode), which can be downloaded from

https://code.visualstudio.com/

After installing the Julia Language Support extension, VSCode will be able to read and execute Julia programs. The extension also comes with a debugger. Apart from the main window for the code, the IDE displays the workspace directory, the REPL window, the system shell, and a plot window. To execute a region with one or more lines in the code, one can highlight the region with the mouse and then press Shift-Enter.

Try out the statements in the following Julia file, either by executing them in the REPL or in VSCode. Running the program via `julia first.jl` in a system shell will provide no output, other than the output from the `println` and `replace` functions.

```julia
first.jl

i = 1          # assignment
println("i has type ", typeof(i))  # type of i
i, j = 2, 8 # assignment via a tuple
k = j/i        # division of (in this case) two integers
typeof(k)      # the result, k, is a float!
div(i,j)       # integer division
```

```julia
i % j           # remainder of integer division
s = "Hello. How are you"
typeof(s)    # String
replace(s, "e" => "a", count = 1)   # string replacement


u = [1, 2, 3]    # vector assignment
typeof(u)        # the vector has integer-type elements
w = u .* u       # elementwise multiplication
x = u + w        # adding two vectors of the same dimension
y = 100 .+ u     # constant plus vector. The . is essential!
sin.(u)          # elementwise computation of sine function
umat = [1 2 3] # 1x3 matrix is not a vector!
umatT = umat'  # transpose is a 3x1 matrix, not the same as u


A = [1 2 3; 4 5 6; 7 8 9]   # 3x3 matrix
u[2]                # second element of u
A[2,3]              # element of A in row 2, column 3
v = A*u             # matrix multiplication
w = u'*A            # premultiply the matrix A with the transpose
   of u
A^2                 # square of matrix A
A.^2                # matrix of elementwise squares
```

A.2 Variables and Their Types

Each *variable* in Julia is a name associated with a *value*, and each value
has a *type*. To find the type of a variable x, use **typeof**(x). The statement
sizeof(x) returns the *size* of the value of x; that is the size in bytes of the
object in computer memory to which x refers.

For example, the statement x = 1 creates a integer variable x, whose value
is 1, with type **Int64**. Its size is 8 bytes in memory. Similarly, the statement
x = 1.0 creates a float variable x, whose value is 1.0, with type **Float64**. Its
size is also 8 bytes in memory. These are the default numerical types (on a
64-bit = 8 bytes) computer.

Types can be *abstract* or *concrete* and form a hierarchy. You can find the
supertypes of a type with **supertypes** and the subtypes with **subtypes**. At
the top of all types is the abstract type **Any**. The number hierarchy is headed
by the abstract type **Number** and lower down the hierarchy are concrete types
such as **Int64** and **Float64**.

For each of the statements below, verify the type and size of the variables.

```
typex.jl
```

```julia
x = [1, 2, 3]        # same as x = Vector{Int64}([1,2,3])
typeof(x)            # 3-element Vector{Int64}
y = Vector{Float64}([1,2,3])
typeof(y)            # 3-element Vector{Float64}
A = [1 2 3]          # Note the absence of commas!
typeof(A)            # 1x3 Matrix{Int64}
b = Vector{Bool}([0,1,1,0])   # 4-element Vector{Bool}
sizeof(b)            # 4 bytes
notb = .~ b          # elementwise NOT operation
typeof(notb)         # 4-element BitVector
tobe = b .| notb     # elementwise OR operation
sizeof(tobe)         # 8 bytes
```

Julia is a *strongly-typed* language, meaning that there are firm restrictions
on mixing different types within a statement. For example, a $1 \times n$ matrix is
not the same as a vector of length n.

```julia
x = [1,2,3]        # a vector of Int64
A = [1 2 3]        # a 1x3 matrix of Int64
z = x + A          # gives an error
```
```
DimensionMismatch: dimensions must match
```

However, when applying mathematical operations such as $+$ or $*$, the
operands are as a rule converted to a common type. For example, adding a
`Int64` variable to a `Float64` results in a `Float64` variable. In the `typex.jl`
program above, although b and **notb** have different types, we can still perform
the elementwise OR operation, as the `VectorBool` object is converted to a
`BitVector` object. We can convert the latter it into a `VectorBool` object via
the `collect` function:

```julia
x = [0.2, 0.6, 0.3, 0.7] . < 0.5  # elementwise comparison
typeof(x)       # 4-element BitVector
y = collect(x)
typeof(x)       # 4-element Vector{Bool}
```

Direct *conversion* between two types can be effected by the function
`convert`. Below is an example that converts a binary vector in `Int64` to
a vector of `Bool`, thus reducing the size of binary vector by a factor of 8.

```julia
x = [1,0,0,1] # 4-element Vector{Int64}
sizeof(x)     # 32 bytes
```

```
bx = convert(Vector{Bool},x)
sizeof(bx)    # 4 bytes
```

Composite data types can be created via the Julia structures, consisting of a collection of field names with (optionally) their types. Here is an example of a `mutable struct` object:

```
mutable struct Person
   name :: String
   age :: Int
   height :: Float64
end
```

A default way to initialize a struct is to specify the values of the field names.

```
p1 = Person("Josh", 39, 1.76)
p2 = Person("Dirk", 60, 1.84)
```

Some functions will return a struct as their output, so it is important to understand how to access the field values. This is done via the dot notation, as is usual in Python and many other languages. For a mutable struct, the field values can not only be read but also be modified. Removing the `mutable` qualifier in the struct definition gives an immutable struct; attempting to change the field values will give an error message. The function `fieldnames` gives the names of the struct.

```
fieldnames(Person)
println(p1.name)     # print the name of person 1
p2.age = 61          # change the age of person 2
println(p2.age)
```
```
(:name, :age, :height)
Josh
61
```

A.3 Vectors, Matrices, and Arrays

Statistical computation often involves the manipulation of vectors and matrices. Julia's syntax for matrix computation is very similar to MATLAB's. In Julia vectors and matrix are special cases of arrays. A vector is a one-dimensional array and a matrix a two-dimensional array. For example, to create a vector a, enter in the REPL or editor:

```
a = [1, 2, 3]
```

The REPL returns:

```
3-element Vector{Int64}:
 1
 2
 3
```

Similarly,

```
A = [1 2 5;  3 4 7; 6 7 9]     # no commas!
```

creates a 3×3 matrix $\mathbf{A}$. It is worth noting that Julia is case sensitive for variable names and built-in functions. That means Julia treats a and $\mathbf{A}$ as different objects. To display the i-th element in a vector x, just type `x[i]`. For example,

```
a[2]
```

refers to the second element of a. Similarly, one can access a particular element of $\mathbf{A}$ by specifying its row and column number (row first followed by column). For instance,

```
A[2,3]
```

displays the $(2, 3)$-entry of the matrix $\mathbf{A}$. To display multiple elements in the matrix, one can use expressions involving colons. For example,

```
A[1,1:2]
```

displays the first and second elements in the first row, whereas

```
A[:,2]
```

displays all the elements in the second column. The elements of a matrix can be stacked into a single vector as follows:

```
v = A[:]
print(v')
```

```
[1 3 6 2 4 7 5 7 9]
```

To perform numerical computation, one needs some basic matrix operations. In Julia, the following matrix operations, among several others, are available:

$+$ addition	$/$ right division
$-$ subtraction	$\char94$ power
$*$ multiplication	$'$ transpose
$\backslash$ left division	

For example,

```
a'
```
```
1x3 adjoint(::Vector{Int64}) with eltype Int64:
 1  2  3
```

returns the transpose of a, whereas

```
a'*A
```
```
1x3 adjoint(::Vector{Int64}) with eltype Int64:
 30 36 42
```

gives the product of a' and $\mathbf{A}$.

Other operations are obvious, except for the matrix divisions $\backslash$ and $/$. If $\mathbf{A}$ is an invertible square matrix and a is a compatible vector, then $x = \mathbf{A}\backslash a$ is the solution of $\mathbf{A}x = a$ and $x = a'/\mathbf{A}$ is the solution of $x\mathbf{A} = a'$. In other words, $\mathbf{A}\backslash a$ gives the same result (in principle) as $\mathbf{A}^{-1}a$, though they compute their results in different ways. Specifically, the former solves the linear system $\mathbf{A}x = a$ for x by Gaussian elimination, whereas the latter first computes the inverse $\mathbf{A}^{-1}$ and then multiplies it by a. As such, the second method is in general slower as computing the inverse of a matrix is time-consuming (and inaccurate).

When using `LinearAlgebra`, Julia reserves the letter I for a "generic" identity matrix object of type `UniformScaling`. The advantage is that this object has negligible memory requirements. For example, the following computes the inverse of the above matrix $\mathbf{A}$.

```
I/A
```
```
-6.5    8.5  -3.0
 7.5  -10.5   4.0
-1.5    2.5  -1.0
```

It is important to note that although addition and subtraction are element-wise operations, the other operations listed above are not—they are matrix operations. For example, $\mathbf{A}^2$ gives the square of the matrix $\mathbf{A}$, not a matrix whose entries are the squares of those in $\mathbf{A}$. One can make the operations $*$, $\backslash$, $/$, and $\verb|^|$ to operate element-wise by preceding them by a full stop. For example, the following returns the square of the matrix $\mathbf{A}$:

```
A^2
```

```
3x3 Matrix{Int64}:
 37   45   64
 57   71  106
 81  103  160
```

On the other hand:

```
A.^2
```

```
3x3 Matrix{Int64}:
  1   4  25
  9  16  49
 36  49  81
```

computes the squares element-wise.

Vectors and matrices are special cases of Julia *arrays*. The following creates an $3 \times 4 \times 2$ array $\mathbf{A}$ that is filled with zeros; these are by default of type `Float64`. The functions `typeof`, `eltype`, `ndims`, `size`, and `length` provide various properties of an array.

```
A = zeros(3,4,2)
typeof(A)      # type of the array
eltype(A)      # type of the elements in the array
ndims(A)       # number of dimensions
size(A)        # dimensions
length(A)      # number of elements
```

```
3x4x2 Array{Float64, 3}:
[:, :, 1] =
 0.0  0.0  0.0  0.0
 0.0  0.0  0.0  0.0
 0.0  0.0  0.0  0.0

[:, :, 2] =
 0.0  0.0  0.0  0.0
 0.0  0.0  0.0  0.0
 0.0  0.0  0.0  0.0

Array{Float64, 3}
Float64
```

```
3
(3, 4, 2)
24
```

Arrays can be accessed in the same way as vectors and matrices, e.g., `A[2,1,1]` is the (2,1,1)th element of **A**, and *slice* operations such as `A[:,:,2]` can also be used. A vector is a one-dimensional array, and a matrix is a two-dimensional array.

Vectors, matrices, and arrays can be added only if they have the same dimensions. However, it possible to add a smaller array to a larger one by the process of *broadcasting*, which involves elementwise duplication of the array elements across the smaller dimension to match the larger dimension. The `.+` operator indicates that addition is carried out via broadcasting. The function **reshape** can be used to reshape an array into an array with different dimensions. Finally, vectors and matrices can be horizontally and vertically concatenated via the **hcat** and **vcat** functions. Here are a few examples.

```
A = [1 2; 3 4];    # matrix (suppress output)
v = [10,20];       # vector (suppress output)
B = v .+ A         # adding the vector to the columns of A
C = 1000 .+ A      # adding a constant to all elements of A
D = hcat(C,B)
E = vcat(B,C,D')
F = reshape(E,4,4)
```

```
2x2 Matrix{Int64}:
 11  12
 23  24

2x2 Matrix{Int64}:
 1001  1002
 1003  1004

2x4 Matrix{Int64}:
 1001  1002  11  12
 1003  1004  23  24

2x8 adjoint(::Matrix{Int64}) with eltype Int64:
 11  23  1001  1003  1001  1002  11  12
 12  24  1002  1004  1003  1004  23  24

4x4 reshape(adjoint(::Matrix{Int64}), 4, 4) with eltype Int64:
 11  1001  1001  11
 12  1002  1003  23
 23  1003  1002  12
 24  1004  1004  24
```

An array can have elements of different types. For example, the following vector has three types of elements.

```julia
x = ["string",  1, 1.0]
typeof(x[1])
typeof(x[2])
typeof(x[3])
```

```
3-element Vector{Any}:
  "string"
 1
 1.0

 String
 Int64
 Float64
```

The common type of these elements is the abstract type **Any**. Finally, note that vectors are different to *tuples* (indicated by round brackets) in that tuples are *immutable*; that is, they cannot be changed.

```julia
x = ("string", 1, 1.0)     # same as x = "string", 1, 1.0
typeof(x)
x[1] = "hello"
```

```
("string", 1, 1.0)
Tuple{String, Int64, Float64}
MethodError: no method matching setindex!(::Tuple{Int64, ... , ::Int64)
```

A.4 Functions

Functions make it easier to divide a complex program into simpler parts. To create a function Julia, the following syntax can be used:

```julia
function <function name>(<parameter_list>)
  <statements>
  return <value>  # this may be omitted
end
```

A shorter way is:

```julia
<function name>(<parameter_list>) = <expression>
```

An expression is any statement that gives a value when executed, such as in `sin(x) + x^2`. Thus,

```julia
f(x) = x^2 + 5*x - 10
```

creates the function with the name **f**, whose value at x is $f(x) = x^2 + 5x - 10$. An alternative way to define **f** is

```julia
f = x -> x^2 + 5*x - 10
```

The function name gives a means of invoking the function. The following evaluates the function for an integer, float, and integer vector argument.

```julia
f(10)
f(10.)
f([1,2,3])
```
```
140
140.0
MethodError: no method matching ^(::Vector{Int64}, ::Int64)
```

Note that the function does not know how to evaluate the square of a vector. We could remedy this by defining the function as

```julia
f(x) = x.^2 .+ 5*x .- 10    # note the three dots!
```

This will take vector and matrix arguments. However, a more elegant approach is to enforce elementwise operations on the function, i.e., broadcasting, by using a dot (.) after the function name:

```julia
f.([1,2,3])        # vector argument
f.([1 2; 3 4])     # matrix argument
```
```
-4
 4
14
-4   4
14  26
```

If the type of function arguments is important, this can be specified in the function definition, using the `::T` syntax, where **T** is the type. For example:

```julia
f(x::Integer) = x^2 + 5*x - 10
f(10)   # 140
f(10.)  # MethodError: no method matching f(::Float64)
```

In fact, one of Julia's strengths is the *multiple dispatch* mechanism, which allows many different versions of the same function to be defined for different types of arguments, similar to function overloading in Python.

Function names can be passed to other functions as inputs. To create a function that takes more than one input is just as easy. For example, the following code takes a column vector of data and computes its mean and standard deviation:

```
function stat(x)
  n = length(x);
  meanx = sum(x)/n;
  stdevx = sqrt(sum(x.^2)/n - meanx.^2);
  return meanx, stdevx
end


meanx,  stdx = stat(randn(100))
```
```
(0.038727242782939215, 1.119568688040557)
```

A function does not make a copy of the values of the names in the parameter list, but only assigns (binds) new names to these values. This means that functions can change the value of input arguments! In most cases, we do *not* want to change the input argument(s) to a function. When a function makes changes to the input, it is common to use an exclamation mark (!) at the end of the function name, as a warning sign. Here is an example:

```
function change2ndto100!(x)
    x[2] = 100
end


y = [1 2 3];
change2ndto100!(y)
print(y)
```
```
[1 100 3]
```

Julia has many in-built functions, and by *using* packages many more functions become available. Because of the multiple dispatch mechanism, there may be many different versions, or *methods*, of the same function. For example, without loading any additional packages, the **rand** function has (currently) 81 different methods.

```
rand
```
```
rand (generic function with 81 methods)
```

One can learn more about a specific function, say, **rand**, by typing ? **rand** in the REPL. Here are some useful matrix-building functions. The functions **diag** and **diagm** are part of the **LinearAlgebra** package.

zeros	create a matrix of zeros
ones	create a matrix of ones
diagm	create a diagonal matrix from a vector
diag	extract the diagonal vector from a matrix
rand	generate $\mathcal{U}(0,1)$ random variables
randn	generate $\mathcal{N}(0,1)$ random variables

Some other useful vector and matrix functions are given below. Note that **exp**, **sqrt**, **sin**, **cos**, and **log** applied to a *matrix* will yield the corresponding matrix function, not the element-wise function. For example, **exp(A)** returns the matrix

$$e^A = \sum_{k=0}^{\infty} \frac{A^k}{k!}.$$

To obtain the elementwise operations for these functions, remember to use broadcasting, e.g., **exp.(A)**. The functions **det** and **cholesky** require the **LinearAlgebra** package.

exp	exponential	**log**	natural log
sqrt	square root	**abs**	absolute value
sin	sine	**cos**	cosine
sum	sum	**prod**	product
maximum	maximum	**minimum**	minimum
cholesky	Cholesky factorization	**inv**	inverse
det	determinant	**size**	dimensions

If x is a vector, **sum(x)** returns the sum of the elements in x. Likewise, for a matrix $\mathbf{X}$, **sum(X)** returns the sum of all elements. For an $m \times n$ matrix $\mathbf{X}$, to obtain the $1 \times n$ matrix consisting of sums of each column, use **sum(X, dims=1)** while **sum(X,dims=2)** returns the $m \times 1$ matrix of sums of each row. For example:

```
A = [1 2 5; 3 4 7]
sum(A)
sum(A, dims=1)
sum(A, dims=2)
```

```
2x3 Matrix{Int64}:
 1  2  5
 3  4  7


22


1x3 Matrix{Int64}:
 4  6  12


2x1 Matrix{Int64}:
  8
 14
```

The function **sum** is an example of a function that has a *keyword argument* (in this case, **dims**). Many plotting functions have such keyword arguments. In general, keyword arguments can be defined via a semicolon in the argument list. For example, the following function **square** has a keyword argument **elw** which is set to **true** by default. The function returns the square of a matrix, unless the **elw** argument is set to **false**, in which case the matrix of elementwise squared values is returned. The function also illustrates the use of a *conditional expression*, as in the C language:

```
<condition> ? <expression1> : <expression2>
```

```julia
function square(A; elw = true)
  elw ? A^2 : A.^2        # conditional expression
end
X = [1 2; 3 4]
square(X)
square(X, elw = false)   # ; instead of , is allowed
```

For a positive definite matrix $\mathbf{A}$, `cholesky(A).L` returns the (lower) Cholesky matrix $\mathbf{B}$ such that $\mathbf{BB}^\top = \mathbf{A}$. Note that **cholesky** returns a **struct** object, which has to be accessed via the dot notation. For example,

```julia
using LinearAlgebra
B = [2 0 0; 3 4 0; 5 1 2]
A = B*B';
cholesky(A).L    # the L field contains the Cholesky matrix
```

returns the lower Cholesky factor of $\mathbf{BB}^\top$, which is, of course, $\mathbf{B}$. For some statistical applications, the current Cholesky implementation gives an error message for matrices that are ill-conditioned but are nevertheless positive definite, e.g., covariance matrices with some very small diagonal elements. For such matrices, the Hermitian nature of the matrix can be enforced via the function **Hermitian**, as in `cholesky(Hermitian(A)).L`. Of course, this stopgap solution should be changed in newer implementations of the **cholesky** function. Examples are given throughout the book, as in Chaps. 3, 8, 10, 12, and 13.

A.5 Flow Control

Julia has the usual control flow statements such as **if-then-else**, **while**, and **for**. For instance, the general form of a simple **if** statement is

```
if <condition1>
   <statements>
elseif <condition2>
   <statements>
else
   <statements>
end
```

Here, `<condition1>` and `<condition2>` are logical conditions that are either `true` or `false`; logical conditions often involve comparison operators (such as `==`, `>`, `<=`, `!=`). In general, there can be more than one `elseif` part, or it can be omitted. The `else` part can also be omitted. For example, the following code simulate rolling a four-sided die:

```
u = rand();
if u <= .25
    print('1');
elseif u <= .5
    print('2');
elseif u <= .75
    print('3');
else
    print('4');
end
```

The `while` loop has the following syntax.

```
while <condition>
   <statements>
end
```

To illustrate the `while` loop syntax, suppose we wish to generate a positive normal random variable (with pdf given in (2.26)). We can do that using the following `while` loop, wrapped in a function.

☞ 56

```
function posrand()
  u = randn();
  while u <= 0
    u = randn();
  end
  return u
end
```

Unlike a `while` loop, the `for` loop executes the statements for a fixed number of times. The `for` loop has the following syntax.

```
for <variable> in <collection>
   <statements>
end
```

Above, `<collection>` is any *iterable* object; that is, an object over which can be iterated. Typically this is a "range" object, such as `start:step:end`, specified by starting value, an optional step size, and an end value. One can also use the function **range** to create range objects. Vectors are natural iterable objects, but note that, in contrast to MATLAB, a range such as $1:10$ is not equal to the vector $[1,\dots,10]$. For one thing, it takes up hardly any computer memory, as only the start and stop values need to be stored. The following shows three equivalent ways to create the same iterable object.

```
r1 = range(start = 0, stop = 1, length =101)
r2 = 0.0:0.01:1.0
r3 = range(start = 0, step = 0.01, stop = 1)
r1 == r2 == r3   # true
```

As an example, the following code generates five draws from the positive normal distribution.

```
x = zeros(5);     # create a storage vector
for i in 1:5      # can also write i=1:5
   x[i] = posrandn()
end
print(round.(x, digits=4)) # print x, rounded to 4 digits
```
```
[0.6404, 0.0033, 0.2557, 1.2712, 2.3754]
```

For further control in `for` and `while` loops, one can use a **break** statement to exit the current loop, and the **continue** statement to continue with the next iteration of the loop, while abandoning any remaining statements in the current iteration.

Similar to Python, Julia has a *list comprehension* syntax:

```
<expression> for <element> in <collection> if <condition>
```

This allows arrays to be constructed via embedded `for` loops. For example, the following produces the vector of squares of the odd numbers from 1 to 10.

```
x = [i^2 for i=1:10 if isodd(i)]
```

When performing loops, speed is important. Consider, for example, the simulation of a billion uniform random numbers, which we want to store in a vector $\boldsymbol{x}$. The following code is one way to fill the vector $\boldsymbol{x}$. Recall that the macro `@time` can be used for timing. In this case we need to wrap the statements inside a begin-end block.

```julia
@time begin
  x = zeros(10^9)
  for i in 1:10^9
    x[i] = rand()
  end
end
28.560135 seconds (2.00 G allocations: 37.253 GiB, 1.75% gc time)
```

We see that the computation takes a long time. However, due to the way Julia's compiler works, it is better to put the loop inside a function. In this case, we refill the vector x by changing its entries one by one.

```julia
function fillrand!(x)
  for i in 1:10^9
    x[i] = rand()
  end
end

@time fillrand!(x)
1.410237 seconds (9.13 k allocations: 578.083 KiB, 0.89% compilation time)
```

Now it only takes a bit more than 1 second! Of course it is much cleaner (easier to read) if we create the vector in one go via the **rand** function, giving a similar performance:

```julia
@time x = rand(10^9)
1.324148 seconds (2 allocations: 7.451 GiB, 0.66% gc time)
```

A.6 Graphics

Julia has several "back-end" plot facilities. The default module is `GR`, which can be accessed via the `Plots` module. It allows users to create various graphical objects including two- and three-dimensional graphs. One can also have a title on a graph, add a legend, change the font and font size, label the axis, etc., by changing the corresponding attributes. A list of plot attributes may be obtained via `plotattr()`. See also

https://docs.juliaplots.org

In Julia the most basic function used to create 2D graphs is **plot**. For example, to make a graph of $y = \sin(x)$ on the interval from $x = 0$ to $x = 2\pi$, we use the following code, which also shows various plotting attributes, how to use LaTeX strings, and how to save a plot as a pdf file.

```julia
using Plots, LaTeXStrings
x = 0:0.01:2*pi
p1 = plot(x,sin.(x), # the . is important! Naming the plot p1
    tickfontsize = 15,              # axis font size
    guidefontsize = 20,             # label font size
    legend = false,                 # legend is on by default
    grid = false,                   # grid is on by default
    linewidth = 3,                  # linewidth is 1 by default
    tickfont = "Computer Modern",   # axis font
    color = "salmon"                # line color
)
xlabel!(L"x")                       # using LaTeX font
ylabel!(L"\sin(x)")
savefig(p1,"sin.pdf")               # saving the figure
```

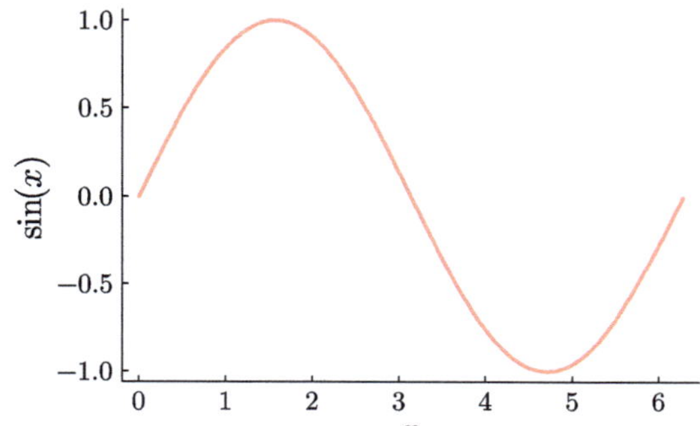

Fig. A.1 A plot of the graph $y = \sin(x)$ from 0 to 2π

The graph produced is given in Fig. A.1. Note that the command `x = 0:.01:2*pi;` creates a iterable grid object of type **StepRangeLen** that ranges from 0 to 2π in steps of 0.01. It is important to note that this is not a vector. As mentioned in the previous section, the function **range** can also be used to create range objects, as in `range(start=0, stop=2*pi, length=100)`.

Another useful function is **histogram**, which allows us to plot histograms. The following Julia script creates standard normal data of size 10000 and makes a histogram with 50 bins. Instead of a histogram, it is often more useful to have a density estimate. The code below uses fast and optimal **theta KDE** of Botev et al. (2010). The corresponding Julia module `.ThetaKDE, Plots` which contains the function `kde`, can be downloaded from the book's website. Note that `plot!` is used to plot the kde and the histogram in the same figure (see Fig. A.2).

```julia
using .ThetaKDE, Plots
data = randn(10000)
histogram(data,bins=50, normalize = true, legend=false)
mindat = minimum(data); maxdat = maximum(data);
h,density,xmesh = kde(data,2^14,mindat,maxdat)
plot!(xmesh[1:2:end],density[1:2:end],linewidth=3)
```

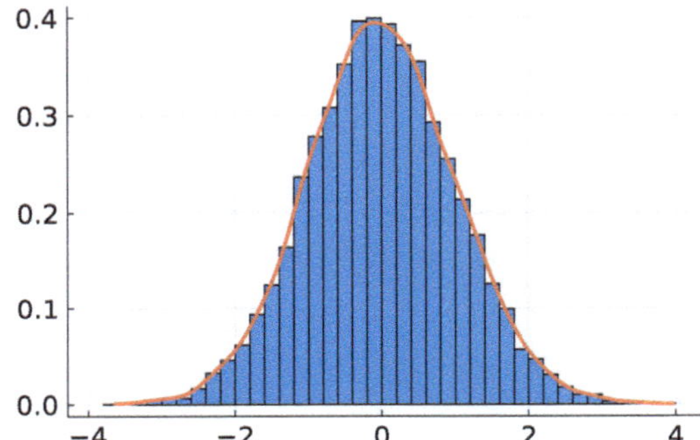

Fig. A.2 A histogram of 10000 standard normal draws and its kernel density estimate

It is often desirable to plot several graphs in the same figure window. For this purpose we can use the **layout** attribute of the **plot** function.

Suppose we wish to make scatterplots of data from the two-dimensional standard normal and uniform distributions in the same figure window (see Fig. A.3). This is accomplished in the code below. The plot attribute **aspectratio** ensures that the x and y scaling is equal. The value of the aspect ratio variable is in this case `:equal`, which is a Julia *symbol*—a unique identifier. The attributes **ms, msw, ma** control the size, linewidth, and alpha value (i.e., transparency) of the marks, respectively. In this case the layout `(1,2)` indicates that the figures are to be plotted next to each other. Finally, **size** determines the size of the plot window.

```julia
x = randn(1000,2)    # 2D standard normal data
y = rand(1000,2)     # 2D standard uniform data
p3 = scatter(x[:,1],x[:,2], aspectratio = :equal, ms = 5,
      msw = 0, ma = 0.3,legend = false)
p4 = scatter(y[:,1],y[:,2], aspectratio = :equal, ms = 5,
```

```
       msw = 0, ma= 0.3, legend = false)
   p34 = plot(p3,p4,layout = (1,2), size = (600,200))
```

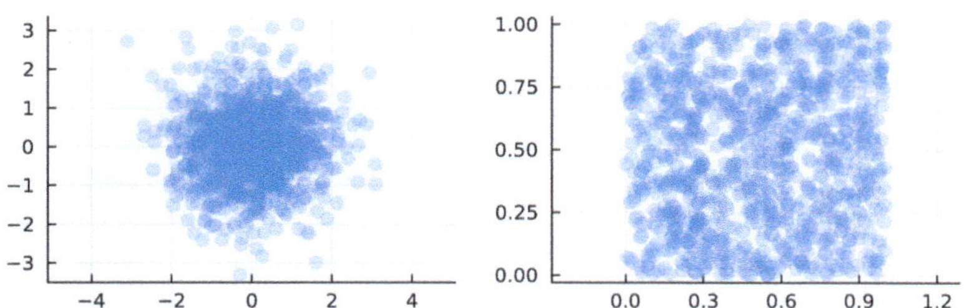

Fig. A.3 Scatterplots for the two-dimensional standard normal and standard uniform distributions

In addition, one can also easily produce 3D graphical objects in Julia. To illustrate various useful routines, suppose we want to plot the density function of the bivariate normal distribution (see Sect. 3.6) given by

☞ 83

$$f(x, y; \varrho) = \frac{1}{2\pi\sqrt{1-\varrho^2}}\, e^{-\frac{1}{2(1-\varrho^2)}\left(x^2 - 2\varrho xy + y^2\right)}\,.$$

As in plotting a 2D graph, we first need to build a grid for x and y, which can be done with the function **range**. For example, we use the following code to plot the bivariate normal density function with $\varrho = 0.8$ in Fig. A.4.

```
using Plots
rho = 0.8
x = range(-3, stop=3, length=100)
y = range(-3, stop=3, length=100)
f(x,y) = 1/(2*pi*sqrt(1-rho^2))*exp(-(x^2 -2*rho*x*y + y^2)
    /(2*(1-rho^2)))
plt = surface(x, y, f,    # surface broadcasts f by default
legend=false,
camera = (75,40)    # azimuth and elevation angles
)
```

By adding the following code, we can even produce an animation that gradually changes the viewing angle

```
anim = @animate for i in 0:180
    plot!(plt, camera = (i, 40))
```

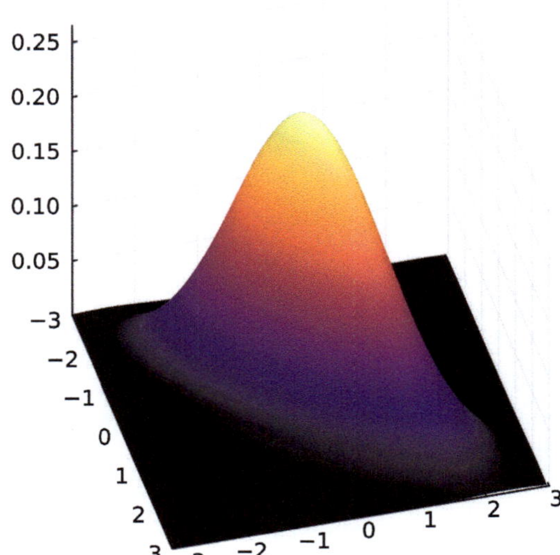

Fig. A.4 The density function of the bivariate normal distribution with $\varrho = 0.6$

```
end
gif(anim, "animsurf.gif", fps = 15)
```

Also, a contour plot can be obtained by using the function **contour**:

```
contour(x,y,f);
```

The result is shown in Fig. A.5.

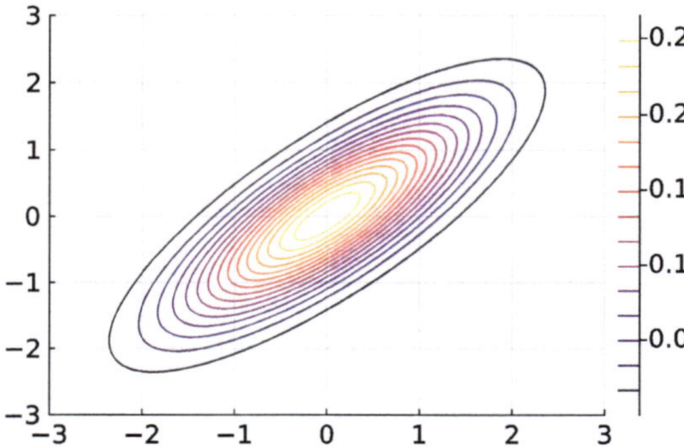

Fig. A.5 A contour plot of the bivariate normal density function with $\varrho = 0.6$

A.7 Optimization Routines

Julia provides various ways to optimize functions. In this section we discuss some of them that are used in the main text. Note that, typically, optimization routines are framed in terms of minimization. In order to perform maximization, some minor changes to the objective function are required. More precisely, suppose we want to maximize the function $f(\boldsymbol{x})$ and find a maximizer $\boldsymbol{x}_{\max} = \operatorname{argmax}_{\boldsymbol{x}} f(\boldsymbol{x})$. Instead of the original maximization problem, consider minimizing $-f(\boldsymbol{x})$ and noting that

$$\boldsymbol{x}_{\max} = \operatorname*{argmax}_{\boldsymbol{x}} f(\boldsymbol{x}) = \operatorname*{argmin}_{\boldsymbol{x}} -f(\boldsymbol{x})\,.$$

Hence, without loss of generality, we will focus on minimization routines. One basic minimization function is **optimize** from the optimization package **Optim**. To illustrate its usage, suppose we wish to minimize the function $f(x) = \sin(x^2)$ over the interval $[0, 3]$ (see Fig. A.6).

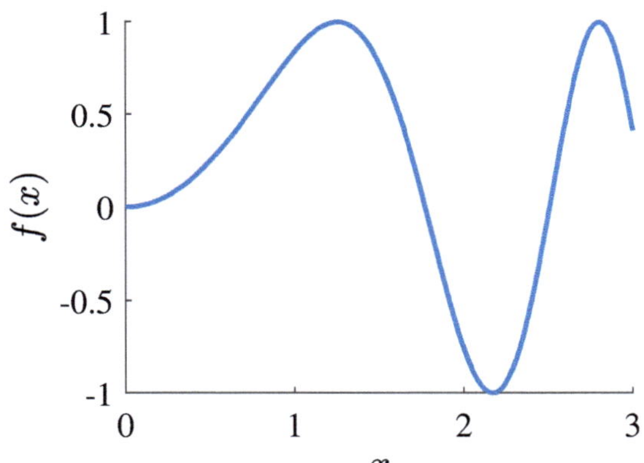

Fig. A.6 A plot of $f(x) = \sin(x^2)$ from 0 to 3

We can define the function in Julia as follows:

```
f(x) =  sin(x^2);
```

or also as

```
f =  x -> sin(x^2);
```

To ensure that we only consider arguments in $[0, 3]$, we could set any function value outside the interval to a very large value, via

```
f(x) = x <= 3 && x >= 0 ? sin(x^2) : 1E50
```

For scalar arguments, **optimize** takes three inputs: the function name and lower and upper bounds of the interval. The minimizer and minimum (i.e., minimum value of the function evaluated at the minimizer) can be found as attributes of the object returned by the function, as illustrated below.

```julia
using Optim
f(x) = x < 3 && x > 0 ? sin(x^2) : 1E50
res = optimize(f,0,3)
println("minimum = ", res.minimum, ";  minimizer = ",
res.minimizer)
```
```
minimum = -1.000000;  minimizer = 2.170804
```

The function **optimize** can also be used to minimize multivariate functions. However, care should be taken with the choice of the starting point for the algorithm. As an example, suppose we wish to minimize the *peaks* function (from MATLAB)

$$S(\boldsymbol{x}) = 3\,(1 - x_1)^2\,\mathrm{e}^{-x_1^2 - (x_2+1)^2} - 10\,\Big(\frac{x_1}{5} - x_1^3 - x_2^5\Big)\,\mathrm{e}^{-x_1^2 - x_2^2}$$

$$-\frac{1}{3}\,\mathrm{e}^{-(x_1+1)^2 - x_2^2}, \quad [x_1, x_2] \in \mathbb{R}^2,$$

with respect to $\boldsymbol{x} = [x_1, x_2]$. A contour plot is given in Fig. A.7.

```julia
function S(x)
  3*(1-x[1])^2*exp(-x[1]^2 - (x[2]+1)^2) - 10*(x[1]/5-x[1]^3
  - x[2]^5)*exp(-x[1]^2-x[2]^2) - 1/3*exp(-(x[1]+1)^2-x[2]^2)
end

x0 = [0.0,0.0];  # starting point
res = optimize(S,x0);
println("minimum = ", res.minimum, ";  minimizer = ",
res.minimizer)
```
```
minimum = -0.064936;    minimizer = [0.296431, 0.320161]
```

This, however, turns out to yield a *local* minimum, rather than a *global* one. If we instead take the starting point x0 = [0.1,-1], we obtain the global minimizer and minimum:

```
minimum = -6.551133;    minimizer = [0.228261, -1.625537]
```

A simple but powerful alternative is to use the *cross-entropy (CE)* method of Rubinstein and Kroese (2004). This is a global optimization function that uses repeated sampling combined with parameter updating, instead of gradient information. Below is a basic implementation. The function makes use of the packages `LinearAlgebra` and `Statistics`.

```julia
function CEmin(f, mu, sigma, N, Nel, tol)
# minimize function f via the CE method
n = length(mu)  # dimension
  while maximum(sigma) > tol
    ds = n == 1 ? sigma : diagm(sigma)  # scalars or vectors?
    X = randn(N,n)*ds .+ mu'  # N rows of n-dim normals
    fX = n==1 ? f.(X) : f.(eachrow(X));  # Function values
    # sort the samples by their function values
    sortfX = sortslices(hcat(X, fX), dims=1, by = x -> x[n
        +1])
    Elite = sortfX[1:Nel, 1:n]; # smallest (= elite) samples
    # update mu and sigma
    mu = n == 1 ? mean(Elite) : vec(mean(Elite,dims=1))
    sigma = n == 1 ? std(Elite) : vec(std(Elite,dims=1))
  end
  return f(mu), mu   # minimum,  minimizer
end
```

To use the function, specify the starting vector (or value for scalar arguments), a vector of standard deviations (initially chosen large enough to sample points from a wide region), the number of samples at each iteration, the number of elite (i.e., best) samples, and a tolerance for stopping.

```julia
using LinearAlgebra, Statistics
mu = [0,0]; sigma = 4.0*ones(2);
N = 1000; Nel = 100; tol = 1E-5;
minS, mu = CEmin(S,mu,sigma,N,Nel,tol);
dig = convert(Int64,-log10(tol))
println("minimum = ",minS, digits = dig),
 " minimizer = ", round.(mu,digits = dig))
```
```
minimum = -6.551130  minimizer = [0.228280, -1.625530]
```

Figure A.7 illustrates that the correct minimizer for this multimodal function is found in a few iterations.

Indeed, the same `CEmin` program can be used to minimize the function f above.

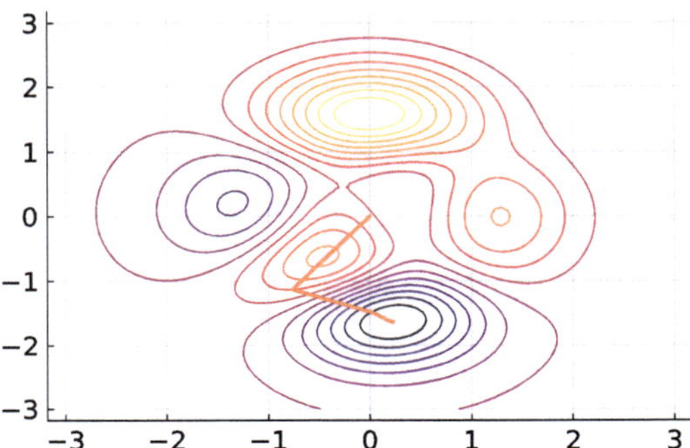

Fig. A.7 Contour plot with the CE minimization path, starting from the origin

```
f(x) = x < 3 && x > 0 ? sin(x^2) : 1E50
minf, mu = CEmin(f,1.0,1.0,100,10,1E-8);
dig = convert(Int64,-log10(tol))
println("minimum = ",round(minf,digits = dig),
"  minimizer = ", round.(mu,digits = dig))
```

```
minimum = -1.000000  minimizer = 2.170804
```

A.8 Handling Sparse Matrices

A **sparse matrix** is simply a matrix that contains a large proportion of zeros. Computation for sparse matrices can typically be done much faster than for full matrices. In addition, as most of the elements in a sparse matrix are zeros, the storage cost of a sparse matrix is also small. In statistics we often need to deal with large sparse matrices. Thus it is useful to learn how to employ them in Julia.

The package `SparseArrays` is necessary for sparse matrix and vector operations, and `LinearAlgebra` is usually also required. A basic function for creating sparse matrices is **sparse**. For example, suppose the matrix

$$\mathbf{W} = \begin{bmatrix} 1 & 0 & 0 & 0 & 0 \\ 0 & 1 & 0 & 0 & 0 \\ 0 & 0 & 2 & 0 & 0 \\ 0 & 0 & 0 & 3 & 1 \end{bmatrix}$$

is stored as a full matrix in Julia. The **sparse** function converts a full matrix to sparse form by squeezing out any zero elements.

```
using SparseArrays
W = [1 0 0 0 0 ;
     0 1 0 0 0
     0 0 2 0 0
     0 0 0 3 1]
S = sparse(W)
```

```
4x5 SparseMatrixCSC{Int64, Int64} with 5 stored entries:
 1  .  .  .  .
 .  1  .  .  .
 .  .  2  .  .
 .  .  .  3  1
```

Notice that only the non-zero elements in $\mathbf{W}$ are stored. To find the indices and values of the nonzero elements, the function **findnz** can be used, which returns a three-tuple of vectors, where the first two vectors identify the indices and the third vector the values. The function **nnz** returns the number of nonzeros of a sparse array.

```
a = findnz(S)
hcat(a[1], a[2], a[3])
nnz(S)
```

```
([1, 2, 3, 4, 4], [1, 2, 3, 4, 5], [1, 1, 2, 3, 1])

 1  1  1
 2  2  1
 3  3  2
 4  4  3
 4  5  1

5
```

In general, we can create a sparse matrix $\mathbf{S}$ by the command

```
S = sparse(i,j,s,m,n)
```

This uses vectors $\boldsymbol{i}$, $\boldsymbol{j}$, and $\boldsymbol{s}$ to generate an $m \times n$ sparse matrix such that $S(\boldsymbol{i}(k), \boldsymbol{j}(k)) = \boldsymbol{s}(k)$. For example, to create the matrix $\mathbf{W}$ above, we first need to build a vector $\boldsymbol{s}$ that stores all the non-zero elements:

```
s = [1, 1, 2, 3, 1];
```

Next, we create a vector $\boldsymbol{i}$ that stores the row position for each element in $\boldsymbol{s}$. For example, the first element in $\boldsymbol{s}$ should be in the first row, the second element in second row, and so on. We then do the same thing for the column positions and store them in the vector $\boldsymbol{j}$:

```
i = [1, 2, 3, 4, 4]
j = [1, 2, 3, 4, 5]
```

To create the 4×5 matrix $\mathbf{W}$ above, write

```
W = sparse(i,j,s,4,5)
```

The function `Array` converts a sparse matrix back to dense form. When using the `LinearAlgebra` package, the command `sparse(I, 100, 100)` creates an $\mathtt{n \times n}$ sparse identity matrix. We can accomplish the same goal via

```
sparse(1:100, 1:100, ones(n))
```

Another useful function is `spdiagm`, the sparse version of `diagm`, which can be used to create sparse diagonal matrices. To extract the (sparse) main diagonal from a sparse matrix, use `Diagonal`; this returns a sparse vector. Notice the syntax of creating diagonal elements below and above the main diagonal.

```
spdiagm(-1 => 1:99, 1 => 1:99) # 100x100 parse matrix with
  # entries on the principal sub and sup diagonals
s = Diagonal(S)   # yields a sparse vector
spdiagm(ones(10))   # 10x10 sparse identity matrix
```

As mentioned earlier, one main advantage of working with sparse rather than full matrices is that computations involving sparse matrices are usually much quicker. For instance, some methods to simulate a Gaussian random process on a grid of 400×400 pixels, as in Fig. A.8, require a Cholesky decomposition of a 160000×160000 matrix, which is impossible to store in CPU memory. However, if each row of the matrix only contains a few nonzero entries, then it is very feasible to compute the Cholesky decomposition quickly; see also Kroese et al. (2011, Section 5.1).

Finally, it should be noted that, currently, the sparse Cholesky method in Julia differs from the ordinary (full-matrix) Cholesky method, in that the sparse method first permutes the rows and columns of the original matrix for efficient storage and retrieval. In particular, if $\mathbf{A}$ is the sparse matrix of interest, Julia determines the Cholesky matrix $\mathbf{L}$ such that

$$\mathbf{LL}^\top = \mathbf{PAP}^\top,$$

for some *permutation matrix* $\mathbf{P}$—a matrix of 0s and 1s with exactly one 1 in each column and row. Note that such a matrix is *orthogonal*; that is, $\mathbf{P}^\top = \mathbf{P}^{-1}$. Hence, defining $\mathbf{B} = \mathbf{P}^\top \mathbf{L}$, we have the matrix decomposition

$$\mathbf{BB}^\top = \mathbf{A}.$$

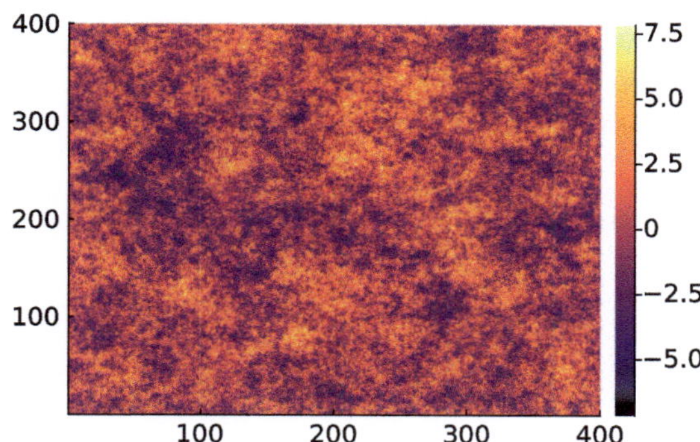

Fig. A.8 A Gaussian
spatial process on a $400 \times$
400 grid

However, the matrix **B** is no longer lower-diagonal! Here is a worked example:

```
a = [1, 2, 3, 1, 2, 4, 1, 3, 4, 2, 3, 4]
b = [1, 1, 1, 2, 2, 2, 3, 3, 3, 4, 4, 4]
c = [1.0, -0.25, -0.25, -0.25, 1.0, -0.25,
     -0.25, 1.0, -0.25, -0.25, -0.25, 1.0]
A = sparse(a,b,c)
R = cholesky(A); # calculate the (sparse) Cholesky matrix
P = sparse(1:4,R.p,ones(4)) # permutation matrix
B = P'*sparse(R.L)  # matrix with B*B' = A
isapprox(B*B', A)   # true
```

A.9 Distributions

We have already encountered the functions **rand** and **randn** from the base
package to generate uniform and standard normal random variables. The
packages **Distributions** and **Random** offer a wide of additional facilities for
probability distributions and random variable simulation. Table A.2 lists
the names of some common distributions available in **Distributions**. See
Sects. 2.5 and 2.6 for various properties of these distributions.

The following illustrates how these distribution types can be used.

```
using Random, Distributions, Plots
Random.seed!(1234)    # set the random seed (optional)
dist = Poisson(5)     # Poisson distribution
mean(dist)            # the expectation for this distribution
var(dist)             # the variance for this distribution
x = rand(dist,10000)  # an iid sample of size 10000
```

Table A.2 Names of common distributions in the `Distributions` package

Name	parameters		Name	parameters
Bernoulli	p		Beta	α, β
Binomial	n, p		Chisq	n
DiscreteUniform	a, b		Exponential	$\theta = 1/\lambda$
Geometric	p		FDist	m, n
Poisson	λ		Gamma	$\alpha, \theta = 1/\lambda$
			Normal	μ, σ
			TDist	n
			Uniform	a, b

```julia
mean(x)                 # the sample mean
var(x)                  # the sample variance
plot(pdf.(dist,0:20), linetype = :scatter,
    line = :stem, marker= :circle) # a plot of the pdf


gammalist = [Gamma(i,4) for i in [0.5,1,2,4]]
                        # 4 different Gamma distributions
mean.(gammalist)        # lists of expectations


xmesh = 0:0.01:20
pdfs = [ pdf.(dist, xmesh) for dist in gammalist ];
plot(xmesh, pdfs, ylims=[0,0.5], linewidth=2)
```

Other useful functions are **cdf**, **quantile**, **std**, and **median**. Note that the latter three can be used to compute the *exact* quantile, standard deviation, and median of a distribution, as well as calculating *approximations* thereof via their sample equivalents.

```julia
dist = TDist(4);
cdf(dist,3.0)
quantile(dist,0.95)  # exact 95% quantile
std(dist)            # exact standard deviation
median(dist)         # exact median


x = rand(TDist(4),100);
quantile(x,0.95)     # sample 95% quantile
std(x)               # sample standard deviation
median(x)            # sample median
```

```
0.9800290159641406
2.1318467863266495
1.4142135623730951
0.0
```

```
2.4844351992270557
1.3846972965065583
-0.07485935730166166
```

A.10 Input/Output

Julia treats input and output as a *stream*: a sequence of data, with a program adding data to one end of the stream and a device taking data from the other end. The devices can either be input devices (e.g., a keyboard or a file) or output devices (e.g., a screen or a file).

The following program writes the prime numbers in the set $\{1, \ldots, 100\}$ into the file **primes.txt**. Note that this file is a *binary* file, as the numbers are written in binary form. To create a human-readable *text* file, the number needs to be written to the file as a string. You can try this out by uncommenting the corresponding lines below.

```julia
using Primes     # import if not already done so
io = open("primes.txt", "w"); # open the stream for writing
for i in 1:100
  if isprime(i) # is the number prime?
  write(io,i)    # write an Int64 object to the file
# write(io,string(i)*"\n") # write a string + newline
# println(io,i) # same as above
    end
end
close(io) # always remember to close the file
```

To read the file thus created, we basically just reverse the stream, making sure the correct data type is read.

```julia
io = open("primes.txt","r")   # open the file for reading
while !eof(io)   # while not the end of the file
    n = read(io,Int64)   # read an Int64 variable
#   n = read(io,String) # read a String variable
    println(n)
end
close(io)
```

To write and read CSV (comma separated values) file, one can use the package **DelimitedFiles**. Here is an example:

```julia
using DelimitedFiles
y = [0.1, 0.2]
X = [1 2 3; 4 5 6]
A = hcat(y,X)
io = open("mydata.csv","w")
writedlm(io,A, ',')  # write A, comma separated
close(io)

A1 = readdlm("mydata.csv",',')  # read A back
A == A1 # true
y1 = A[:,1]
X1 = A[:,2:end]
```

Finally, the following illustrates some dictionary and string operations on a large text file. A dictionary is a data structure that stores (key,value) pairs in an efficient way—via a hash-table, similar to an old-fashioned telephone book. The output of the script is a list of words consisting of at least five letters that appear at least 250 times in the text file.

```julia
io = open("ataleof2cities.txt")
d = Dict()  # create a new dictionary
for line in readlines(io)
    words = lowercase.(split(strip(line)))
    for w in words
        w = replace.(w, ['.', ',',';'] => "") # ignore punct.
        if !haskey(d,w) # is the word already in the dictionary
          ?
            d[w] = 1  # if not, add it
        else
            d[w] +=1
        end
    end
end
close(io)
sortd = sort(collect(d),by=last,rev=true)
for w in sortd
    if length(w[1]) >= 5 && w[2] >=250
        println(w[1],"    ",w[2])
    end
end
```

```
there    499
which    388
would    335
lorry    320
```

```
their    317
could    280
defarge    265
little    263
```

A.11 Other Aspects of the Language and Caveats

The previous sections cover most of the elements of the Julia language that are relevant for this book. However, there are many more language aspects to discover for the interested reader.

One thing we have not yet discussed is the *scoping* of variables, i.e., the way in which variable names are known or unknown within different regions of the code. Like in most other languages, functions have their own namespace. That is, any variable defined inside the function is not accessible outside the function. In general, code in Julia is organized in *modules*—regions of code that have their own namespace, and every time a module or package is loaded, a new namespace is created. The default modules are **Main, Core,** and **Base.** The function `varinfo` gives a summary of all the variables in a module. For example, to find the variables in the scope of the REPL, type `varinfo(Main)`. Likewise, the many variables and functions in the base module can be viewed with `varinfo(Base)`. As we have no need for user-defined modules in this book, we will say no more about this topic. Another feature of Julia that is out of the scope of this book is *metaprogramming*, i.e., writing a program that modifies a Julia program. The only encounter we will have with metaprogramming is via macros such as `@time` that measure the running time of a function or block of code.

We next list a number of caveats of which the reader should be aware, especially if they are familiar with MATLAB. Some of the issues have already been discussed in earlier sections, but it is prudent to emphasize them.

- Like most other computing languages, Julia uses square brackets [ ] to access arrays, in contrast to MATLAB, which uses parentheses ( ).
- In Julia, the type of a variable matters, much more than is the case in MATLAB. Nevertheless, variables of different types can often be combined in a natural way. Consider, for example, the following code, where the variables x, y, and z refer to different types of objects.

```julia
x = 1:3                # range object 1:3
y = [1.0,2.0,3.0]      # 3-element vector of Float64
z = [1 2 3]'           # 3x1 matrix of Int64
x + z                  # 3x1 matrix of Int64
x + 1                  # ERROR
```

```julia
x + y                   # 3-element vector of Float64
x .+ 1                  # range object 2:4
x/x                     # 3x3 matrix of Float64
x./x                    # 3-element vector of 1.0s
A = [1 2 3 ; 4 5 6]# 2x3 matrix of Int64
A*x                     # 2-element vector of Int64
x + y                   # 3-element vector of Float64
A*z                     # 2x1 matrix of Int64
```

- Elementwise operations on arrays in Julia are generally carried out via
  broadcasting, and this needs to be explicitly specified via the dot operator.
  For example:

```julia
using Plots
x = 1:0.1:3             # range object
y = sin.(x) .- 1        # 21-element Float64 vector
plot(x,y)               # plotting y against x
```

- It is important to realize that assigning a new name to an existing object
  does not create another instance of that object. Consider, for example,

```julia
x = [1 2 3 4];      # x refers to a matrix object
y = x;              # y refers to the SAME matrix object
z = copy(x);        # z refers to a NEW matrix object
y[2] = 0;           # same as x[2] = 0
z[2] = 0;           # now the new object is changed
println(x - y)      # x and y still refer to the same
println(x - z)
```
```
[0 0 0 0]
[0 2 0 0]
```

In contrast, in MATLAB the assignment y = x will automatically create a
new copy of the object to which x refers.

- A main difference with the scoping in MATLAB is that for and while
  loops introduce their own *local* scope. For example, the following common
  construction in MATLAB gives a warning and error message in Julia:

```julia
a = 0;
for i=1:10
    a = a + 1
end
```
```
Warning: Assignment to `a` in soft scope is ambiguous ...
ERROR: UndefVarError: `a` not defined
```

Instead we need to let Julia know that `a` is a global variable.

```julia
a = 0;
for i=1:10
  global a = a + 1
end
```

Another, rather bothersome, issue is that it is not possible to reset or clear various variables from the workspace. The easiest way to "clear" the workspace is to restart/delete the REPL.

- Punctuation in Julia is applied in many different ways. For example, a semicolon (`;`) at the end of a statement is used to suppress output, but a semicolon in an argument list of a function indicates a keyword argument. A colon (`:`) in front of a name indicates a *symbol*. For example if `f` refers to a function (i.e., a numerical recipe that maps input to output), `:f` refers to the symbol/letter `f` that represents this recipe. This is similar to the Lisp `quote` syntax which returns an expression without evaluating it. The different rules for punctuation are summarized in https://docs.julialang. org/en/v1/base/punctuation/

- Because Julia uses *just in time compilation*, first-time compilation or the "using" of a package or module can be slow. Subsequent running of the (now compiled) code will be much faster.

- As Julia is still in development (currently version 1.11.1), various scientific computing applications are not as well developed as in more mature computing platforms. For example, the plotting routines in Julia are still inferior to MATLAB's, especially for 3D plotting. Also the optimization packages have limited functionality.

- Although Julia has corrected various quirks of other languages (such as the use of parentheses to access matrices in MATLAB, and the strange R syntax for vector/matrix operations), it has itself introduced some idiosyncrasies, which perhaps may disappear in later versions. An example is the local scope within `for` loops and the required use of the `global` qualifier for certain global variables within the loop. We also mentioned the different results that the `cholesky` method yields when applied to sparse and dense matrices and use of the function `Hermitian` to force the method to accept certain positive definite matrices without throwing a (false) error message. Here are some more unexpected results:

```julia
"hello" * "hello"   # * for string concatenation,  not +
"hello"^2
10*10^6             # Int64
1e6                 # Float64
60^20               # gives a negative integer
80^60               # results in 0
```

```
max(1,2,3)              # maximum of 3 arguments
x = [1,2,3]
max(x)                  # ERROR
maximum(x)              # different function name required
```

```
"hellohello"
"hellohello"
10000000
1.0e7
-6450068360557232128
0
3
ERROR
3
```

A.12 Further Reading and References

Recent books that use Julia for statistics and decision-making include Nazarathy
and Klok (2021), Chan (2021), and Kochenderfer et al. (2022). Another useful
resource for learning Julia is

https://juliateachingctu.github.io/Julia-for-Optimization-and-Learning/
stable/

Finally, all programs and (large) data files in this book may be downloaded
from the homepage

https://people.smp.uq.edu.au/DirkKroese/statbook/

To accommodate the users of MATLAB and R, we have mirrored each Julia
program with its equivalent in MATLAB and R.

Appendix B
Mathematical Supplement

B.1 Multivariate Differentiation

For a real-valued multivariate function $f(x_1, \ldots, x_n)$, the **partial derivative** with respect to x_i, denoted $\frac{\partial f}{\partial x_i}$ or simply $\partial_i f$, is the derivative taken with respect to x_i, while all other variables are held constant. The partial derivative of $\partial_i f$ with respect to x_j is denoted $\frac{\partial^2 f}{\partial x_i \, \partial x_j}$ or simply $\partial_{ij} f$.

Let $\boldsymbol{f}$ be a multivariate function taking values in $\mathbb{R}^m$, defined by

$$
\boldsymbol{x} = \begin{bmatrix} x_1 \\ x_2 \\ \vdots \\ x_n \end{bmatrix} \mapsto \begin{bmatrix} f_1(\boldsymbol{x}) \\ f_2(\boldsymbol{x}) \\ \vdots \\ f_m(\boldsymbol{x}) \end{bmatrix} = \boldsymbol{f}(\boldsymbol{x}) .
$$

The **derivative** of $\boldsymbol{f}$ at $\boldsymbol{x}$ is defined as the matrix of partial derivatives

$$
J_{\boldsymbol{f}}(\boldsymbol{x}) = \begin{bmatrix} \partial_1 f_1(\boldsymbol{x}) & \cdots & \partial_n f_1(\boldsymbol{x}) \\ \vdots & \cdots & \vdots \\ \partial_1 f_m(\boldsymbol{x}) & \cdots & \partial_n f_m(\boldsymbol{x}) \end{bmatrix} , \tag{B.1}
$$

and is called the **matrix of Jacobi** of $\boldsymbol{f}$ at $\boldsymbol{x}$; sometimes written as $\frac{\partial \boldsymbol{f}}{\partial \boldsymbol{x}}(\boldsymbol{x})$.

Example B.1 (Differentiating a Linear Function). Let $\boldsymbol{f}(\boldsymbol{x}) = \mathbf{A}\boldsymbol{x}$ for some $m \times n$ constant matrix $\mathbf{A}$. Then,

$$
\frac{\partial \boldsymbol{f}(\boldsymbol{x})}{\partial \boldsymbol{x}} = \mathbf{A} . \tag{B.2}
$$

To see this, let a_{ij} denote the (i,j)-th element of $\mathbf{A}$, so that

© The Author(s), under exclusive license to Springer Science+Business Media, LLC, part of Springer Nature 2025
J. C. C. Chan, D. P. Kroese, *Statistical Modeling and Computation,*
Springer Texts in Statistics, https://doi.org/10.1007/978-1-0716-4132-3

$$f(\boldsymbol{x}) = \mathbf{A}\boldsymbol{x} = \begin{bmatrix} \sum_{k=1}^{n} a_{1k}x_k \\ \vdots \\ \sum_{k=1}^{n} a_{mk}x_k \end{bmatrix} .$$

To find the (i,j)-th element of the $m \times n$ Jacobian matrix $\mathbf{J}_{\boldsymbol{f}}$, we differentiate the i-th element of $\boldsymbol{f}$ with respect to x_j:

$$\frac{\partial f_i(\boldsymbol{x})}{\partial x_j} = \frac{\partial}{\partial x_j} \sum_{k=1}^{n} a_{ik}x_k = a_{ij} .$$

In other words, the (i,j)-th element of $\mathbf{J}_{\boldsymbol{f}}$ is a_{ij}, the (i,j)-th element of $\mathbf{A}$.

For a real-valued multivariate function, that is, $f : \mathbb{R}^n \to \mathbb{R}$, the **gradient** of f is the transpose of the Jacobian matrix, that is, the *column* vector

$$\nabla f(\boldsymbol{x}) = \begin{bmatrix} \partial_1 f(\boldsymbol{x}) \\ \vdots \\ \partial_n f(\boldsymbol{x}) \end{bmatrix} . \tag{B.3}$$

The derivative of the function $\boldsymbol{x} \mapsto \nabla f(\boldsymbol{x})$ is called the **Hessian matrix** of f, denoted $\mathbf{H}_f(\boldsymbol{x})$ or $\nabla^2 f(\boldsymbol{x})$. In other words, the Hessian is the matrix of second derivatives:

$$\nabla^2 f(\boldsymbol{x}) = \begin{bmatrix} \partial_{11} f(\boldsymbol{x}) & \cdots & \partial_{1n} f(\boldsymbol{x}) \\ \vdots & \ldots & \vdots \\ \partial_{n1} f(\boldsymbol{x}) & \cdots & \partial_{nn} f(\boldsymbol{x}) \end{bmatrix} . \tag{B.4}$$

If the partial derivatives are *continuous* in a region around $\boldsymbol{x}$, then $\partial_{ij} f(\boldsymbol{x}) = \partial_{ji} f(\boldsymbol{x})$ and, hence, the Hessian matrix $\mathbf{H}_f(\boldsymbol{x})$ is *symmetric*.

Example B.2 (Differentiating a Quadratic Function). Let $f(\boldsymbol{x}) = \boldsymbol{x}^\top \mathbf{A}\boldsymbol{x}$ for some $n \times n$ constant matrix $\mathbf{A}$. Then,

$$\nabla f(\boldsymbol{x}) = (\mathbf{A} + \mathbf{A}^\top)\boldsymbol{x} . \tag{B.5}$$

It follows immediately that if $\mathbf{A}$ is *symmetric*, i.e., $\mathbf{A} = \mathbf{A}^\top$, then $\nabla(\boldsymbol{x}^\top \mathbf{A}\boldsymbol{x}) = 2\mathbf{A}\boldsymbol{x}$ and $\nabla^2 (\boldsymbol{x}^\top \mathbf{A}\boldsymbol{x}) = 2\mathbf{A}$.

To prove (B.5), first observe that the quadratic function $f(\boldsymbol{x}) = \boldsymbol{x}^\top \mathbf{A}\boldsymbol{x}$ is real-valued, and therefore the Jacobian $\mathbf{J}_f$ is a $1 \times n$ vector (and its transpose is the gradient). Specifically,

$$f(\boldsymbol{x}) = \sum_{i=1}^{n} \sum_{j=1}^{n} a_{ij}\, x_i x_j ,$$

and the k-th element of $\mathbf{J}_f$ is obtained by differentiating $f(\boldsymbol{x})$ with respect to x_k:

$$\frac{\partial f(\boldsymbol{x})}{\partial x_k} = \frac{\partial}{\partial x_k} \sum_{i=1}^{n} \sum_{j=1}^{n} a_{ij} x_i x_j = \sum_{j=1}^{n} a_{kj} x_j + \sum_{i=1}^{n} a_{ik} x_i \; .$$

The first term on the right-hand side is equal to the k-th element of $\mathbf{A}\boldsymbol{x}$, whereas the second term equals the k-th element of $\boldsymbol{x}^\top \mathbf{A}$, or equivalently the k-th element of $\mathbf{A}^\top \boldsymbol{x}$.

Gradients and Hessian matrices feature prominently in multidimensional Taylor expansions.

Theorem B.1. (Multidimensional Taylor Expansions). Let $\mathscr{X}$ be an open subset of $\mathbb{R}^n$ and let $\boldsymbol{a} \in \mathscr{X}$. If $f : \mathscr{X} \to \mathbb{R}$ is a continuously twice differentiable function with gradient $\nabla f(\boldsymbol{x})$ and Hessian matrix $\mathbf{H}_f(\boldsymbol{x})$, then for every $\boldsymbol{x} \in \mathscr{X}$ we have the following first- and second-order Taylor expansions

$$f(\boldsymbol{x}) = f(\boldsymbol{a}) + [\nabla f(\boldsymbol{a})]^\top (\boldsymbol{x} - \boldsymbol{a}) + \mathcal{O}(\|\boldsymbol{x} - \boldsymbol{a}\|^2)$$

and

$$f(\boldsymbol{x}) = f(\boldsymbol{a}) + [\nabla f(\boldsymbol{a})]^\top (\boldsymbol{x} - \boldsymbol{a}) + \frac{1}{2}(\boldsymbol{x} - \boldsymbol{a})^\top \mathbf{H}_f(\boldsymbol{a}) (\boldsymbol{x} - \boldsymbol{a}) + \mathcal{O}(\|\boldsymbol{x} - \boldsymbol{a}\|^3)$$

as $\|\boldsymbol{x} - \boldsymbol{a}\| \to 0$. By dropping the $\mathcal{O}$ remainder terms, one obtains the corresponding Taylor approximations.

B.2 Proof of Theorem 2.6 and Corollary 2.2

The proof makes use of two fundamental properties of the expectation $\mathbb{E}$:   ☞ 34 the *monotone convergence theorem* and the *dominated convergence theorem*. The first states that if $X_1 \le X_2 \le X_3 \le \ldots$ is a sequence of positive random variables that increases to a random variable X, then the corresponding expectations $\mathbb{E}X_1 \le \mathbb{E}X_2 \le \mathbb{E}X_3 \ldots$ converge to $\mathbb{E}X$. The second theorem states that the same holds true for any positive sequence $X_1, X_2, \ldots$ converging to X, if there exists a Y with $\mathbb{E}Y < \infty$ such that $X_n \le Y$ for all n. An accessible account of these theorems may be found, for example, in Williams (1991).

We prove Theorem 2.6 for the case $k = 1$ only. Let $G(z) = \mathbb{E}z^X$. Take a fixed z with $|z| < R$ and any $r < R$ such that $r < |z| < R$. Let (h_n) be any sequence converging to 0, such that $|z + h_n| < r$. By definition, the derivative of G at z is $\lim_{n \to \infty} \mathbb{E}C_n$, where $C_n = h_n^{-1}[(z + h_n)^X - z^X]$. Observe that

1. $|C_n|$ is dominated by $X\, r^{X-1}$,

2. $\mathbb{E}Xr^{X-1} < \infty$, because the power series $\sum_{x=0}^{\infty} xz^{x-1}f(x)$ has again radius of convergence R,
3. $\lim_{n\to\infty} C_n = Xz^{X-1}$.

It follows by the dominated convergence theorem that

$$\lim_{n\to\infty} \mathbb{E}C_n = \mathbb{E}\lim_{n\to\infty} C_n = \mathbb{E}Xz^{X-1}\,.$$

Next, let (z_n) be a sequence of real numbers that is converging to 1, where $|z_n| < 1$ for all n. The sequence of random variables (Y_n) defined by $Y_n = X(X-1)\cdots(X-k+1)z_n^k$ is increasing to $Y = X(X-1)\cdots(X-k+1)$. Hence, by the monotone convergence theorem $\lim_{n\to\infty} \mathbb{E}Y_n = \mathbb{E}Y$. This shows (2.11). The second statement of the corollary is left as an exercise.

B.3 Proof of Theorem 2.7

If the moment generating function of a random variable X is finite in an open interval containing 0, then for all $n = 0, 1, \ldots$,

$$\mathbb{E}X^n = M^{(n)}(0)\,,$$

where $M^{(n)}$ is the n-th derivative of the MGF M evaluated at 0.

Proof. Let $R > 0$ be such that $M(s) < \infty$ for all $|s| < R$. Choose any numbers r and s such that $0 < r < R$ and $|s| < r$. Let (h_n) be a sequence converging to 0 satisfying $|h_n| < \varepsilon$ and $|s + h_n| < r$ for some $\varepsilon > 0$. Let $C_n = h_n^{-1}[\mathrm{e}^{(s+h_n)X} - \mathrm{e}^{sX}] = \mathrm{e}^{sX}(\mathrm{e}^{h_n X} - 1)/h_n$, which converges to $X\mathrm{e}^{sX}$. Also, $|C_n| \le H(X) \stackrel{\text{def}}{=} \mathrm{e}^{(|s|+\varepsilon)|X|}|X|$, because $0 \le (\mathrm{e}^t - 1)/t \le \mathrm{e}^{|t|}$ for all t. Moreover, because $|s| + \varepsilon < r$ and x grows at a lesser rate than e^{ax} for any $a > 0$, there must exist an $M > 0$ such that for all $|x| > M$, $H(x) < \mathrm{e}^{r|x|}$. It follows that

$$\mathbb{E}H(X) \le \mathbb{E}H(X)\,\mathbb{1}_{\{|X|>M\}} + \mathbb{E}H(X)\,\mathbb{1}_{\{|X|\le M\}}$$
$$\le \mathbb{E}\mathrm{e}^{r|X|} + \max_{|x|\le M} H(x) < \infty\,.$$

By the dominated convergence theorem, we have $M'(s) = \lim_{n\to\infty} \mathbb{E}C_n = \mathbb{E}\lim_{n\to\infty} C_n = \mathbb{E}[X\mathrm{e}^{sX}]$. Finally, take a monotone sequence (s_n) converging to 0 and apply the monotone convergence theorem to the sequence $(X\mathrm{e}^{s_n X})$ to find $M'(0) = \mathbb{E}X$. The proof for higher moments is similar. $\qquad\square$

B.4 Proof of Theorem 3.10

Let $\boldsymbol{v}_1, \ldots, \boldsymbol{v}_n$ be an orthonormal basis of $\mathbb{R}^n$ such that $\boldsymbol{v}_1, \ldots, \boldsymbol{v}_k$ spans $\mathscr{V}_k$ and $\boldsymbol{v}_1, \ldots, \boldsymbol{v}_m$ spans $\mathscr{V}_m$. We can write the orthogonal projection matrices onto $\mathscr{V}_j$, as $\mathbf{P}_j = \sum_{i=1}^{j} \boldsymbol{v}_i \boldsymbol{v}_i^\top$, $j = k, m, n$, where $\mathscr{V}_n$ is defined as $\mathbb{R}^n$. Note that $\mathbf{P}_n$ is simply the identity matrix. Let $\mathbf{V} = [\boldsymbol{v}_1, \ldots, \boldsymbol{v}_n]$ and define $\boldsymbol{Z} = [Z_1, \ldots, Z_n]^\top = \mathbf{V}^\top \boldsymbol{X}$. Recall that any orthogonal transformation such as $\boldsymbol{z} = \mathbf{V}^\top \boldsymbol{x}$ is *length preserving*; that is $\|\boldsymbol{z}\| = \|\boldsymbol{x}\|$.

To prove the first statement of the theorem, note that $\mathbf{V}^\top \boldsymbol{X}_j = \mathbf{V}^\top \mathbf{P}_j \boldsymbol{X} = [Z_1, \ldots, Z_j, 0, \ldots, 0]^\top$, $j = k, m$. It follows that $\mathbf{V}^\top (\boldsymbol{X}_m - \boldsymbol{X}_k) = [0, \ldots, 0, Z_{k+1}, \ldots, Z_m, 0, \ldots, 0]^\top$ and $\mathbf{V}^\top (\boldsymbol{X} - \boldsymbol{X}_m) = [0, \ldots, 0, Z_{m+1}, \ldots, Z_n]^\top$. Moreover, being a linear transformation of a normal random vector, $\boldsymbol{Z}$ is also normal, with covariance matrix $\mathbf{V}^\top \mathbf{V} = \mathbb{I}$; see also Problem 3.13. In particular, the $\{Z_i\}$ are *independent*. This shows that $\boldsymbol{X}_k$, $\boldsymbol{X}_m - \boldsymbol{X}_k$ and $\boldsymbol{X} - \boldsymbol{X}_m$ are independent as well. ☞ 95

Next, observe that $\|\boldsymbol{X}_k\| = \|\mathbf{V}^\top \boldsymbol{X}_k\| = \|\boldsymbol{Z}_k\|$, where $\boldsymbol{Z}_k = [Z_1, \ldots, Z_k]^\top$. The latter vector has independent components with variances 1, and its squared norm has therefore (by definition) a $\chi_k^2(\theta)$ distribution. The non-centrality parameter is $\theta = \|\mathbb{E}\boldsymbol{Z}_k\| = \|\mathbb{E}\boldsymbol{X}_k\| = \|\boldsymbol{\mu}_k\|$, again by the length-preserving property of orthogonal transformations. This shows that $\|\boldsymbol{X}_k\|^2 \sim \chi_k^2(\|\boldsymbol{\mu}_k\|)$. The distributions of $\|\boldsymbol{X}_m - \boldsymbol{X}_k\|^2$ and $\|\boldsymbol{X} - \boldsymbol{X}_m\|^2$ follow by analogy. $\qquad\square$

B.5 Proof of Theorem 5.2

First, observe that, by Theorem 5.1, ☞ 13

$$\frac{(m-1)S_X^2}{\sigma^2} \sim \chi_{m-1}^2 \quad \text{and} \quad \frac{(n-1)S_Y^2}{\sigma^2} \sim \chi_{n-1}^2 .$$

Because these random variables are independent of each other, their sum, V say, can be written as the sum of $m + n$ independent squared standard normal random variables and has therefore a χ_{m+n-2}^2 distribution. Thus,

$$V = \frac{(m+n-2)S_p^2}{\sigma^2} \sim \chi_{m+n-2}^2 .$$

Second, let

$$Z = \frac{\overline{X} - \overline{Y} - (\mu_X - \mu_Y)}{\sigma / \sqrt{\frac{1}{m} + \frac{1}{n}}}.$$

Then, $Z \sim \mathcal{N}(0, 1)$ and the square of the pivot T in Theorem 5.2 can be written as

$$T^2 = \frac{Z^2}{V/(m+n-2)} \, ,$$

where Z and V are independent, because $\overline{X}$ and $\overline{Y}$ are independent of each other, and are both independent of S_X^2 and S_Y^2; see Theorem 5.1. The random variable T^2 is thus the independent quotient of a χ_1^2 and a χ_{m+n-2}^2 random variable. Hence, by Theorem 3.11, $T^2 \sim \mathsf{F}(1, m+n-2)$. It follows now from Theorem 2.19 (and the fact that the pdf of T is symmetric around 0) that $T \sim \mathsf{t}_{m+n-2}$. $\qquad\square$

☞ 88
☞ 51

References

Bishop, C. M. (2006). *Pattern Recognition and Machine Learning*. Springer, New York.

Botev, Z. I., Grotowski, J. F., and Kroese, D. P. (2010). Kernel density estimation via diffusion. *Annals of Statistics*, 38(5):2916–2957.

Botev, Z. I., Kroese, D., and Taimre, T. (2025). *Data Science and Machine Learning: Mathematical and Statistical Methods*. Chapman & Hall/CRC, Boca Raton, 2nd edition.

Boyd, S., Parikh, N., Chu, E., Peleato, B., and Eckstein, J. (2010). Distributed optimization and statistical learning via the alternating direction method of multipliers. *Foundations and Trends in Machine Learning*, 3:1–122.

Boyd, S. and Vandenberghe, L. (2004). *Convex Optimization*. Cambridge University Press, Cambridge. Seventh printing with corrections, 2009.

Carter, C. K. and Kohn, R. (1994). On Gibbs sampling for state space models. *Biometrika*, 81:541–553.

Chan, J. C. C. (2013). Moving average stochastic volatility models with application to inflation forecast. *Journal of Econometrics*, 176(2):162–172.

Chan, J. C. C. and Jeliazkov, I. (2009). Efficient simulation and integrated likelihood estimation in state space models. *International Journal of Mathematical Modelling and Numerical Optimisation*, 1(1):101–120.

Chan, S. H. (2021). *Introduction to Probability for Data Science*. Michigan Publishing Services, Ann Arbor.

Chib, S. (1995). Marginal likelihood from the Gibbs output. *Journal of the American Statistical Association*, 90:1313–1321.

Chib, S. and Jeliazkov, I. (2001). Marginal likelihood from the Metropolis-Hastings output. *Journal of the American Statistical Association*, 96:270–281.

Cox, D. R. and Snell, E. J. (1981). *Applied Statistics: Principles and Examples*. Chapman & Hall/CRC, London.

Del Negro, M. and Primiceri, G. E. (2015). Time-varying structural vector autoregressions and monetary policy: A corrigendum. *Review of Economic Studies*, 82(4):1342–1345.

Durbin, J. and Koopman, S. J. (2002). A simple and efficient simulation smoother for state space time series analysis. *Biometrika*, 89:603–615.

Efron, B. and Hastie, T. (2016). *Computer Age Statistical Inference*. Cambridge University Press, Cambridge.

Fair, R. C. (1978). A theory of extramarital affairs. *Journal of Political Economy*, 86:45–61.

Feller, W. (1970). *An Introduction to Probability Theory and Its Applications*, volume I. John Wiley & Sons, New York, second edition.

Gelfand, A. E., Hills, S., Racine-Poon, A., and Smith, A. F. M. (1990). Illustration of Bayesian inference in normal data models using Gibbs sampling. *Journal of American Statistical Association*, 85:972–985.

Green, P. J. and Silverman, B. W. (1993). *Nonparametric Regression and Generalized Linear Models: A Roughness Penalty Approach*. Chapman & Hall/CRC.

Harvey, A. C. (1985). Trends and cycles in macroeconomic time series. *Journal of Business and Economic Statistics*, 3(3):216–227.

Harvey, A. C. (1990). *Forecasting, Structural Time Series Models and the Kalman Filter*. Cambridge University Press.

Hastie, T., Tibshirani, R., Friedman, J. H., and Friedman, J. H. (2009). *The Elements of Statistical Learning*. Springer, second edition.

James, W. and Stein, C. (1961). Estimation with quadratic loss. In *Proc. Fourth Berkeley Symp. Math. Statist. Prob.*, volume 1, pages 361–379.

Kim, S., Shepherd, N., and Chib, S. (1998). Stochastic volatility: Likelihood inference and comparison with ARCH models. *Review of Economic Studies*, 65(3):361–393.

Kochenderfer, M. J., Wheeler, T. A., and Wray, K. H. (2022). *Algorithms for Decision Making*. MIT Press, Cambridge.

Kolassa, J. (2020). *An Introduction to Nonparametric Statistics*. Chapman & Hall/CRC, Boca Raton.

Koop, G., Poirier, D. J., L., J., and Tobias (2007). *Bayesian Econometric Methods*. Cambridge University Press.

Kroese, D. P. and Botev, Z. I. (2023). *An Advanced Course in Probability and Stochastic Processes*. Chapman & Hall/CRC.

Kroese, D. P., Botev, Z. I., Taimre, T., and Vaisman, R. (2019). *Data Science and Machine Learning: Mathematical and Statistical Methods*. Chapman & Hall/CRC, Boca Raton.

Kroese, D. P., Taimre, T., and Botev, Z. I. (2011). *Handbook of Monte Carlo Methods*. John Wiley & Sons, New York.

L'Ecuyer, P. (1999). Good parameters and implementations for combined multiple recursive random number generators. *Operations Research*, 47(1):159 – 164.

McCausland, W. J., Miller, S., and Pelletier, D. (2011). Simulation smoothing for state-space models: A computational efficiency analysis. *Computational Statistics and Data Analysis*, 55(1):199–212.

McLachlan, G. J. and Krishnan, T. (2008). *The EM Algorithm and Extensions*. John Wiley & Sons, Hoboken, NJ, second edition.

Metropolis, M., Rosenbluth, A. W., Rosenbluth, M. N., Teller, A. H., and Teller, E. (1953). Equations of state calculations by fast computing machines. *J. of Chemical Physics*, 21:1087–1092.

Nazarathy, Y. and Klok, H. (2021). *Statistics with Julia: Fundamentals for Data Science*. Springer, New York.

Pratt, J. W. and Gibbons, J. D. (1981). *Concepts of Nonparametric Theory*. Springer, New York.

Rubinstein, R. Y. and Kroese, D. P. (2004). *The Cross-Entropy Method: A Unified Approach to Combinatorial Optimization Monte-Carlo Simulation, and Machine Learning*. Springer, New York.

Rue, H. (2001). Fast sampling of Gaussian Markov random fields with applications. *Journal of the Royal Statistical Society: Series B (Methodological)*, 63(2):325–338.

Shawe-Taylor, J. and Cristianini, N. (2004). *Kernel Methods for Pattern Analysis*. Cambridge University Press, Cambridge.

Stock, J. H. and Watson, M. W. (2007). Why has U.S. inflation become harder to forecast? *Journal of Money Credit and Banking*, 39(s1):3–33.

Verdinelli, I. and Wasserman, L. (1995). Computing Bayes factors using a generalization of the Savage-Dickey density ratio. *Journal of the American Statistical Association*, 90(430):614–618.

Wald, A. and Wolfowitz, J. (1944). Statistical tests based on permutations of the observations. *Annals of Mathematical Statistics*, 15:358–372.

Watson, M. W. (1986). Univariate detrending methods with stochastic trends. *Journal of Monetary Economics*, 18(1):49–75.

Williams, D. (1991). *Probability with Martingales*. Cambridge University Press, Cambridge.

Index

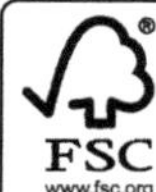